Equine Hematology, Cytology, and Clinical Chemistry

Equine Hematology, Cytology, and Clinical Chemistry

Edited by

Raquel M. Walton *VMD, MS, PhD, DACVP (Clinical Pathology)*
Senior Veterinary Clinical Pathologist
IDEXX Laboratories, Inc.
Langhorne, PA, USA

Rick L. Cowell *DVM, MS, DACVP (Clinical Pathology)*
Retired
Stillwater, OK, USA

Amy C. Valenciano *DVM, MS, DACVP (Clinical Pathology)*
Senior Veterinary Clinical Pathologist
IDEXX Laboratories, Inc.
Dallas, TX, USA

Second Edition

WILEY Blackwell

This edition first published 2021

Edition History
John Wiley & Sons (1e, 2013)

Registered Office
John Wiley & Sons, Inc., 111 River Street, Hoboken, NJ 07030, USA

Editorial Office
111 River Street, Hoboken, NJ 07030, USA

For details of our global editorial offices, customer services, and more information about Wiley products visit us at www.wiley.com.

Wiley also publishes its books in a variety of electronic formats and by print-on-demand. Some content that appears in standard print versions of this book may not be available in other formats.

Library of Congress Cataloging-in-Publication Data

Names: Walton, Raquel M., editor. | Cowell, Rick L., editor. | Valenciano, Amy C., editor.
Title: Equine hematology, cytology, and clinical chemistry / edited by, Raquel M. Walton, Rick Cowell, Amy Valenciano.
Other titles: Equine clinical pathology
Description: Second edition. | Hoboken, NJ : Wiley-Blackwell, 2021. | Preceded by Equine clinical pathology / edited by Raquel M. Walton. 2014. | Includes bibliographical references and index.
Identifiers: LCCN 2020004372 (print) | LCCN 2020004373 (ebook) | ISBN 9781119500247 (hardback) | ISBN 9781119500223 (adobe pdf) | ISBN 9781119500193 (epub)
Subjects: MESH: Horse Diseases–pathology | Hematologic Diseases–veterinary | Hematologic Tests–veterinary | Cytodiagnosis–veterinary | Pathology, Clinical–methods
Classification: LCC SF951 (print) | LCC SF951 (ebook) | NLM SF 951 | DDC 636.1/089–dc23
LC record available at https://lccn.loc.gov/2020004372
LC ebook record available at https://lccn.loc.gov/2020004373

Cover Design: Wiley
Cover Images: Blue microscopic images Courtesy of Amy Valenciano, Gray horse © GeptaYs/Shutterstock

Set in 9.5/12.5pt STIXTwoText by SPi Global, Pondicherry, India

Printed in Singapore

M WEP348362 170325

I would like to thank my parents, Bryce and Elmira, for instilling in me a love of the biological world and all in it; my sisters, Judy and Laurel, for their guidance and love; and my friends, colleagues, and mentors who give life purpose and zest. I owe my colleagues and managers at IDEXX Laboratories a debt of gratitude and respect for their support, participation, and encouragement in the pursuit of knowledge and advancement in veterinary clinical pathology.

This book is dedicated to my fellow veterinary clinical pathologists and to veterinarians, veterinary students and technologists, who wander, never lost, pursuing answers but, more importantly, the questions preceding all answers.

Raquel

I dedicate this beautiful text to God and my family: my dear parents Norman Ross and Mary Ann, my twin sister Bonny, my husband Daniel, daughter Avery and son Ty. I thank my wonderful mentors especially Drs Dave Fisher, Sonjia Shelly, Carol Grindem, Jan Andrews, Mary Jo Burkhard, Gregg Dean, Christine Stanton, Lon Rich, and especially Rick Cowell. I also thank IDEXX Laboratories for supporting academic growth and for promoting excellence in veterinary pathology.

Amy

To my parents who taught me the value of honesty and instilled in me a work ethic that has served me well through the years. To my wife (Annette) and daughter (Anne) who have continually given support, meaning, and inspiration to my life. To my daughter (Rebecca) who showed me the face of true courage and taught me to laugh and love even in the worst of times. While she lost her battle with cancer at the age of 11, her memories and life lessons will forever be remembered. To the many outstanding veterinary clinical pathologists I have had the opportunity to learn from, especially Drs Ronald D. Tyler, James Meinkoth, Dennis DeNicola, and Amy Valenciano. To the many veterinary practitioners, residents, and students who taught me much more than I could ever have hoped to teach them and have become colleagues and friends.

Rick

Contents

List of Contributors

Jill Beech, VMD, DACVIM (LAIM)
Emeritus Professor of Medicine and Reproduction
Georgia E. and Philip B. Hofmann New Bolton Center
School of Veterinary Medicine
University of Pennsylvania
Kennett Square, PA, USA

Allison Billings, VMD, DACVP (Clinical Pathology)
Veterinary Clinical Pathologist
IDEXX Laboratories, Inc.
Portland, OR, USA

Melissa Blauvelt, DVM, MS, DACVP (Clinical Pathology)
Veterinary Clinical Pathologist
IDEXX Laboratories, Inc.
Worthington, OH, USA

Andrea A. Bohn, DVM, PhD, DACVP (Clinical Pathology)
Associate Professor
Department of Microbiology, Immunology, and Pathology
College of Veterinary Medicine and Biomedical Sciences
Colorado State University
Fort Collins, CO, USA

Angela Borchers, DVM, DACVIM (LAIM), DACVECC
Associate Veterinarian in Small Animal Emergency and Critical Care
School of Veterinary Medicine
University of California
Davis, CA, USA

Andrew Burton, BVSc (Hons), DACVP (Clinical Pathology)
Veterinary Clinical Pathologist
IDEXX Laboratories, Inc.
North Grafton, MA, USA

Rick L. Cowell, DVM, MS, DACVP (Clinical Pathology)
Retired
Stillwater, OK, USA

Susan E. Fielder, DVM, MS, DACVP (Clinical Pathology)
Clinical Assistant Professor
Department of Veterinary Pathobiology
College of Veterinary Medicine
Oklahoma State University
Stillwater, OK, USA

Camilo Hernández-Avilés, DVM
Graduate Research Assistant, PhD candidate in Equine Theriogenology
Large Animal Clinical Sciences
College of Veterinary Medicine and Biomedical Sciences
Texas A&M University
College Station, TX, USA

Karen V. Jackson, BVSc (Hons I), MANZCVS (Internal Medicine), DACVP (Clinical Pathology)
Senior Lecturer in Veterinary Clinical Pathology
School of Veterinary Science
University of Queensland
Gatton, Queensland, Australia

Kathryn Jacocks, DVM, DACVP (Clinical Pathology)
Veterinary Clinical Pathologist
IDEXX Laboratories, Inc.
Dallas, TX, USA

Cheryl A. Lawson, DVM, MS, DACVP (Clinical Pathology)
Assistant Professor
Department of Veterinary Pathology
College of Veterinary Medicine
Iowa State University
Ames, IA, USA

Chelsea Makloski-Cohorn, DVM, MS, DACT
Pinnacle Equine Veterinary Services, PLLC
Whitesboro, TX, USA

Maggie R. McCourt, DVM
Resident, Veterinary Clinical Pathology
Department of Veterinary Pathobiology
College of Veterinary Medicine
Oklahoma State University
Stillwater, OK, USA

Joanne B. Messick, VMD, PhD, DACVP (Clinical Pathology)
Professor of Veterinary Clinical Pathology
Department of Comparative Pathobiology
College of Veterinary Medicine
Purdue University
West Lafayette, IN, USA

Dennis J. Meyer, DVM, DACVIM (SAIM), DACVP (Clinical Pathology)
Executive Director, Navigator Services
Senior Veterinary Clinical Pathologist
Charles River Laboratories
Reno, NV, USA

Julie Piccione, DVM, MS, Diplomate ACVP (Clinical Pathology)
Clinical Pathology Section Head
Texas A&M Veterinary Medical Diagnostic Laboratory
College Station, TX, USA

Martina Piviani, DVM, SPCAA, MSc, DACVP (Clinical Pathology), MRCVS
Senior Lecturer in Clinical Pathology
Department of Small Animal Clinical Science
University of Liverpool
Liverpool, UK

Jennifer K. Quinn, BVM&S
Resident, Veterinary Clinical Pathology
IDEXX Laboratories, Inc.
Wetherby, UK

Luisa Ramírez-Agámez, DVM
Animal Reproductive Services Bogotá, Colombia

Andrea Siegel, DVM, DACVP (Clinical Pathology)
Veterinary Clinical Pathologist
IDEXX Laboratories, Inc.
New York, NY, USA

Melanie S. Spoor, DVM, MS, DACVP (Clinical Pathology)
Veterinary Clinical Pathologist
IDEXX Laboratories, Inc.
Wetherby, UK

Amy C. Valenciano, DVM, MS, DACVP (Clinical Pathology)
Senior Veterinary Clinical Pathologist
IDEXX Laboratories, Inc.
Dallas, TX, USA

Lucien Vallone, DVM, DACVO
Assistant Clinical Professor of Comparative Ophthalmology
Department of Small Animal Clinical Sciences
College of Veterinary Medicine
Texas A&M University
College Station, TX, USA

Koranda A. Walsh, VMD, DACVIM (SAIM), DACVP (Clinical Pathology)
Clinical Assistant Professor
Department of Pathobiology
School of Veterinary Medicine
University of Pennsylvania
Philadelphia, PA, USA

Raquel M. Walton, VMD, MS, PhD, DACVP (Clinical Pathology)
Senior Veterinary Clinical Pathologist
IDEXX Laboratories, Inc.
Langhorne, PA, USA

Preface

Veterinary clinical pathology is the study of disease in the living animal and encompasses hematology, clinical chemistry, cytopathology, endocrinology, urinalysis, coagulation, immunohematology, laboratory management, and general pathophysiology. The interpretation of clinical pathological data often leads to a disease diagnosis, from which treatment and prognosis are derived. Thus, as a discipline, clinical pathology is integral to the practice of veterinary medicine and is essential to the training of veterinary students, technicians, clinicians, and specialists.

While there are general pathophysiological principles that carry across most genera, species-dependent deviations exist. Disease pathogenesis is a consequence of individual physiology and species differences produce unique disease characteristics. Significant differences between equids and other common domestic species exist and yet a comprehensive equine clinical pathology textbook has been lacking. The authors of this book present equine disease from a clinicopathological perspective, which is systems based rather than problem based. We hope that this book will fill an important need and serve as a valuable resource for all those engaged in the care of equids, from students to specialists.

1

General Laboratory Medicine

Raquel M. Walton

IDEXX Laboratories, Inc., Langhorne, PA, USA

Acronyms and abbreviations that appear in this chapter include: Hb, hemoglobin; MCH, mean cell Hb; MCHC, mean cell Hb concentration; MCV, mean cell volume; PCV, packed cell volume; POC, point of care; POCT, point-of-care testing; RBC, red blood cells; TP, total protein; TP_{Ref}, refractometer total protein; TS, total solids.

1.1 Introduction to Laboratory Medicine

Laboratory medicine, more commonly referred to as clinical pathology (or bioanalytical pathology), is a distinct specialty that overlaps other medicine specialties such as internal medicine and oncology in the area of diagnostics. In contrast to internists, clinical pathologists practice a systems-based rather than problem-based approach when interpreting hematological and biochemical results. However, in addition to recognizing disease-associated changes, two other phenomena contribute to test interpretation: how test results are generated and how "normal" is defined. Artifacts due to sample preparation, sample condition or disease processes need to be identified and distinguished from true disease-associated changes. Similarly, test interpretation is always performed in context – the context of health. The accuracy and sensitivity of tests and the use of appropriately established reference intervals are essential to the ability to diagnose disease.

This chapter will provide selected information on hematological and biochemical test methodologies and validation, and will discuss the basic knowledge needed for generating and/or using reference intervals. The remainder of the book will address test interpretation using a systems-based approach.

1.2 Preanalytical Factors

Preanalytical factors that may affect test results should be minimized in order to ensure result accuracy [1]. Specimens should be collected according to standard practices and transported to the laboratory in a timely manner under conditions appropriate for the type of specimen and its stability. The minimum information on a specimen label for laboratory evaluation should include the full name of the patient (animal and owner), the patient signalment, and the specimen type (e.g., whole blood, serum or plasma). Especially for hematological evaluation, it is important that the patient's signalment be correct as analyzer settings vary with respect to species.

Anticoagulated specimens for hematology that have visible macroclots in the tube will produce variably erroneous results. Because the degree of inaccuracy cannot be predicted, clotted specimens are unsuitable for analyzis and these specimens should not be analyzed or submitted for analysis.

Blood films and cytology smears should not be refrigerated and should be protected from condensation and freezing during transport to the laboratory to avoid condensation artifact (Figure 1.1). Failure to fully dry blood films or cytology preparations before placing them into slide holders can also result in moisture artefact.

Equine Hematology, Cytology, and Clinical Chemistry, Second Edition.
Edited by Raquel M. Walton, Rick L. Cowell, and Amy C. Valenciano.

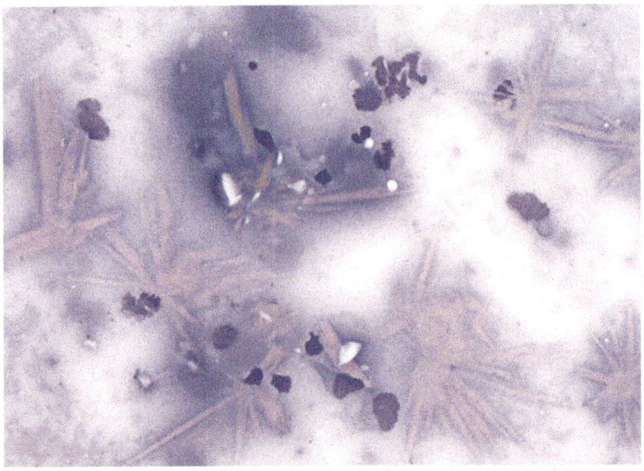

Figure 1.1 Condensation artifact caused by exposure of unfixed slides to moisture. The nucleated cells are lyzed and many hemoglobin crystals are present, formed from erythrocytes.

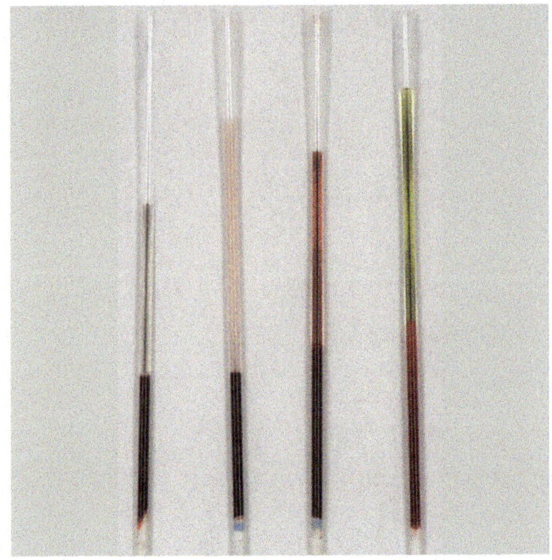

Figure 1.2 Evaluation of plasma. From left to right: normal plasma color and consistency; lipemic and slightly hemolyzed plasma; hemolyzed plasma; icteric plasma.

1.3 Basic Hematological Techniques

1.3.1 Packed Cell Volume and Plasma Evaluation: Disease and Artifacts

Measurement of the percentage of red blood cells in whole blood can provide more information than simply the packed cell volume (PCV). In addition to the packed erythrocytes at the bottom of a microhematocrit tube, there is the white buffy coat layer and a plasma layer. The size of the buffy coat is related to the white blood cell (WBC) (and platelet) count; a thick buffy coat would indicate a high leukocyte (and/or platelet) count, whereas a scant buffy coat suggests leukopenia. The character of the plasma can also yield valuable information pertaining to a disease process, as well as contributing to spurious results. The plasma can appear hemolyzed, icteric or lipemic (Figure 1.2).

Hemolysis in samples from horses usually indicates an *in vivo* phenomenon due to toxins or immune-mediated disease (see Chapter 4). However, hemolysis can also occur during blood collection if excessive force or too small needle gauge is used in phlebotomy. Whether *in vivo* or *in vitro*, hemolysis produces a color change that can make refractometer readings difficult or interfere with spectrophotometric tests.

Icterus indicates hyperbilirubinemia that usually exceeds 1.5 mg/dL (see Chapter 5). However, in herbivorous animals yellow-colored plasma is not a reliable indicator of hyperbilirubinemia due to the presence of diet-associated carotene pigments, which impart a yellow color to plasma. Icterus has not been demonstrated to interfere with refractometer readings [2]. Depending upon the chemistry analyzer, icterus can cause interference with some serum chemistry tests.

Lipemia is visible to the eye as increased turbidity in plasma or serum at triglyceride concentrations >300 mg/dL. Whether physiological (postprandial) or pathological (see Chapter 9), lipemia can cause spuriously high refractometer readings and will interfere with many chemistry tests.

1.3.2 Protein Measurement by Refractometer

Protein can be rapidly and accurately measured by handheld refractometers. Because refractometers measure protein via a total solids-based technique, the total dissolved solids in the sample affect light refraction. In addition to protein, total solids include electrolytes, glucose, urea, and lipids. The term "total solids" has caused much confusion in the reporting of refractometric protein results. Total protein (TP) and total solids (TS) are not synonymous. Currently, the vast majority of refractometers incorporate a conversion factor in their design so that the scales report TP and not TS. Contributing to the confusion is the fact that at least one refractometer is named the "TS meter" (AO Corporation) when it is in fact calibrated to report TP. While the altered refraction of plasma is mostly due to protein content, increases in lipid, glucose or urea content interfere with refractometric protein measurements. However, marked increases in urea or glucose (273 and 649 mg/dL, respectively) are needed to increase protein measurement by 0.4–0.5 g/dL. Increases in plasma cholesterol of 39 mg/dL are shown to increase the refractometer TP (TP_{Ref}) by 0.14 g/dL [2].

Another potential cause of erroneous refractometer readings is the addition of EDTA from K_3EDTA anticoagulant tubes. At the standard concentration of EDTA (5 µmol/mL), K_3EDTA by itself has minimal effect on the plasma's refraction (≤0.1 g/dL increase). This is not true for peritoneal fluid, however, where overestimation of TP_{Ref} by 0.7 +/− 0.1 g/dL was reported in one study (see Chapter 18). At higher concentrations of EDTA (10 and 20 µmol/mL), EDTA can increase TP_{Ref} by 0.9–1.0 g/dL. Underfilling of EDTA tubes has the effect of increasing the EDTA concentration and will cause spurious increases in the TP_{Ref} [3]. Some commercial tubes with K_3EDTA anticoagulant may also contain additives to prevent crystallization of the EDTA. Tubes that contain the additive may increase TP_{Ref} readings by up to 0.9 g/dL, even when properly filled. In general, polypropylene (plastic) tubes are more likely to include additives to prevent evaporation than glass tubes [4]. While sodium heparin anticoagulant has no effect on TP_{Ref}, heparin has deleterious effects on cellular morphology and is not recommended for samples that will be evaluated cytologically.

1.4 Point-of-Care Testing

Point-of-care testing (POCT) is defined as testing done at or near the patient with the expectation that results will be available quickly to facilitate immediate diagnosis and/or clinical intervention [5]. Whilst POCT provides quick, relatively inexpensive results with small volumes of blood, it also comes with its own set of risks. The major sources of error associated with POCT were categorized in one study as most often due to operator incompetence, nonadherence to test procedures, and the use of uncontrolled reagents and testing equipment [6]. Instrument calibrations and quality control measures may be omitted due to ignorance or the need for fast results. And, in veterinary medicine, analyzers may be used with species for which the instrument has not been validated. It should also be noted that diagnostic instruments for veterinary use are not subject to government regulations as they are for human use, which means that devices may not have been independently evaluated or tested [7]. Finally, poorly maintained instruments that are carried from one area to another may be a source of nosocomial infection or may transmit antibiotic-resistant bacterial strains [5].

As part of the process of ensuring accuracy in an analytical method, calibrators and controls are used. A *calibrator* is a material of known or assigned characteristics that is used to correlate instrument readings with the expected results from the calibrator (or standard). A *control* is a preparation of human or animal origin intended for use in assuring the quality control of the measurement procedure, not for calibration. Controls usually represent abnormal and normal concentrations of the measured analyte. Currently, there are some POC analyzers marketed as "maintenance free" that do not come with controls and some that do not have calibrators. These instruments should be used with caution as there is no way to verify assay accuracy.

1.4.1 Hematology Analyzers

1.4.1.1 Impedance Technology

Many POC hematology analyzers are based upon impedance methodology. Examples include the HM series (Abaxis, Union City, CA), the HemaVet 950 (Drew Scientific, Oxford, CT), the HemaTrue® (Heska, Loveland, CO), and the scil Vet abc™ (Scil, Gurnee, IL). Impedance technology employs an electric current that flows through a conductive liquid. When cells, which are nonconductive, pass through an aperture containing this fluid, there is an electrical impedance created for each cell that is proportional to the size of the cell. The impedance method facilitates measurement of the mean RBC and platelet volumes, as well as enumeration of WBCs, RBCs, and platelets. The WBCs (and any nucleated red blood cells) are counted separately from RBCs and platelets after cell lysis. Hemoglobin (Hb) concentration is also measured after RBC lysis. In the isotonic solution, nucleated cells are prevented from being counted along with RBCs and platelets because they are too big to pass through the aperture (Figure 1.3).

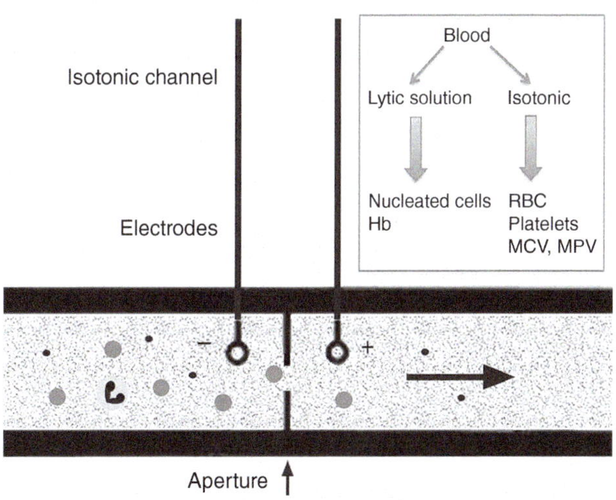

Figure 1.3 Schematic representing standard impedance methodology. Blood is directed into two chambers. In one chamber, a lytic solution is used to obtain the WBC count by evaluating bare nuclei and measuring the hemoglobin released from erythrocytes. The second chamber contains isotonic solution and an aperture of limited size through which erythrocytes and platelets are enumerated.

Failure of RBCs to lyze may result in their being counted as WBCs, thereby falsely increasing the WBC count. Similarly, large platelet aggregates may be erroneously counted as WBCs, resulting in spuriously low platelet and high WBC counts. Very large platelets may be miscounted as erythrocytes.

1.4.1.2 Centrifugal Hematology Analyzers

Centrifugal analyzers operate by taking quantitative measurements on the cell layers below and within the buffy coat. The quantitative buffy coat (QBC) VetAutoread™ (IDEXX Laboratories Inc., Westbrook, ME) is an example of a centrifugal hematology analyzer. Granulocytes, mononuclear cells (monocytes and lymphocytes), erythrocytes, and platelets are separated into layers in an enlarged microhematocrit-like tube using a cylindrical float to further expand the buffy coat layer. Cells separate into layers upon centrifugation according to relative density and fluorescent staining differentiates layers. Centrifugal analyzers can also provide fibrinogen concentrations by re-reading the sample after incubating in a precipitator.

Only the spun hematocrit is measured with centrifugal analyzers. Since erythrocyte counts are not determined, the MCV cannot be calculated. The Hb can be estimated assuming a constant relationship between hematocrit and Hb. From Hb and hematocrit, MCHC can be calculated. Estimated WBC counts are obtained from the thickness of layers by assuming an average cell size.

1.4.1.3 Laser Technology

Laser hematology analyzers generate both cell counts and differentials using light scatter. Single cells pass through a laser beam and scatter light at forward and side angles from the cell, which is picked up by photoreceptors (Figure 1.4). Forward, right-angle, and side light scatter represent cell size and complexity.

While this technology affords the opportunity to generate leukocyte differentials, in general there is not good precision with differential leukocyte counts [7, 8]. The presence of band neutrophils, toxic change or reactive lymphocytes can result in poor separation between leukocyte groups, adversely affecting the instrument differential (Figure 1.5). A manual differential from a blood film is still recommended to verify instrument differentials. Examples of POC hematology analyzers using light scatter are the ProCyte® and LaserCyte® (IDEXX) and ElementHT5® (Heska).

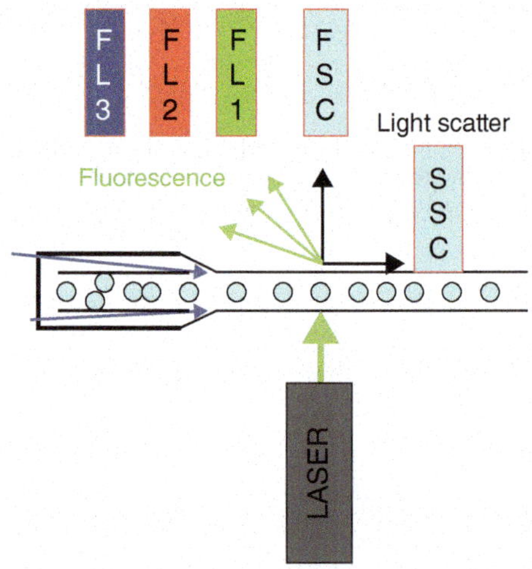

Figure 1.4 Schematic representing the principle of hematological analysis using laser methodology. Light passing directly through the cells (forward scatter; FSC) and light deflected 90° (side scatter; SSC) is captured by detectors. FSC and SSC correspond to cell size and complexity, respectively. Complexity refers to the character of the cytoplasm (e.g., presence or absence of granules). Fluorescence detectors capture fluorescence from dyes that stain RNA, myeloperoxidase or reticulum to differentiate leukocytes or to count reticulocytes.

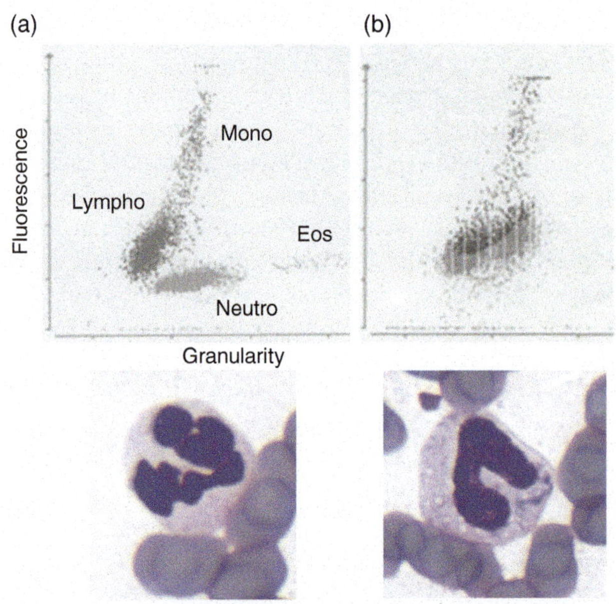

Figure 1.5 Laser-generated leukocyte differentials from the ProCyte Dx POC hematology analyzer (Idexx). The scatterplot is based upon side scatter (granularity) and fluorescence from a fluorescent polymethine dye that stains nucleic acids. (a) Scatterplot from a healthy horse. Neutrophils have the least amount of cytoplasmic RNA, thus are located at the base of the y-axis. (b) Scatterplot from a horse with toxic change in neutrophils and a left shift to band neutrophils. Neutrophils with toxic change and bands both have increased RNA content relative to normal mature neutrophils. Note how the increased RNA staining causes the neutrophil plot area to move upwards on the y-axis, blending into the lymphocyte region.

1.4.2 Clinical Chemistry Analyzers

1.4.2.1 Dry Reagent Analyzers

The majority of in-clinic chemistry analyzers are based upon dry reagent technology, which uses reflectance photometry. Similar to absorbance photometry, a chemical reaction (occurring within a dry fiber pad or multilayer film) results in a product that absorbs a portion of the light that illuminates it. The remaining reflected light reaches a photodetector that measures its intensity relative to the original illuminating light or a reference surface. There is an inverse relationship between reflected light (transmittance) and absorbance, where T is the percent transmittance (Equation 1.1). Analyzers will convert transmittance into absorbance because of the linear relationship between concentration and absorbance. Thus, concentration can be directly calculated from the absorbance.

$$\text{Absorbance} = 2 \quad \log \%T \tag{1.1}$$

Dry reagent technology has the advantage of minimal interference from hemolysis, lipemia, and icterus relative to wet chemistry analyzers. While most of the common chemistry analytes can be measured with dry chemistry systems, electrolytes cannot. Common in-clinic analyzers using this methodology include the Spotchem® (Heska), VetTest® (IDEXX), and RefloVet® Plus (Scil Animal Care Company, Grayslake, IL).

1.4.2.2 Reconstituted Liquid Chemistry Analyzers

Liquid chemistry analyzers operate via absorbance photometry. Reconstituted liquid systems use lyophilized rather than liquid reagents in cuvettes attached to rotors so that centrifugation mixes the sample with the reagent. Similar to reflectance photometry, when the sample is added to the reagents a chemical reaction occurs, manifesting as a color change in the liquid. Light of a specific wavelength is then passed through the liquid; the wavelength used is usually the one at which maximum absorbance for the substance being measured occurs. The light transmitted through the fluid post reaction is measured and converted into absorbance. Liquid chemistry systems are affected by hemolysis, lipemia, and bilirubinemia more than dry reagent systems. If not already known, determining the effect of substances such as these on the measurement of specific analytes should be part of the validation of a methodology.

Examples of this type of chemistry analyzer include VetScan® (Abaxis) and Hemagen Analyzt® (Hemagen Diagnostics, Columbia, MD). Just as with dry reagent systems, most common chemistry analytes, with the exception of electrolytes, can be measured.

1.4.2.3 Electrochemistry

In order to measure ion concentration, electrochemistry (also known as ion selective electrode [ISE] methodology) is employed in POC analyzers. Examples include the VitalPath™ (Heska), VetLyte® and VetStat® (IDEXX), and

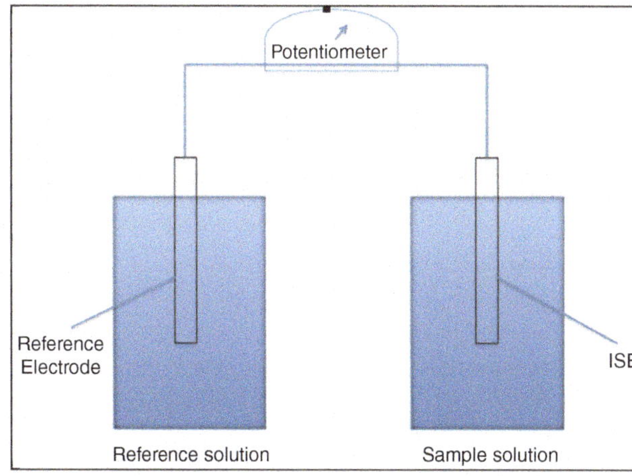

Figure 1.6 Ion selective electrode (ISE) methodology. When a sample is in contact with the membrane selective for the ion to be measured, a membrane potential proportional to the activity of the ion develops. The ion concentration is calculated using the Nernst equation by comparing the sample potential to the potential generated from a reference electrode in a reference solution.

EasyLyte® Plus (Hemagen). ISE technology relies upon development of a membrane potential for the ion being measured. This is achieved by using an electrode with a membrane selective for the ion being measured. The membrane potential that develops when the membrane is in contact with the sample is then proportional to the activity of the ion of interest (Figure 1.6). This is compared to the reference electrode to calculate the ion concentration using the Nernst equation. Unlike flame photometry methods to measure electrolytes, ISE is not affected by lipemia or hyperproteinemia.

1.5 Test Validation and Reference Values

1.5.1 Test Validation

Laboratory test method validation refers to the multitiered process of evaluating the performance of a new instrument or test methodology, often in relation to an instrument or methodology that is currently in use. In its broadest sense, method validation comprises the evaluation of test performance following a change in reagents, instruments, methodology, or – unique to veterinary clinical laboratories – introduction of a new species. The importance of test validation for different species cannot be overstated. As a result of the interspecies structural differences in any given analyte, a methodology that is adequate for one species may be inappropriate for another. Differences in expected reference values may affect whether a test has an appropriate detection limit and analytical range. Species differences exist also in how lipid, hemoglobin or bilirubin interfere with analyte measurements [9]. Certainly, drug interferences could also be species specific. Thus, in the age of POC instrumentation, it is essential that the instrument be validated for the species in which it is used.

Before evaluating a test for a novel species, it is important to know whether the analyte to be measured is clinically relevant. For example, in equids there is little need to validate an alanine aminotransferase (ALT) assay for clinical purposes (see Chapters 5 and 10). The ultimate goal of method validation is to provide objective evidence that the evaluated method will show acceptable reproducibility and accuracy so as to be clinically applicable.

The major steps in test validation consist of estimating the following.

1) Precision
2) Accuracy
3) Sensitivity
4) Specificity
5) Reference intervals

Reproducibility of results is referred to as *precision*. Precision is measured as a coefficient of variation and reflects the amount of variation inherent in the method and is estimated by repeating measurements of the same sample at least 20 times (intraassay precision). Estimating day-to-day precision (interassay precision) requires running aliquots of the same sample over 20 days [10].

Accuracy or *bias* measures the amount of closeness in agreement between the measured value of an analyte and its "true" value. Accuracy is estimated by comparing the performance of the candidate method with that of a definitive or reference method (gold standard), by performing a recovery experiment, or by comparing the candidate method with the established method that is being replaced. Recovery experiments estimate the ability of an analytical method to correctly measure an analyte when a known amount of the analyte is added to authentic biological samples.

Sensitivity is related to precision and refers to a test's ability to detect both small quantities of the analyte and small differences between samples. A "sensitive" methodology has a high level of analytical sensitivity and a low detection limit. The detection limit and analytical sensitivity are related but not synonymous. The detection limit is defined by the International Union of Pure and Applied Chemistry (IUPAC) as the smallest quantity or concentration that can be detected with reasonable certainty. The detection limit depends on the magnitude of the blank measurements and is related to their imprecision [11].

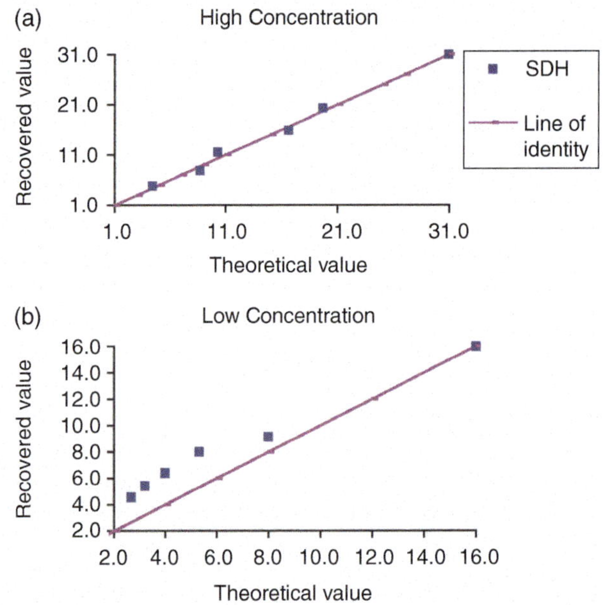

Figure 1.7 Serial dilutions of high and low concentrations of sorbitol dehydrogenase (SDH) to determine assay sensitivity. (a) There is very good correlation between the expected and recovered values in dilutions made from high SDH concentrations. (b) In contrast, at low concentrations of SDH the assay is less sensitive.

Sensitivity measures the change in signal relative to a defined change in the quantity or concentration of an analyte. This is usually accomplished by measuring a series of dilutions of a known amount of analyte (Figure 1.7).

Analytical specificity refers to the ability of a method to detect only the analyte of interest and is related to accuracy. Specificity may be affected by factors such as hemolysis, icterus or lipemia of serum or plasma, or by drugs and other substances that compete for reagents or affect the physical properties of the sample. Interference studies are performed by adding the interfering material directly and measuring its effects or by comparing measurements from hemolyzed, icteric or lipemic samples using the candidate method and one that is not affected by these factors.

Reference values are typically generated at the end of the method validation process and should be included with an instrument after the manufacturer has validated the methodology. When considering a POC instrument for purchase, if the manufacturer has truly validated the instrument for horses, species-specific reference values should be available.

1.5.2 Reference Values

The use of reference values to diagnose or screen for disease implies that health is a relative concept; clinical examination, evaluation of laboratory data, and diagnostic imaging findings all require comparison to a "normal" standard. "Normality" itself is also relative. What would be considered usual values for a racehorse may vary significantly from values from a cold-blooded working horse. Because health and disease are defined against "normal" or reference standards, the importance of appropriate reference values cannot be overstated. A few general principles regarding the use of reference values should be common knowledge for all veterinary practitioners.

1) When laboratory-specific or instrument-specific reference values are not available, published reference intervals (RI) should be used with caution. Published reference values should provide basic information regarding how health was defined for the population, as well as the general characteristics of the population (including number of animals sampled) and the instrumentation from which the values were derived. The practitioner should attempt to match the population and instruments from which the values were generated as closely as possible to the patient to which they are being applied.
2) Reference values obtained from one type of POC instrument should not be used interchangeably with those for another instrument, especially when different methodologies are involved. Similarly, using RIs generated from diagnostic laboratories analyzers to interpret data from your POC analyzer can be like comparing apples and oranges. If your POC analyzer does not come with RIs provided by the company from which you bought it, look for published RIs which are for similar POC analyzers. If your POC analyzer *does* have RIs provided from the manufacturer, take the time to find information on where the RIs came from. Some POCs may be designed for humans and the RIs provided may not even be from a veterinary species or may pertain only to a given species.
3) If you plan to replace a POC analyzer with a similar but different instrument and want to use the old RIs from your original analyzer, the old RIs should be validated for the new instrument. Validation can be achieved using a small sample (n = 20) of "normal" individuals. The values obtained from these healthy individuals can be tested against the RI to be used with the new instrument; if two or fewer subjects are outside the candidate RI, it is considered transferable. If three or four values fall outside the RI, another 20 patients can be tested and interpreted in the same manner as the original 20 samples. If >4 of the original 20 values fall outside the candidate RI, transference is rejected for that analyte and an alternative RI must be used [10].

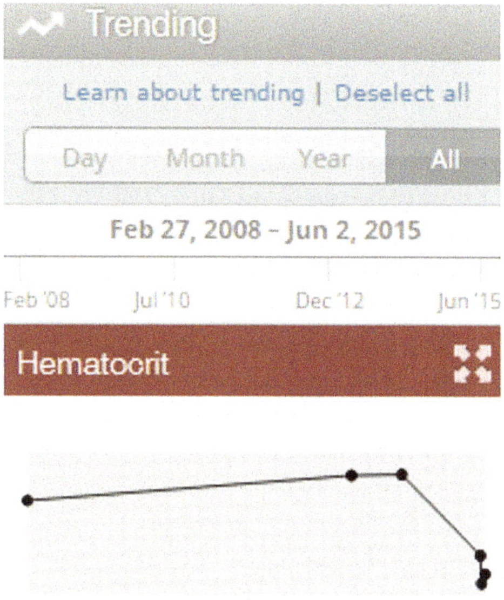

Figure 1.8 A graph from Idexx Laboratories' VetConnect® platform depicting a patient's hematocrits over the course of seven years. The gray zone represents the reference limits for hematocrit. Although the last three values on the graph are within the reference limits for "normal," these values are clearly abnormal for this individual.

Reference intervals used for interpretation of laboratory data are population based, using cross-sectional data typically representing 95% of the population chosen. Thus, by definition, any given RI implies that there will always be about 2.5% of the population whose values will normally fall above or below the RI. This fact should be considered when interpreting abnormal data that do not fit the clinical picture.

A population-based RI may not be sensitive enough to detect change in an individual if it is not marked. While this can be true for any analyte, some analytes are much more prone to this effect than others [12]. For these analytes, using the individual as its own normal can be much more effective in identifying abnormalities, especially with particular analytes (Figure 1.8). Patient-based RIs are generated from the individual patient's longitudinal data, if available, and can be assessed by looking at how the data trend from that patient in health. Some diagnostic laboratories and practice information systems provide graphing tools to follow patient data over time. In this manner, significant changes in an analyte can be detected before the values fall outside the RI.

References

1 Vap, L.M., Harr, K.E., Arnold, J.E. et al. (2012). ASVCP quality assurance guidelines: control of preanalytical and analytical factors for hematology for mammalian and nonmammalian species, hemostasis, and crossmatching in veterinary laboratories. *Vet. Clin. Pathol.* 41: 8–17.

2 George, J.W. (2001). The usefulness and limitations of hand-held refractometers in veterinary laboratory medicine: an historical and technical review. *Vet. Clin. Pathol.* 30: 201–210.

3 Dubin, S. and Hunt, P. (1978). Effect of anticoagulants and glucose on refractometric estimation of protein in canine and rabbit plasma. *Lab. Anim. Sci.* 28: 541–544.

4 Estepa, J.C., Lopez, I., Mayer-Valor, R. et al. (2006). The influence of anticoagulants on the measurement of total protein concentration in equine peritoneal fluid. *Res. Vet. Sci.* 80: 5–10.

5 Plebani, M. (2009). Does POCT reduce the risk of error in laboratory testing? *Clin. Chim. Acta* 404: 59–64.

6 Meier, F.A. and Jones, B.A. (2005). Point-of-care testing error: sources and amplifiers, taxonomy, prevention strategies, and detection monitors. *Arch. Pathol. Lab. Med.* 129: 1262–1267.

7 Weiser, M.G., Vap, L.M., and Thrall, M.A. (2007). Perspectives and advances in in-clinic laboratory diagnostic capabilities: hematology and clinical chemistry. *Vet. Clin. North Am. Small Anim. Pract.* 37: 221–236.

8 Giordano, A., Rossi, G., Pieralisi, C., and Paltrinieri, S. (2008). Evaluation of equine hemograms using the ADVIA 120 as compared with an impedance counter and manual differential count. *Vet. Clin. Pathol.* 37: 21–30.

9 Jacobs, R.M., Lumsden, J.H., and Grift, E. (1992). Effects of bilirubinemia, hemolysis, and lipemia on clinical chemistry analytes in bovine, canine, equine, and feline sera. *Can. Vet. J.* 33: 605–608.

10 Westgard, J.O., Barry, P.L., Carey, R.N. et al. (2008). *Basic Method Validation*, 3e. Madison: Westgard QC, Inc.

11 Koch, D.D. and Peters, T. (2001). Evaluation of methods-with an introduction to statistical techniques. In: *Tietz Fundamentals of Clinical Chemistry*, 5e (eds. E.R. Ashwood and C.A. Burtis), 234–250. Philadelphia: Elsevier.

12 Walton, R.M. (2012). Subject-based reference values: biological variation, individuality, and reference change values. *Vet. Clin. Pathol.* 41: 175–181.

2

Equine Hematology

Raquel M. Walton[1] and Cheryl A. Lawson[2]

[1] *IDEXX Laboratories, Inc., Langhorne, PA, USA*
[2] *Department of Veterinary Pathology, College of Veterinary Medicine, Iowa State University, Ames, IA, USA*

2.1 CBC Interpretation

The complete blood count (CBC) provides information beyond the concentrations of blood cells. Insight into disease processes, their severity, and even diagnoses can be gleaned from a complete evaluation of the CBC, especially in conjunction with a peripheral blood film. A single CBC is merely a "snapshot" in time; therefore, serial CBCs are often beneficial in better understanding a progressing or improving disease process.

Blood submitted for a CBC should be collected and immediately mixed with EDTA, which is the preferred anticoagulant for mammalian blood. Ideally, analysis of the sample should occur promptly to prevent the formation of cellular changes such as swelling and degeneration, which can affect both blood smear analysis and the evaluation of the blood sample with an automated hematology analyzer.

It is not uncommon in equine medicine for delays in sample analysis up to 24 hours to occur as a result of restricted access to diagnostic laboratories. Characteristic changes in blood parameters associated with delayed analysis of equine blood samples using a common hematology analyzer (Advia 120, Bayer Corporation, Tarrytown, NY) include increased numbers of normocytic, hypochromic red blood cells (RBCs), increased numbers of macrocytic, hypochromic RBCs, misclassification of granulocytes as mononuclear cells using the basophil reagent method, and a pseudothrombocytosis due to the categorization of lyzed erythrocytes as platelets. These changes are mitigated by storage at 24 °C rather than at 4 °C [1]. In general, equine blood differential leukocyte counts obtained from the Advia 120 show less precision compared with classic impedance methods and it is recommended that these instrument-derived counts should be verified with manual differentials [2].

It is also suggested that blood samples be warmed to 37 °C prior to analysis. Warming EDTA blood samples reduces pseudothrombocytopenia secondary to platelet clumping, a common preanalytical error for platelet counts [3].

2.1.1 The Erythrogram

In health, erythrocyte lifespan in horses appears to vary between breeds, but is approximately 140–160 days [4]. After a hemorrhagic event, erythrocyte lifespan is shortened to an average of approximately 139 days [5] and 144 days after a hemolytic event [6]. The erythrogram typically comprises the following elements: RBC count ($\times 10^6/\mu L$); hematocrit or packed cell volume (PCV) (%); hemoglobin (Hb) concentration (pg/dL); mean cell volume (MCV) (fL); mean cell Hb (MCH) (pg); mean cell Hb concentration (MCHC) (g/dL).

Calculated indices:

$$\textbf{Hematocrit}(\%) = \frac{\text{MCV} \times \text{RBC}}{10} \quad (2.1)$$

$$\textbf{MCH}(\text{pg}) = \frac{\text{Hb} \times 10}{\text{RBC}} \quad (2.2)$$

$$\textbf{MCHC}(\text{g/dL}) = \frac{\text{MCH}}{\text{MCV}} \text{ or } \frac{\text{Hb}}{\text{PCV}} \quad (2.3)$$

The indices that are measured by the hematology analyzer include RBC count, Hb, MCV, and PCV. Knowledge of which indices are calculated and which are measured will help to determine possible artifacts in the erythrogram. For example, a discrepancy between the hematocrit and PCV (>2% difference) will point to a spurious MCV or RBC measurement. When there is agglutination, the hematocrit may be spuriously low as a result of the measured RBC count being lower than the true RBC count due to the

Equine Hematology, Cytology, and Clinical Chemistry, Second Edition.
Edited by Raquel M. Walton, Rick L. Cowell, and Amy C. Valenciano.

presence of RBC aggregates that are not detected by the hematology analyzer. However, agglutination also may spuriously increase the MCV measurement when RBC doublets are measured as individual RBCs. If the spuriously increased MCV is in proportion to the spuriously decreased RBC count, the hematocrit may not be significantly different from the PCV.

Another example of artifact-associated change that may not affect measured values would be erythrocyte swelling associated with lithium heparin anticoagulant. Lithium heparin anticoagulant may cause spuriously high hematocrits as a result of RBC swelling causing spuriously high MCV [7]. However, the increased MCV will similarly affect the centrifuged hematocrit so there may not be a mismatch between the calculated hematocrit and PCV.

As a control for the accuracy of the analyzer hematocrit, a spun hematocrit (PCV) should always be run for comparison with the hematocrit. In the absence of a PCV, the universal relationship between the mammalian Hb concentration and hematocrit can be used to determine the accuracy of the hematocrit; for mammals other than camelids, the hemoglobin should be one-third of the hematocrit. For example, if the Hb concentration is 11 pg/dL, the hematocrit should be approximately 33%.

2.1.1.1 Erythrocytosis

Erythrocytosis is defined as an increased hematocrit and may be relative or absolute. Transient, absolute erythrocytosis in horses may occur as a result of splenic contraction (see Section 2.1.1.6). Hemoconcentration produces a relative erythrocytosis secondary to dehydration. Erythrocytosis due to hemoconcentration will produce concomitant increases in both the PCV and plasma protein concentration, whereas erythrocytosis from splenic contraction is not accompanied by alterations in plasma protein concentration [8].

Paraneoplastic erythrocytosis is rare in horses and has been reported with lymphoma, hepatoblastoma, hepatocellular carcinoma, and a carcinoma of unknown origin as a result of autonomous erythropoietin excretion by the neoplastic cells [9–12]. Neoplastic erythrocytosis (primary erythrocytosis or polycythemia vera) is very rare in equids with only a single confirmed case report in a 2-year old Arabian gelding [34].

2.1.1.2 Anemia

2.1.1.2.1 Regenerative Anemia Similar to other species, equids release erythropoietin in response to hypoxemia caused by decreased erythrocyte circulating mass due to loss or hemolysis. Thus, regenerative anemias in horses occur as a result of hemorrhage or hemolysis from immune-mediated damage, toxins, or oxidative damage. During immune-mediated hemolytic anemia (IMHA), antibodies with or without complement accelerate erythrocyte destruction [13]. Immune-mediated hemolytic anemia may be idiopathic or secondary to medications, neoplasia, or infectious disease. Oxidative damage in horses has been associated with red maple leaf toxicity, glucose-6-phosphate dehydrogenase deficiency, erythrocyte flavin adenine dinucleotide deficiency, onion ingestion, phenothiazine, and equine infectious anemia viral infection (EIAV).

2.1.1.2.2 Nonregenerative Anemia In horses, nonregenerative anemias are most often attributable to decreased erythropoiesis associated with inflammation or disease due to inflammatory cytokine effects, often referred to as "anemia of chronic disease." This type of anemia is now more appropriately termed "anemia of inflammation." The net effects of inflammatory cytokines result in decreased iron availability for erythropoiesis and direct suppression of erythropoiesis (Figure 2.1) [14].

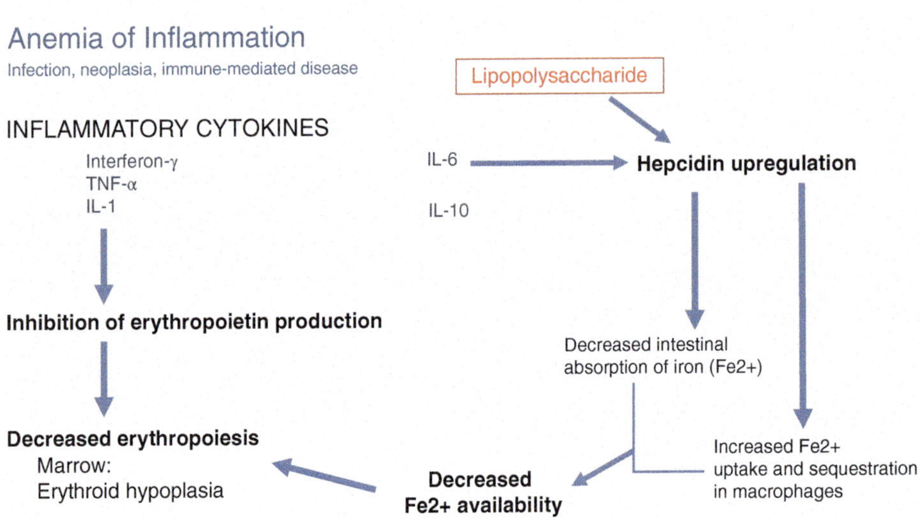

Figure 2.1 Simplified overview of the mechanisms in anemia of inflammation that result in erythroid hypoplasia and nonregenerative anemia.

Decreased plasma iron concentration was shown to have good sensitivity as a marker of systemic inflammation in horses [15]. The decrease in iron is a relative rather than absolute deficiency due to sequestration in macrophages. Absolute iron deficiency in adult horses is very rare.

Inflammation can be associated with neoplasia, infectious disease, and immune-mediated disease, resulting in nonregenerative anemia. However, these diseases can also cause hemolysis or hemorrhage, so some neoplasms, infectious agents, or immune-mediated disease may be associated with regenerative anemia depending upon the net effect of stimulatory and inhibitory forces. Impaired renal function may result in anemia due to decreased production of erythropoietin, but also as a result of inflammation [14, 16].

2.1.1.3 Changes in Erythrocyte Indices in Response to Anemia

The response to increased erythropoietin from most mammalian species is to release marrow reticulocytes into circulation, which can primarily affect MCV, MCH, and MCHC. The classic change in RBC parameters in regenerative anemia is therefore macrocytic and hypochromic in most species. In contrast, the typical regenerative response to anemia in horses is macrocytic and normochromic. Horses are unique amongst domestic mammalian species with respect to the lack of release of reticulocytes following mild to moderate anemia. While reticulocytes are produced within the marrow and increases in marrow reticulocytes are associated with regenerative erythroid responses, too few reticulocytes are released into circulation to be useful as an indicator of regeneration.

Until the advent of automated reticulocyte enumeration methods that evaluate more than 40 times the number of erythrocytes evaluated by manual methods, reticulocytosis was not thought to occur in equine blood. Using laser methodology (Advia 120), small numbers of circulating reticulocytes (0.5–$85 \times 10^3/\mu L$) can be detected in health [2]. Reticulocyte numbers vary slightly depending on breed and age, with cold-blooded horses having approximately 20% fewer reticulocytes compared to other breeds and Thoroughbred foals with approximately 50% more reticulocytes compared to adults. Nonblood diseases such as colic or dysproteinemia resulted in approximately 36% greater numbers of reticulocytes while marked anemia resulted in 120% greater numbers of reticulocytes [17]. However, since there are only low circulating numbers of reticulocytes overall, the clinical use of reticulocyte numbers is limited to severe anemias in select situations such as anemia associated with immune-mediated hemolysis [18] or with high-dose erythropoietin administration [19].

A regenerative response to blood loss anemia in horses is reported to take about four days from the onset of RBC loss, with a maximal response seen at nine days [20]. Recovery to normal values after a hemolytic event takes about 1–2 months [6], whereas recovery from hemorrhagic anemia is of the order of 2–3 months [5]. Historically, the best indicator of a regenerative response in horses prior to increasing hematocrit is evaluation of bone marrow. However, erythrocyte indices can show characteristic changes indicative of a regenerative response, especially in severe hemorrhagic or hemolytic anemias.

2.1.1.3.1 Mean Cell Volume Macrocytosis, characterized by the release of macrocytes that are roughly twice normal size, is part of the maximal erythrocyte regenerative response. This macrocytosis is not strictly related to reticulocytosis as regenerative macrocytosis in horses and other species does not correlate with reticulocytosis [19]. Macrocytosis is one of the first and most consistent parameters to show change following anemia in horses and is a more sensitive indicator of regeneration than hematocrit. However, horses with effective regenerative responses do not always have macrocytosis as defined by increases above reference values, especially with mild blood loss or hemolytic anemias. In these cases, serial evaluation of individual MCVs was more sensitive in detecting macrocytosis than comparison with a population-based reference interval [21]. Widening in the red cell distribution width (RDW) (discussed later) can also identify macrocytic subpopulations before the MCV increases above reference values.

In horses, macrocytosis subsequent to anemia is associated with a decrease in the number of normocytes, which suggests that macrocytes remain large and do not contribute to the normocyte population [22]. Macrocytes persist after hematocrit and RBC counts have returned to preanemia levels, so macrocytosis in the presence of other normal erythrocyte values in horses may be an indicator of a recent regenerative response [21, 22].

Microcytosis is typically associated with absolute or functional iron deficiency or portosystemic shunting in many species. In horses, the most common cause of microcytosis is physiological and age associated, necessitating separate reference values for MCV in horses less than 9 months of age. In horses, microcytosis associated with absolute iron deficiency has not been reported. Documented iron deficiency anemia in a foal was characterized as normocytic and normochromic [23]. Functional iron deficiency attributable to iron sequestration (i.e., anemia of inflammation) may result in microcytosis and does appear to occur in horses. Reported cases of larval cyathostominosis associated with microcytosis attributed the finding to systemic inflammation and/or protein exudation associated with intestinal parasitism [24].

2.1.1.3.2 RDW and the Distribution Histogram Most hematology analyzers will report the RDW with the erythrocyte indices. The RDW is a calculated value assessing the coefficient of variance of the erythrocyte volumes. In other words, it evaluates the amount of variation in the erythrocyte volumes and reflects the degree of anisocytosis.

Increases in RDW are associated with blood loss and hemolytic anemias, as well as with erythropoietin administration [19, 21]. Similar to the MCV, increases in RDW due to macrocytosis are detectable in serial comparisons of individuals, but may not exceed population-based reference intervals. Because the RDW can increase as a result of the emergence of smaller and/or larger erythrocyte populations, the distribution histogram itself can better identify the cause of increases in RDW. The impedance method (see Chapter 1) generates a histogram depicting the distribution of erythrocyte volumes (Figure 2.2). The RBC histogram is valuable in detecting the emergence of macrocytic and microcytic erythrocyte subpopulations. This is best accomplished by comparing serial histograms from a patient at weekly intervals. In horses, the histogram is especially useful because macrocytic subpopulations representing a regenerative response to anemia can be detected before the MCV rises above the reference interval [22]. Moreover, as discussed previously, not all horses with regenerative responses show changes in MCV above the reference interval, but macrocytic subpopulations are detectable on the histogram.

2.1.1.3.3 MCH and MCHC The mean cell hemoglobin (MCH) and mean cell hemoglobin concentration (MCHC) represent the quantity and the concentration of Hb, respectively, per average erythrocyte. Any increase in MCH and/or MCHC indicates artifact since it is not physiologically possible for these indices to increase outside the upper reference limit because Hb synthesis halts when the optimal amount of Hb is present within the erythrocyte cytoplasm.

Mean cell hemoglobin and MCHC are indices calculated from RBC and Hb concentrations, thus increases are associated with spurious RBC or Hb measurements. RBC

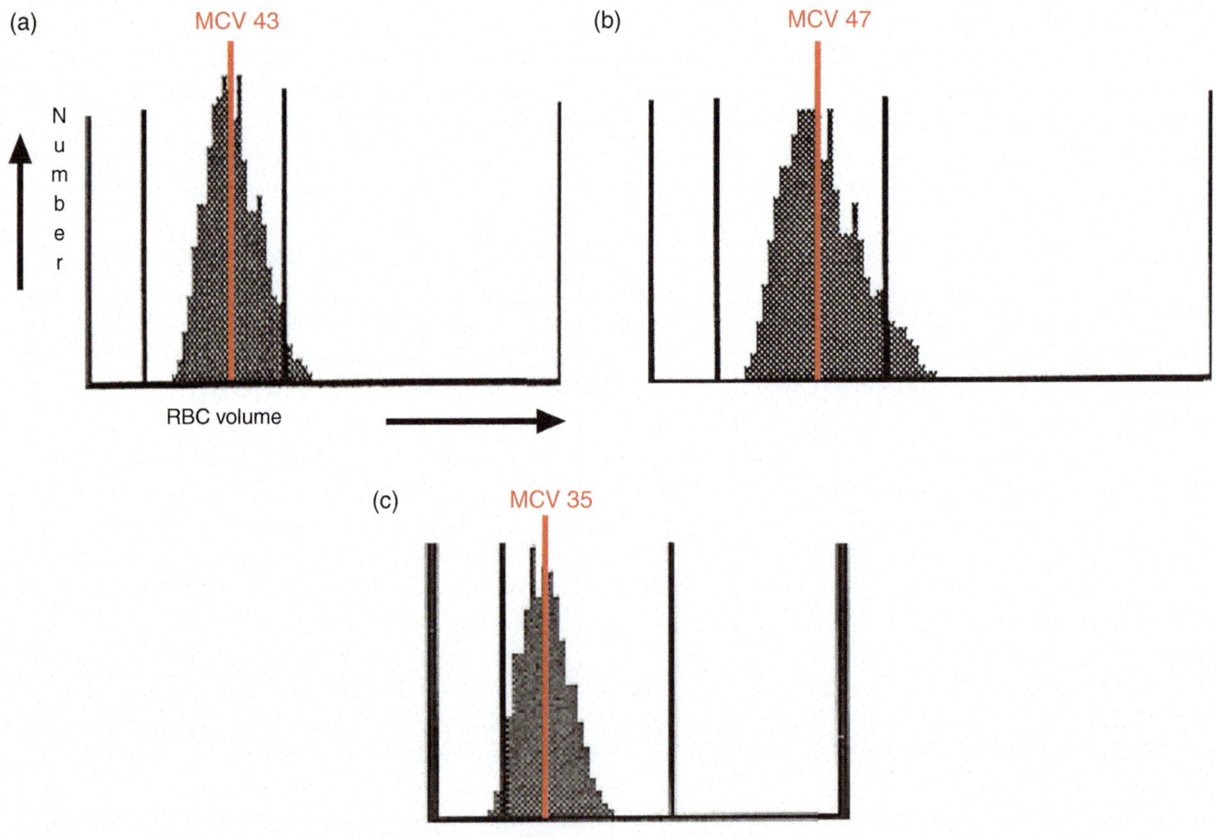

Figure 2.2 Red blood cell (RBC) histograms from the Advia 120 (Bayer Corporation) hematology analyzer. (a) Histogram from a hematologically normal horse. The red line shows the mean cell volume (MCV) in femtoliters; the black lines represent the instrument's preset range of equine RBC volume. (b) Histogram from a horse with a macrocytic anemia. Note the widening of the histogram to include a right shoulder. The MCV is still within the reference limits established for this instrument (38–55 fL), but there is an emerging population of macrocytes suggesting a regenerative response. (c) Histogram from a horse with a microcytic anemia. The whole population of RBCs is microcytic, resulting in a shift of the entire histogram to the left. This horse had an anemia of chronic disease.

agglutination may cause increases in MCH or MCHC due to a spuriously low RBC count. However, as discussed previously, decreases in RBC count due to agglutination may be countered by spuriously increased MCV measurements, resulting in minimal impact on the MCH and/or MCHC. Another common cause of increased MCH and/or MCHC is the presence of lipemia, which results in spurious increases in the Hb measurement. Heinz bodies will also falsely increase MCH and MCHC when determined by laser hematology analyzers and will spuriously increase the Hb measurement with spectrophotometric methods. *In vitro* hemolysis will also increase the MCH and MCHC because the number of intact RBCs is disproportionately low for the amount of Hb measured.

Decreases in MCH and/or MCHC are typically associated with regenerative responses to anemia in species that release reticulocytes in large numbers. Since horses do not usually release substantial numbers of reticulocytes into circulation in a regenerative response, the regenerative response is often normochromic. In other species, decreased hemoglobin concentration as a result of iron deficiency causes hypochromic (and microcytic) anemia, but in horses iron deficiency anemia is reported to be normochromic [23].

2.1.1.4 Age and Breed Effects on RBC Parameters

Relative to adults, erythrocyte number, Hb, and hematocrit (Hct) are increased at birth, decline sharply within 12–24 hours, and then show a gradual decline over the subsequent two weeks to levels at the lower end of adult reference intervals. This change is suspected to be due to the transfusion of placental blood to the foal with subsequent catecholamine release and fluid balance adjustment due to osmotic effects from absorption of immunoglobulins in colostrum [25]. Continued decline is thought to be due to factors such as decreased erythrocyte circulating lifespan, decreased iron delivery to the bone marrow, and reduced stimulation for erythropoietin production from higher hemoglobin saturation.

The MCV is high at birth and decreases to reach a nadir at 3–5 months of age; values are microcytic relative to adult reference intervals until 9 months to 1 year of age [26]. The microcytosis is thought to be due to a relative iron deficiency from limited storage of body iron or low concentration of iron in the dam's milk [23].

Breed effects on erythrocyte indices are reflected in higher Hct, Hb, and RBC counts in "hot-blooded" breeds (Arabians and Thoroughbreds) compared with the "cold-blooded" draught horse and pony breeds. In addition, Thoroughbreds have a smaller reported MCV compared to draught horses [26]. The use of breed-appropriate and age-specific reference values is therefore very important.

2.1.1.5 Splenic Effects

The equine spleen can store up to a third of the RBC mass and rapidly transfer large numbers of erythrocytes into the systemic circulation following epinephrine-induced splenic contraction [25, 27]. Epinephrine-induced splenic contraction is associated with excitement or strenuous exercise. Depending upon the baseline PCV, splenic contraction may result in erythrocytosis or a normal PCV. The time taken for the PCV to return to baseline following contraction may be 40–60 minutes to up to several hours, depending upon the magnitude of the stimulus.

In contrast, splenic RBC sequestration and congestion following barbiturate, alpha-2 agonist, or halothane anesthesia may drop the PCV below baseline values [28]. Thus, the spleen's large storage capacity may impact significantly on the circulating RBC mass. Anemia could potentially be masked following splenic contraction or simulated secondary to anesthetic-induced splenic congestion and RBC sequestration.

2.1.2 The Leukogram

The leukogram includes the numeric and morphological data pertaining to white blood cells. The leukogram, like erythrocyte indices, can provide information regarding the presence of a pathological or pathophysiological process, but rarely leads to a specific diagnosis. There are distinct leukogram profiles associated with inflammation, corticosteroids, and epinephrine.

2.1.2.1 Leukogram Patterns

2.1.2.1.1 Inflammation Acute inflammation results in the release of mature neutrophils and bands from the marrow storage and maturation pools, so neutrophilia with a left shift is characteristic of an active need for neutrophils. The marrow responds to inflammatory cytokines released into the blood by replenishing the storage and maturation pools from the stem cell and proliferation pools, resulting in a chronic or compensated inflammatory leukogram characterized by a mature neutrophilia. Inflammatory mediators stimulate neutropoiesis and subsequent granulocytic hyperplasia in the bone marrow. The total 7–9 days neutrophil transit time in health decreases to 3–4 days with inflammatory cytokine stimulation. When there is peracute, severe inflammation, neutropenia may occur as marked tissue demand depletes the storage pool before enhanced neutropoiesis can replenish the storage and maturation pools. A simplified depiction of the growth factors responsible for stimulation of neutrophil production and release is presented in Figure 2.3.

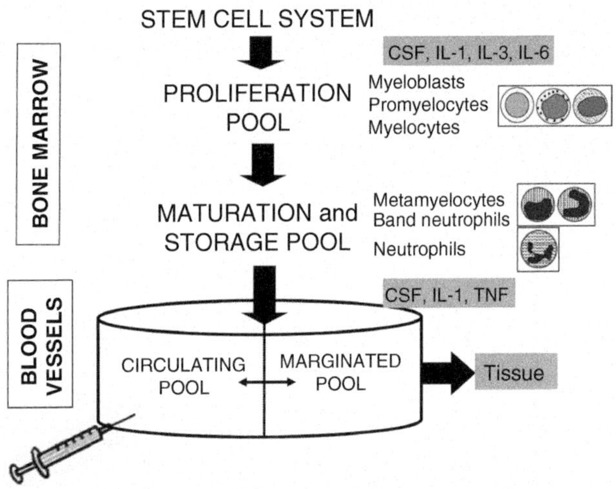

Figure 2.3 Schematic diagram of bone marrow and blood neutrophil pools. Inflammatory mediators released into the blood stimulate the marrow to produce neutrophils via an increase in growth factors and cytokines, mainly colony-stimulating factors (CSF) and interleukins (IL). G-CSF, GM-CSF, and IL-1, IL-3, and IL-6 are the most prominent in neutropoiesis. Inflammatory mediators and cytokines such as tumor necrosis factors (TNF), IL-1, and CSF increase neutrophil release from marrow sinuses and migration from blood into tissue. The most mature neutrophil forms preferentially leave the marrow; these forms also preferentially migrate into tissue.

The equine neutrophil storage pool is intermediate in size compared to the canine and bovine pools, which have the largest and smallest pools, respectively. Horses may have little to no neutrophilia or left shift during inflammation. Inflammatory neutrophilias in horses only occasionally exceed 20,000/μL and it is uncommon to see neutrophilias greater than 30,000/μL.

Monocytosis may be a feature of both acute and compensated (chronic) inflammation and generally reflects a need for macrophages. Thus, inflammatory processes that elicit histiocytic responses are associated with monocytosis.

2.1.2.1.2 Corticosteroid Response Endogenous and exogenous glucocorticoids produce a characteristic leukogram pattern consisting of a mature neutrophilia and lymphopenia. Unlike dogs and cats, horses do not have monocytosis as part of the glucocorticoid response. The neutrophilia is caused by release of marginated neutrophils into circulation. The ratio of marginated to circulating neutrophils in horses is 1:1, thus the maximum increase in neutrophil concentration due to demargination does not exceed twofold. Lymphopenia is considered the hallmark of the glucocorticoid response and is attributed to margination and emigration of lymphocytes to tissues and lymph nodes; chronic glucocorticoid effects include lymphoid hypoplasia, which contributes to the lymphopenia.

2.1.2.1.3 Physiological (Catecholamine) Response A physiological leukogram results from catecholamine release due to excitement, fear, or vigorous exercise. Catecholamine-associated leukocytosis occurs more often in young horses and stallions. A physiological leukogram, promoted by the effects of catecholamines, is characterized by lymphocytosis and a mature neutrophilia. Catecholamines promote an increase in circulating lymphocytes via demargination, especially from the spleen. The concomitant mature neutrophilia is also due to demargination. A modest mature neutrophilia and a lymphocytosis are characteristic of this leukogram. A lymphocytosis of 6000–14,000/μL is not uncommon. Physiological leukogram responses are transient (20–30 minutes) [29].

2.1.2.2 Changes in Individual Leukocyte Parameters

Sometimes, the changes to the leukogram do not correspond with a particular pattern and an abnormality must be assessed individually.

2.1.2.2.1 Neutropenia Neutropenia is clinically significant since it predisposes the patient to infection. In horses, neutropenia is most often due to increased distribution into tissues and/or rapid margination of circulating neutrophils secondary to overwhelming inflammation and endotoxemia, respectively. Less commonly, neutropenia is due to decreased neutrophil production in the bone marrow, which has been reported due to displacement of marrow by neoplastic cells (myelophthisis), myelonecrosis, and possible immune-mediated disease [29–32]. A rare cause of cyclic neutropenia was reported in related Standardbred horses believed to be caused by bone marrow microenvironment or growth factor defects [33].

2.1.2.2.2 Lymphocytosis Antigenic stimulation may produce lymphocytosis, but lymphocytosis in horses is more commonly attributable to epinephrine-associated responses than to antigenic stimulation. The presence of reactive lymphocytes supports an interpretation of antigenic stimulation even in the absence of absolute lymphocytosis.

Leukemias are rare in horses, though lymphocytic leukemia is the most common leukemia reported [34]. Leukemias are characterized as acute or chronic and by the cell line affected. Acute leukemias are represented by blast-like cells, whereas neoplastic cells in chronic leukemias appear fully differentiated. Chronic lymphocytic leukemia (CLL) manifests as peripheral mature lymphocytosis. Both B- and T-cell chronic lymphoid leukemias have been described [35–37]. Reported lymphocyte counts in blood range from 30,000 to 492,300/μL.

Immunophenotyping of CLL can be accomplished via flow cytometric analysis of the blood [35, 37, 38].

Small cell lymphoma (SCL) typically arises within tissue (lymph nodes and viscera), and peripheral blood involvement may occur in advanced stages when the marrow is infiltrated (secondary leukemia). In primary leukemia, neoplastic lymphocytes originate in the bone marrow and secondarily spread into the peripheral blood. In advanced cases of CLL, neoplastic lymphocytes may infiltrate lymph nodes and other tissues, making differentiation between CLL and SCL difficult or impossible. However, in most species, the distinction between SCL and CLL is not important. In the WHO classification of hematopoietic tumors of domestic animals, small cell lymphocytic leukemias and lymphomas derived from the same neoplastic clone are classified in the same category (i.e., B/T-cell SCL/CLL). By convention, if the neoplastic cells are predominantly in blood and bone marrow, the disease is referred to as leukemia, whereas if the neoplastic proliferation manifests primarily in tissue, the disease is referred to as lymphoma. CLL and SCL are indolent diseases with prolonged survival.

2.1.2.2.3 Lymphopenia In addition to corticosteroid affects from stress or administration of steroids or acute inflammation, lymphopenia (including both B- and T-cells) may also be seen with combined immunodeficiency. Combined immunodeficiency has been described in Arabian and Arabian-cross foals and results in a severe lymphopenia (<1000/μL) and the lack of IgM production [39]. Severe combined immunodeficiency has also been described in a Caspian filly [40]. Lymphopenia has also been noted with infections with *Anaplasma* spp. and with early viral infections such as herpesvirus type I (HV-1).

2.1.2.2.4 Eosinophilia Production of eosinophils from the bone marrow takes 2–6 days. Eosinophilia is uncommon in horses but is most often inflammatory, associated with parasitic, fungal, and allergic (hypersensitivity) conditions, and the degree can be variable depending on the organ(s) affected. Eosinophilic myeloproliferative disease is rare but has been reported [41]. Paraneoplastic eosinophilia has been reported with intestinal lymphoma in a horse [42]. Multisystemic eosinophilic epitheliotropic disease, while associated with eosinophilic abdominal effusions and eosinophilic marrow hyperplasia, is not usually associated with peripheral eosinophilias [43, 44].

2.1.2.2.5 Monocytopenia, Eosinopenia, and Basopenia Monocytopenia, eosinopenia, and basopenia are difficult to document due to relatively low numbers being present in healthy animals. These conditions are not considered to be clinically significant, though eosinopenia may be appreciated with exposure to corticosteroids.

2.1.2.2.6 Pancytopenia Pancytopenia refers to reduced numbers of all three cell lines (anemia, neutropenia, and thrombocytopenia). Pancytopenia may occur secondary to myelophthisis, defined as crowding of the bone marrow, usually by neoplastic cells. Pancytopenia may also occur due to destruction or suppression of early multipotential hematopoietic stem cells from viral infections, necrosis, medications (e.g., trimethoprim; sulfa drugs; pyrimethamine) [45], or toxins.

2.1.3 The Thrombogram

In horses, platelet number and size are shown to be directly proportional rather than inversely proportional as in some species. Normal platelet counts in horses are the lowest of the common domestic species. Equine platelets are also smaller compared to dog and cat platelets with a mean platelet volume of approximately 5.0 fL [46].

2.1.3.1 Thrombocytopenia

The causes of thrombocytopenia are increased platelet utilization, decreased production, and increased destruction and/or sequestration. Of these etiologies, equine thrombocytopenia is most commonly attributable to consumptive processes related to inflammation and endotoxemia [47]. Prothrombotic stimuli, especially potent platelet activators such as thrombin and platelet activating factor (PAF), are produced subsequent to endotoxemia and with severe inflammation. Systemic activation of the coagulation system associated with severe inflammation and/or endotoxemia may result in thrombocytopenia from platelet activation and consumption [48]. Thrombocytopenia may be present in colic horses with or without disseminated intravascular coagulation (DIC) [49]. Thrombocytopenia is a common sequela of snake envenomation, likely through consumption and sequestration due to inflammation caused by venom components [50, 51].

A less frequent cause of equine thrombocytopenia is immune-mediated destruction (IMT). Etiologies associated with IMT include infectious, neoplastic and idiopathic. In equine infectious anemia (EIA), infection immune complexes consisting of EIA virus particles and antibodies deposit on platelets, targeting them for destruction. In addition, EIA-induced IMT shows a lack of compensatory megakaryocytopoiesis, which contributes to the development of thrombocytopenia [52, 53]. The mechanism of thrombocytopenia in *A. phagocytophilum* infection may also be immune mediated [54]. IMT has also been reported in horses with lymphoma, secondary to drugs (e.g., trimethoprim, penicillin) and as an idiopathic disorder [47, 53, 55]. Intermittent thrombocytopenia attributable to decreased production is unusual, but has been reported in conjunction with myeloid and megakaryocytic hypoplasia in related Standardbreds [33].

Pseudothrombocytopenia occurs when platelets are not counted in a blood sample. This may be the result of traumatic venipuncture resulting in platelet aggregation and clumping or EDTA-associated platelet clumping [56]. If the latter is suspected, reevaluation of the blood using lithium heparin anticoagulant is recommended.

2.1.3.2 Thrombocytosis

Thrombocytosis in most species is most commonly attributable to physiological or reactive processes. Physiological thrombocytosis occurs secondary to epinephrine-induced splenic contraction. Reactive thrombocytosis is reported secondary to inflammation, infection, or neoplasia. In one study population, thrombocytosis was reported in 1% of horses over a five-year period and was highly associated with inflammatory/infectious disease [57]. Thrombocytosis was also more likely to occur in younger horses and stallions.

2.2 Blood Film Evaluation

A blood film can be dissected into three parts: the body, the monolayer, and the feathered edge (Figure 2.4). The general approach to a blood film can be summed up as follows.

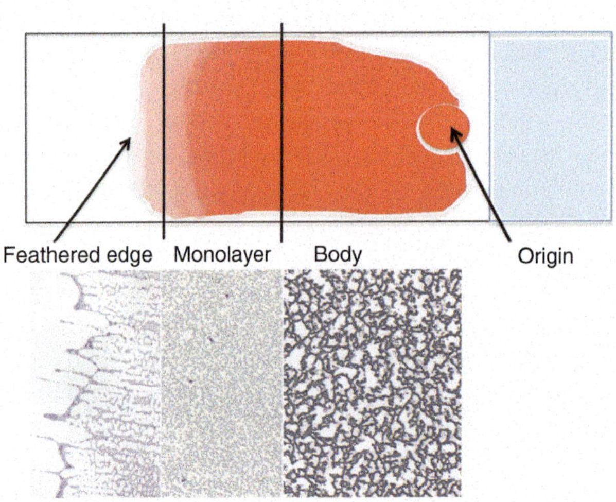

Figure 2.4 Anatomy of a blood smear. The feathered edge and monolayer should be scanned at first low power (4–10×) and the monolayer then evaluated at high magnification (50–100×). Note that leukocytes and erythrocytes cannot be evaluated adequately in the smear body due to the thickness of the preparation in this area.

1) Low-power scan (4× or 10×) of the feathered edge for platelet clumps, large cells, or microorganisms (Figure 2.5).
2) Low-power scan (10×) of the monolayer to estimate RBC and WBC density (Figure 2.6).
3) High-power (40× or 100×) scan of the monolayer to evaluate cellular morphology and perform leukocyte differential and platelet estimation. Note that the 40× objective was designed for use with coverslipped samples and will not focus properly unless the slide has a coverslip. A coverslip may be temporarily placed on the slide for viewing purposes or permanently fixed to the slide with mounting medium.

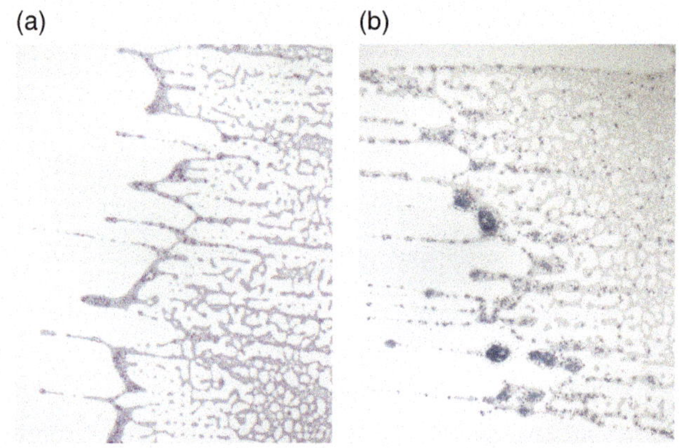

Figure 2.5 Comparison of the feathered edge from two different blood smears. (a) Normal blood smear feathered edge. (b) Note the presence of large platelet clumps that can interfere with both the automated platelet count and manual platelet estimation.

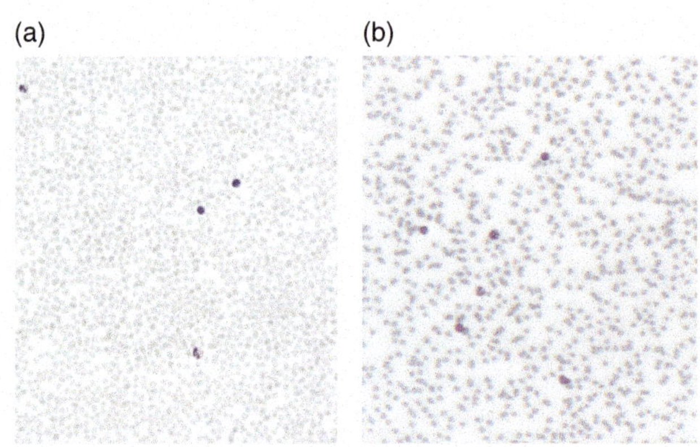

Figure 2.6 Evaluation of red blood cell density at low magnification (10×). (a) Monolayer of a normal blood smear. (b) Monolayer from an anemic blood smear. Note the difference in the concentration of erythrocytes in the monolayers.

2.2.1 Erythrocytes and Platelets

2.2.1.1 Erythrocyte Morphology

More than any other domestic species, equine erythrocytes have a strong tendency for rouleaux formation that is characterized by "coin-stacking." The prominent rouleaux is likely a result of the unique RBC glycocalyx glycoprotein composition of equids [58]. Rouleaux must be distinguished from agglutination, which also occurs in horses and has been associated with IMHA, unfractionated heparin therapy, and red maple leaf toxicosis [18, 59–61]. Agglutination on a blood film is characterized by the formation of grape-like RBC clusters in contrast to the "coin-stacking" associated with rouleaux (Figure 2.7). Distinction between agglutination and rouleaux can be difficult on a blood film, but is readily determined using a saline dilution test. When RBCs are diluted in saline (1:10 dilution), the rouleaux will disperse, but not agglutinated RBCs.

The umbrella term for variability in erythrocyte morphology is *poikilocytosis*, from the Greek *poikilos* meaning varied. The types of poikilocytosis encountered in equine hematology are similar to other species. Abnormal erythrocyte morphologies reported for the horse include eccentrocytes, spherocytes, and ecchinocytes [18, 60–63]. Morphological abnormalities such as keratocytes, acanthocytes, ovalocytes, and schistocytes are less common and have been reported in association with iron deficiency anemia in a foal [23].

2.2.1.1.1 Eccentrocytes Eccentrocytes are dense, spherocyte-like RBCs with a semilunar cytoplasmic clear area with irregular edges (Figure 2.8). They occur as a result of oxidative injury to erythrocyte membranes causing fusion of opposing areas of the cytoplasmic face of the erythrocyte membrane. Pyknocytes, which need to be distinguished from spherocytes, develop from eccentrocytes following the loss of much of the fused membrane (see Figure 2.8) [64]. Eccentrocytes likely represent a more severe form of oxidative damage than Heinz bodies [61]. Hemolytic anemia with eccentrocytosis has been associated with red maple leaf toxicity, glucose-6-phosphate dehydrogenase deficiency, and erythrocyte flavin adenine dinucleotide deficiency [61, 63, 65]. Hemolytic anemia with eccentrocytosis has also been reported in horses after ingestion of leaves from *Pistacia* species [66].

2.2.1.1.2 Heinz Bodies Heinz bodies are the result of oxidative denaturation and precipitation of the globin portion of hemoglobin into large aggregates, which are more readily seen using a vital stain such as brilliant cresyl blue (Figure 2.9) [64]. Hemolytic anemia with Heinz bodies has been reported with copper-associated hepatic toxicity, red maple leaf toxicosis, onion ingestion, phenothiazine and EIAV infection [61, 67, 68]. Heinz bodies should not be confused with Howell-Jolly bodies, which represent nuclear remnants remaining in the cytoplasm after mitosis.

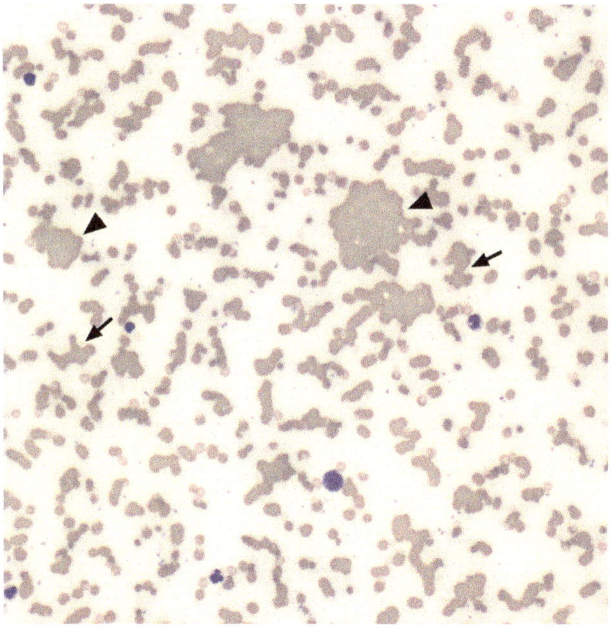

Figure 2.7 Equine blood film showing agglutination (*arrowheads*) and prominent rouleaux (*arrows*). There is some overlap in morphology between grape-like agglutination and coin-stacking rouleaux formation.

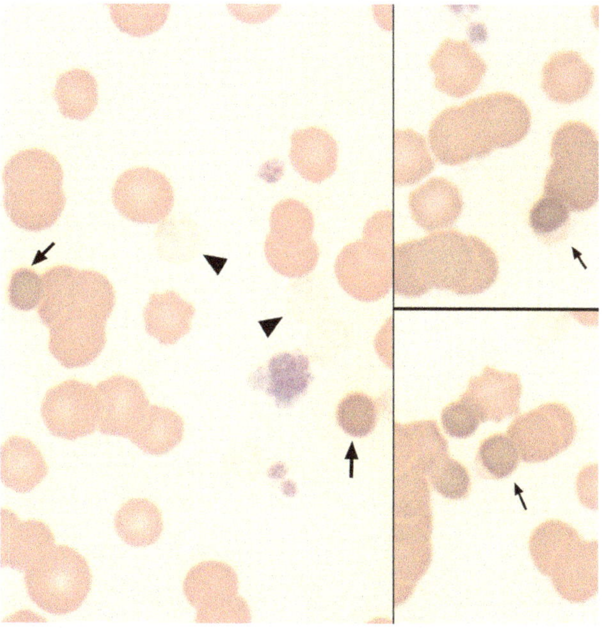

Figure 2.8 Equine blood film showing evidence of erythrocyte oxidative damage. Note the eccentrocytes (*right panels; small arrows*) and pyknocytes (*left panel; large arrows*). Ghost cells, indicating intravascular hemolysis, are also present (*left panel; arrowheads*).

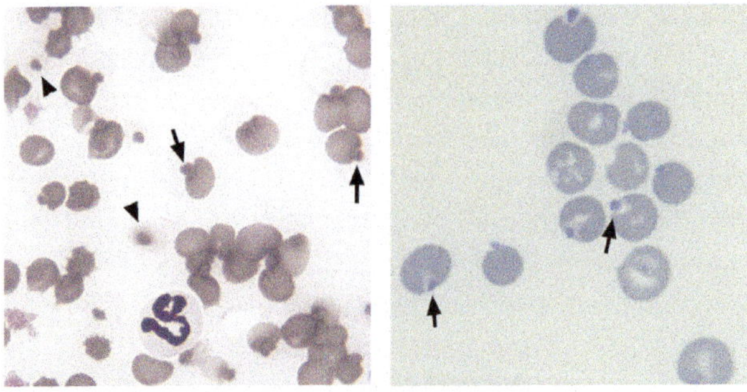

Figure 2.9 Heinz body hemolytic anemia. (*Left panel*) Heinz bodies are evident as dense round bodies that stain the same color as hemoglobin with Wright–Giemsa stain (*arrows*). Note the presence of ghost cells with Heinz bodies (*arrowheads*). (*Right panel*) A vital stain such as brilliant cresyl blue stains Heinz bodies blue (*arrows*).

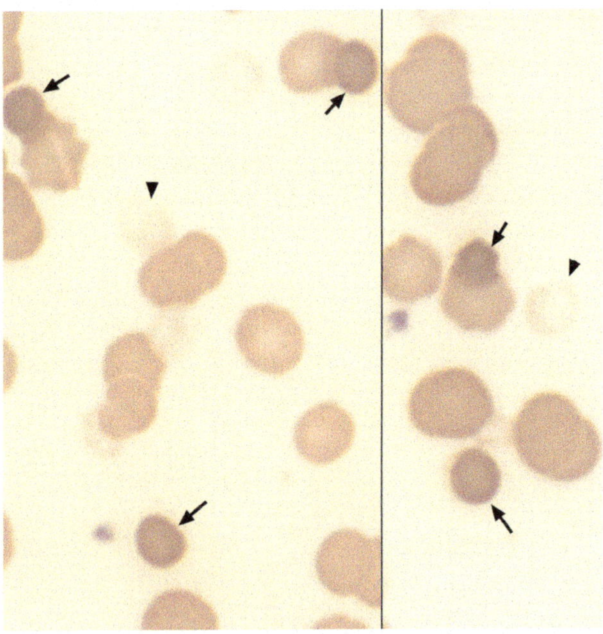

Figure 2.10 Spherocytes can be identified as dense, darkly staining erythrocytes (*arrows*) that appear smaller than normal erythrocytes. Note the presence of ghost cells (*arrowheads*).

These can be seen in small numbers in healthy horses (see Figure 2.14).

2.2.1.1.3 Spherocytes In species with small erythrocytes and a lack of central pallor, identification of spherocytes is difficult, but not impossible. Spherocytes are dense RBCs that appear smaller than average RBCs, although volume is not decreased (Figure 2.10). Spherocytes are morphologically similar to pyknocytes, but accurately distinguishing between the two is clinically important. Spherocytosis is the result of macrophage phagocytosis of bits of RBC membrane opsinized with immunoglobulin or complement. Thus, the presence of spherocytes usually indicates IMHA. In contrast, pyknocytes are derived from eccentrocytes following the loss of much of the fused membrane, thus represent oxidative damage to RBCs. Hemolytic anemia with spherocytosis has been reported in EIAV and IMHA [60].

2.2.1.1.4 Echinocytes Echinocytes are characterized by multiple undulations or spicules uniformly distributed around the erythrocyte circumference (Figure 2.11). This morphology can be an artifact associated with slow drying of blood smears or represent a true morphology associated with *in vitro* or *in vivo* conditions. Echinocytosis in horses has been strongly associated with hyponatremia, as a result of either disease or diuretic administration [62, 69]. Echinocytosis is a common sequela immediately following snakebite envenomation in dogs, but this does not seem to be the case in horses, likely because of venom dilution with the horse's relatively large circulating blood volume [70]. Aged blood may also have echinocytosis as a result of *in vitro* adenosine triphosphate (ATP) depletion and accumulation of lysolecithin in the RBC membrane. Thus, an interpretation of *in vivo* echinocytosis should only be made when fresh blood is evaluated and the smear has been properly prepared.

Spheroechinocytes have been reported in association with *Clostridium perfringens* IMHA [18]. It is thought that these spiculated spherocytes may represent true

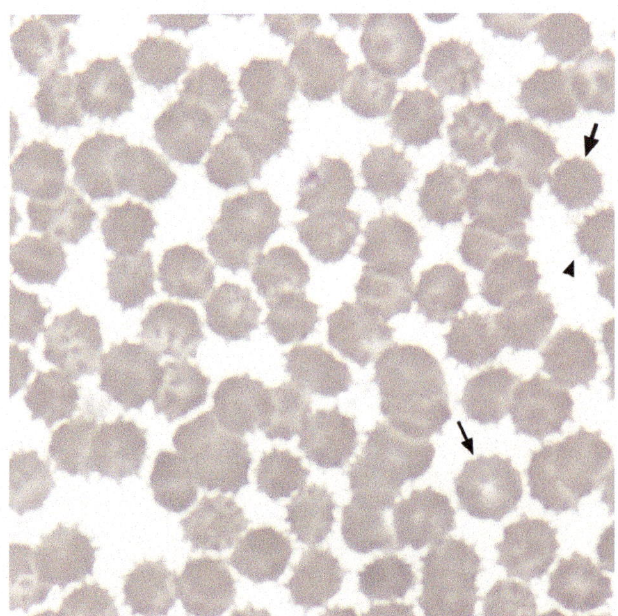

Figure 2.11 Echinocytes can range from erythrocytes with symmetrically undulating membrane (*small arrow*) to erythrocytes with symmetrical spiculated projections (*arrowhead*). A small, dense, darkly staining erythrocyte with sharp projections is a spheroechinocyte (*large arrow*).

spherocytes that have been modified by the echinocytic effects of the *C. perfringens* type A alpha toxin.

2.2.1.1.5 Schistocytes Schistocytes are erythrocyte membrane fragments resulting from shearing by mechanical or physical forces. They may be comma-shaped, triangular, or round to irregular bits of membrane (Figure 2.12). Fibrin strands from microthrombi, such as occurs with DIC or with vasculitis, can shear off RBC fragments. Schistocytes are not as consistently noted in horses with DIC as in dogs. Schistocytes can also be associated with iron deficiency, likely due to oxidative membrane damage or increased susceptibility to trauma in iron-deficient erythrocytes, and have been reported with iron deficiency in a foal [23].

2.2.1.1.6 Keratocytes Keratocytes are also grouped as products of membrane fragmentation injury. They are erythrocytes that contain a blister-like vesicle or vacuole at the cell periphery that ruptures to form a cell with a crescent-shaped defect and 1–2 horn-like projections (see Figure 2.12). Like schistocytes, they are associated with iron deficiency and microangiopathic disease (e.g., DIC or vasculitis). In the horse, it is unusual to see keratocytes, although they have been reported in association with iron deficiency in a foal [23].

2.2.1.1.7 Acanthocytes Acanthocytes are defined as cells with irregular, asymmetrically spaced projections, often with a paddle-like end (see Figure 2.12). The etiopathogenesis of acanthocytes is unknown in domestic animals, but in humans is due to lipid membrane changes, such as occurs with liver disease. They are associated with hemangiosarcoma in dogs and hepatic lipidosis in cats. These are rarely seen or reported in horses [23].

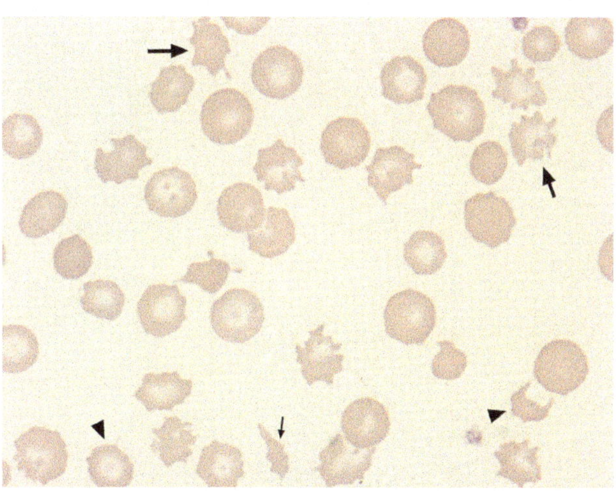

Figure 2.12 Schistocytes (*small arrow*), keratocytes (*arrowheads*), and acanthocytes (*large arrows*) in peripheral blood. These are uncommon in equine blood, but have been reported in association with iron deficiency in a foal.

2.2.1.2 Platelet Evaluation

Of the common domestic species, horses have the lowest platelet counts [46]. Thus, an adequate platelet estimation using oil immersion magnification (100× objective) is an average of 7–20 platelets per 100× field [71]. Equine platelets are smaller than dog and cat platelets, with a mean platelet volume around 5.0 fL [46]. Giant forms, approaching the size of erythrocytes, are indicative of increased platelet consumption or destruction.

2.2.2 Leukocytes

2.2.2.1 Neutrophils

Neutrophils are the predominant leukocyte in blood in healthy horses. Neutrophils circulate about 5–10 hours before entering tissues and do not return to circulation. Mature equine neutrophils have a segmented nucleus with 3–5 segmentations and cytoplasm that is pale pink to nonstaining (Figure 2.13). Fine magenta granules may be evident with Wright–Giemsa staining. Band neutrophils (Figure 2.14) have a nucleus with a uniform diameter that is U-shaped or S-shaped, whereas metamyelocytes have a reniform nucleus.

2.2.2.1.1 Toxic Change Toxic change is the result of altered bone marrow neutropoiesis and is associated with severe inflammation. Neutrophils and neutrophil precursors have increased amounts of organelles that are normally minimal to absent at later maturation stages, imparting characteristic morphological changes. Despite these morphological changes, the cells have normal function. Toxic change is characterized by any or all of the following (Figure 2.15): cytoplasmic basophilia, diffuse or focal (Döhle bodies); foamy cytoplasm; giant size; and less mature nuclei (more open chromatin pattern with segmented nuclei). The suspected cause for giant neutrophils is skipped mitosis at the myelocyte stage due to accelerated myelopoiesis [72]. Döhle bodies should not be mistaken for *Anaplasma phagocytophilum*, which are dark purple to black granular inclusions rather than blue (see Figure 2.14).

Cytoplasmic purple granules have been noted in foals up to 30 days of age without any other evidence of toxic change. Up to 70% of the neutrophils in 38 healthy newborn Thoroughbred foals were noted to display this change (Figure 2.16). Similarly, purple granules have been noted in a Paso Fino mare with hyperlipidemia and hepatic lipidosis that also had no other evidence of toxic change. These granules are suspected to be primary

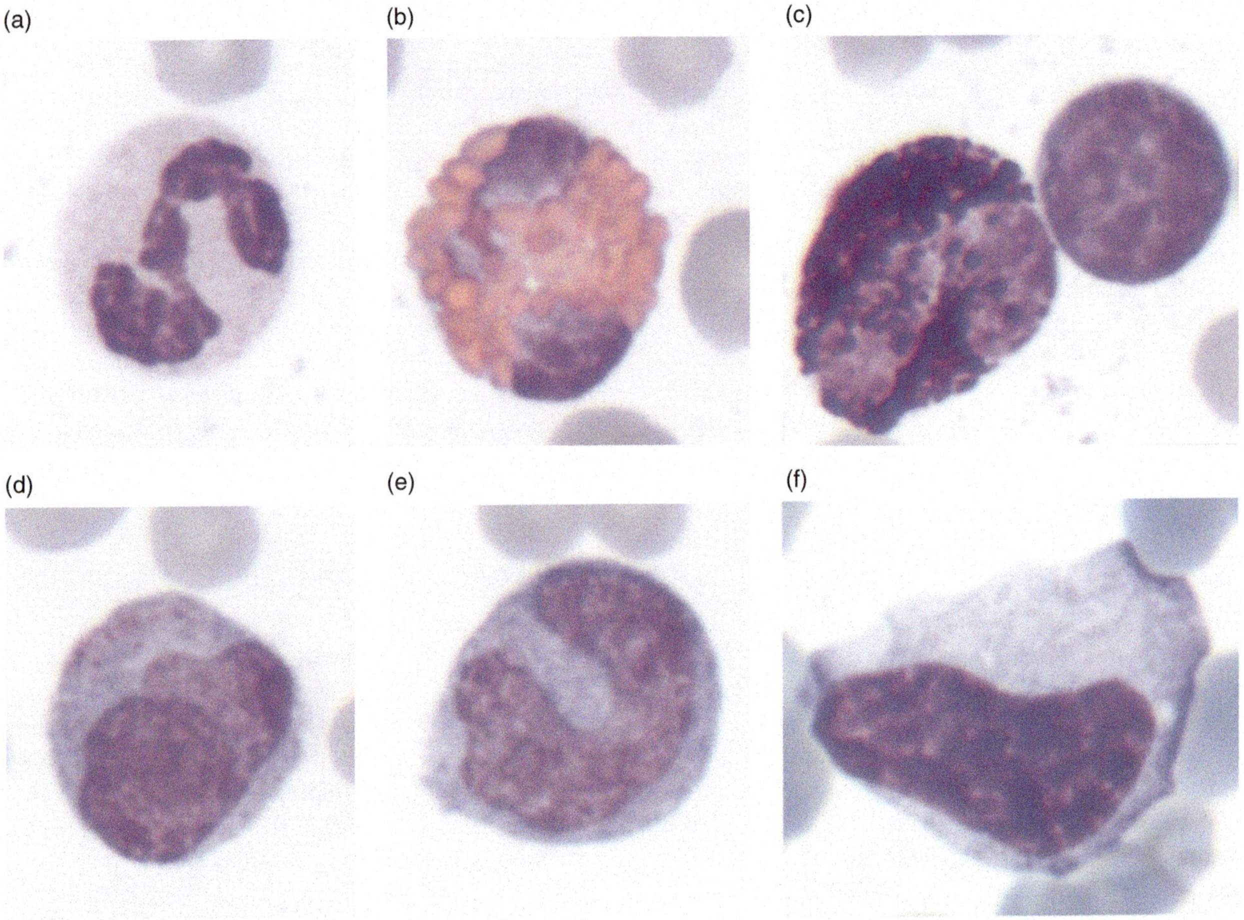

Figure 2.13 Equine blood leukocytes (Wright–Giemsa stain). (a) Mature neutrophil. (b) Eosinophil. (c) Basophil and small lymphocyte (on right). (d–f) Monocytes.

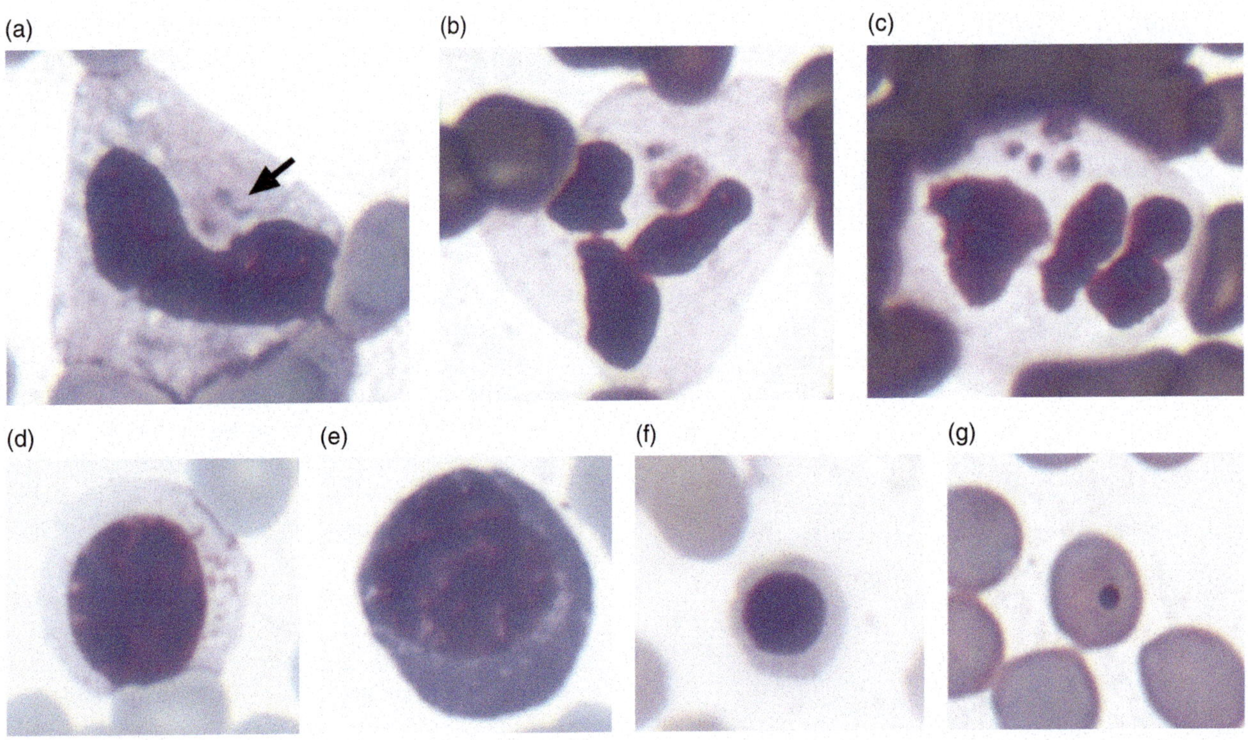

Figure 2.14 (a) Neutrophil band with linear to globular basophilic Döhle bodies (*arrow*). (b,c) *Anaplasma phagocytophilum* morulae in neutrophils (Diff-Quik stain). (d) Granulated lymphocyte. (e) Reactive lymphocyte. (f) Metarubricyte. (g) Howell–Jolly body in an erythrocyte.

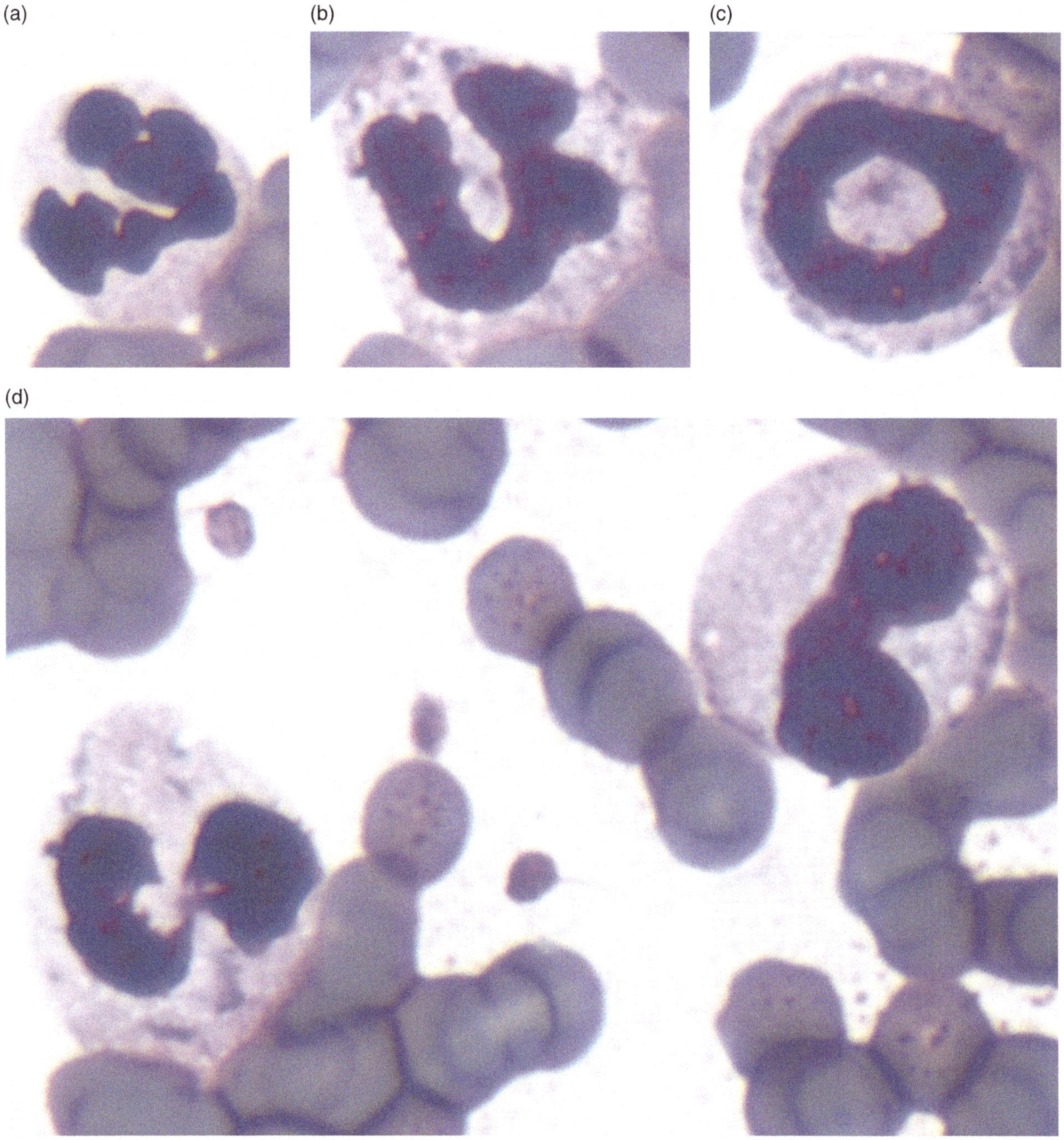

Figure 2.15 Toxic changes in neutrophils (Diff-Quik stain). (a) Normal neutrophil. (b) Neutrophil with toxic changes characterized by large size, presence of Döhle bodies, increased cytoplasmic basophilia, and less condensed chromatin. (c) The "donut" neutrophil is also considered a toxic morphology. (d) Toxic neutrophils with linear Döhle bodies (*left*) and generalized cytoplasmic basophilia with vacuolization (*right*).

granules with retained staining intensity similar to promyelocytes in the bone marrow.

Neutrophil hypersegmentation (defined by five or more nuclear lobes) can occur secondary to exposure to corticosteroids (endogenous or exogenous) due to delayed emigration of neutrophils from vessels into tissues. Pelger–Huet anomaly, a congenital defect resulting in hyposegmentation of granulocytes (neutrophils, eosinophils, and basophils), has been described in Arabian horses and must be differentiated from a degenerate left shift (Figure 2.17). Although neutrophils are hyposegmented, neutrophil function is not impaired [73, 74].

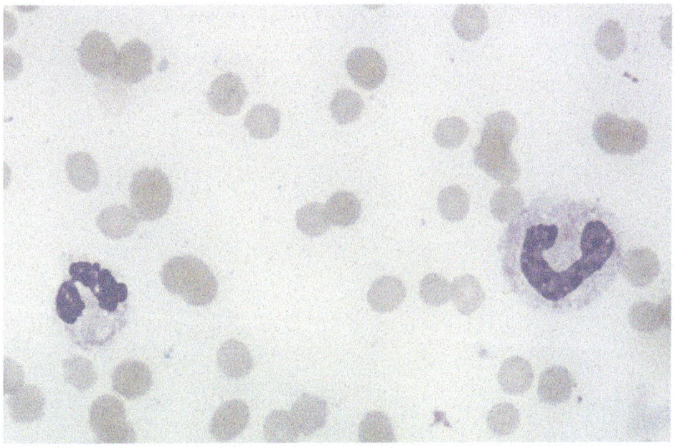

Figure 2.16 Two neutrophils from an Arab foal. Note the fine magenta granulation in the cytoplasm. Although the neutrophil on the right is slightly larger and less segmented, no other morphological changes associated with toxicity are present in the neutrophil population.

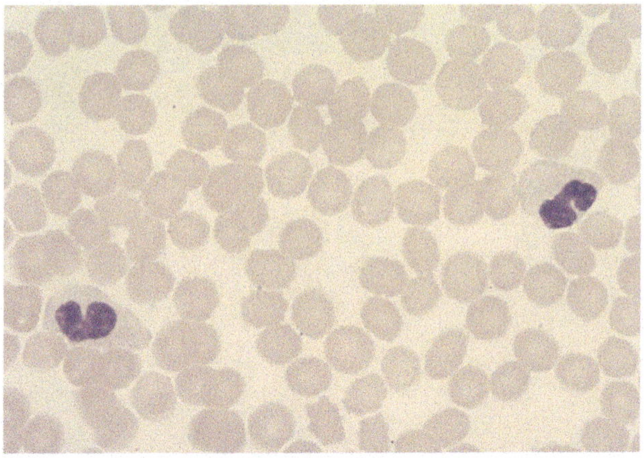

Figure 2.17 Hyposegmented, band-shaped neutrophils with no evidence of toxic change in Pelger–Huet anomaly.

2.2.2.2 Lymphocytes

Lymphocytes are the second most plentiful blood leukocyte in health. The ratio of circulating neutrophils to lymphocytes is about 1.5:1. The majority of circulating lymphocytes consist of T-cells (about 60%). B-cells comprise about 35% of lymphocytes and natural killer (NK) cells the remaining 5% [75].

Lymphocytes in blood are morphologically mature. Mature lymphocytes are the smallest of the blood leukocytes (7–9 μm diameter) and have a round nucleus, condensed chromatin, and scant basophilic rim of cytoplasm (see Figure 2.13). In comparison, nucleated RBCs (metarubricytes) have a nucleus with much more condensed chromatin and either gray or hemoglobinized cytoplasm (see Figure 2.14). The presence of circulating large lymphocytes (12–14 μm diameter) with less condensed, granular chromatin is abnormal and suggests a lymphoproliferative process (Figure 2.18).

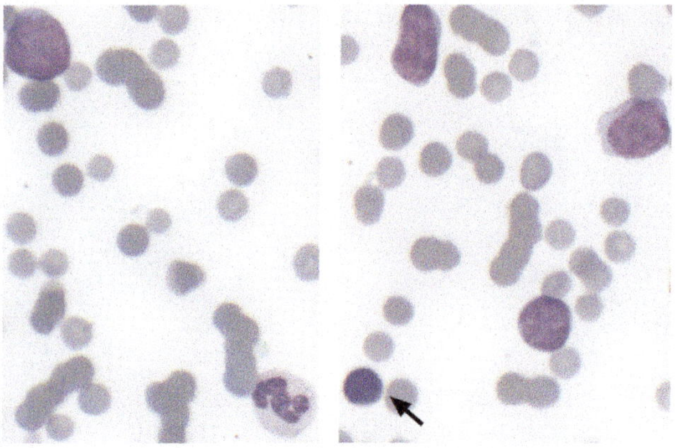

Figure 2.18 Two fields from a peripheral blood film from a horse with large cell lymphoma (Wright–Giemsa stain). The majority of lymphocytes are intermediate to large (10–16 μm diameter) with immature, granular chromatin. A normal small, mature lymphocyte is indicated by the arrow.

Reactive lymphocytes are slightly larger than mature lymphocytes with a mature, condensed chromatin and an increased amount of cytoplasm that is deeply basophilic. Granulated lymphocytes typically contain fine, magenta cytoplasmic granules (see Figure 2.14). Reactive lymphocytes and granulated lymphocytes are associated with antigenic stimulation. Granulated lymphocytes represent either T-cell or NK cell phenotypes.

Foals up to 6 months of age have increased numbers of circulating B-cells compared to adult horses and absolute and proportional B-cell concentrations are even greater in foals infected with *Rhodococcus equi* pneumonia [76]. Circulating numbers of CD4+ and CD8+ T-cells and B-cells increase linearly from birth to 3 months of age.

2.2.2.3 Monocytes

Monocytes are the third most common peripheral leukocyte, the largest in size, and usually comprise less than 10% of blood leukocytes. Monocytes have a reniform to lobate nucleus with abundant gray-blue cytoplasm that may or may not contain few punctate vacuoles. Monocytes have varied morphologies, and can resemble toxic neutrophils or even large lymphocytes (see Figure 2.13).

2.2.2.4 Eosinophils

Unlike neutrophils, the half-life of circulating eosinophils is days rather than hours. Eosinophils have a segmented nucleus and prominent round pink-orange secondary granules filling the cytoplasm (see Figure 2.13). Equine eosinophil granules are the largest of the common domestic species.

2.2.2.5 Basophils

Basophils are uncommon in the peripheral blood of horses (see Figure 2.13). The segmented nucleus, when visible under the dark blue to purple cytoplasmic granules, distinguishes the basophil from the mast cell, which has similar granules but an oval to round nucleus.

2.2.2.6 Neoplastic Cells

Neoplastic cells, identifiable as large, blast-like cells, may be observed on peripheral blood smear evaluation in horses with leukemia or lymphoma (see Figure 2.18). Blast-like cells are characterized by a high nuclear to cytoplasmic ratio, round to oval nucleus with finely dispersed chromatin, and ≥1 nucleoli.

Lymphoma, which originates in tissue other than bone marrow, is the most prevalent equine hematopoietic neoplasm, with 14 subtypes categorized using the World Health Organization classification system [77]. Neoplastic large lymphocytes may be seen in peripheral blood in lymphoma with or without bone marrow involvement [38, 78].

Acute leukemias, which originate in bone marrow, usually present with blast-like neoplastic cells in circulation. The diagnosis of acute leukemia requires bone marrow evaluation, and current criteria for diagnosis stipulate ≥20% blast cells in the bone marrow (see Chapter 3). Acute leukemias of lymphoid and myeloid origin are reported in horses [79, 80]. In horses with acute leukemia, the hemogram is typically characterized by bicytopenia or pancytopenia with the presence of neoplastic blasts; leukocytosis was not a feature of most reported cases of acute leukemia. Because large, blast-like cells do not generally show morphological characteristics of lineage, cellular identity cannot be definitively determined via morphology alone. Additional diagnostic tests such as immunophenotyping, immunohistochemistry, or immunocytochemistry are often necessary for definitive characterization of acute leukemia [81].

References

1 Clark, P., Mogg, T.D., Tvedten, H.W., and Korcal, D. (2002). Artifactual changes in equine blood following storage, detected using the Advia 120 hematology analyzer. *Vet. Clin. Pathol.* 31: 90–94.

2 Giordano, A., Rossi, G., Pieralisi, C., and Paltrinieri, S. (2008). Evaluation of equine hemograms using the ADVIA 120 as compared with an impedance counter and manual differential count. *Vet. Clin. Pathol.* 37: 21–30.

3 Williams, T.L. and Archer, J. (2016). Effect of prewarming EDTA blood samples to 37°C on platelet count measured by Sysmex XT-2000iV in dogs, cats, and horses. *Vet. Clin. Pathol.* 45: 444–449.

4 Carter, E.I., Valli, V.E., McSherry, B.J. et al. (1974). The kinetics of hematopoiesis in the light horse. I. The lifespan of peripheral blood cells in the normal horse. *Can. J. Comp. Med.* 38: 303–313.

5 Lumsden, J.H., Valli, V.E., McSherry, B.J. et al. (1975). The kinetics of hematopoiesis in the light horse. II. The hematological response to hemorrhagic anemia. *Can. J. Comp. Med.* 39: 324–331.

6 Lumsden, H.J., Valli, V.E., McSherry, B.J. et al. (1975). The kinetics of hematopoiesis in the light horse. III. The hematological response to hemolytic anemia. *Can. J. Comp. Med.* 39: 332–339.

7 Weiser, M.G., Vap, L.M., and Thrall, M.A. (2007). Perspectives and advances in in-clinic laboratory diagnostic capabilities: hematology and clinical chemistry. *Vet. Clin. North Am. Small Anim. Pract.* 37: 221–236.

8 Lording, P.M. (2008). Erythrocytes. *Vet. Clin. North Am. Equine Pract.* 24: 225–237.

9 Cook, G., Divers, T.J., and Rowland, P.H. (1995). Hypercalcemia and erythrocytosis in a mare associated with a metastatic carcinoma. *Equine Vet. J.* 27: 316–318.

10 Koch, T.G., Wen, X., and Bienzle, D. (2006). Lymphoma, erythrocytosis, and tumor erythropoietin gene expression in a horse. *J. Vet. Intern. Med.* 20: 1251–1255.

11 Roby, K.A., Beech, J., Bloom, J.C., and Black, M. (1990). Hepatocellular carcinoma associated with erythrocytosis and hypoglycemia in a yearling filly. *J. Am. Vet. Med. Assoc.* 196: 465–467.

12 Lennox, T.J., Wilson, J.H., Hayden, D.W. et al. (2000). Hepatoblastoma with erythrocytosis in a young female horse. *J. Am. Vet. Med. Assoc.* 216: 718–721.

13 Wilkerson, M.J., Davis, E., Shuman, W. et al. (2000). Isotype-specific antibodies in horses and dogs with immune-mediated hemolytic anemia. *J. Vet. Intern. Med.* 14: 190–196.

14 Weiss, G. and Goodnough, L.T. (2005). Anemia of chronic disease. *N. Engl. J. Med.* 352: 1011–1123.

15 Borges, A.S., Divers, T.J., Stokol, T., and Mohammed, O.H. (2007). Serum iron and plasma fibrinogen concentrations as indicators of systemic inflammatory diseases in horses. *J. Vet. Intern. Med.* 21: 489–494.

16 Grimes, C.N. and Fry, M.M. (2015). Nonregenerative anemia: mechanisms of decreased or ineffective erythropoiesis. *Vet. Pathol.* 52: 298–311.

17 Balan, M., McCullough, M., and O'Brien, P.J. (2018). Equine blood reticulocytes: reference intervals, physiological and pathological changes. *Comp. Clin. Pathol.* 28: 53–62.

18 Moritz, A. (2003). Equine immune-mediated hemolytic anemia associated with *Clostridium perfringens* infection. *Vet. Clin. Pathol.* 32: 22–26.

19 Cooper, C., Sears, W., and Bienzle, D. (2005). Reticulocyte changes after experimental anemia and erythropoietin treatment of horses. *J. Appl. Physiol.* 99: 915–921.

20 Malikides, N., Kessell, A., Hodgson, J. et al. (1999). Bone marrow response to large volume blood collection in the horse. *Res. Vet. Sci.* 67: 285–293.

21 Radin, M.J. and Eubank, M.C. (1986). Electronic measurement of erythrocyte volume and volume heterogeneity in horses during erythrocyte regeneration associated with experimental anemias. *Vet. Pathol.* 23: 656–660.

22 Weiser, G., Kohn, C., and Vachon, A. (1983). Erythrocyte volume distribution analysis and hematologic changes in two horses with immune-mediated hemolytic anemia. *Vet. Pathol.* 20: 424–433.

23 Fleming, K.A., Barton, M.H., and Latimer, K.S. (2006). Iron deficiency anemia in a neonatal foal. *J. Vet. Intern. Med.* 20: 1495–1498.

24 Peregrine, A.S., McEwen, B., Bienzle, D. et al. (2006). Larval cyathostominosis in horses in Ontario: an emerging disease? *Can. Vet. J.* 47: 80–82.

25 Hanson, C.M., Kline, K.H., Foreman, J.H. et al. (1995). Heart and spleen mass related to blood parameter changes after epinephrine injection. *Equine Vet. J.* 27 (S18): 113–116.

26 Harvey, J.W., Asquith, R.L., McNulty, P.K. et al. (1984). Hematology of foals up to one year old. *Equine Vet. J.* 16: 347–353.

27 Persson, S. (1967). On blood volume and working capacity in horses. Studies of methodology and physiological and pathological variations. *Acta Vet. Scand.* Suppl 19: 9–189.

28 Kullmann, A., Sanz, M., Fosgate, G.T. et al. (2014). Effects of xylazine, romifidine, or detomidine on hematology, biochemistry, and splenic thickness in healthy horses. *Can. Vet. J.* 55: 334–340.

29 Lester, G.D., Alleman, A.R., Raskin, R.E., and Meyer, J.C. (1993). Pancytopenia secondary to lymphoid leukemia in three horses. *J. Vet. Intern. Med.* 7: 360–363.

30 Kelton, D.R., Holbrook, T.C., Gilliam, L.L. et al. (2008). Bone marrow necrosis and myelophthisis: manifestations of T-cell lymphoma in a horse. *Vet. Clin. Pathol.* 37: 403–408.

31 Lavoie, J.P., Morris, D.D., Zinkl, J.G. et al. (1987). Pancytopenia caused by bone marrow aplasia in a horse. *J. Am. Vet. Med. Assoc.* 191: 1462–1464.

32 Spier, S.J., Madewell, B.R., Zinkl, J.G., and Ryan, A.M. (1986). Acute myelomonocytic leukemia in a horse. *J. Am. Vet. Med. Assoc.* 188: 861–863.

33 Kohn, C.W., Swardson, C., Provost, P. et al. (1995). Myeloid and megakaryocytic hypoplasia in related standardbreds. *J. Vet. Intern. Med.* 9: 315–323.

34 Muñoz, A., Riber, C., Trigo, P., and Castejón, F. (2009). Hematopoietic neoplasias in horses: myeloproliferative and lymphoproliferative disorders. *J. Equine Sci.* 20: 59–72.

35 Cian, F., Tyner, G., Martini, V. et al. (2013). Leukemic small cell lymphoma or chronic lymphocytic leukemia in a horse. *Vet. Clin. Pathol.* 42: 301–306.

36 Dascanio, J.J., Zhang, C.H., Antczak, D.F. et al. (1992). Differentiation of chronic lymphocytic leukemia in the horse: a report of two cases. *J. Vet. Intern. Med.* 6: 225–229.

37 Rendle, D.I., Durham, A.E., Thompson, J.C. et al. (2007). Clinical, immunophenotypic and functional characterisation of T-cell leukemia in six horses. *Equine Vet. J.* 39: 522–528.

38 McClure, J.T., Young, K.M., Fiste, M. et al. (2001). Immunophenotypic classification of leukemia in 3 horses. *J. Vet. Intern. Med.* 15: 144–152.

39 Crisman, M.V. and Scarratt, W.K. (2008). Immunodeficiency disorders in horses. *Vet. Clin. North Am. Equine Pract.* 24: 299–310.

40 Larson, J., Maxwell, V.B., Crisman, M.V. et al. (2011). Severe combined immunodeficiency in a Caspian filly. *J. Vet. Intern. Med.* 25: 954–958.

41 Morris, D.D., Bloom, J.C., Roby, K.A. et al. (1984). Eosinophilic myeloproliferative disorder in a horse. *J. Am. Vet. Med. Assoc.* 185: 993–996.

42 Duckett, W.M. and Matthews, H.K. (1997). Hypereosinophilia in a horse with intestinal lymphosarcoma. *Can. Vet. J.* 38: 719–720.

43 Bosseler, L., Verryken, K., Bauwens, C. et al. (2013). Equine multisystemic eosinophilic epitheliotropic disease: a case report and review of literature. *N. Z. Vet. J.* 61: 177–182.

44 La Perle, K.M., Piercy, R.J., Long, J.F., and Blomme, E.A. (1998). Multisystemic, eosinophilic, epitheliotropic disease with intestinal lymphosarcoma in a horse. *Vet. Pathol.* 35: 144–146.

45 Cudmore, L., Jalim, S., Williamson, M.M., and McKinnon, A.O. (2015). Pancytopenia in two horses following administration of potentiated sulfonamide antimicrobials. *Equine Vet. Educ.* 27: 519–523.

46 Boudreaux, M. and Ebbe, S. (1998). Comparison of platelet number, mean platelet volume and platelet mass in five mammalian species. *Comp. Hematol. Intl.* 8: 16–20.

47 Sellon, D.C., Levine, J., Millikin, E. et al. (1996). Thrombocytopenia in horses: 35 cases (1989–1994). *J. Vet. Intern. Med.* 10: 127–132.

48 Weyrich, A.S., Lindemann, S., and Zimmerman, G.A. (2003). The evolving role of platelets in inflammation. *J. Thromb. Hemost.* 1: 1897–1905.

49 Dolente, B.A., Wilkins, P.A., and Boston, R.C. (2002). Clinicopathologic evidence of disseminated intravascular coagulation in horses with acute colitis. *J. Am. Vet. Med. Assoc.* 220: 1034–1038.

50 Fielding, C.L., Pusterla, N., Magdesian, K.G. et al. (2011). Rattlesnake envenomation in horses: 58 cases (1992–2009). *J. Am. Vet. Med. Assoc.* 238: 631–635.

51 Goddard, A., Schoeman, J.P., Leisewitz, A.L. et al. (2011). Clinicopathologic abnormalities associated with snake envenomation in domestic animals. *Vet. Clin. Pathol.* 40: 282–292.

52 Clabough, D.L., Gebhard, D., Flaherty, M.T. et al. (1991). Immune-mediated thrombocytopenia in horses infected with equine infectious anemia virus. *J. Virol.* 65: 6242–6251.

53 McGovern, K.F., Lascola, K.M., Davis, E. et al. (2011). T-cell lymphoma with immune-mediated anemia and thrombocytopenia in a horse. *J. Vet. Intern. Med.* 25: 1181–1185.

54 Granick, J.L., Reneer, D.V., Carlyon, J.A., and Borjesson, D.L. (2008). Anaplasma phagocytophilum infects cells of the megakaryocytic lineage through sialylated ligands but fails to alter platelet production. *J. Med. Microbiol.* 57: 416–423.

55 McGurrin, M.K.J., Arroyo, L.G., and Bienzle, D. (2004). Flow cytometric detection of platelet-bound antibody in three horses with immune-mediated thrombocytopenia. *J. Am. Vet. Med. Assoc.* 224: 83–87.

56 Hinchcliff, K.W., Kociba, G.J., and Mitten, L.A. (1993). Diagnosis of EDTA-dependent pseudothrombocytopenia in a horse. *J. Am. Vet. Med. Assoc.* 203: 1715–1716.

57 Sellon, D.C., Levine, J.F., Palmer, K. et al. (1997). Thrombocytosis in 24 horses (1989–1994). *J. Vet. Intern. Med.* 11: 24–29.

58 Bäumler, H., Neu, B., Mitlöhner, R. et al. (2001). Electrophoretic and aggregation behavior of bovine, horse and human red blood cells in plasma and in polymer solutions. *Biorheology* 38: 39–51.

59 Feige, K., Schwarzwald, C.C., and Bombeli, T. (2003). Comparison of unfractioned and low molecular weight heparin for prophylaxis of coagulopathies in 52 horses with colic: a randomised double-blind clinical trial. *Equine Vet. J.* 35: 506–513.

60 Messer, N.T. and Arnold, K. (1991). Immune-mediated hemolytic anemia in a horse. *J. Am. Vet. Med. Assoc.* 198: 1415–1416.

61 Reagan, W.J., Carter, C., and Turek, J. (1994). Eccentrocytosis in equine red maple leaf toxicosis. *Vet. Clin. Pathol.* 23: 123–127.

62 Geor, R.J., Lund, E.M., and Weiss, D.J. (1993). Echinocytosis in horses: 54 cases (1990). *J. Am. Vet. Med. Assoc.* 202: 976–980.

63 Harvey, J.W., Stockham, S.L., Scott, M.A. et al. (2003). Methemoglobinemia and eccentrocytosis in equine erythrocyte flavin adenine dinucleotide deficiency. *Vet. Pathol.* 40: 632–642.

64 Harvey, J.W. (2006). Pathogenesis, laboratory diagnosis, and clinical implications of erythrocyte enzyme deficiencies in dogs, cats, and horses. *Vet. Clin. Pathol.* 35: 144–156.

65 Stockham, S.L., Harvey, J.W., and Kinden, D.A. (1994). Equine glucose-6-phosphate dehydrogenase deficiency. *Vet. Pathol.* 31: 518–527.

66 Bozorgmanesh, R., Magdesian, K.G., Rhodes, D.M. et al. (2015). Hemolytic anemia in horses associated with ingestion of Pistacia leaves. *J. Vet. Intern. Med.* 29: 410–413.

67 Ankringa, N., Wijnberg, I.D., Boerma, S., and Ijzer, J. (2012). Copper-associated hepatic cirrhosis in a Friesian horse. *Tijdschr. Diergeneeskd.* 137: 310–314.

68 McGuire, T.C., Henson, J.B., and Keown, G.H. (1970). Equine infectious anemia: the role of Heinz bodies in the pathogenesis of anemia. *Res. Vet. Sci.* 11: 354–357.

69 Weiss, D.J., Geor, R., Smith, C.M., and McClay, C.B. (1992). Furosemide-induced electrolyte depletion associated with echinocytosis in horses. *Am. J. Vet. Res.* 53: 1769–1772.

70 Walton, R.M., Brown, D.E., Hamar, D.W. et al. (1997). Mechanisms of echinocytosis induced by Crotalus atrox venom. *Vet. Pathol.* 34: 442–449.

71 Weiss, D.J. (1984). Uniform evaluation and semiquantitative reporting of hematologic data in veterinary laboratories. *Vet. Clin. Pathol.* 13: 27–31.

72 Lilliehöök, I., Tvedten, H.W., Bröjer, J. et al. (2016). Time-related changes in equine neutrophils after experimental endotoxemia: myeloperoxidase staining, size, and numbers. *Vet. Clin. Pathol.* 45: 66–72.

73 Gill, A.F., Gaunt, S., and Sirninger, J. (2006). Congenital Pelger–Huët anomaly in a horse. *Vet. Clin. Pathol.* 35: 460–462.

74 Grondin, T.M., DeWitt, S.F., and Keeton, K.S. (2007). Pelger–Huët anomaly in an Arabian horse. *Vet. Clin. Pathol.* 36: 306–310.

75 Satue, K., Hernandez, A., Lorente, C., and O'Connor, J.E. (2010). Immunophenotypical characterization in Andalusian horse: variations with age and gender. *Vet. Immunol. Immunopathol.* 133: 219–227.

76 Flaminio, M.J., Rush, B.R., and Shuman, W. (1999). Peripheral blood lymphocyte subpopulations and immunoglobulin concentrations in healthy foals and foals with Rhodococcus equi pneumonia. *J. Vet. Intern. Med.* 13: 206–212.

77 Durham, A.C., Pillitteri, C.A., San Myint, M., and Valli, V.E. (2013). Two hundred three cases of equine lymphoma classified according to the World Health Organization (WHO) classification criteria. *Vet. Pathol.* 50: 86–93.

78 Meichner, K., Kraszeski, B.H., Durrant, J.R. et al. (2017). Extreme lymphocytosis with myelomonocytic morphology in a horse with diffuse large B-cell lymphoma. *Vet. Clin. Pathol.* 46: 64–71.

79 Barrell, E.A., Asakawa, M.G., Felippe, M.J.B. et al. (2017). Acute leukemia in six horses (1990–2012). *J. Vet. Diagn. Invest.* 29: 529–535.

80 Cooper, C.J., Keller, S.M., Arroyo, L.G. et al. (2018). Acute leukemia in horses. *Vet. Pathol.* 55: 159–172.

81 Raskin, R.E. (2018). Diagnostic tools and dilemmas with equine leukemias. *Vet. Pathol.* 55: 11–13.

3

Bone Marrow Evaluation

Joanne B. Messick

Department of Comparative Pathobiology, College of Veterinary Medicine, Purdue University, West Lafayette, IN, USA

3.1 Indications, Technique, and Evaluation of Equine Bone Marrow Cytology

Bone marrow, the primary site of hematopoiesis, is one of the most widely distributed organs in the equine body. While hematopoiesis in the horse is similar to that described in humans, it is much less well studied and we rely heavily on extrapolation to understand this process in the horse. It is well established that hematopoietic stems cells (HSC), found mainly in the bone marrow, give rise to all the cells in the peripheral blood [1, 2]. In addition, the bone marrow serves as an important component of the reticuloendothelial system. Clusters of HSCs and their progeny in the marrow are nurtured and develop in the extravascular spaces between a vast network of vascular channels known as sinusoids. A support lattice for the developing hematopoietic cells is formed by cytoplasmic extensions from reticular cells that cover the surface of the sinusoids.

Additional components of the bone marrow stroma include vascular endothelial cells, macrophages, and adipocytes, as well as associated extracellular matrix molecules that regulate and control the process of hematopoiesis and provide an adhesive framework for the developing precursors. These components are collectively referred to as the microenvironment of the bone marrow.

The regenerative capacity and plasticity of bone marrow is extraordinary, with millions of red cells, platelets, and leukocytes produced every second of life. In times of hematopoietic stress or challenge, such as with blood loss, hemolysis, or infections, the marrow has tremendous reserve capacity and can increase production to 5–10 times normal [3].

The skeleton of the horse is mainly composed of two types of bony tissue that are important to our understanding of the bone marrow and collection of marrow for cytological or histological evaluation. Cortical or compact bone, which forms a dense, hard osseous shell around the bone, makes up about 80% of bone mass in the adult animal. Its outer surface is covered by a fibroelastic tissue known as periosteum, while a thin vascular membrane of connective tissue, the endosteum, lines its inner surface. Cavities within the cortical bone (medullary cavities) contain a meshwork of bony plates and rods, known as trabecular or cancellous bone, which are lined by endosteal cells, a continuum of their cortical counterpart [4]. The thickness and strength of the cortical bone that surrounds the trabecular meshwork vary depending on the location, as well as inherent stresses applied to that area [5]. Trabecular bone makes up much of the enlarged ends of long bones and it is within the spaces formed in this trabecular meshwork that hematopoietically active bone marrow tissue is found.

A large portion of the medullary cavity of bones is filled with active blood-forming tissue at the time of birth. However, in the adult horse, active marrow is found only in the axial skeleton, including the sternum, ribs, vertebrae, pelvis, and proximal ends of the femur and humerus. The most accessible of these sites for collection of bone marrow in the horse are sternum, dorsal ribs, and tuber coxae of the ileum [6]. The various bone marrow sites, it is assumed, have relatively uniform cellularity and proportions of hematopoietic cells under normal physiological conditions. Thus, generalization about hematopoiesis can be made from collection of bone marrow from a single site. The diagnostic accuracy for most hematological disorders does not appear to be improved by collecting samples from multiple bone marrow sites.

Equine Hematology, Cytology, and Clinical Chemistry, Second Edition.
Edited by Raquel M. Walton, Rick L. Cowell, and Amy C. Valenciano.

It is essential that bone marrow evaluation, whether an aspiration or core biopsy, should be preceded by an extensive review of all pertinent historical information and clinical features. Meticulous assessment of the blood film, complete blood count (CBC) data, and other laboratory tests, as well as any imaging studies, are essential to making an accurate diagnosis.

3.2 Indications

When a routine blood smear evaluation and other diagnostic testing fail to uncover the reason for an observed abnormality on the CBC, a bone marrow evaluation is indicated. The most common indication for this procedure is the presence of peripheral cytopenia in one or several hematopoietic cell lines for which an etiology cannot be found. However, unexplained elevations in blood cell numbers, abnormal cellular morphology, suspicion of marrow malignancy, and other clinical or laboratory abnormal findings, such as fever of unknown origin, hypercalcemia, hyperproteinemia, and presence of a lytic bony lesion, may also warrant a bone marrow evaluation [7].

There are few contraindications for obtaining a bone marrow sample. Marrow aspiration or core biopsies can be safely obtained even in horses with thrombocytopenia. However, in horses with an abnormal coagulation profile or platelet dysfunction [8, 9], severe thrombocytopenia ($<30\times10^3/\mu L$), and when there is concomitant use of anticoagulants, these procedures should be approached with great caution. The most frequent adverse events reported in humans are hemorrhage, persistent pain at the marrow site, and infection [10]. It was concluded in one study that bone marrow aspiration from the sternum of the horse did not elicit a measurable pain response during, or in the two hours following, the procedure [11]. While the collection of a bone marrow sample from the sternum is considered an innocuous procedure, there have been case reports of fatal cardiac puncture and nonfatal pneumopericardium in the horse [12]. This emphasizes the need for a thorough understanding of the anatomy of the equine sternum as well as the exact site and depth of needle placement before attempting the collection of bone marrow samples from this site.

3.3 Technique for Bone Marrow Collection

The two most commonly used sites for bone marrow collection in horses are the sternum and the tuber coxae. While the sternum is not covered by thick muscle and is often the preferred site, the awkward and somewhat unsafe position the person must assume when performing this procedure, and the possibility of severe complications, cannot be dismissed. These sites have been compared relative to the adequacy of samples obtained for harvesting the mononuclear cell fraction to be used for *in vitro* culture expansion of mesenchymal stem cells (MSC). MSC are shown to have high osteogenic capacity and may be used to treat tendon, ligament, and meniscal injuries, as well as enhancing the healing of cartilage defects and subchondral bone cystic lesions in the horse. For collection of multipotent mononuclear cells, the amount of bone marrow sample obtained and MSC yield were greatest from the sternal site [13]. The tuber coxae of the ilium may be used for collection of a bone marrow sample in younger horses, but it is doubtful whether an adequate sample can be obtained from this site in the adult horse, particularly as it relates to the collection of cells for therapeutic purposes. A bone marrow sample can also be obtained from the iliac crest in adult horses, but the needle must penetrate deeply through the overlaying layer of muscle to reach this site and needle placement appears to be more critical [14].

The bone marrow aspiration is typically done on the standing horse that has been sedated. Recent evidence suggests that the fifth sternebra is the most consistent and safe site for aspiration of bone marrow in horses. It is usually located just caudal to the point of the elbow, but identification of the correct site and accurate placement of the bone marrow needle into its medullary cavity can be greatly facilitated by the use of ultrasonography [12, 15]. The fourth sternebra may also be used for collection of bone marrow. Both the fourth and fifth sternebrae are somewhat spherical in shape and possess a dorsoventral extension of at least 2 inches [15]. Care must be taken to avoid moving more caudally as the sixth and seventh sternebrae are thinner and closer to the apex of the heart. It is this author's experience that moving too far caudally and penetrating too deeply are major mistakes that may result in a catastrophic outcome.

The bone marrow needles most commonly used for sample collection in the horse include the Illinois sternal/iliac bone marrow needle for aspirates and Jamshidi bone marrow biopsy needle for core bone marrow samples. It is suggested the bone marrow needle should be positioned substantially cranial to the most caudal aspect of bony structures of the sternum, which are also identified by this imaging modality; while this is a rather gross indication of "where not to tread," it may help to avoid a catastrophic outcome. The reader is referred to Kasashima et al. [12] for photographs, as well as ultrasonographic and radiographic images that delineate the topographical anatomy of the sternum and the appropriate sternebrae for obtaining a bone marrow aspiration or core biopsy.

A wide band of hair overlying the sternal site that is approximately 8 cm wide and 10 cm long and centered on the mid-line is clipped. The skin is over the fifth sternebra is aseptically prepared, cleaning the intended biopsy site outward in increasingly large concentric circles with surgical scrub and alcohol. Sterile gloves should be worn and aseptic technique maintained throughout the procedure to avoid the possibility of infection. Several 12 mL syringes should be preloaded with the appropriate anticoagulant. For therapeutic bone marrow harvesting, syringes are preloaded with 0.5 mL of 5000 IU/mL heparin solution, which gives a final concentration of 250 IU/mL of heparin after the addition of 9.5 mL of bone marrow [12].

Dipotassium ethylenediamine tetraacetic acid (K2 EDTA) is the anticoagulant of choice for bone marrow to be used for morphological evaluations. Syringes should be preloaded with 20 mg of K2 EDTA per each 10 mL of bone marrow volume collected; thus, three drops of a 15% K2 EDTA solution should be added to each 12 mL syringe.

The skin at the entry point for a bone marrow aspiration is infiltrated with local anesthetic, extending the injection of anesthetic to all tissues down to and including the periosteum of the bone. Following a second surgical scrub, a small stab incision is made through the skin and the bone marrow needle with its stylet in place is inserted to the level of the bone. The ventral surface of the sternebra is usually contacted at a depth of about 1.5–2 inches; the needle is advanced an additional 0.5–0.75 inches through the cortical bone into the marrow cavity using steady pressure and a gentle forward and backward rotation of the needle. For an aspiration sample, the stylet is removed once the needle is in place, a 12 mL syringe preloaded with K2 EDTA is attached, and rapid, strong negative pressure is applied to obtain approximately 7–10 mL of bone marrow. If necessary, additional syringes may be attached to the needle hub and the aspiration repeated to obtain more bone marrow. A sterile cap is placed on the syringe and marrow samples are immediately mixed by gentle inversion for, at the least, several minutes. The needle is removed after checking to make certain that an adequate bone marrow aspiration sample has been obtained, and pressure is applied to the site to control any bleeding that may occur following the procedure.

Smears from bone marrow aspirates for microscopic examination may be prepared using either the wedge-spread or crush techniques. There are advantages to each of these techniques; since particles are collected after the well-mixed aspiration sample is poured into a Petri dish, slides prepared by the crush technique of the transferred particles have less blood dilution and assessment of megakaryopoiesis appears to be more accurate. On the other hand, the wedge-spread may be more beneficial for the assessment of total cellularity. Whilst this author prefers the crush technique, there may be merit to routinely making slides using both of these techniques [16]. The prepared slides are air-dried and at least 2–3 slides, representing each of these techniques, are stained with a Romanowsky type stain such as Wright–Giemsa for cytological evaluation. Any remaining marrow sample in K2 EDTA and unstained slides should also be sent to the laboratory. This sample may be useful for additional studies such as cytochemistry, immunocytochemistry, or polymerase chain reaction evaluation, as well as automated hematology analysis.

The core biopsy sample can be collected through the same stab incision in the skin, but the needle should be directed in a slightly different direction to avoid the disrupted marrow spaces resulting from the aspiration procedure. As previously mentioned, the ventral surface of the sternebra is typically contacted at a depth of about 1.5–2 inches; the needle is then advanced through the cortical bone using firm pressure with an alternating clockwise and counterclockwise motion. It is suggested to position the forefinger on the Jamshidi needle about 0.5 inches from the skin surface to limit the depth of penetration of the needle through the cortex into the marrow space [6]. Once in the marrow space, the stylet is removed and the Jamshidi needle is advanced about 1–1.25 inches before rotating it several times in place to ensure that the core sample is detached. The needle is withdrawn and the core sample removed from its shaft and placed into 10% formalin for fixation. Notice the total depth of the needle penetration should not exceed 0.5 inches through cortical bone and 1.25 inches into the marrow space or 1.75 inches total, which is slightly less than the dorsoventral extension of this bone.

3.4 Bone Marrow Evaluation

Bone marrow aspiration and core biopsy samples must be interpreted in the context of a current CBC and should be evaluated by an experienced veterinary pathologist (see Cases 1 and 2). The CBC should be collected at the same time or within 24 hours of bone marrow collection. A careful review of the peripheral blood smear may reveal important clues that are directly related to an underlying hematological problem or provide information to help direct marrow evaluation and other diagnostics. In general, the bone marrow aspirate examination includes an overall assessment of cellularity and iron stores, as well as evaluation of the myeloid to erythroid ratio and judging whether maturation of the myeloid, erythroid, and megakaryocytic lineages is orderly and their morphology is normal. Further, other cell types such as lymphocytes, plasma cells, histiocytes (macrophages and dendritic cells), mast cells, stroma cells, and putative neoplastic cells must be characterized in terms of their abundance, distribution, and morphology.

3.4.1 Bone Marrow Aspirate

3.4.1.1 Cellularity

Bone marrow cellularity can be estimated on preparations of an aspirated sample, but should be verified by a determination made from a good-quality core biopsy section. The assessment of cellularity on slides prepared from an aspirated sample is subjective and can be influenced by adequacy of specimen collection, as well as hemodilution of the aspirated sample.

The overall cellularity in multiple bone marrow fragments or particles is evaluated. Cellularity is expressed in terms of the hematopoietic tissue as a percentage of total tissue within the particle, including hematopoietic and adipose tissue. The percentage of hematopoietic tissue within several particles should be estimated and this should be done on several slides before calculating an average. If the cellularity is highly variable amongst the particles, more particles should be assessed to provide as accurate an estimate as possible. An average particle cellularity varies from about 25% to 75%, but the age of the horse must be taken into consideration. The younger the animal, the higher the cellularity; it is not unusual in animals less than 6 months of age to have greater than 75% cellularity within particles and for the neonate, this may approach 100%. Cellularity decreases with age and senior horses (>25 years of age) may have as little as 20% cellularity within particles. This is considered normal cellularity given the young or advanced age of the animal, respectively. In an adult horse (~2–20 years), bone marrow cellularity is considered hypocellular when the percentage of hematopoietic cells within particles is on average less than 25%, whereas hypercellularity is defined when marrow particles have greater than 75% cellularity (see Case 1) (Figure 3.1a,b).

3.4.1.2 Myeloid to Erythroid Ratio and Marrow Reticulocyte Count

The orderliness and completeness of erythroid maturation in the bone marrow, determination of a myeloid to erythroid (M:E) ratio, and percentage of marrow reticulocytes are critical components for assessing the erythroid lineage in horses. To calculate the M:E ratio, a minimum of 500 nucleated cells should be classified as belonging to either the myeloid or erythroid lineage; it should be evaluated in several areas of the bone marrow slide and on several different slide preparations and should be correlated to the overall marrow cellularity. The range for the M:E ratio in healthy adult horses is 0.5–2.4 whereas the marrow reticulocyte count, which is a reflection of erythroid activity, is typically less than 3% [6]. In the horse, these parameters should be assessed concurrently in order to classify an anemia as regenerative or nonregenerative. The anemia is regenerative when the M:E ratio is <0.5 and the reticulocyte count >3%, whereas a low reticulocyte percentage in the bone marrow and a normal or increased M:E ratio support a nonregenerative erythroid response. In an intensely regenerative erythroid response, reticulocytosis in the bone marrow may increase dramatically and values as high as 60% have been reported [17, 18].

The presence of a peripheral regenerative response is difficult to assess in horses, since they do not tend to release reticulocytes into the blood but rather the vast majority of these cells mature in the marrow or spleen [19]. In addition to assessing the bone marrow components as discussed above, an increase in the red cell distribution width (RDW) and mean corpuscular volume (MCV) of circulating red cells may be subtle indicators of a regenerative response [6]. A clearer indication that the horse has mounted a regenerative response is sequential packed cell volume (PCV) measurements over time that show a steady increase, provided the hydration status of the horse is unchanged. It has been suggested that the reticulocyte count using an automated hematology analyzer, where thousands of the horse's erythrocytes are counted in assessing this response, may be a sensitive way to establish the presence of a regenerative response in some hemolytic anemias [18, 20].

3.4.1.3 Erythroid Lineage, Iron, and Abnormalities

An assessment of the morphology of erythroid precursors in the marrow is also essential. The nucleus and cytoplasm should be individually evaluated for any abnormalities and for the synchronicity of their maturation. Morphological irregularities or dysplastic changes of erythroid cells may present as abnormally large erythroid precursors, bizarre nuclear shapes, nuclear fragments, multiple nuclei, and asynchronous maturation of nucleus relative to its cytoplasm. While these changes are uncommon in horses, erythroid hyperplasia with a left shift in maturation and concurrent dysplasia eventually progressing to severe erythroid hypoplasia in the bone marrow of foals with fell pony syndrome or foal immunodeficiency syndrome (FIS) has been reported [21]. Iron stores should be easy to find in the bone marrow of horses (see Case 1) (Figure 3.1c), and a tendency for stores to be more prominent in older animals is reported. In some instances, Prussian blue staining of the bone marrow may be indicated to assess the presence or absence of iron stores. This procedure may be particularly useful if an anemia due to iron deficiency is suspected, although this is an extremely rare condition in horses [22].

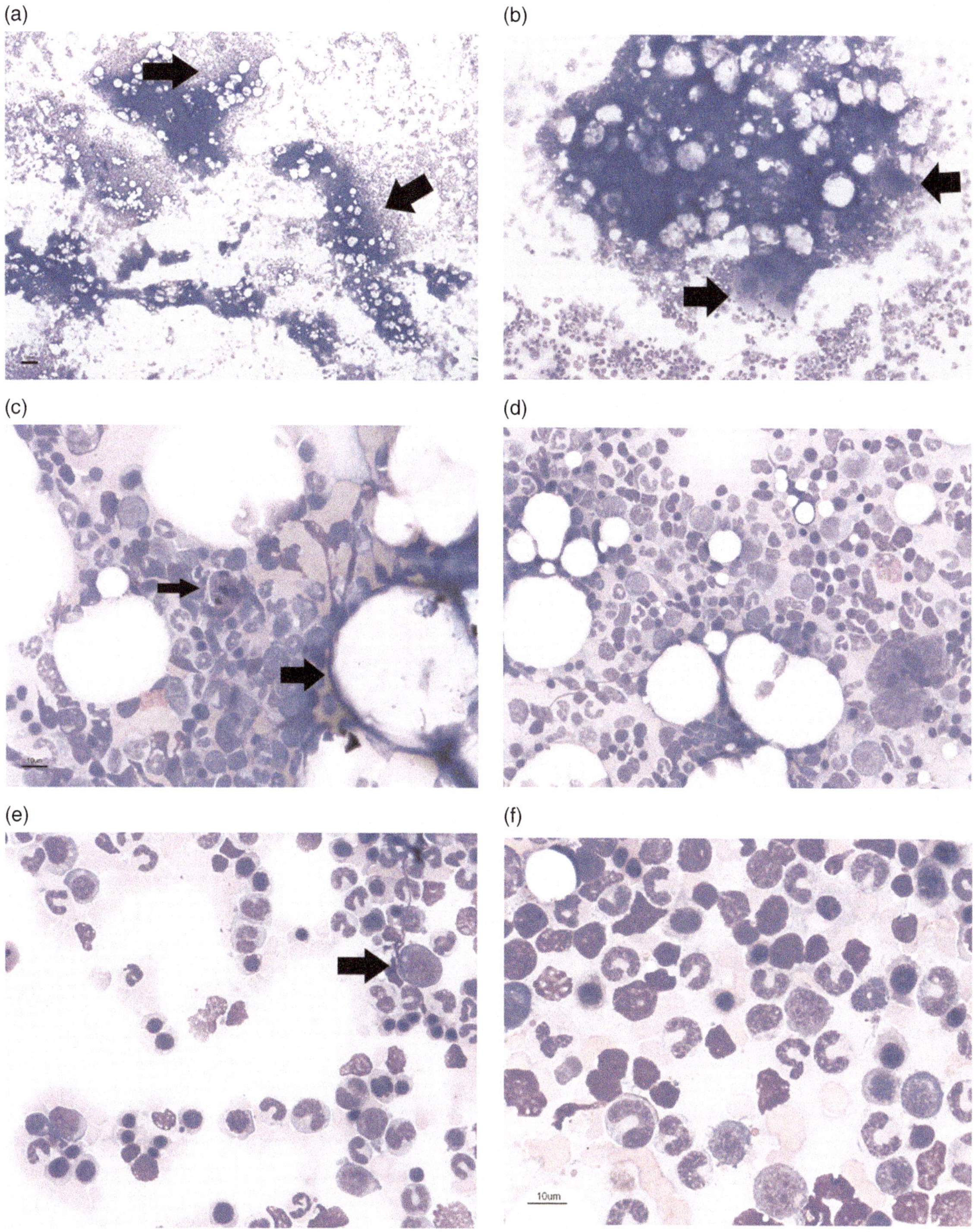

Figure 3.1 Bone marrow aspirate. (a) Many hypercellular particles are shown in this photomicrograph; adjacent to the particles, the cells are nicely spread out (*arrows*) and there are appropriate areas for individual cell identification and making morphological assessments (Wright, 10×). (b) This particle is composed of dense cellular aggregates with about 25% fat (clear spaces or balloon-like adipocytes). Hypercellular particles suggest increased hematopoiesis, but to exclude an infiltrative disease (primary or metastatic neoplasia), the cellular composition must be examined at a higher power. At the edge of this particle, several mature megakaryocytes can be seen (*arrows*). There are several more within the thicker portions of the particle, but these are more difficult to appreciate (Wright, 20×). (c) While iron is not abundant in this marrow aspirate, a few macrophages containing hemosiderin (*top arrow*) are observed. A Prussian blue stain could be performed on the aspirate to better assess the iron stores in this case. Nevertheless, there are no established guidelines for quantifying marrow iron; the assessment is very subjective. A typical balloon-like adipocyte is also seen in this field (*lower arrow*) (Wright, 60×). (d) In the area adjacent to this particle, the cytomorphological details of individual cellular elements are nicely preserved. However, these cells should be evaluated at a higher magnification to determine if the smaller, dense nuclei are erythroid or lymphoid and to evaluate finer details (Wright, 60×). (e) The M:E ratio is 1:1 with appropriate maturation of the erythroid lineage. The majority of the nucleated red blood cells in this image are metarubricytes, but rare erythroblasts are also noted (*arrow*). A new methylene blue staining of the bone marrow revealed there were 8% reticulocytes (Wright, 100×). (f) The maturation of the myeloid lineage does not go to completion. There is a paucity of segmented neutrophils and the bands, which are the most frequent cell in this lineage, have a more open chromatin pattern and their cytoplasm is slightly more basophilic than normal (Wright, 100×).

In horses with immune-mediated hemolytic anemia, phagocytosis of nonnucleated red cells and occasionally erythroid precursors may be observed [23]. Thus, prominent erythrophagocytosis, as well as increased macrophage iron as demonstrated by Prussian blue staining of bone marrow aspirates, are evidence of possible immune-mediated destruction of red cells. A regenerative response as indicated by a decrease in the M:E ratio and concurrent increase in marrow reticulocytes are anticipated findings for both blood loss and hemolytic anemias. However, with concurrent myeloid hyperplasia, the M:E ratio may be normal. The myeloid hyperplasia in this case increases the ratio while erythroid hyperplasia causes it to decrease and thus the ratio is normal (see Case 1) (Figure 3.1d,e).

In contrast, the finding of a prominent population of neoplastic cells or significant fibrosis and/or necrosis may indicate the underlying cause of a nonregenerative anemia. Anemia of chronic inflammation/inflammatory disease (AID) is the most common cause of nonregenerative anemia in the horse, although the anemia is typically mild. AID occurs as bone marrow production is unable to compensate for the reduced life span of red blood cells in inflammatory conditions (see Chapter 2). The sequestration of iron in macrophages and failure to mobilize stored iron for erythropoiesis is the major marrow defect leading to decreased erythropoiesis in this condition [24]. Thus, while marrow stores of iron are replete in AID, the production of red blood cells is decreased.

Horses infected with the equine infectious anemia (EIA) virus also typically have decreased erythroid production. It is believed that the production of tumor necrosis factor (TNF) alpha by infected macrophages may participate in the suppression of erythropoiesis in EIA [25]. However, both peripheral destruction of mature red blood cells and phagocytosis of erythroid precursors in the bone marrow are also likely to play a role in the pathogenesis of anemia for this disease [22]. It is important to correlate any dysplastic or other marrow changes to a possible underlying cause as well as to peripheral blood morphological findings. This also means that historical and clinical information, in addition to any drug treatment, should be carefully reviewed to determine if they might be implicated in these changes.

The sequence of maturation for the erythroid lineage typically shows fewer than 5% rubriblasts with progressively greater numbers of the more mature erythroid precursors. The maturation index or ratio between proliferating erythroid precursors (erythroblasts and prorubricytes) versus maturing, nonproliferating precursors (late-stage polychromatophilic rubricytes and metarubricytes) is approximately 1:4 [26, 27]. Thus, in a normal bone marrow, most of the nucleated erythroid precursors in the aspirate are late-stage rubricytes and metarubricytes. Several patterns of disrupted maturation may be recognized, such as a paucity of certain erythroid precursors due to enhanced cell death or destruction, particularly evident in association with immune-mediated destruction, myelodysplastic syndromes, and FIS; increased early precursors due to a reactive proliferative process; and a neoplastic proliferative process associated with increased blasts [17, 21, 23, 28]. The total number of erythroid cells must ultimately be correlated with bone marrow cellularity to provide meaningful information about overall erythropoietic activity.

3.4.1.4 Myeloid Lineage and Abnormalities

As with the erythroid lineage, the M:E ratio, maturation sequence of the myeloid lineage and the completeness of its maturation, as well as the overall cellularity of marrow particles, are important components in evaluating this lineage. The myeloid lineage usually predominates in an aspiration cytology of bone marrow from horses, but the numbers of these cells sometimes equal that of the erythroid precursors and may approach an M:E ratio of 1:1. The majority of the granulocytes in the marrow are mature segmented neutrophils with progressively fewer of the less mature myeloid precursors. In general, the number of myeloid cells in the mitotic (myeloblasts, promyelocytes, and myelocytes) to postmitotic pool (metamyelocyte, band, and segmented granulocytes) is about 1:4 [27]. Three patterns of myeloid response commonly observed that define a disrupted sequence of maturation are: (i) paucity of segmented neutrophils and bands due to depletion of the maturation/storage pool (see Case 1) (Figure 3.1f); (ii) increased promyelocytes and myelocytes (promyelocyte/myelocyte bulge) due to a reactive proliferative response; and (iii) increased blasts due to a neoplastic proliferative response [23, 29].

A rare, inherited condition in a family of Standardbred horses showing severe depletion of myeloid and megakaryocytic precursors in the bone marrow is also reported. The disruption of the myeloid response is related to an almost complete absence of this lineage in the marrow. The affected horses have a moderate to profound neutropenia as well as intermittent thrombocytopenia. It appears that a bone marrow microenvironment or growth factor defect is involved in the pathogenesis of this condition [30]. As with the erythroid lineage, the total number of myeloid cells must ultimately be correlated with bone marrow cellularity to provide meaningful information about overall myelopoietic activity.

It is essential to review the CBC as well as historical and clinical data to determine whether an etiology for the observed response can be established. Further, the presence of toxic or dysplastic changes are important morphological characteristics that must be addressed. Enhanced cytoplasmic basophilia and discrete, clear vacuoles in myeloid precursors are strong indicators of toxicity, whereas nuclear changes such as hypolobulation or hyperlobulation are morphological changes more commonly associated with dysplasia. However, neither of these changes is pathognomonic for a reactive versus a neoplastic process. An integrated review of all the pertinent data is essential to provide the most informed determination of which process is most likely. It also may be necessary to assess the numbers of cells in the mitotic versus postmitotic pool if the sequence of maturation appears disrupted and a blast cell count is indicated if the number of myeloblasts appears subjectively increased.

3.4.1.5 Megakaryocytic Lineage and Abnormalities

The number of megakaryocytes, their sequence of maturation, and morphology are aspects of this lineage that should be assessed in cytological specimens. Although megakaryocytes are the largest cell in normal bone marrow, they account for less than 1% of all nucleated hematopoietic cells. In general, there are 1–4 megakaryocytes in each low-power 10× or 20× field [23]. The majority of the megakaryocytes are mature forms with a large amount of granular, weakly basophilic cytoplasm and a multilobulated nucleus (see Case 2) (Figure 3.2a,b). Megakaryoblasts are often difficult to identify, but blebbing of cytoplasmic margins is a characteristic that may aid in identifying them. Increased numbers of megakaryocytes (megakaryocytic hyperplasia) may be seen in the bone marrow aspirates of horses with peripheral platelet destruction (immune-mediated thrombocytopenia) or consumption (disseminated intravascular coagulation) [6]. On the other hand, decreased numbers of bone marrow megakaryocytes or megakaryocytic hypoplasia, such as that reported in a family of Standardbred trotters, suggests the likelihood of a production problem [30].

Ineffective production has been implicated in the moderate to severe thrombocytopenia that occurs in horses infected with EIA virus, given the normal numbers and morphology of marrow megakaryocytes. It is hypothesized that the impairment of platelet production may be due to suppressive factors released by infected macrophages [25]. Thrombocytopenia is also a consistent finding in horses infected with *Anaplasma phagocytophilum*, in addition to moderate leukopenia (lymphopenia and neutropenia) and mild anemia, although the mechanism of these cytopenias is largely unknown. Studies in mice have shown that *A. phagocytophilum* infections induced a significant decrease in bone marrow proliferation involving all cell lines. The production of powerful chemokines in the bone marrow capable of suppressing hematopoiesis is thought to be responsible for these myelosuppressive effects [31].

Dysplastic megakaryocytes usually have single or multiple separate nuclei. Their cytoplasm is typically granulated, although pale gray or water clear cytoplasm and spare granulation may be observed. These dysplastic cells must be distinguished from young megakaryocytes. When significant dysplastic changes are identified, the reason behind these changes needs to be investigated. Reports of dysplastic changes involving this cell lineage are rare in the horse.

3.4.1.6 Lymphocytes, Plasma Cells, Mast Cells, and Abnormalities

Small lymphocytes with a condensed nuclear chromatin pattern and lacking nucleoli may comprise up to 10% of all the nucleated cells in the bone marrow of horses. The majority of lymphocytes in normal bone marrow are T-cells. It is common to find increased percentages of both lymphocytes and plasma cells and sometimes mast cells in an aspirate from a marrow in which hematopoiesis is severely reduced. These cells are usually associated with marrow particles. Plasma cells and mast cells generally represent less than 1–3% of the marrow cells.

The most common neoplastic lymphoproliferative disorders with bone marrow involvement in horses are acute and chronic lymphocytic leukemia, multiple myeloma (MM), and lymphoma. As in other species, the occurrence of acute lymphoblastic leukemia (ALL) in the horse is rapid in onset and associated with severe cytopenias, as well as short survival time. The overall bone marrow cellularity may be variable, but the percentage of bone marrow blasts often accounts for ≥80% of all the nucleated cells, and blasts are consistently found in the peripheral blood. Blasts are typically medium in size with fine nuclear chromatin pattern, indistinct nucleoli, and scant, agranular cytoplasm. However, in some cases, the lymphoblasts have larger nuclei with variable fine to clumped chromatin pattern and distinct nucleoli, and their cytoplasm is more abundant. Whilst the majority of reported cases in horses are subclassified as B-cell ALL, T-cell ALL is also recognized. The total peripheral blood leukocyte numbers in ALL are not typically elevated and in many cases, leukopenia is reported. A moderate to severe, normocytic, normochromic anemia and thrombocytopenia are also common findings in horses with ALL [32, 33].

Chronic lymphocytic leukemia (CLL) is rare in the horse, but appears to be associated with a more indolent course, and marked lymphocytosis with extensive tissue infiltrates are hallmarks of this disease. Most of the documented cases have a T-cell phenotype. The majority of the lymphocytes are small to medium in size with a clumped nuclear

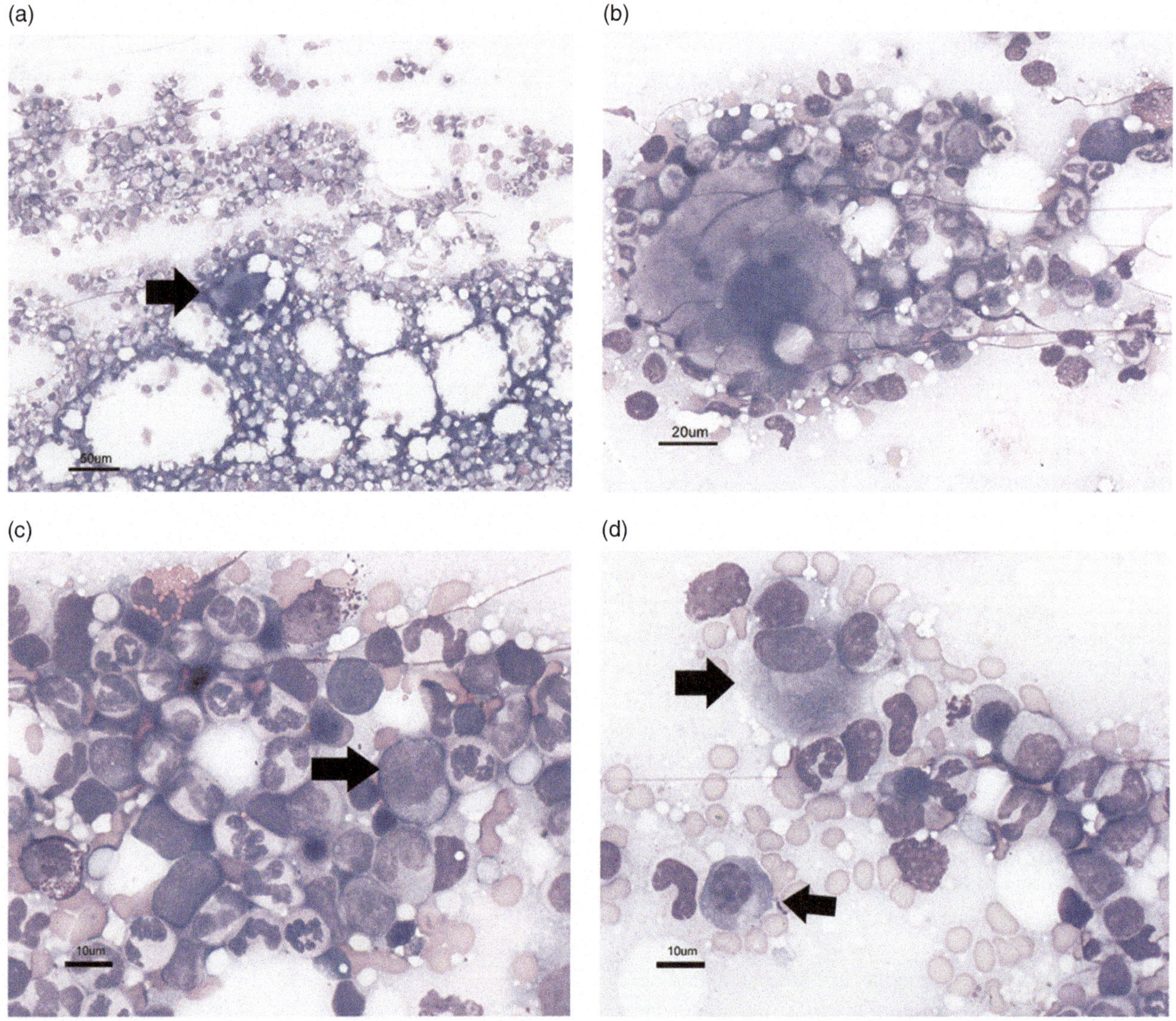

Figure 3.2 Bone marrow aspirate. (a) While the cellularity of the particles varies from 40% to 60%, it is overall considered normocellular. On average, one to four megakaryocytes (*arrow*) are seen within or in close proximity to the particles (Wright, 10×). (b) As shown in this photomicrograph, the majority of the megakaryocytes have hyperlobulated nuclei and voluminous, lightly basophilic granular cytoplasm (Wright, 10×). (c) The M:E ratio is 2.5:1 with a synchronous maturation of both myeloid and erythroid precursors. However, a few large putative lymphoblasts (*arrow*) are scattered throughout these preparations. These cells have prominent nucleoli, a fine chromatin pattern, and a moderate amount of agranular, moderately basophilic cytoplasm (Wright, 100×). (d) Individual osteoblasts (*top arrow*) and a few clumps of these cells, as well as occasional plasma cells (*lower arrow*), are identified during examination of the bone marrow aspirate (Wright, 100×).

chromatin pattern and scant to moderately abundant cytoplasm. However, a few larger lymphocytes with variably prominent nucleoli may be present in both the blood and bone marrow. The presence of anemia and other cytopenias is variable but despite extensive marrow involvement, these decreases tend to be less severe than those reported in horses with ALL [34–36].

Multiple myeloma or plasma cell myeloma is a rare lymphoid disorder in the horse that involves the neoplastic proliferation of plasma cells, primarily in the bone marrow [37, 38]. The proliferation of plasma cells is sometimes focal and in other cases the bone marrow is diffusely involved. Overproduction of a monoclonal immunoglobulin by the neoplastic plasma cells is the hallmark of this disease and, as with CLL, it most frequently affects older animals. Plasma cell myeloma may rarely present as a nonsecretory neoplastic entity in horses. Other criteria that are useful for diagnosis of MM include excessive clonal plasma cells in the bone marrow, monoclonal proteins in the urine, and osteolytic bone lesions. In the presence of at least one myeloma attributable event – bone lesions, monoclonal gammopathy, hypercalcemia, renal insufficiency, or anemia – clonal plasma cells ≥10% of all the nucleated bone marrow cells is considered sufficient to diagnose MM. If no myeloma attributable event is recognized, the presence of clonal bone marrow plasma cells must be ≥60% to establish a diagnosis [39]. Anemia is a consistent finding in affected horses, while leukopenia, thrombocytopenia, and presence of circulating plasma cells are variable [37, 38].

Reactive plasmacytosis is a relatively common bone marrow finding and occasionally the number of these cells may reach a frequency that raises concern for a plasma cell myeloma. Chronic infections, autoimmune diseases, and hypersensitivity reactions may be associated with varying degrees of polyclonal plasmacytosis in the bone marrow. The occurrence of atypical forms including enlarged forms, bi- or multinucleation, prominent nucleoli, and centrally placed nuclei are features that favor a neoplastic plasma cell population. However, in many cases the neoplastic plasma cells have a classic morphology characterized by distinct light to dark blue cytoplasm with an eccentrically placed nucleus. Their chromatin pattern is coarse or clumped, nucleoli are not prominent, and adjacent to the nucleus there may be a clearing, which represents the Golgi apparatus of the cell. The absence of any myeloma attributable events would strengthen concerns for a reactive process. Carefully looking over the other laboratory data and conversing with the attending veterinarian are important steps to follow in these cases to avoid making an incorrect diagnosis.

Lymphoma is a heterogeneous group of neoplastic disorders involving the clonal proliferation of a population of lymphocytes. The neoplastic cells arise from lymphoid tissues that may include lymph nodes, spleen, thymus, or gut-associated lymphoid tissue. Infiltration of bone marrow occurs late in this neoplastic process and in the horse, bone marrow involvement appears to be an uncommon event (see Case 2) (Figure 3.2c). Tumor infiltration of the bone marrow leading to myelophthisis and necrosis, resulting in pancytopenia in a 14-year-old Paint mare with T-cell lymphoma, has been reported [40].

3.4.1.7 Other Bone Marrow Cells

A variety of other cells may be found in the bone marrow aspirate including osteoblasts and osteoclasts, histiocytes (macrophages and dendritic cells), fibroblasts, and adipocytes. Macrophages usually comprise <1% of the marrow cells and may be more easily visualized by staining for the presence of iron in their cytoplasm with Prussian blue. Macrophages usually have a bland nuclear morphology and lack nucleoli and if there is significant atypia, erythrophagocytosis, and high numbers, the possibility of a neoplastic histiocytic disorder should be investigated. A single case report of malignant histiocytosis, involving the proliferation of atypical histiocytes in the bone marrow and lymph nodes of a 16-month-old Arabian filly, is found in the literature. This filly presented with pancytopenia [41].

Stromal components such as adipocytes and fibroblasts may be occasionally observed in cytological preparations. Adipocytes are particularly prominent when the hematopoietic cellularity is low, whereas they are sparse in a highly cellular bone marrow. Fat cell atrophy with the loss of hematopoietic cells and deposition of an extracellular, gelatinous material are characteristic findings associated with severe starvation. Fibroblasts are infrequently observed in an aspiration cytology and when present, the likelihood of myelofibrosis must be considered.

Osteoblasts and osteoclasts are rare on aspirate smears from adult horses, but in young animals they may be occasionally encountered. Osteoblasts are mononuclear cells; they have an eccentrically placed nucleus and abundant, lightly basophilic to grayish cytoplasm (see Case 2) (Figure 3.2e). In contrast, osteoclasts are multinucleated cells which have multiple, discrete, round to oval nuclei and abundant cytoplasm that may range from basophilic to eosinophilic and contains many coarse granules. The presence of these cells in a bone marrow aspirate from an adult horse likely indicates bone pathology, which should be further investigated by evaluation of a core biopsy specimen. Again, other clinical information should be carefully reviewed to determine if the reason for the presence of these cells is apparent.

3.4.2 Additional Diagnostics

Specialized techniques such as cytochemistry, immunohistochemistry, flow cytometry, and molecular methods are not routinely used in bone marrow evaluation in the work-up of hematopoietic disorders of horses. However, these procedures may provide valuable information, particularly for diagnosis and classification of hematopoietic neoplasms. Enzymatic cytochemical stains such as myeloperoxidase (MPO) are useful in identifying cells of the granulocytic lineage. MPO is a lysosomal enzyme found in primary granules of myelocytic precursors. The intensity of MPO is strongest for granulocytes, much less intense for monocytes, and negative for erythroid and lymphoid precursors. However, Sudan black B (SBB), a neutral stain for lipids, may be more sensitive for identification of myeloblasts than MPO. It is particularly useful for distinguishing positive-staining acute myeloid leukemias (AML) from acute leukemias of lymphoid origin, which are negative. Alpha-naphthyl butyrate esterase is another enzymatic staining procedure, which has been used to identify precursors of the monocytic lineage. All enzymatic procedures must be performed on unfixed/unstained blood or bone marrow slides and some variability in the specificity of these staining patterns has been recognized [6].

Immunophenotyping of leukemic cells may be relevant to cell identification and often provides valuable clues about the biological behavior of the neoplasm as well as the prognosis and treatment for the patient. Immunohistochemistry, performed on paraffin-embedded bone marrow tissue, identifies the cell lineage by using monoclonal antibodies for specific cell surface antigens. The monoclonal antibodies that have been validated for use in horses include CD3, CD79α, CD20, and MPO. MPO is a robust procedure developed specifically for use in fixed tissues. CD3 is a lineage-specific protein and is considered a pan-T-lymphocyte marker, whereas CD79α is part of the B-cell receptor complex. CD20 is a lineage-restricted molecule, expressed on B-lymphocytes throughout B-cell differentiation. Flow cytometric analysis also may be used to immunophenotype cell populations of the horse. CD4 and CD8 monoclonal antibodies may be used to enumerate and identify neoplastic cells using this technique, recognizing helper and cytotoxic T-lymphocytes, respectively. B-lymphocyte markers, B29A and E18A, are similarly validated for flow cytometric use [36].

The reported use of polymerase chain reaction for clonality testing (PARR) to assess lymphoid malignancies in horses is limited at this time [6]. PARR relies on detection of a clonal rearrangement in either the immunoglobulin or T-cell receptor gene. Because normal or reactive lymphocytes should have a polyclonal rearrangement of these genes, detection of a clonal population with PARR would suggest the cells are neoplastic. Data that address the sensitivity and specificity of this testing in horses are not currently available, so care must be taken in interpreting these results.

In summary, it is important to remember that these specialized techniques were developed using normal cell populations, and neoplastic cells sometimes do not follow all the rules. Thus, the neoplastic population may stain differently from normal cells, making interpretation of their precise lineage problematic at times. Despite these limitations, special staining and molecular techniques used as adjuncts to the baseline evaluation of cell morphology should provide lineage assignment in most cases of acute leukemia.

3.5 Case Examples

3.5.1 Case 1

A 5-year-old quarter horse was presented to a teaching hospital after sustaining a severe leg laceration three days previously. The clients reported that there was a large amount of blood in the area where the accident happened. They cleaned the wound, treated it topically with antibiotics, and bandaged the leg. However, the horse was now febrile and inappetent. A complete blood count (Table 3.1) showed a normocytic, normochromic anemia with a leukocytosis characterized by a regenerative left shift and toxicity. Hypoproteinemia was also present.

A bone marrow aspirate (Figure 3.1) was obtained to assess whether there was appropriate response to the presumed blood loss anemia.

Table 3.1 Case 1.

Erythron, total protein, platelets					
	Hct (%)	**MCV (fL)**	**MCHC (g/dL)**	**TP (g/dL)**	**Plts**
RI	35–55	35–55	30–36	5.7–8.1	100–600 K/μL
Horse	20	51	34.5	4.7	252 K
Leukon					
	WBC	**Neuts**	**Bands**	**Lymphs**	**Monos**
RI	5.5–12.5 K/μL	3–7 K/μL	0–100/μL	1.5–5.5 K/μL	50–800/μL
Horse	21.5 K	18.7 K moderate toxicity	860	1.9 K	0

RI, reference interval; Hct, hematocrit; TP, total protein; Plts, platelets; Neuts, neutrophils; Lymphs, lymphocytes; Monos, monocytes; MCV, mean cell volume; MCHC, mean corpuscular hemoglobin concentration; WBC, white blood cells.

Table 3.2 Case 2.

Erythron, TP, platelets					
RI	Hct (%) 35–55	MCV (fL) 35–55	MCHC (g/dL) 30–36	TP (g/dL) 5.7–8.1	Plts 100–600 K/μL
Horse	44.7	44.4	36.0	5.6	344 K
Leukon					
	WBC	**Neuts**	**Bands**	**Lymphs**	**Monos**
RI	5.5–12.5 K/μL	3–7 K/μL	0–100/μL	1.5–5.5 K/μL	50–800/μL
Horse	10.8 K	6.5 K	0	3.9 K Blasts 2%	430

RI, reference interval; Hct, hematocrit; TP, total protein; Plts, platelets; Neuts, neutrophils; Lymphs, lymphocytes; Monos, monocytes; MCV, mean cell volume; MCHC, mean corpuscular hemoglobin concentration; WBC, white blood cells.

3.5.1.1 Marrow Aspirate Interpretation

The 'normal' M:E ratio in this case was due to both myeloid hyperplasia (driving the ratio up) and erythroid hyperplasia (driving the ratio down). Peripheral leukocytosis due to neutrophilia and a mild increase in bands further supported an interpretation of an effective inflammatory response by the bone marrow. The marrow reticulocyte count of 8% confirmed that a regenerative response to the anemia had been mounted.

3.5.1.2 Follow-Up

The wound was cleaned and debrided, bandaged, and allowed to heal by second intention. On a second recheck visit, which was three weeks later, all results on the CBC were normal.

3.5.2 Case 2

A 10-year-old Thoroughbred stallion was presented to the teaching hospital with unilateral conjunctival swelling and exophthalmos. On physical examination, there was a mild peripheral lymphadenopathy and abdominal ultrasonography revealed a massive splenomegaly. A biopsy of the spleen confirmed a diagnosis of diffuse large cell lymphoma. While erythrocyte, leukocyte, and platelet counts were within the established reference intervals for horses (Table 3.2), the presence of low numbers of blasts prompted the clinician to pursue a bone marrow evaluation.

3.5.2.1 Marrow Aspirate Interpretation

A bone marrow aspirate (Figure 3.2) was obtained. Bony remodeling and metastatic lymphoma were suspected due to the presence of osteoblasts and putative lymphoblasts, respectively.

3.5.2.2 Follow-Up

Mild bony remodeling was identified on histological evaluation of the bone marrow core biopsy section and CD20 staining confirmed the presence of several interstitial foci of large, neoplastic lymphocytes.

References

1 Dunn, C.D. (1971). The differentiation of hemopoietic stem cells. *Ser. Hematol.* 4 (4): 1–71.

2 Lim, W.F., Inoue-Yokoo, T., Tan, K.S. et al. (2013). Hematopoietic cell differentiation from embryonic and induced pluripotent stem cells. *Stem Cell Res. Ther.* 4 (3): 71.

3 Riley, R.S., Williams, D., Ross, M. et al. (2009). Bone marrow aspirate and biopsy: a pathologist's perspective. II. Interpretation of the bone marrow aspirate and biopsy. *J. Clin. Lab. Anal.* 23 (5): 259–307.

4 Clarke, B. (2008). Normal bone anatomy and physiology. *Clin. J. Am. Soc. Nephrol.* 3 (Suppl 3): S131–S139.

5 Firth, E.C. (2006). The response of bone, articular cartilage and tendon to exercise in the horse. *J. Anat.* 208 (4): 513–526.

6 Tornquist, S.J. (2008). Bone marrow and lymph node evaluation. *Vet. Clin. North Am. Equine Pract.* 24 (2): 261–283.

7 Raskin, R.E. and Messick, J.B. (2012). Bone marrow cytologic and histologic biopsies: indications, technique, and evaluation. *Vet. Clin. North Am. Small Anim. Pract.* 42 (1): 23–42.

8 Brooks, M., Leith, G.S., Allen, A.K. et al. (1991). Bleeding disorder (von Willebrand disease) in a quarter horse. *J. Am. Vet. Med. Assoc.* 198 (1): 114–116.

9 Brooks, M.B. (2008). Equine coagulopathies. *Vet. Clin. North Am. Equine Pract.* 24 (2): 335–355.

10 Abla, O., Friedman, J., and Doyle, J. (2008). Performing bone marrow aspiration and biopsy in children: recommended guidelines. *Paediatr. Child Health* 13 (6): 499–501.

11 Rowland, A.L., Navas de Solis, C., Lepiz, M.A. et al. (2018). Bone marrow aspiration does not induce a measurable pain response compared to sham procedure. *Front. Vet. Sci.* 5: 233.

12 Kasashima, Y., Ueno, T., Tomita, A. et al. (2011). Optimisation of bone marrow aspiration from the equine sternum for the safe recovery of mesenchymal stem cells. *Equine Vet. J.* 43 (3): 288–294.

13 Delling, U., Lindner, K., Ribitsch, I. et al. (2012). Comparison of bone marrow aspiration at the sternum and the tuber coxae in middle-aged horses. *Can. J. Vet. Res.* 76 (1): 52–56.

14 Bohn, A. (2019). Collection and analysis of bone marrow. In: *Large Animal Internal Medicine*, 6e (eds. B.P. Smith, D. van Metre and N. Pusterla), 449–461. St Louis: Mosby.

15 Eydt, C., Geburek, F., Schröck, C. et al. (2016). Sternal bone marrow derived equine multipotent mesenchymal stromal cells (MSCs): investigations considering the sampling site and the use of different culture media. *Vet. Med. Sci.* 2 (3): 200–210.

16 Lewandowski, K., Kowalik, M.M., Pawlaczyk, R. et al. (2012). Microscopic examination of bone marrow aspirate in healthy adults – comparison of two techniques of slide preparation. *Int. J. Lab. Hematol.* 34 (3): 254–261.

17 Malikides, N., Kessell, A., Hodgson, J. et al. (1999). Bone marrow response to large volume blood collection in the horse. *Res. Vet. Sci.* 67 (3): 285–293.

18 Weiss, D.J. and Moritz, A. (2003). Equine immune-mediated hemolytic anemia associated with *Clostridium perfringens* infection. *Vet. Clin. Pathol.* 32 (1): 22–26.

19 Cooper, C., Sears, W., and Bienzle, D. (2005). Reticulocyte changes after experimental anemia and erythropoietin treatment of horses. *J. Appl. Physiol.* 99 (3): 915–921.

20 Balan, M., McCullough, M., and O'Brien, P.J. (2018). Equine blood reticulocytes: reference intervals, physiological and pathological changes. *Comp. Clin. Pathol.* 28 (1): 53–62.

21 Tallmadge, R.L., Stokol, T., Gould-Earley, M.J. et al. (2012). Fell pony syndrome: characterization of developmental hematopoiesis failure and associated gene expression profiles. *Clin. Vaccine Immunol.* 19 (7): 1054–1064.

22 Sellon, D.C., Fuller, F.J., and McGuire, T.C. (1994). The immunopathogenesis of equine infectious anemia virus. *Virus Res.* 32 (2): 111–138.

23 Latimer, K.S. and Andreasen, C.B. (2002). Bone marrow. In: *Diagnostic Cytology and Hematology of the Horse*, 2e (eds. R. Cowell and R. Tyler), 217–226. St Louis: Mosby.

24 Grimes, C.N. and Fry, M.M. (2015). Nonregenerative anemia: mechanisms of decreased or ineffective erythropoiesis. *Vet. Pathol.* 52 (2): 298–311.

25 Leroux, C., Cadoré, J.-L., and Montelaro, R.C. (2004). Equine infectious anemia virus (EIAV): what has HIV's country cousin got to tell us? *Vet. Res.* 35 (4): 485–512.

26 Dörmer, P., Schalhorn, A., Wilmanns, W., and Hershko, C. (1987). Erythroid and myeloid maturation patterns related to progenitor assessment in the myelodysplastic syndromes. *Br. J. Hematol.* 67 (1): 61–66.

27 Valli, V.E., McGrath, J.P., and Chu, I. (2002). Hematopoietic system. In: *Handbook of Toxicologic Pathology* (eds. W.M. Haschek, C.G. Rousseaux and M.A. Wallig), 666–672. San Diego: Academic Press.

28 Forbes, G., Feary, D.J., Savage, C.J. et al. (2011). Acute myeloid leukemia (M6B: pure acute erythroid leukemia) in a thoroughbred foal. *Aust. Vet. J.* 89 (7): 269–272.

29 Miglio, A., Pepe, M., Felippe, M.J.B., and Antognoni, M.T. (2019). Subleukaemic acute myeloid leukemia with myelodysplasia in a horse. *Equine Vet. Educ.* 31 (6): e39–e46.

30 Kohn, C.W., Swardson, C., Provost, P. et al. (1995). Myeloid and megakaryocytic hypoplasia in related standardbreds. *J. Vet. Intern. Med.* 9 (5): 315–323.

31 Borjesson, D., Macnamara, K., Johns, J., and Winslow, G. (2009). Anaplasma phagocytophilum and Ehrlichia muris induce cytopenias and global defects in hematopoiesis. *Clin. Microbiol. Infect.* 15 (Suppl 2): 66–67.

32 Barrell, E.A., Asakawa, M.G., Felippe, M.J.B. et al. (2017). Acute leukemia in six horses (1990–2012). *J. Vet. Diagn. Investig.* 29 (4): 529–535.

33 Cooper, C.J., Keller, S.M., Arroyo, L.G. et al. (2018). Acute leukemia in horses. *Vet. Pathol.* 55 (1): 159–172.

34 Cian, F., Tyner, G., Martini, V. et al. (2013). Leukemic small cell lymphoma or chronic lymphocytic leukemia in a horse. *Vet. Clin. Pathol.* 42 (3): 301–306.

35 Dascanio, J.J., Zhang, C.H., Antczak, D.F. et al. (1992). Differentiation of chronic lymphocytic leukemia in the horse: a report of two cases. *J. Vet. Intern. Med.* 6 (4): 225–229.

36 Rendle, D.I., Durham, A.E., Thompson, J.C. et al. (2007). Clinical, immunophenotypic and functional characterisation of T-cell leukemia in six horses. *Equine Vet. J.* 39 (6): 522–528.

37 Edwards, D.F., Parker, J.W., Wilkinson, J.E., and Helman, R.G. (1993). Plasma cell myeloma in the horse. A case report and literature review. *J. Vet. Intern. Med.* 7 (3): 169–176.

38 Pusterla, N., Stacy, B.A., Vernau, W. et al. (2004). Immunoglobulin A monoclonal gammopathy in two horses with multiple myeloma. *Vet. Rec.* 155 (1): 19–23.

39 Rajkumar, S.V., Dimopoulos, M.A., Palumbo, A. et al. (2014). International Myeloma Working Group updated criteria for the diagnosis of multiple myeloma. *Lancet Oncol.* 15 (12): e538–e548.

40 Kelton, D.R., Holbrook, T.C., Gilliam, L.L. et al. (2008). Bone marrow necrosis and myelophthisis: manifestations of T-cell lymphoma in a horse. *Vet. Clin. Pathol.* 37 (4): 403–408.

41 Lester, G.D., Alleman, A.R., Raskin, R.E., and Mays, M.B. (1993). Malignant histiocytosis in an Arabian filly. *Equine Vet. J.* 25 (5): 471–473.

4

Immunohematology and Hemostasis

Karen V. Jackson

School of Veterinary Science, University of Queensland, Gatton, Queensland, Australia

Acronyms and abbreviations that appear in this chapter include: RBC, red blood cell; NI, neonatal isoerythrolysis; pRBC, packed red blood cells; EDTA, ethylenediamine tetraacetic acid; ACD, acid citrate dextrose; PBS, phosphate buffered saline; DS, 2% dextrose in 0.9% saline; IMHA, immune-mediated hemolytic anemia; JFA, jaundiced foal agglutination; MAC, membrane-attack complex; IgG, immunoglobulin class G; IgM, immunoglobulin class M; IgA, immunoglobulin class A; EIA/EIAV; equine infectious anemia/equine infectious anemia virus; CBC, complete blood count; UA, urinalysis; PCV, packed cell volume; DIC, disseminated intravascular coagulation; PGI_2, prostacyclin; PCR, polymerase chain reaction; NO, nitric oxide; FV/FVa, factor V/activated factor V; FVIII/FVIIIa, factor VIII/activated factor VIII; TFPI, tissue factor pathway inhibitor; TF, tissue factor; tPA, tissue plasminogen activator; vWF, von Willebrand factor; PAI-1, plasminogen activator inhibitor-1; PAF, platelet activating factor; PDGF, platelet-derived growth factor; PF4, platelet factor 4; ADP, adenosine diphosphate; ATP, adenosine triphosphate; GPIb, glycoprotein Ib; GPIIb-IIIa, glycoprotein IIb-IIIa; FXII/FXIIa, factor XII/activated factor XII; FXI/FXIa, factor XI/activated factor XI; HMWK, high molecular weight kininogen; PK, prekallikrein; FIX/FIXa, factor IX/activated factor IX; FX/FXa, factor X/activated factor X; FII, factor II or prothrombin; FIIa, activated factor II or thrombin; PL, phospholipid; FDPs, fibrin(ogen) degradation products; ATIII, antithrombin III; TAT, thrombin-antithrombin complex; EPCR, endothelial cell protein C receptor; aPC, activated protein C; TAFI/TAFIa, thrombin-activatable fibrinolysis inhibitor/activated thrombin-activatable fibrinolysis inhibitor; BMBT, buccal mucosal bleeding time; TBT, template bleeding time; PT, prothrombin time; aPTT, activated partial thromboplastin time; ACT, activated clotting time.

4.1 Immunohematology Testing

Blood types are surface red blood cell (RBC) antigens that are genetically coded and therefore inherited. Benchtop blood typing uses specialized antisera to identify these RBC antigens. In the horse, their clinical significance has historically lain in parentage testing but now parentage testing via blood type is genetic in basis and benchtop blood typing is more often used in the transfusion setting for blood donor and recipient typing and in the investigation of neonatal isoerythrolysis (NI) cases. Cross-matching is used to detect potential transfusion incompatibilities between donor sera and RBCs and recipient sera and RBCs to ensure optimal RBC survival post transfusion. It is often used directly prior to transfusion for selection of a compatible donor for packed RBC (pRBC) and plasma transfusions. Antibody screening and the jaundiced foal agglutination (JFA) test are most often used combined with blood typing for investigation or prediction of NI. Antibody screening alone can also be used in the transfusion setting for blood donor screening and patients at risk for previous development of antibodies (i.e., previous transfusions or pregnancies).

4.1.1 Blood Typing

4.1.1.1 Blood Types and Clinical Relevance

Horses have eight RBC groups or systems: A, C, D, K, P, Q, U, and T. The first seven are recognized by the International Society of Animal Blood Grouping Research and the remaining T blood group is mainly of research interest [1]. Recently, new nomenclature has been proposed for standardization, with the two letters 'EA' for erythrocyte antigen preceding the traditional groups above. Within these groups there are more than 30 factors, which are designated by a

Equine Hematology, Cytology, and Clinical Chemistry, Second Edition.
Edited by Raquel M. Walton, Rick L. Cowell, and Amy C. Valenciano.

lowercase letter that follows the uppercase group/system. A summary of the horse blood groups and factors is presented in Table 4.1. As the equine blood group systems are complex with many factors, identification of a blood donor with an identical blood group profile is difficult, if not impossible. This is why blood typing and/or antibody screening is recommended to select blood donors with a high likelihood of being compatible to other horses although cross-matching is always recommended prior to transfusion.

Although there are many blood groups and factors in horses and these can be overwhelming when viewed together, the majority of clinically significant transfusion reactions and/or NI cases relate to factor incompatibilities associated with blood groups *EAA* and *EAQ*. Incompatibilities occur when RBC antigens on the surface of one horse's RBC (e.g., anemic patient, NI foal) encounter plasma antibodies from another horse against these same antigens (e.g., antibodies from donor plasma or colostrum). In practice, blood donors are blood typed to best predict compatible patient–donor pairings for cross-matching and mares are blood typed to determine if they lack A^a and/or Q^a as they are then considered at risk of having a foal with NI.

4.1.1.2 Methodology

Blood typing in horses is a time-intensive process requiring 2.5–3.0 hours to complete. It is also specialized and only performed by select laboratories as the reagents are not commercially available. A list of some laboratories which perform equine blood typing is provided in Table 4.2; however, please note other veterinary laboratories may offer equine blood typing if contacted. Either an ethylenediamine tetraacetic acid (EDTA) (purple top) or acid citrate dextrose (ACD) (yellow top) whole blood sample is recommended for submission to the laboratory.

Table 4.1 Internationally recognized horse blood groups, factors, and alleles.

Blood groups	Factors	Alleles[a]
EAA	a b c d e f g	A^a, A^{adf}, A^{adg}, A^{abdf}, A^{abdg}, A^b, A^{bc}, A^{bce}, A^c, A^{ce}, A^e, A^-
EAC	a	C^a, C^-
EAD	a b c d e f g h i j k l m n o p q r	D^{adl}, D^{adlnr}, D^{adlr}, D^{bcmq}, D^{cefgmq}, $D^{cegimnq}$, D^{cfgkm}, D^{cfmqr}, D^{cgm}, D^{cgmp}, D^{cgmq}, D^{cgmqr}, D^{cgmr}, D^{deklr}, D^{deloq}, D^{delq}, D^{dflkr}, D^{dghmp}, D^{dghmq}, D^{dghmqr}, D^{dkl}, D^{dlnq}, D^{dlnqr}, D^{dlqr}, D^q, D^-
EAK	a	K^a, K^-
EAP	a b c d	P^a, P^{ac}, P^{acd}, P^{ad}, P^b, P^{bd}, P^d, P^-
EAQ	a b c	Q^{abc}, Q^{ac}, Q^a, Q^b, Q^c, Q^-
EAU	a	U^a, U^-

[a] The absence of a factor is denoted as a dash (–).

Table 4.2 Equine blood typing laboratories (United States).

University of California, Davis Hematology Laboratory Room 1012, Veterinary Teaching Hospital One Garrod Drive University of California, Davis Davis, CA, 95616 +1–530–752-1303 www.vetmed.ucdavis.edu/hospital/support-services/lab-services/clinical-laboratory-services/equine-blood-type-and-antibody-screen
University of Kentucky Animal Genetic Typing and Research Laboratory 108 Gluck Equine Research Centre University of Kentucky Lexington, KT, 40546 +1–859–218-1212 www.ca.uky.edu/gluck/AGTRL.asp
Rood and Riddle Veterinary Laboratory 2150 Georgetown Road Lexington, KY, 40511 +1–859–233-0331 www.roodandriddle.com/laboratory.html
Hagyard Equine Medical Institute 4520 Iron Works Pike Lexington, KY, 40511 +1–859–259-3685 www.hagyard.com/

Briefly, the procedure involves incubating aliquots of 2% washed RBC saline suspension with aliquots of each specific antisera at 37 °C. A positive reaction, visualized as either hemolysis or agglutination depending on the known reaction of each antisera, indicates the presence of a blood factor. A negative reaction, visualized as a lack of hemolysis or agglutination, indicates the absence of a blood factor. This has to be performed for each blood factor individually. The hemolytic reactions require addition of complement before incubation. This complement is from rabbit serum that has been adsorbed at 4 °C with equine RBCs to remove nonspecific hemolysins.

More recent blood typing methods include a rapid agglutination method for equine blood typing for equine RBC blood types/antigens A^a and C^a which requires only 15–30 minutes and is performed a room temperature [2] and an immunochromatographic method for C^a which requires approximately three minutes at room temperature [3]. These may be more practical for pretransfusion testing but particularly as they cannot assess for blood group *EAQ*, as a hemolysin reagent (not agglutination) is used for this blood group, these methods cannot replace cross-matching or complete blood typing and antibody screening for donor–patient compatibility testing before transfusion.

4.1.2 Cross-matching

4.1.2.1 Clinical Relevance

Cross-matching is used to detect incompatible antibodies in plasma/serum of the donor and patient that will react with RBC antigens/blood types of the patient and donor, respectively. Cross-matching does not specify to which RBC blood types/antigens the incompatibility occurs and does not predict all transfusion reactions (e.g., platelet or leukocyte antibodies, pRBC bacterial contamination, urticarial reactions, hypocalcemia secondary to excessive citrate administration); however, even in patients that have been blood typed, cross-matching should be performed prior to transfusion to minimize the likelihood of a transfusion reaction secondary to antibody incompatibilities.

All horses can develop antibodies to RBC antigens/blood types they do not have themselves if they are sensitized; however, sensitization even with incompatible blood transfusions is uncommon [4]. These antibodies are called *acquired* alloantibodies. They develop if a horse is exposed to RBC antigens/blood types it does not recognize as self (e.g., incompatible transfusion, mare with Q^a or A^a foal when they are Q^- or A^- themselves). Approximately 10% of Thoroughbred horses and 20% of Standardbred horses have *naturally* occurring RBC alloantibodies (i.e., without sensitization they have antibodies present in their plasma that target RBC antigens that they do not have themselves) [5]. Whether these acquired or naturally occurring alloantibodies cause transfusion reactions or NI depends on their action and strength. Antibodies can be either agglutinins (i.e., causing agglutination of RBCs) or hemolysins (i.e., causing hemolysis of RBCs), or both. Anti-A^a and anti-C^a alloantibodies are both agglutinins and hemolysins whereas anti-Q^a alloantibodies are solely hemolysins. This is important to understand mainly for interpreting blood typing and cross-matching results.

The majority of alloantibodies present in horses are either anti-A^a or anti-C^a, with fewer anti-Q^a alloantibodies [5]. Anti-A^a and anti-Q^a alloantibodies are likely to cause clinically significant transfusion reactions and/or NI whereas anti-C^a alloantibodies cause blood typing and cross-match reactions that may not cause a significant transfusion reaction and have not been reported to cause NI. Other alloantibodies that have been reported to rarely cause NI include anti-A^b, Q^b, Q^c, Q^{rs}, D^a, D^b, D^c, D^g, K^a, P^a, and U^a [6–10]. Based on this information, blood typing and antibody screening for A^a, C^a, and Q^a blood types/antigens and anti-A, anti-C, and anti-Q antibodies should be performed as a minimum on blood donors and when managing NI cases or at-risk pregnancies. Cross-matching should, wherever possible, be used prior to transfusion as transfused RBC life span is markedly reduced with tube cross-match incompatible transfusions (5d vs 11d vs 35d for ≥2+ incompatible, ≥1+ incompatible and compatible cross-match reactions respectively) [4].

4.1.2.2 Methodology

As horses have naturally occurring and acquired alloantibodies that are both hemolysins and agglutinins, cross-matching should be performed with both a saline-agglutinating technique and a technique that can detect hemolysis. The hemolysis technique requires the addition of complement usually from rabbit serum that has been adsorbed at 4 °C with equine RBCs to remove nonspecific hemolysins. Although the saline-agglutinating technique is often performed by many veterinary practices and is a good screening test prior to transfusion, a hemolytic technique should also be performed as clinically significant transfusion reactions often occur secondary to the presence of anti-Q antibodies that are hemolysins and will not be detected with an agglutinating cross-match alone.

Patient and donor(s) anticoagulated blood (either EDTA or ACD samples) and serum are required for cross-matching. It has recently been shown that the patient and donor blood samples need to be fresh rather than stored for accurate cross-matching and the best chance of finding a compatible donor [11]. If blood typing cannot be performed prior to donor selection, consider untransfused geldings of the same breed as the recipient as the best donor options. As blood types are hereditary, being of the same breed will help to minimize blood type incompatibilities whilst being untransfused and a gelding avoids any acquired alloantibodies (i.e., transfusion or pregnancy-induced alloantibodies). Donkeys should not be used as donors for horses as they have a donkey-specific RBC antigen that will cause sensitization [12].

The cross-match procedures are outlined in Table 4.3. Briefly, in the agglutination cross-match, aliquots of saline washed RBCs and serum from both the recipient and donor are mixed for the major and minor cross-matches and incubated at 37 °C for 15 minutes. For the hemolysin cross-match, an aliquot of rabbit complement is also added and the incubation is at 37 °C for longer, 90 minutes. Autocontrols are also performed for both the agglutination and hemolysin cross-matches. The tubes are then centrifuged and assessed for agglutination (macroscopically and microscopically) and hemolysis. The agglutination can be graded (0–4+ for macroscopic [see Table 4.4], and positive or negative for microscopic) whereas hemolysis is either positive or negative [2, 13]. It has recently been shown that

Table 4.3 Cross-matching procedure.

1) Obtain anticoagulated blood (EDTA or ACD, i.e., purple top or yellow top) and serum (coagulated blood, i.e., red top) from the recipient and donor(s).
2) Centrifuge and separate the samples into multiple tubes:[a]
   a) Patient RBCs
   b) Patient serum
   c) Donor(s) RBCs
   d) Donor(s) serum
3) Wash patient and donor(s) RBCs separately by adding saline, phosphate buffered saline (PBS), or 2% dextrose in 0.9% saline solution (DS) to a small amount of pRBCs from each. Mix, then centrifuge and pour off supernatant. Repeat at least 3 times.
4) After the last wash, resuspend the pRBCs in saline, PBS, or DS to a 2–4% RBC suspension. This can be subjectively judged on color (i.e., "Kool-Aid" or weak tomato juice in color) or calculated (i.e., 0.05 mL pRBCs in 2.4 mL saline gives a 2% suspension).
5) Have a source of complement that has been adsorbed at 4 °C on equine RBCs to remove nonspecific hemolysins
6) Make the following mixtures in appropriately labeled tubes (label abbreviations given in parentheses).

Agglutination cross-match

a) Major agglutination (MaA) cross-match: 2 drops patient serum, 2 drops donor 2–4% RBC
b) Minor agglutination (MiA) cross-match: 2 drops donor serum, 2 drops patient 2–4% RBC
c) Autocontrol 1 (CTL1A): 2 drops patient serum, 2 drops patient 2–4% RBC
d) Autocontrol 2 (CTL2A): 2 drops donor serum, 2 drops donor 2–4% RBC
e) Incubate at 37 °C for **15 min**
f) Centrifuge for 15–20 sec (3400 rpm/1000× g)
g) Read and record results.
   a) First examine tubes for hemolysis and record if present. Then gently rotate and shake the tube to cause RBCs to swirl off the RBC "button" at the bottom of the tube. Evaluate the suspension for the presence of aggregates/agglutinates:
   i) Macroscopically: Grade 0–4+ (see Table 4.4) depending on the strength of the agglutination.
   ii) Microscopically: Place a drop of the mixture on a slide with a coverslip and examine unstained. If rouleaux is present, recentrifuge the original sample and try again with the pRBC and saline. This is either negative or positive.

Hemolysin cross-match

a) Major hemolysin (MaH) cross-match: 2 drops patient serum, 2 drops donor 2–4% RBC, 2 drops complement
b) Minor hemolysin (MiH) cross-match: 2 drops donor serum, 2 drops patient 2–4% RBC, 2 drops complement
c) Autocontrol 3 (CTL1H): 2 drops patient serum, 2 drops patient 2–4% RBC, 2 drops complement
d) Autocontrol 4 (CTL2H): 2 drops donor serum, 2 drops donor 2–4% RBC, 2 drops complement
e) Incubate at 37 °C for **90 min**
f) Centrifuge for 15–20 sec (3400 rpm/1000× g)
g) Read and record results.
   a) Positive or negative for hemolysis.

[a] Tubes are 12 × 75 mm glass test tubes.
Note: If autocontrols are positive for either hemolysis or agglutination, that portion of the cross-match is invalidated.

there is unlikely to be a need for concurrent micro- and macroscopic assessment for agglutination as the two findings are highly correlated [3]. The same study also evaluated a novel gel column cross-matching method which requires some specialized equipment, whose results were well correlated with the agglutination but not the hemolysis component of the gold-standard tube cross-match [3]. Another study also correlated this novel gel method with a stall-side gel method, showing adequate correlation and concluding that if a reference laboratory was not open to test, the stall-side method is recommended [14]. Further studies have yet to be performed to determine the clinical accuracy of these new methods as these studies did not evaluate posttransfusion clinical information.

4.1.3 Antibody Screening and Jaundiced Foal Agglutination Test

Antibody screening and the JFA test are modified cross-match procedures. Antibody screening uses patient serum added to washed RBCs of known blood types (i.e., stock samples kept at the laboratory) to determine if the patient serum causes agglutination or hemolysis of the known blood type RBCs (as per the cross-match procedure detailed

Table 4.4 Macroscopic agglutination.

0	No visible agglutination
Weak	Few small aggregates of RBCs
1+	Many small aggregates of RBCs
2+	Large aggregates with some smaller aggregates of RBCs
3+	Several large aggregates of RBCs
4+	Single solid aggregate of RBCs

above). Which of the mixtures are positive indicates the antibodies that are present within the patient's serum. Horses without antibodies to *EAA*, *EAC*, and *EAQ* are good plasma donors and if they are negative for these antibodies within the final four weeks of pregnancy, they are unlikely to have a foal with NI.

The JFA test is a modified agglutination cross-match procedure mixing colostrum from the mare in various saline dilutions with RBCs from the foal. Anticoagulated blood (e.g., EDTA or ACD samples) from the foal and colostrum from the mare are required for this test. Colostrum is used as it contains the mare's antibodies that are transferred to the foal for immunity, which may include an alloantibody for the foal's RBCs. If there is a blood type mismatch between the mare and foal and the mare either has naturally occurring alloantibodies or has acquired alloantibodies (from a previous pregnancy or transfusion), then one of the antibodies transferred could also act as an agglutinin to the foal's RBCs and cause NI. This test is considered clinically significant if there is agglutination at or greater than a dilution of 1:16 in horse foals and 1:64 in mule foals [15, 16]. NI will be further discussed in the next section.

4.2 Immune-Mediated Hemolytic Anemia

Immune-mediated hemolytic anemia (IMHA) is the premature destruction of RBCs due to the presence of antibodies directed against RBC antigens. This can be either a primary (i.e., autoimmune) or secondary (e.g., to RBC parasites, infection, neoplasia, drugs) process. As opposed to dogs and cats, IMHA in horses is not considered common and when it occurs, it is most often a secondary disease process. Excluding NI cases, approximately 45 cases of IMHA have been reported in the horse [17–38] and the most common causes were clostridial infection in approximately 20–29% of reported cases [22–25, 28, 30, 33, 36], penicillin administration in approximately 13% of reported cases [28, 29, 31, 32], and lymphoma in approximately 13% of reported cases [20, 21, 34].

Regardless of whether the cause is primary or secondary, the mechanism of destruction of the RBCs is the same and occurs through antibody binding to the surface of the RBCs causing either intravascular or extravascular hemolysis. Extravascular hemolysis is most common and occurs when the RBC-bound antibody binds to the Fc receptors on tissue macrophages, predominantly in the spleen but also liver and other organs, causing premature removal and breakdown of the RBCs within the macrophages. Intravascular hemolysis is less common and a more severe clinical entity that requires the binding of complement to the antibody-bound RBC surface with subsequent activation of the complement cascade and formation of the membrane-attack complex (MAC) on the RBC surface, causing lysis within the vascular space. Extravascular hemolysis is clinically associated with icterus, hyperbilirubinemia, and bilirubinuria due to the excessive hemoglobin breakdown. Intravascular hemolysis is clinically similar except there is also hemoglobinemia and hemoglobinuria as the RBCs are lyzed within the vascular space and the free hemoglobin is cleared directly by the kidneys. Most often, the antibody type responsible for IMHA in the horse is immunoglobulin class G (IgG) with rare cases involving immunoglobulin class M (IgM) and as yet no immunoglobulin class A (IgA) reported but this is potentially due to the difficulty in identifying this antibody class in horses [28].

Primary and secondary IMHA cannot be clinically or diagnostically distinguished except if no secondary causes of IMHA can be found then primary IMHA is assumed. Common clinical signs associated with IMHA are due to the anemia and RBC breakdown and include fever, depression, pallor, icterus, hemoglobinuria (if intravascular), tachycardia, and weakness. IMHA is diagnosed if multiple of the following criteria are present: (i) an anemia (often regenerative); (ii) autoagglutination after RBC washing (i.e., persistent autoagglutination); (iii) a positive Coombs test; (iv) RBC morphological changes reported with equine IMHA (e.g., spheroechinocytes, type III echinocytes, agglutination) [36]; and (v) elimination of other causes (e.g., blood loss, oxidative damage).

Laboratory testing in cases of suspect IMHA should start with complete blood count (CBC), biochemical panel, and urinalysis (UA). If the CBC is supportive of an immune-mediated process (i.e., anemia with concurrent hyperbilirubinemia without evidence of oxidative damage and with agglutination, spheroechinocytes, or type III echinocytes) then consider Coombs' testing. Although IMHA is most often regenerative, this is difficult to determine on a single CBC in horses as reticulocytes are only very rarely noted in the peripheral blood of horses, even in severe anemia. Regeneration is therefore confirmed either through bone marrow aspiration or rising packed cell volume (PCV) with stable plasma/total protein.

Coombs' testing (otherwise called direct antiglobulin testing) is used to confirm the presence of anti-RBC antibodies and it does so by incubating washed patient RBCs with antiserum specific to equine IgG, IgM, and/or complement. If IgG, IgM, or complement is present on the washed RBCs, there will be agglutination of the RBCs and a positive result. This same method of incubating washed RBCs with specific antiserum has also been reported successful using flow cytometry instead of positive agglutination to detect the bound antibody; however, there were too few cases to determine if this is a more sensitive or specific method than the traditional Coombs' test and this test is not easily accessible clinically. Flow cytometry was shown to accurately document reducing antibody in a foal with NI, so it may also have a use in disease monitoring [28].

Although a positive result often indicates an immune-mediated process, negative results via conventional Coombs' testing are relatively common in cases in which all other causes of anemia are ruled out or another method is used to confirm IMHA (e.g., flow cytometry, antipenicillin antibodies) [20, 39, 40]. Unfortunately, a defined sensitivity for Coombs' testing is not known in equine IMHA given the low number of overall cases; however, this test is still recommended, as a positive result indicates immune-mediated anemia is the most likely cause.

Other testing to consider is based on assessment for secondary causes of IMHA and would include targeted investigation of body systems for infection or neoplasia depending on clinical signs and presentation (e.g., abdominal or thoracic imaging, rectal examination, aspiration of lymph nodes, fluid analysis, any drug administration history) and serology and/or polymerase chain reaction (PCR) for infectious diseases with known associations with IMHA (e.g., equine infectious anemia [EIA], PCR for leptospirosis, PCR/culture for *Streptococcus equi*/*Clostridium* spp.). Differential diagnoses for anemia in horses include blood loss, oxidative hemolysis (e.g., red maple toxicity, hereditary diseases), infectious diseases (e.g., EIA, *Babesia* spp., ehrlichiosis, leptospirosis), and anemia of chronic or inflammatory disease.

4.2.1 Neonatal Isoerythrolysis

Neonatal isoerythrolysis is the most common cause for icterus and hemolytic anemia in the neonatal foal and is caused by the reaction of antibodies transferred in the colostrum of the mare that are directed against antigens present on the foal's RBCs that are not present on the mare's RBCs (i.e., immunogenic RBC antigens inherited from the stallion). Studies have shown that RBC incompatibilities between mare and foal are common (up to 14%) [41] and that antibody development by the mare is also common and breed specific, with 10% of Thoroughbred and 20% of Standardbred mares having detectable antibodies in serum [5]. However, despite this, the occurrence of NI is much lower and a simple answer for why this is the case has not yet been found. In the same study that documented the presence of serum antibodies against RBC antigens in 10% and 20% of Thoroughbred and Standardbred horses, respectively, there were only 1% in Thoroughbreds and 2% in Standardbreds of incompatibilities between mare and foal that were associated with NI [5]. The rate of NI is much higher in mules (donkey sire with horse dam) at 8–10% as donkeys have a unique RBC antigen to which the mare becomes sensitized during prior pregnancies [12].

4.2.1.1 Pathogenesis

Neonatal isoerythrolysis is caused by alloantibodies produced in the mare that are directed against RBC antigens that are only present on the foal's RBCs. These alloantibodies are produced during pregnancy or delivery if there is leakage of blood across the placenta (e.g., placentitis or difficult delivery) or produced secondary to a previous mismatched blood transfusion. Alloantibodies can persist for years and are often strongest in late-term pregnancy, so if antibody screening is to be performed to predict NI, it is recommended in late-term pregnancy (i.e., the final four weeks). These alloantibodies are usually IgG and do not cross the placenta but rather are transmitted to the foal in colostrum.

Passive transfer of immunity is the transfer of immunoglobulins from the mare's colostrum to the foal's plasma via uptake of whole immunoglobulin through the gastrointestinal mucosa, which can occur only in the first 24 hours of life and provides the foal with immunity to environmental pathogens until its own immune system is fully functional. Unfortunately, if the mare has developed antibodies to foal-specific RBC antigens (i.e., through this pregnancy, previous pregnancies, or blood transfusion) then these will also be transmitted in the colostrum and could cause hemolysis and/or hemagglutination, depending on whether the antibody is a hemolysin or agglutinin or both. Anti-A^a alloantibodies are agglutinins and hemolysins whereas anti-Q^a alloantibodies are solely hemolysins. There are eight known blood groups and within these groups 35 known RBC antigens (see Table 4.1) to which alloantibodies could be developed, yet the RBC antigens and serum antibody incompatibilities that commonly cause NI are mostly related to blood groups *EAA* and *EAQ*. Anti-A^a and anti-Q^a alloantibodies are most commonly implicated in NI with anti-A^b, Q^b, Q^c, Q^{rs}, D^a, D^b, D^c, D^g, K^a, P^a, and U^a also reported rarely [6–10].

4.2.1.2 Clinical Features

As the alloantibodies are transferred in colostrum, the foals are normal at birth with signs developing after alloantibody absorption. Hemolysis and associated clinical signs can develop as early as five hours after birth but more commonly within 12–48 hours and as late as 12 days after birth [7, 9]. Clinical presentation is associated with the severity of anemia and rapidity of hemolysis and varies from lethargy and icterus to weakness, tachypnea, tachycardia, hemoglobinuria, and hypovolemic shock that can result in death through multiorgan failure and disseminated intravascular coagulation (DIC). Liver failure ± kernicterus have been noted as the major cause of death in NI patients with complications of sepsis noted as the other common cause [9, 42]. The development of liver failure ± kernicterus was found to be statistically associated with the volume of blood products administered (>4.0 L resulted in a 19.5 times higher likelihood of liver failure) and the maximum total bilirubin (>27.0 mg/dL resulted in a 17.0 times higher likelihood of kernicterus) during hospitalization [42]. A recent publication has shown the success of plasma exchange as an intervention to decrease marked hyperbilirubinemia and avoid kernicterus in two foals [43].

4.2.1.3 Diagnosis

As other causes of IMHA are considered very uncommon in the neonate, any neonate (i.e., less than 2 weeks old) presenting with a hemolytic anemia should be considered to have NI until proven otherwise. The CBC should be considered essential as a first step in diagnosis and if an anemia ± hyperbilirubinemia/hemoglobinemia with normal total/plasma protein is found, this is considered supportive. Definitive tests include cross-matching (between the mare serum and foal RBCs – submit serum from the mare and EDTA/ACD from the foal); JFA test (submit EDTA/ACD from the foal with colostrum from the mare); direct Coombs' test of the foal (submit EDTA/ACD from the foal); and/or antibody screening of the mare with concurrent blood typing of the mare and foal or stallion if prefoaling (submit EDTA/ACD from mare and foal with serum from the mare). See earlier in this chapter for methodologies, but recognize that the alloantibodies associated with NI are often stronger hemolysins than agglutinins, so if cross-match or antibody screening is performed, they should include an incubation with complement to assess for hemolysins so need to be performed by a reference laboratory (see Table 4.2). Confirmation of NI occurs if there is proof of mare alloantibodies of sufficient titer directed against foal RBC antigens.

4.2.1.4 Prevention

Prevention is best achieved by identifying mares that are at risk of producing NI-inducing alloantibodies and breeding them accordingly; however, if this is not possible or the mare is already pregnant, then prevention of NI involves determining if the foal is at risk and protecting the foal from exposure to alloantibody.

Blood typing of the mare prior to mating can help to choose appropriate stallions (i.e., if the mare is Q^a or A^a negative then only breed the mare to stallions that are also negative for these blood group factors) and this is recommended in any mare with a history of NI. Blood typing during pregnancy, if not performed before, can be used to identify mares that are at risk and would benefit from antibody screening during the last 3–4 weeks of pregnancy. Antibody screening will identify whether the mare has alloantibodies to RBC antigens she does not carry (either developed during this/previous pregnancies or due to previous blood transfusion); however, determination of whether this will cause NI will require cross-matching and/or blood typing of the foal or stallion with the mare. Antibody screening ± blood typing of the stallion is recommended prefoaling in mares with a history of NI. Unless hemolysis-based cross-matching is available where the foal is delivered, cross-matching the foal and mare is unlikely to be clinically useful for prevention as it would need to be performed after delivery but before colostrum ingestion (i.e., within the first 2–3 hours of life). More often, cross-matching is performed to diagnose NI as the cause for anemia and illness in a foal. The JFA test, however, can be used stall-side and has been shown to correlate well with the hemolysis-based cross-match if performed by trained personnel [16]. As this is stall-side, it can be used before the foal ingests colostrum to predict if the foal would develop NI as well as being used as a confirmatory test in diagnosing NI as the cause for a foal presenting hyperbilirubinemic and anemic.

If the foal and mare have incompatible RBC antigens and alloantibodies, it is recommended that the foal be muzzled to prevent colostrum ingestion for the first 36–48 hours postpartum. The mare should be stripped to ensure milk production for when the foal is allowed to return to nursing. The foal needs to receive colostrum from another source to ensure passive transfer of immunity. If a transfusion is required in a clinical NI case, washed pRBCs from the mare is considered the transfusion of choice. Blood from the stallion should never be used as it is his RBC antigens, which the foal has inherited, that are causing the mismatch.

4.2.2 Infection-Associated (Clostridial, EIA, *Rhodococcus equi*, *S. equi*)

4.2.2.1 Pathogenesis

The mechanisms of clostridial-associated, *R. equi*-associated, and *S. equi*-associated IMHA are unknown. Proposed mechanisms in clostridial-associated IMHA in horses include that the clostridial toxins damage the RBC membrane, exposing new antigens to which the body develops autoantibodies [33], and/or that the clostridial toxins (specifically alpha toxin, a phospholipase) cause RBC damage, echinocyte/spheroechinocyte formation, hemolysis, and autoagglutination [36].

Equine infectious anemia is caused by a retrovirus for the *Lentivirus* genus that infects tissue macrophages. Infection occurs through transmission of blood from horse to horse by biting flies. After infection, the virus replicates in tissue macrophages, causes intermittent viremia, and infects the patient lifelong, allowing for further transmission. The mechanism of anemia in EIA is threefold. There is rarely intravascular immune-mediated hemolysis in acute disease, more commonly there is extravascular immune-mediated hemolysis in acute and chronic disease paired with an impaired bone marrow response. The immune-mediated hemolysis is associated with complement binding to the surface of RBCs causing activation of the intravascular complement cascade (intravascular hemolysis) and phagocytosis by tissue macrophages (extravascular hemolysis). The complement binding in EIA is thought to be secondary to a hemagglutinin, one of the surface proteins of EIAV, or circulating virus–antibody immune complexes attaching to the RBCs and attracting and activating complement [44].

4.2.2.2 Clinical Features

Patients with clostridial-associated IMHA have features of both IMHA (i.e., anemia often with echinocytes/spheroechinocytes, high total/plasma protein, lethargy, icterus) and clostridial disease which in horses is most often a clostridial myositis (i.e., recent deep, penetrating wound with swelling, pain, marked fever, and minimal inflammatory cells) [36, 45]. *R. equi*-associated IMHA is rare with patients having clinical signs associated both with IMHA (i.e., anemia, high total/plasma protein, lethargy, icterus) and pulmonary abscesses, neutrophilic inflammation in respiratory wash samples, fever, and occasionally concurrent extrapulmonary lesions [18, 46]. *S. equi*-associated IMHA is also rare with patients having clinical signs associated both with IMHA (i.e., anemia, high total/plasma protein, lethargy, icterus) and retropharyngeal lymph node abscessation with positive *S. equi* culture +/− PCR. Occasionally, the *S. equi* cases can also develop purpura hemorrhagica (i.e., aseptic vasculitis) that is thought to be secondary to precipitation of IgA immune complexes in the blood vessel walls to a protein associated with *S. equi* [17].

One of the major features of EIA is anemia and this is most often seen in the chronic disease form as an extravascular IMHA. The clinical presentation of EIA can be categorized into three forms: acute, chronic, and inapparent carrier status. The acute disease form is often not noticed clinically as there is usually only a transient, 3–5-day fever and thrombocytopenia associated with the original viremia. Whether the patient develops the chronic form or becomes an inapparent carrier relates to the host–virus immune interaction. The chronic form is seen when the patient experiences multiple relapses in fever associated with recurrent viremia. Classic symptoms of the chronic form include recurrent fevers, ventral edema and edema of the hindlimbs, depression, and weight loss that are found concurrently with marked thrombocytopenia, occasionally causing petechiation and ecchymoses, and anemia ± hyperbilirubinemia. As the anemia is complement mediated, the patient is Coombs' positive during the recurrent febrile episodes. Most horses develop a strong cell-mediated and humoral response to the virus and eventually cease to have recurrent viremia and fever; however, they never clear the virus.

4.2.2.3 Diagnosis

For clostridial-associated, *R. equi*-associated, and *S. equi*-associated IMHA, the presence of IMHA (anemia, icterus, high plasma protein, Coombs' positivity, certain morphological features) combined with confirmed bacterial infection (culture and sensitivity testing, PCR analysis, or toxin quantification [clostridial]) is diagnostic. Often, the response to therapy for the bacterial infection is also used to support the diagnosis of infection-associated IMHA.

Diagnosis of IMHA associated with EIAV infection requires a combination of antibody positivity, appropriate clinical signs (i.e., edema, weight loss), and the hallmarks of IMHA (i.e., anemia, icterus, high total/plasma protein, Coombs' positivity). As the virus is never cleared and there is a good immune response to the virus, affected animals are assured to be antibody positive if tested >45d after exposure via the AGID test (i.e., Coggins test). If the patient is negative via AGID and thought to be an acute case (i.e., exposed <45d), consider other testing methods (e.g., ELISA, PCR); however, these more sensitive tests are prone to false positives, so an AGID should always be used to confirm >45d after original exposure [44].

4.2.3 Drug-Associated

Drug-associated IMHA in the horse is most commonly reported secondary to penicillin [28, 29, 31, 32, 40] but has also been reported with trimethoprim-sulfamethoxazole administration [39]. In the case of penicillin, it is known that the penicillin coats the surface of RBCs and that in a small number of patients, an antibody develops either to the penicillin itself or to an antigen that represents a combination of the penicillin and RBC membrane (i.e., penicillin is acting as a hapten). Ultimately, as the penicillin is bound to the RBC, the presence of an antibody, usually IgG, to either penicillin or a combination of penicillin and RBC membrane causes immune-mediated hemolysis, most often through extravascular hemolysis [31, 32]. It is hypothesized that the method of antibody development was the same in the case of trimethoprim-sulfamethoxazole-induced IMHA [39].

Clinically, drug-associated IMHA is indistinguishable from other causes of IMHA except for the temporal association with drug administration. The diagnosis of drug-induced IMHA involves the presence of classic IMHA components (i.e., anemia, high total/plasma protein, icterus, Coombs' positivity, persistent agglutination) with a history of drug administration in the previous 5–10 days without other causes of IMHA found. Often, this diagnosis is supported by the cessation of hemolysis with removal of the drug and occasionally further supported by recrudescence of the hemolysis with readministration of the drug [39]. In cases where penicillin is suspected as the cause, specialized laboratory tests can be performed which involve performing a Coombs test using both untreated and penicillin-coated RBCs from the patient and from healthy horses and assessing for the ability of the patient's serum to cause agglutination of these altered RBCs.

4.2.4 Neoplasia-Associated

Neoplasia-associated IMHA is most often reported secondary to lymphoma [20, 21, 25, 34, 47, 48] but has also been associated with other neoplasms (e.g., melanoma). Anemia is considered one of the most common hematological abnormalities in equine patients with lymphoma, with anemia present in 30–60% of reported cases [47, 48]. The anemia can be due to chronic/inflammatory disease, blood loss, immune-mediated hemolysis, and myelophthisis. Depending on the study, 10–30% of anemias reported with lymphoma are due to IMHA [47, 48]. The antibodies directed against RBCs are hypothesized to be produced due to inappropriate activation or inactivation of T-cells, autoantibodies produced by the neoplastic cells themselves, and/or the presence of a common genetic rearrangement in the patient associated with both lymphoma and immune system dysregulation allowing immune-mediated disease [20]. Clinically, the presentation of neoplasia-associated IMHA is indistinguishable from other IMHAs except there may be evidence of neoplasia (e.g., cutaneous lymphoma lesions, mediastinal mass lesions, gastrointestinal (GI) lesions, leukemia on CBC evaluation). Confirmation of an immune-mediated anemia requires the presence of an anemia with normal total/plasma protein, icterus, and possibly positive Coombs' testing. As with all secondary IMHA, ruling out other causes (e.g., infection-associated or drug-associated) is required.

4.3 Coagulation Testing

4.3.1 Physiology of Hemostasis

Hemostasis is the arrest of bleeding or stoppage of blood flow through a vessel that is required for the control of bleeding associated with daily trauma or surgery. It also refers to the intricate processes involved in maintaining blood flow in healthy vessels (i.e., without clotting) and the reestablishment of vessel patency once the damage that caused the original bleeding has been resolved. It results from a delicate balance between procoagulant components (vasoconstriction, exposed tissue factor [TF], activated platelets, coagulation proteins), anticoagulant components (normal vessel endothelium, vasodilation, anticoagulant proteins), and fibrinolytic components (fibrinolytic proteins). The importance of the cellular components of hemostasis as well as the proteins has been noted in the more recently proposed cell-based model of hemostasis; however, comprehending the more classic description of hemostasis is useful to understand coagulation testing, so both will be discussed in this chapter.

4.3.1.1 Blood Vessels

The vascular endothelial cells are the primary components of the vessel wall involved in maintenance of normal blood flow through antiplatelet, anticoagulation, and fibrinolytic activities in healthy vessels. They are also essential in inducing and maintaining coagulation when there is vessel damage, so are considered dynamic and pivotal in hemostasis.

During homeostasis, endothelial cells produce prostacyclin (PGI2), adenosine, and nitric oxide (NO) that inhibit platelet–platelet and platelet–endothelial binding whilst also ensuring vasodilation. Physically, the electronegative charges on both endothelium and platelets also help to prevent adhesion. Endothelial cells also express thrombomodulin on the luminal surface that binds any thrombin formed, thereby inhibiting platelet activation, coagulation cascade initiation, and coagulation cascade amplification whilst also activating protein C to downregulate the amplification effects of any activated factors V (FVa) and VIII (FVIIIa). Tissue pathway factor inhibitor (TFPI) is synthesized by endothelial cells and prevents colocalization of TF and FVII (i.e., prevents activation of the extrinsic cascade or initiation, depending on the hemostasis model). Tissue plasminogen activator (tPA) from endothelial cells activates plasmin, the start of the fibrinolytic cascade, ensuring that any fibrin produced is quickly broken down and does not form a clot. Proteoglycans (e.g., heparin, heparan sulfate, and dermatan sulfate) expressed on the endothelial surface inhibit clotting factors and platelet aggregation.

During vessel damage, the initial reaction of the vessel is transient vasoconstriction to restrict blood flow, which both reduces blood loss and aids in fibrin formation. Vasoconstriction is mediated by an autonomic neurogenic reflex, vasoactive mediators, and potentially reduced production of normal vasodilators. As the endothelium is metabolically active, environmental changes associated with damage cause the homeostatic anticoagulant effect of the endothelium to alter and become procoagulant so that fibrin clot formation occurs. The alterations include increased expression of TF on the luminal surface causing activation of the extrinsic cascade/initiation; loss of thrombomodulin and heparan sulfate expression, allowing platelet and coagulation protein adherence; release of von Willebrand factor (vWF) from within the endothelium, aiding platelet adherence to exposed subendothelial collagen; release of plasminogen activator inhibitor-1 (PAI-1) which negates the plasmin activation by tPA, stopping fibrinolysis and allowing the fibrin formation to build up; release of thromboxane A_2 and platelet-activating factor (PAF), encouraging platelet aggregation and activation; and expression of P-selectin and other adhesion molecules is increased to aid in platelet tethering. Note that the endothelium can alter from anticoagulant to procoagulant due to stimuli other than direct damage (e.g., systemic inflammation, certain viral infections, gram-negative bacterial infections, some rickettsial agents, vasculitis) with the same effects. When this is inappropriate or excessive, this procoagulant effect can result in localized or even disseminated intravascular coagulation.

4.3.1.2 Primary Hemostasis

Primary hemostasis provides primary hemostatic plugs to repair small vascular defects. Platelet interaction with activated endothelium or subendothelial collagen is the basis of primary hemostasis. The activated platelets are also then involved in secondary hemostasis as binding sites for coagulation factors (discussed later). Platelets are anuclear, cytoplasmic fragments from megakaryocytes within the bone marrow and contain dense granules, alpha-granules, and lysosomal granules, which store most of the proteins and ions required for platelet function in hemostasis. The largest population of granules is the alpha-granules, which contain proteins which are either synthesized by the megakaryocyte or endocytosed during circulation. The proteins that are predominantly involved in platelet aggregation, adhesion, and vascular repair include fibrinogen, FV, fibronectin, thrombospondin, platelet-derived growth factor (PDGF), and platelet factor 4 (PF4). Dense granules contain predominantly ions and amines rather than proteins and those involved in platelet aggregation, adhesion, and vascular repair include calcium, magnesium, adenosine diphosphate (ADP), adenosine triphosphate (ATP), serotonin, and histamine. Lysosomal granules contain hydrolases similar to neutrophils that are responsible for degradation of unwanted cell debris after fibrin formation [49].

Platelet involvement in primary hemostasis is split into three major categories: adhesion, aggregation, and granule release. Platelets are the first responders to vessel damage through adhesion to either P-selectin on activated endothelium or, more often, to vWF that bridges between the subendothelial collagen and platelet glycoprotein Ib (GPIb). When platelets adhere, they can flatten to form a monolayer that effectively halts blood loss. If the damage is minor (e.g., daily trauma) this adhesion alone may be adequate for hemostasis; however, if the damage is more major, platelet aggregation and granule release occur with subsequent activation of secondary hemostasis. Platelet aggregation is stimulated by ADP, thrombin, and collagen. Unlike other species, ADP stimulation is reversible in horses [50]. The stimulation causes a conformational membrane change that allows glycoprotein IIb-IIIa (GPIIb-IIIa) expression, which then binds fibrinogen, allowing cross-linking or aggregation of the platelets, firming the platelet plug. With platelet aggregation, the granules release their contents (e.g., ADP, Ca, fibrinogen, FV, fibronectin), amplifying the platelet aggregation and activation, which combined with the activated platelet membrane allows for secondary hemostasis where the platelet plug has formed.

4.3.1.3 Secondary Hemostasis

Secondary hemostasis is a series of enzyme activations and reactions that ultimately cause soluble fibrinogen to form a stable, insoluble fibrin clot. Until recently, this was described in the traditional cascade model with intrinsic, extrinsic, and common pathways which is useful when interpreting and understanding coagulation testing; however, the more recent cell-based model of hemostasis shows that these cascades are very interconnected *in vivo* and should not be thought of as separate [51].

The coagulation cascade model (Figure 4.1a) is centered around the soluble factors and describes a series of interconnected enzyme and cofactor activations resulting in fibrin formation that is now best used to understand *in vitro* coagulation testing rather than *in vivo* hemostasis. The intrinsic pathway starts with the activation of FXII through contact with a negatively charged surface (e.g., activated phospholipid [PL] membrane, collagen, glass tube, and kaolin). Contact proteins including high molecular weight kininogen (HMWK) and prekallikrein (PK) interact with FXII to

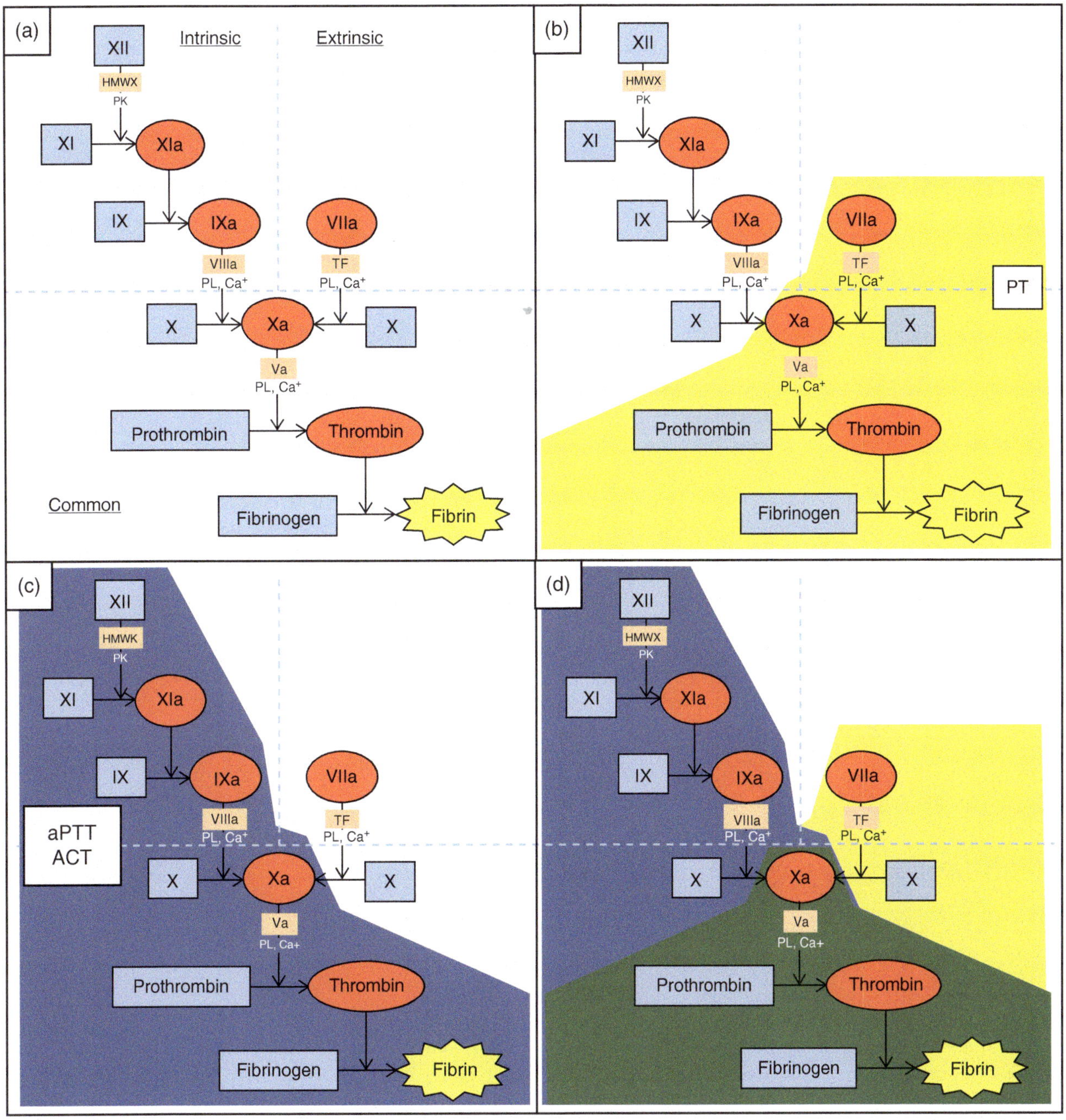

Figure 4.1 (a) The coagulation cascade model: intrinsic, extrinsic, and common pathways. (b) Shaded area represents the pathway tested with the PT assay. (c). Shaded area represents the pathway tested with the aPTT and ACT assays. (d) If only PT or aPTT is prolonged, the common pathway (*middle shaded area*) is not affected, leaving only the factors in the upper shaded areas as potential deficiencies (i.e., PT prolonged, aPTT not prolonged → FVII deficiency; aPTT prolonged, PT not prolonged → FXII, FXI, FIX, or FVIII deficiency). Roman numerals indicate factors. HMWK, high molecular weight kininogen; PK, prekallikrein; PL, phospholipid; Ca^{++}, calcium; TF, tissue factor.

accelerate its activation. Activated FXII causes activation of FXI, which in the presence of free calcium and an activated PL membrane (often platelet) causes activation of FIX. Activated FVIII, a cofactor, in the presence of free calcium and an activated PL membrane (often platelet), binds FIXa and activates FX, which heralds the start of the common pathway.

The extrinsic pathway is simpler and starts with activation of FVII by TF, which is either exposed due to tissue damage or is upregulated on the surface of activated leukocytes, platelets, and endothelium. The TF–FVIIa complex then activates FX in the presence of free calcium and an activated PL membrane (often platelet), starting the common pathway.

The common pathway starts with FXa, which in the presence of FVa, a cofactor, calcium, and an activated PL membrane (often platelet) activates prothrombin (FII) to thrombin (FIIa). Thrombin is central to hemostasis as it has both procoagulant and anticoagulant effects, of which the most important is the conclusion of the common cascade: conversion of fibrinogen to fibrin. Factor XIIIa then stabilizes the fibrin clot through cross-linking of the fibrin strands.

The cell-based model (Figure 4.2), which is better used to understand *in vivo* hemostasis compared to the coagulation cascade model, occurs in three overlapping phases: initiation, amplification, and propagation [51]. The same factors are involved but the importance of the activated PL membrane localization, the overlapping activation of the intrinsic, extrinsic, and common pathways from the cascade model, and the concept of a point of no return within the coagulation model are highlighted.

Initiation occurs due to TF, which is either present on damaged or exposed tissue (e.g., fibroblasts) or upregulated on activated endothelium, leukocytes, and other cells, often associated with systemic inflammation. FVII is circulating in plasma and when it binds to tissue-bound TF, it is activated. If the procoagulant stimulus is strong enough, this complex, TF–FVIIa–PL, in the presence of calcium, activates FX and FIX. Activated FX that is tissue bound with FVa, a cofactor, causes the generation of small amounts of thrombin. The free FXa generated in plasma is rapidly cleared to avoid systemic coagulation and to localize coagulation to where it is needed. This small amount of thrombin allows the movement of coagulation to the platelet surface and subsequent *amplification* of coagulation through platelet activation, activation of cofactors, and localization of the activated cofactors on the platelet surface at the site of tissue damage. Platelet activation occurs through thrombin, which moves platelet proteins and ions to the surface and causes the platelet membrane to flip, exposing the negatively charged phosphatidylserine. After platelet granule release, FV is one protein that is now available on the platelet surface in a partially activated form (directly from platelet alpha-granules). It is fully activated in the presence of thrombin and FXa. The vWF that has bound the platelet to the site is also bound to FVIII, which the thrombin now cleaves, releasing FVIII to the platelet surface for activation and vWF to encourage more platelet adhesion. Thrombin also activates FXI using the platelet surface as an activated PL membrane cofactor.

The third phase, *propagation*, occurs on the activated platelet membrane and involves localization of the

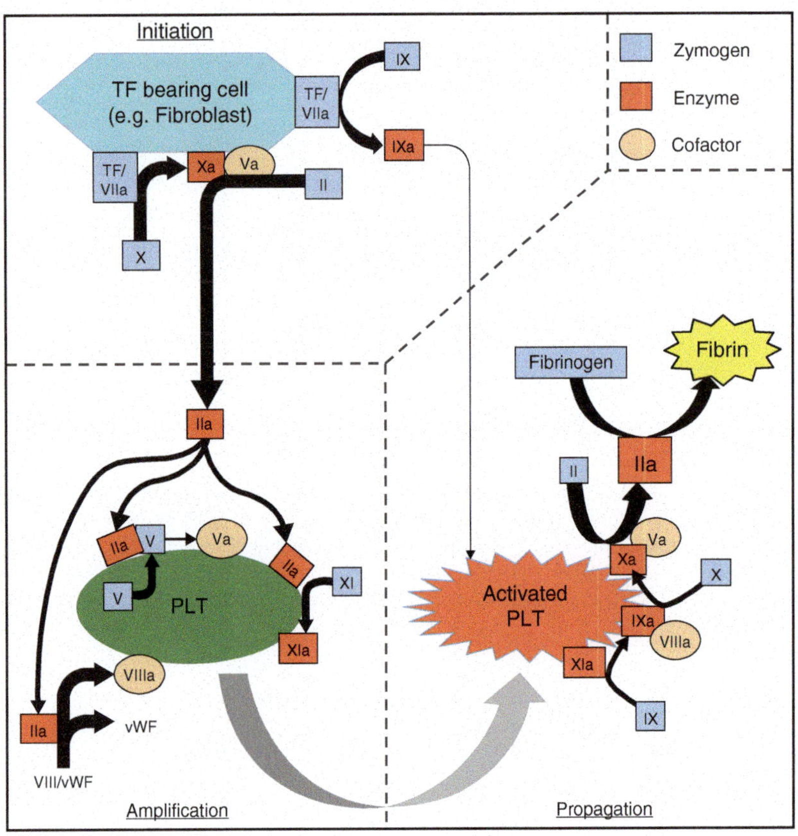

Figure 4.2 The cell-based model of hemostasis showing initiation, amplification, and propagation phases. Roman numerals indicate factors. TF, tissue factor; PLT, platelet; vWF, von Willebrand factor.

coagulation complexes (i.e., FIXa with FVIIIa = tenase complex which then activates FX which then binds FVa = prothrombinase complex) and the generation of large amounts of thrombin (i.e., thrombin burst). FIXa can either be activated on the platelet surface (through FXIa from the amplification phase) or directly diffuse to the platelet surface from the initiation phase as there is no soluble inactivator for FIXa. The larger amounts of thrombin generated in the thrombin burst are required for fibrin polymerization whereas the small amounts generated during the initiation phase can only activate platelets and start activating the coagulation factors. This is a feature of physiological hemostasis that ensures fibrin polymerization only occurs where it is needed (i.e., where there is an activated PL membrane and all the appropriate hemostatic factors). Table 4.5 summarizes the coagulation factors, their abbreviations, and their role within each hemostasis model.

Table 4.5 Coagulation factors, abbreviations, and roles within each hemostasis model.

Factor	Name	Cascade model	Cell-based model	Function
I	Fibrinogen	Common	Propagation	Substrate for thrombin – converted to fibrin
II	Prothrombin	Common	Initiation Amplification Propagation	Proenzyme: IIa (thrombin) cleaves fibrinogen to fibrin, activates V, VIII, XI, XIII, protein C, platelets, plasmin
(III)	Tissue factor (TF), tissue thromboplastin factor	Extrinsic	Initiation	Cofactor: TF binds and activates VII, and the TF/VIIa complex activates IX and X
(IV)	Free ionized Ca	Extrinsic Intrinsic Common	Initiation Amplification Propagation	Cofactor for IIa, VIIa, IXa, Xa, and XIIIa
V	Proaccelerin	Common	Initiation Amplification Propagation	Pro-cofactor for Xa; cofactor after activation to Va
VII	Proconvertin, stable factor	Extrinsic	Initiation	Proenzyme: VIIa activates IX and X
VIII	Antihemophilic factor	Intrinsic	Amplification Propagation	Pro-cofactor for IXa; cofactor after activation to VIIIa
IX	Christmas factor	Intrinsic	Initiation Amplification Propagation	Proenzyme: IXa activates X
X	Stuart factor, Stuart–Prower factor	Common	Initiation Amplification Propagation	Proenzyme: Xa activates II
XI	Plasma thromboplastic antecedent	Intrinsic	Amplification Propagation	Proenzyme: XIa activates IX
XII	Hageman factor	Intrinsic	Unnecessary for coagulation	Proenzyme: XIIa activates XI, PK, HMWK, and plasminogen
XIII	Fibrin-stabilizing factors, fibrinase	Common	Propagation	Proenzyme: XIIIa cross-links fibrin and protects it from plasmin degradation
HMWK	Fitzgerald factor	Intrinsic	Unnecessary for coagulation	Cofactor for activation of XII and XI
PL	Phospholipid membrane	Intrinsic Common	Initiation Amplification Propagation	Negatively charged plt mmb lipoproteins important for *in vivo* activation of X and II and localization of hemostasis to sites of injury
PK	Fletcher factor	Intrinsic	Unnecessary for coagulation	Proenzyme: kallikrein activates XII and PK, generates bradykinin from HMWK, and leads to plasmin generation

4.3.1.4 Fibrinolysis

At the same time as the coagulation system is activated, so is the fibrinolytic system. This is another in-built balance ensuring thrombus formation occurs exactly where it is needed and only for the time it is needed, with quick restoration of blood flow through clot dissolution once the damage is repaired. Plasminogen, an inactive zymogen produced mostly in the liver and present in circulating blood, binds to fibrin. Plasminogen activators, tPA and urokinase plasminogen activator (uPA), are released from damaged or activated endothelial or circulating cells, and activate plasmin, which then degrades fibrinogen and fibrin to soluble fibrin(ogen) degradation products (FDPs). Note thrombin is a cofactor for plasmin activation, which is yet another way to localize the fibrinolysis to the areas of active coagulation. Kallikrein and FXIIa can also activate plasmin. Plasmin also degrades the amplifiers of coagulation (i.e., FVa and FVIIIa) as well as PK, HMWK, and vWF, so downregulating coagulation whilst also playing its major role in fibrinolysis.

FDPs are the plasmin generated fragments of fibrinogen and the fibrin monomer (i.e., fragment X, fragment Y, fragment D, and fragment E). When plasmin degrades cross-linked fibrin polymers, D-dimers are generated. Both are cleared through the liver. Increased FDPs and D-dimers are therefore used as indicators of increased coagulation and fibrinolysis, with D-dimers being thought of as more specific for clinically significant coagulation (e.g., DIC, thrombotic disease); however, they can also elevate with hemorrhage, surgery, and inflammatory disease. Horses have higher FDPs and D-dimers in health than companion animals and humans [52].

4.3.1.5 Inhibitors of Coagulation and Fibrinolysis

Physiological inhibitors of coagulation help to prevent excessive coagulation. They include a group of proteins that complex with and enzymatically inactivate many enzymatic coagulation factors as well as causing the degradation and removal of activated cofactors. The main inhibitors of coagulation are antithrombin III (ATIII), heparin, protein C, and tissue factor pathway inhibitor (TFPI).

Antithrombin III is the major inhibitor of coagulation enzymes. Its most important anticoagulant function lies in its ability to inhibit thrombin. It inactivates thrombin through binding and forming a stable, measurable, inactivated complex (thrombin–antithrombin complex – TAT), which is cleared by the reticuloendothelial system primarily in the liver and spleen. ATIII's thrombin binding capacity is markedly enhanced, up to 1000-fold, by its cofactors heparin and heparan sulfate, which are present due to exogenous administration (heparin), endogenously from mast cells (heparin), or on the endothelial cells (heparan sulfate). As well as binding thrombin, ATIII is also able to bind and inactivate factors IXa, Xa, XIa, and XIIa. The horse has higher concentrations of ATIII than humans and other companion species [53].

Heparin, as well as enhancing ATIII's ability to bind thrombin, releases the membrane-bound TFPI from endothelial cells. TFPI is also produced by monocytes, macrophages, and hepatocytes with most body TFPI within the endothelial cells of the microvasculature and a small amount bound to circulating lipoproteins. TFPI inhibits coagulation by forming a stable quaternary complex (TF–VIIa–Xa–TFPI), which prevents further FIXa and FXa generation by TF-VIIa, so dramatically reducing initiation of coagulation. The complex is cleared by receptor-mediated endocytosis.

Protein C is a vitamin K-dependent proenzyme that when activated has both anticoagulant and profibrinolytic action. Activation of protein C occurs through thrombomodulin–thrombin complexes. Thrombomodulin is a thrombin receptor present on most endothelial cell membranes. The concurrent presence of endothelial cell protein C receptor (EPCR) on the endothelial membrane accelerates thrombin-mediated activation of protein C and concentrates the activated protein C (aPC) near the surface of the vessel wall. More EPCR is expressed in large than small vessels, centering aPC's action in large vessels. When aPC is released into circulation, it becomes associated with membrane-bound protein S, another vitamin K-dependent cofactor produced by endothelial cells, hepatocytes, and megakaryocytes, which in combination with aPC and inactive FV inactivates factors Va and VIIIa, the cofactors associated with amplification and propagation.

Activated protein C's profibrinolytic action is through inhibition of PAI-1 which normally blocks the conversion of plasminogen to plasmin by tPA or uPA. PAI-1 is synthesized and secreted by endothelial cells in its active form. Once plasmin is formed, its major inhibitor is alpha-2-antiplasmin which acts by binding and clearing plasmin from the circulation. These two methods prevent premature fibrinolysis and clot dissolution. Thrombin–thrombomodulin complexes as well as activating protein C cause activation of thrombin-activatable fibrinolysis inhibitor (TAFI), which is another fibrinolytic inhibitor. TAFI can also be activated by thrombin itself (although more slowly), plasmin, and trypsin. TAFIa cleaves plasminogen binding sites from fibrin and as such inhibits fibrinolysis. Table 4.6 summarizes the major inhibitors of coagulation and fibrinolysis and their actions.

Table 4.6 Major inhibitors of coagulation and fibrinolysis and their functions.

Factor	Function
ATIII	Major anticoagulant associated with thrombin inhibition. Binds, inactivates, and removes most coagulation enzymes from circulation. Specifically binds IIa, IXa, Xa, XIa, XIIa, kallikrein, plasmin, urokinase. Action markedly enhanced by heparin or heparan sulfate
aPC	Major anticoagulant and profibrinolytic that is vitamin K dependent. Activated by thrombin bound to thrombomodulin (often large vessels). Anticoagulant through inactivation Va and VIIIa. Profibrinolytic through inhibition of PAI-1
TFPI	Major anticoagulant through inhibition of TF–VIIa and Xa by forming a quaternary complex (TF–VIIa–Xa–TFPI). Heparin can increase TFPI in circulation by releasing the membrane-bound TFPI from endothelial cells
Heparin	Anticoagulant. Cofactor in ATIII action – increases the binding affinity of ATIII for thrombin by up to 1000×. Increased TFPI concentrations in circulation
Alpha-2-antiplasmin	Major inhibitor of fibrinolysis. Binds, inhibits, and clears plasmin from circulation
Alpha-2-macroglobulin	Minor inhibitor of fibrinolysis. Binds, inhibits, and clears plasmin from circulation
PAI-1	Inhibitor of fibrinolysis through decreasing production of plasmin. Produced by endothelial cells. Inactivates tPA and uPA
TAFI	Inhibitor of fibrinolysis. Zymogen activated by thrombin and thrombomodulin; TAFIa cleaves plasminogen-binding sites from fibrin, thus inhibiting fibrinolysis

ATIII, antithrombin III; aPC, activated protein C; TFPI, tissue factor pathway inhibitor; PAI-1, plasminogen activator inhibitor; tPA, plasminogen activator, tissue type; uPA, plasminogen activator, urokinase type; TAFI, thrombin activatable fibrinolysis inhibitor.

4.3.2 Coagulation Testing and Disorders Causing Abnormalities

Coagulation testing is used clinically when a patient is bleeding without obvious trauma, bleeding excessively from a surgical/traumatic wound, suspected of being in a hypercoagulable or hypocoagulable state associated with inflammation or DIC, or has an underlying disease that can predispose to bleeding. The tests requested will depend on the clinical signs and which component(s) of hemostasis are thought to be affected. Most coagulation testing is designed to assess for disorders associated with excessive bleeding (i.e., hypocoagulable states); however, more recently developed tests are also helping to investigate hypercoagulable states (i.e., procoagulant state of inflammation and/or DIC, protein-losing enteropathy).

Disorders of primary hemostasis often present with mucosal/small vessel bleeding (e.g., petechiation, ecchymoses, epistaxis, melena, hematuria, bleeding from the gums). Disorders of secondary hemostasis often present with large vessel or cavitary bleeding (e.g., hematomas, hemarthrosis, hemothorax, hemoperitoneum, excessive bleeding post surgery). Disorders of fibrinolysis (i.e., hypercoagulable states) are more difficult to detect on physical examination but can be expected in patients with systemic inflammatory conditions that may lead to DIC.

4.3.2.1 Primary Hemostasis

If the patient presents with mucosal bleeding (e.g., petechiation, ecchymoses, epistaxis, melena, hematuria, bleeding from the gums), testing for primary hemostatic disorders should be considered first. Testing should commence with a CBC to evaluate for thrombocytopenia as this is the most common cause for a primary hemostatic defect. Thrombocytopenia must be marked to cause bleeding (i.e., <50 000/μL) and as platelet clumping is common in horses, a blood smear should always be evaluated in concert with the machine CBC results to confirm the machine platelet count is accurate.

Causes of marked thrombocytopenia include vasculitis, certain infectious causes (e.g., EIAV, *Anaplasma phagocytophilum*), immune-mediated thrombocytopenia, neoplasia, and rarely idiosyncratic drug reactions [54]. If platelet numbers are not markedly decreased and/or within or above reference interval, yet the bleeding is definitively mucosal, platelet function tests should be considered. The most clinically available test of platelet function is the template bleeding time (TBT), which can be performed on the buccal mucosa (BMBT) or a shaved region of skin on the medial forelimb, and involves a commercial device which uses a spring-loaded blade to cause multiple small cuts of defined length and depth (5 mm long and 1 mm deep). Venostasis is required prior to instituting the cuts. The length of time until the cuts stop bleeding is the template or BMBT. This will be prolonged if there is thrombocytopenia, thrombopathia, or vWF deficiency, and might be prolonged with vasculitis. Unfortunately, the variation between horses and within the same horse at different times has been shown to be too wide to determine a sufficiently narrow reference interval for clinical use. Only if the test is repeatedly markedly prolonged (i.e., >860 seconds) can a diagnosis of primary hemostatic defect be made [55]. Other platelet function assays are available primarily at referral institutions and include the PFA-100, platelet aggregation studies, and flow cytometry assessing platelet activation and membrane protein and glycoprotein expression [50, 56].

Hereditary primary hemostatic disorders reported in the horse include Glanzmann thrombasthenia [57, 58], atypical equine thrombasthenia [59–61], and vWF deficiency [54, 62]; however, they are all considered rare and should only be considered a differential if there is mucosal bleeding or prolonged postsurgical bleeding and a normal platelet count and other functional assays.

4.3.2.2 Secondary Hemostasis

If the patient presents with large vessel or cavitary bleeding (e.g., hematomas, hemarthrosis, hemothorax, hemoperitoneum) without surgery or significant trauma or there is excessive bleeding post surgery or trauma, then consider testing for secondary hemostatic defects. Most of the tests used for secondary hemostatic disorders are functional tests of the coagulation proteins and involve the addition of free calcium ± activators to platelet-poor citrated plasma with an incubation step and then measurement of the time to fibrin clot formation. These measurements can be manual (i.e., to visible fibrin formation), mechanical (i.e., steel ball with a magnetic sensor that notes when the ball is not moving freely within the sample), or optical (i.e., turbidimetry [light transmittance through the fluid] or nephelometry [detection of light scatter through a fluid]). The automated assays (i.e., mechanical and optical) have increased the precision and decreased operator error.

Sample collection and processing techniques are critical to retain protein function and so derive clinically useful information from the results of the coagulation testing. First, blood sampling should be minimally traumatic with the samples representing a "clean stick." This reduces the activation of platelets, coagulation, and/or fibrinolytic systems prior to placement within the tube. Second, it was recently shown that it does not alter results if you collect the blood sample from an indwelling catheter compared to a direct jugular venipuncture [63]. Third, most coagulation assays involve citrate as the anticoagulant with the ratio of citrate to whole blood being important for accurate results. Citrate causes anticoagulation by reversibly binding calcium, which allows for the subsequent readdition of calcium in the laboratory to reverse the anticoagulation. The ratio of citrate to blood is critical at 1:9, with either 3.2% or 3.8% citrate tubes, depending on the laboratory. If the tubes are over- or underfilled, the ratio will not be accurate and this can cause falsely shortened or prolonged coagulation testing results, respectively.

After confirming the absence of any clots in the sample, the citrated blood should be centrifuged for 10–15 minutes at 1500× g. It is recommended to centrifuge and remove the plasma within one hour and test within six hours if refrigerated and 24 hours if frozen at −20 °C [64]. In humans and dogs, it has been shown that transport times of up to 48 hours at ambient temperature of whole blood (i.e., without plasma separation) had no significant effects on prothrombin time (PT) and activated partial thromboplastin time (aPTT) in humans and no significant effects on PT and only mildly shortened aPTT measurements in dogs, allowing for the possibility of accurate measurements even without rapid sample processing. However, this has been disproven with equine plasma samples [64] with whole blood not yet evaluated [65, 66].

Once the blood sample has been collected, commonly used screening tests include PT, aPTT, and activated clotting time (ACT). The PT and aPTT tests are performed predominantly on citrated plasma but some machines, often point of care, can perform this on citrated whole blood.

The aPTT and ACT measure the function of the intrinsic and common pathways (Figure 4.1c), so deficiencies in FXI, FIX, FVIII, FX, FV, prothrombin, and fibrinogen will cause prolongations. Note that both aPTT and ACT will also be prolonged with PK, HMWK, and FXII deficiencies; however, in the majority of cases, even if the patient is deficient in these factors, this should not cause a bleeding tendency and is likely an incidental finding. The original study outlining PK deficiency in a family of Belgian horses did show clinical hemorrhage in one patient secondary to their deficiency [67].

The ACT is performed as a bedside test on nonanticoagulated whole blood. The whole blood is added to a tube containing an intrinsic pathway activator, often diatomaceous earth, but other materials including kaolin and celite have also been used. The tube is maintained at 37 °C and the time to first clot formation is measured as the ACT. It is expected to be between two and three minutes in healthy horses [54]. The ACT can be performed patient side which is its major benefit; however, it is less sensitive than the aPTT for detection of deficiencies, so is often not useful unless used as a quick screening test to guide potential further investigation.

The aPTT test is performed by mixing excess procoagulant PLs (partial thromboplastin) and a surface activator (e.g., kaolin, silicates, or ellagic acid) with platelet-poor citrated plasma and measuring the time to clot formation when incubated at 37 °C.

The PT measures the function of the extrinsic and common pathways (Figure 4.1b), so deficiencies in FVII, FX, FV, prothrombin, and fibrinogen will cause prolongations. Platelet-poor plasma is mixed with thromboplastin (containing PL and excess TF) and calcium and the time to clot formation at 37 °C incubation is reported as the PT result.

Both PT and aPTT results should be interpreted in light of the reference interval provided with either the results from the reference laboratory or the point-of-care machine being used, as different activators and methodologies result in markedly different reference intervals. Also be aware during interpretation of results that both PT and aPTT are relatively insensitive for the detection of factor deficiencies, with a requirement to have a 50–75% deficiency in an individual factor before a prolongation is noted.

The PT and aPTT should be interpreted together to help narrow the cause for any prolongation (Figure 4.1d). If only one of the two is prolonged, the common pathway factors (i.e., FX, FV, prothrombin, and fibrinogen) can be ruled out as the cause for the prolongation, leaving FVII as the cause if only the PT is prolonged and any or multiple of PK, HMWK, FXII, FXI, FIX, and FVIII as the cause if only the aPTT is prolonged. If solely the aPTT or ACT is prolonged with a normal PT, the exact factor deficiency causing the prolongation cannot be determined. In these circumstances, individual factor analysis could be considered for further evaluation; however, usually this is performed only at referral institutions. Also individual factor deficiencies (i.e., inherited secondary defects) are very uncommon in the horse and should not be thought of as the likely cause for any prolongations. Reported inherited defects include deficits in PK [67], factors VIII [68, 69], IX, and XI [70], which would all cause prolongations in aPTT and/or ACT without a prolongation in PT.

Acquired secondary hemostatic defects are much more likely as the cause for any prolongations. Causes to consider for acquired secondary hemostatic defects include inappropriate heparin administration, severe liver disease/hepatic insufficiency (e.g., secondary to hepatic necrosis, cirrhosis, or acute hepatitis), vitamin K deficiency (e.g., secondary to biliary obstruction, chronic oral antibiotic administration, severe infiltrative bowel disease, rodenticide toxicity, and sweet clover mold ingestion), DIC, or severe systemic inflammation. Most often, the coagulation panel abnormalities associated with acquired secondary hemostatic disease will cause prolongations in both PT and aPTT/ACT as many factors are affected. With vitamin K deficiency, only the vitamin K-dependent factors (i.e., II, VII, IX, and X) are affected; however, this will prolong both PT and aPTT while leaving fibrinogen concentration and function unaffected.

Fibrinogen measurement as part of a coagulation profile is an attempt to document hypofibrinogenemia, which is seen with DIC due to consumption and hepatic insufficiency due to decreased production. Most often in horses, fibrinogen is being measured as a sign of inflammatory disease as fibrinogen is a positive acute-phase protein. Severe inflammatory disease is a common cause of DIC in horses so true hypofibrinogenemia (i.e. <150 mg/dL) is often masked with an inflammatory rise in fibrinogen. However, horses with subclinical DIC from colitis have been documented to have lower than expected fibrinogen and a precipitous drop in fibrinogen (>100 mg/dL) which in this same patient population was associated with poor prognosis, so perhaps serial measurement of fibrinogen could be useful in assessment for DIC [71]. Fibrinogen can be measured by heat precipitation, von Clauss method, or detection of fibrinogen antigen (i.e., nonfunctional assay). Heat precipitation is not accurate enough for hemostasis testing as precision is too low at low measurement values.

Anticoagulant testing can also be performed although this is done less commonly as anticoagulants are often only able to be measured at specialized coagulation laboratories due to the requirement for species-specific standards and controls [72–75]. Their clinical utility lies in detection of the subclinical or hypercoagulable state of DIC. The most commonly measured would be ATIII and aPC, with TAT measurement also reported. Decreases in ATIII have been associated with DIC, protein loss (often renal and GI), or with failure of production (i.e., hepatic insufficiency). ATIII has been shown to be a sensitive test for the diagnosis of DIC whilst also being prognostic for outcome [76–79]. Decreases in aPC are also associated with DIC and a hypercoagulable state but as with fibrinogen, aPC is a positive acute-phase protein, so true decreases are often masked when there is concurrent inflammation [72].

4.3.2.3 Fibrinolysis

Fibrinogen degradation products and D-dimers are formed after plasmin-mediated degradation of fibrinogen, fibrin monomers, fibrin polymers, and cross-linked fibrin polymers and as such are used to diagnose excessive clot formation (i.e., hypercoagulable state). Excessive clot formation in the horse is most often associated with the procoagulant state associated with inflammation and leading into DIC but can also be seen with hemorrhage and postsurgically. FDPs have been evaluated but the sensitivity for detection of DIC is low and due to this and a limited availability, they have been predominantly replaced by the measurement of

D-dimers [52, 71, 77, 80]. D-dimers are formed solely from cross-linked fibrin polymer degradation and are therefore thought to be more specific for clinically significant thrombosis or DIC in humans and other companion species [81, 82]. When evaluated in horses with severe inflammatory conditions and ischemic disease, they have been shown to be significantly elevated, supporting their clinical significance in the horse as well [83, 84].

4.3.2.4 Global Hemostasis Testing

As previously discussed, the coagulation cascade model, although helpful for understanding coagulation testing, is recognized as not highlighting the importance of the cellular components of coagulation and for falsely separating the intrinsic, extrinsic, and common coagulation pathways, which is not the case *in vivo*. The cell-based model of hemostasis attempts to correct these misconceptions. Along similar lines, there has been a movement to evaluate global hemostasis rather than individual coagulation assays with the advent of viscoelastic hemostatic testing.

Available viscoelastic testing devices include thromboelastography (TEG), rotational thromboelastometry (ROTEM), automated thromboelastometer (TEM-A), and Sonoclot analyzers. These analyzers evaluate all phases of clot formation and retraction with all cellular components present and therefore are a better assessment of global hemostasis (i.e., primary and secondary hemostasis as well as fibrinolysis). Theoretically, they are able to detect hypercoagulable as well as the more commonly assessed hypocoagulable states which, if this proves true in the horse, will help to identify early DIC patients. Briefly, a small (~350 μL) whole blood aliquot (either anticoagulated or nonanticoagulated if the machine is patient side) is placed in a cup with a central metal pin or wire. Activators are added, with calcium if required, and the cup is oscillated in a small rotation left to right. As the blood clots, the metal pin is held away from the center of the cup and a tracing is formed whose dimensions are defined by the rate and strength of clot formation and retraction. The main differences between the machines are whether the cup or the pin/wire are rotating or whether the pin/wire moves up and down within the sample. Measurements from the tracing (e.g., in TEG: time to first clot formation (R); time to a clot amplitude of 20 mm (K); maximum amplitude (MA); and angle (α)) are used to evaluate not only for hypocoagulable states but also platelet plug formation, hypercoagulable states, and, if the test is run to completion (i.e., two hours, until clot dissolution), for disorders associated with fibrinolysis.

Discussing TEG abnormalities with disease states in detail is beyond the scope of this chapter but this has been well reviewed by Mendez-Angulo et al. and readers are referred there for more information [85]. TEG in the horse has shown good precision when run in duplicate; however, marked interindividual variation, significant overlap between healthy and sick horses, and moderate interoperator variability indicate that the main use of viscoelastic studies will likely be in serial monitoring of cases to determine changes from baseline/admission and response to therapy [84, 86–90]. Of all the TEG variables, MA has been shown to have the lowest variability, perhaps suggesting this will be the most reliable variable to compare between horses [88].

4.3.2.5 Laboratory Diagnosis of DIC

Disseminated intravascular coagulation is a common condition in the horse, with studies showing up to 32% of horses with colitis [71], 40% horses with ischemic/inflammatory gastrointestinal disease [91], 70% of horses with large colon volvulus [92] and 70% of septic foals [93] having either clinicopathological or histopathological evidence of DIC. DIC is an acquired coagulopathy characterized by overactivation of the coagulation system (i.e., procoagulant state) which when it overwhelms the natural inhibitory systems causes exaggerated intravascular fibrin formation with widespread fibrin deposition and microvascular thrombus formation in different tissues with mild consumption of platelets, coagulation factors, and inhibitors of coagulation (i.e., hypercoagulable state or subclinical DIC). The microvascular thrombus formation can lead to ischemic tissue lesions and multiorgan dysfunction/failure. With time and in a small subset of equine patients, if the fibrin formation is not halted by the inhibitory systems, significant consumption of platelets, coagulation factor depletion, and consumption of coagulation inhibitors occur, leading to a consumptive coagulopathy (i.e., clinical or fulminant DIC), which presents clinically with signs of spontaneous hemorrhage. Spontaneous hemorrhage is uncommon as the clinical presentation of DIC in the horse, with most patients presenting in subclinical DIC (i.e., some coagulation panel abnormalities but no overt signs of bleeding). Also, clinical evidence of hypercoagulability is not common in the horse except for jugular thrombophlebitis [94, 95].

Disseminated intravascular coagulation always develops secondary to an underlying disease that induces systemic activation of coagulation combined with depression of the anticoagulant system. A common example is sepsis with gram-negative bacteria (often from GI disease), in which endotoxemia is thought to trigger DIC by the induction of TF expression within the vascular space (i.e., on circulating monocytes and endothelial cells).

The diagnosis of DIC is based on the presence of a disease that can cause increased coagulation combined with clinical and laboratory abnormalities consistent with DIC.

Laboratory test results which are considered features of DIC include thrombocytopenia (usually mild to moderate, i.e. <100 000/μL), prolonged PT, prolonged aPTT, low fibrinogen (i.e. <150 mg/dL), low ATIII activity (if available), and increased FDPs or D-dimers. In clinical reports, DIC is diagnosed if at least three of the six features are present. Reports have shown that with this diagnostic system, the presence of DIC is a negative prognostic indicator, with one study reporting an 8× higher likelihood of death in patients with DIC compared to those without and many studies providing evidence of increased morbidity and mortality associated with coagulation alterations, particularly in horses with gastrointestinal disease and foals with sepsis [71, 76, 78, 79, 96, 97]. Other laboratory tests that have been reported to be prognostic for survival include increased TATs, decreased ATIII, decreased protein C, and increased PAI-1 [75–77, 98].

In summary, a coagulation panel and/or global assessment of hemostasis at admission/first consult and then serially throughout hospitalization would be recommended in any equine patient presented due to gastrointestinal disease and/or sepsis. This recommendation is based on the fact that these disease states commonly cause DIC, DIC has been shown to be prognostic for length of hospitalization and survival to discharge, and prompt intervention is associated with better outcomes.

References

1 The International Society for Animal Blood Group Research (1987). *Proceedings of the 20th International Conference on Animal Blood Groups and Biochemical Polymorphisms, Helsinki, Finland (28 July–1 August 1986). Anim. Genet.* 18(s1):1–145.

2 Owens, S.D., Snipes, J., Magdesian, K.G., and Christopher, M.M. (2008). Evaluation of a rapid agglutination method for detection of equine red cell surface antigens (Ca and Aa) as part of pretransfusion testing. *Vet. Clin. Pathol.* 37 (1): 49–56.

3 Luethy, D., Owens, S.D., Stefanovski, D. et al. (2016). Comparison of tube, gel, and immunochromatographic strip methods for evaluation of blood transfusion compatibility in horses. *J. Vet. Intern. Med.* 30 (6): 1864–1871.

4 Tomlinson, J.E., Taberner, E., Boston, R.C. et al. (2015). Survival time of cross-match incompatible red blood cells in adult horses. *J. Vet. Intern. Med.* 29 (6): 1683–1688.

5 Bailey, E. (1982). Prevalence of anti-red blood cel antibodies in the serum and colostrum of mares and its relationship to neonatal isoerythrolysis. *Am. J. Vet. Res.* 43 (11): 1917–1921.

6 Cox, L. (1984). *A survey of equine red blood cell antibody frequencies and their relevance to neonatal isoerythrolysis*. MS thesis. Genetics Laboratory, University of California, Davis.

7 MacLeay, J.M. (2001). Neonatal isoerythrolysis involving the Qc and Db antigens in a foal. *J. Am. Vet. Med. Assoc.* 219 (1): 79–81.

8 Zaruby, J.F., Hearn, P., and Colling, D. (1992). Neonatal isoerythrolysis in a foal, involving anti-Pa alloantibody. *Equine Vet. J.* 24 (1): 71–73.

9 Boyle, A.G., Magdesian, K.G., and Ruby, R.E. (2005). Neonatal isoerythrolysis in horse foals and a mule foal: 18 cases (1988–2003). *J. Am. Vet. Med. Assoc.* 227 (8): 1276–1283.

10 O'Neil, E., Horney, B., and Burton, S. (2014). What is your diagnosis? Blood smear from a foal. *Vet. Clin. Pathol.* 43 (2): 287–288.

11 Harris, M., Nolen-Walston, R., Ashton, W. et al. (2012). Effect of sample storage on blood crossmatching in horses. *J. Vet. Intern. Med.* 26 (3): 662–667.

12 McClure, J.J., Koch, C., and Traub-Dargatz, J. (1994). Characterization of a red blood cell antigen in donkeys and mules associated with neonatal isoerythrolysis. *Anim. Genet.* 25 (2): 119–120.

13 Marsh, W.L. (1972). Scoring of hemagglutination reactions. *Transfusion* 12 (5): 352–353.

14 Casenave, P., Leclere, M., Beauchamp, G., and Blais, M.-C. (2019). Modified stall-side crossmatch for transfusions in horses. *J. Vet. Intern. Med.* 33 (4): 1775–1783.

15 Sprayberry, K.A. (2003). Neonatal transfusion medicine: the use of blood, plasma, oxygen-carrying solutions, and adjunctive therapies in foals. *Clin. Tech. Equine Pract.* 2 (1): 31–41.

16 Axon, J.E. and Palmer, J.E. (2008). Clinical pathology of the foal. *Vet. Clin. North Am. Equine Pract.* 24 (2): 357–385.

17 Heath, S.E., Geor, R.J., Tabel, H., and McIntosh, K. (1991). Unusual patterns of serum antibodies to *Streptococcus equi* in two horses with purpura hemorrhagica. *J. Vet. Intern. Med.* 5 (5): 263–267.

18 Johns, I.C., Desrochers, A., Wotman, K.L., and Sweeney, R.W. (2011). Presumed immune-mediated hemolytic anemia in two foals with Rhodococcus equi infection. *J. Vet. Emerg. Crit. Care* 21 (3): 273–278.

19 Underwood, C. and Southwood, L.L. (2008). Hemolytic anemia as a complication following colic surgery in a 10-year-old Arabian stallion. *Equine Vet. Educ.* 20 (8): 422–426.

20 McGovern, K.F., Lascola, K.M., Davis, E. et al. (2011). T-cell lymphoma with immune-mediated anemia and thrombocytopenia in a horse. *J. Vet. Intern. Med.* 25 (5): 1181–1185.

21 Raidal, S.L., Clark, P., and Raidal, S.R. (2006). Angiotrophic T-cell lymphoma as a cause of regenerative anemia in a horse. *J. Vet. Intern. Med.* 20 (4): 1009–1013.

22 Cottle, H.J. and Hughes, K.J. (2010). Hemolytic anemia in a pony associated with a perivascular abscess caused by *Clostridium perfringens*. *Equine Vet. Educ.* 22 (1): 13–19.

23 Weiser, G. and O'Grady, M. (1983). Erythrocyte volume distribution analysis and hematologic changes in dogs with iron deficiency anemia. *Vet. Pathol.* 20 (2): 230–241.

24 Rebhun, W.C., Shin, S.J., King, J.M. et al. (1985). Malignant edema in horses. *J. Am. Vet. Med. Assoc.* 187 (7): 732–736.

25 Mair, T.S., Taylor, F.G., and Hillyer, M.H. (1990). Autoimmune hemolytic anemia in eight horses. *Vet. Rec.* 126 (3): 51–53.

26 Lokhorst, H.M. and Breukink, H.J. (1975). Auto-immune hemolytic anemia in two horses. *Tijdschr. Diergeneeskd.* 100 (14): 752–757.

27 Taylor, F.G. and Cooke, B.J. (1990). Use of erythrocyte fragility profiles for monitoring immune-mediated hemolysis in horses. *Res. Vet. Sci.* 48 (1): 138–140.

28 Wilkerson, M.J., Davis, E., Shuman, W. et al. (2000). Isotype-specific antibodies in horses and dogs with immune-mediated hemolytic anemia. *J. Vet. Intern. Med.* 14 (2): 190–196.

29 McConnico, R.S., Roberts, M.C., and Tompkins, M. (1992). Penicillin-induced immune-mediated hemolytic anemia in a horse. *J. Am. Vet. Med. Assoc.* 201 (9): 1402–1403.

30 Perdrizet, J.A., Callihan, D.R., Rebhun, W.C., and Shin, S.J. (1987). Successful management of malignant edema caused by Clostridium septicum in a horse. *Cornell Vet.* 77 (4): 328–338.

31 Blue, J.T., Dinsmore, R.P., and Anderson, K.L. (1987). Immune-mediated hemolytic anemia induced by penicillin in horses. *Cornell Vet.* 77 (3): 263–276.

32 Step, D.L., Blue, J.T., and Dill, S.G. (1991). Penicillin-induced hemolytic anemia and acute hepatic failure following treatment of tetanus in a horse. *Cornell Vet.* 81 (1): 13–18.

33 Reef, V.B. (1983). Clostridium perfringens cellulitis and immune-mediated hemolytic anemia in a horse. *J. Am. Vet. Med. Assoc.* 182 (3): 251–254.

34 Reef, V.B., Dyson, S.S., and Beech, J. (1984). Lymphosarcoma and associated immune-mediated hemolytic anemia and thrombocytopenia in horses. *J. Am. Vet. Med. Assoc.* 184 (3): 313–317.

35 Messer, N.T. and Arnold, K. (1991). Immune-mediated hemolytic anemia in a horse. *J. Am. Vet. Med. Assoc.* 198 (8): 1415–1416.

36 Weiss, D.J. and Moritz, A. (2003). Equine immune-mediated hemolytic anemia associated with *Clostridium perfringens* infection. *Vet. Clin. Pathol.* 32 (1): 22–26.

37 Beck, D.J. (1990). A case of primary autoimmune hemolytic anemia in a pony. *Equine Vet. J.* 22 (4): 292–294.

38 Sockett, D.C., Traub-Dargatz, J., and Weiser, M.G. (1987). Immune-mediated hemolytic anemia and thrombocytopenia in a foal. *J. Am. Vet. Med. Assoc.* 190 (3): 308–310.

39 Thomas, H.L. and Livesey, M.A. (1998). Immune-mediated hemolytic anemia associated with trimethoprim-sulphamethoxazole administration in a horse. *Can. Vet. J.* 39 (3): 171–173.

40 Robbins, R.L., Wallace, S.S., Brunner, C.J. et al. (1993). Immune-mediated hemolytic disease after penicillin therapy in a horse. *Equine Vet. J.* 25 (5): 462–465.

41 Becht, J.L. and Semrad, S.D. (1985). Hematology, blood typing, and immunology of the neonatal foal. *Vet. Clin. North Am. Equine Pract.* 1 (1): 91–116.

42 Polkes, A.C., Giguère, S., Lester, G.D., and Bain, F.T. (2008). Factors associated with outcome in foals with neonatal isoerythrolysis (72 cases, 1988–2003). *J. Vet. Intern. Med.* 22 (5): 1216–1222.

43 Broux, B., Lefère, L., Deprez, P., and van Loon, G. (2015). Plasma exchange as a treatment for hyperbilirubinemia in 2 foals with neonatal isoerythrolysis. *J. Vet. Intern. Med.* 29 (2): 736–738.

44 Sellon, D.C., Fuller, F.J., and McGuire, T.C. (1994). The immunopathogenesis of equine infectious anemia virus. *Virus Res.* 32 (2): 111–138.

45 Peek, S.F., Semrad, S.D., and Perkins, G.A. (2003). Clostridial myonecrosis in horses (37 cases 1985–2000). *Equine Vet. J.* 35 (1): 86–92.

46 Reuss, S.M., Chaffin, M.K., and Cohen, N.D. (2009). Extrapulmonary disorders associated with Rhodococcus equi infection in foals: 150 cases (1987–2007). *J. Am. Vet. Med. Assoc.* 235 (7): 855–863.

47 Meyer, J., Delay, J., and Bienzle, D. (2006). Clinical, laboratory, and histopathologic features of equine lymphoma. *Vet. Pathol.* 43 (6): 914–924.

48 Mair, T.S. and Hillyer, M.H. (1992). Clinical features of lymphosarcoma in the horse: 77 cases. *Equine Vet. Educ.* 4 (3): 108–113.

49 Boudreaux, M.K. (2008). Characteristics, diagnosis, and treatment of inherited platelet disorders in mammals. *J. Am. Vet. Med. Assoc.* 233 (8): 1251–1259.

50 Segura, D., Monreal, L., Pérez-Pujol, S. et al. (2006). Assessment of platelet function in horses: ultrastructure, flow cytometry, and perfusion techniques. *J. Vet. Intern. Med.* 20 (3): 581–588.

51 Hoffman, M. and Monroe, D.M. (2001). A cell-based model of hemostasis. *Thromb. Hemost.* 85 (6): 958–965.

52 Stokol, T., Erb, H.N., de Wilde, L. et al. (2005). Evaluation of latex agglutination kits for detection of fibrin(ogen) degradation products and D-dimer in healthy horses and horses with severe colic. *Vet. Clin. Pathol.* 34 (4): 375–382.

53 Johnstone, I.B., Petersen, D., and Crane, S. (1987). Antithrombin III (ATIII) activity in plasmas from normal and diseased horses, and in normal canine, bovine and human plasmas. *Vet. Clin. Pathol.* 16 (1): 14–18.

54 Brooks, M.B. (2008). Equine coagulopathies. *Vet. Clin. North Am. Equine Pract.* 24 (2): 335–355.

55 Segura, D. and Monreal, L. (2008). Poor reproducibility of template bleeding time in horses. *J. Vet. Intern. Med.* 22 (1): 238–241.

56 Segura, D., Monreal, L., Espada, Y. et al. (2005). Assessment of a platelet function analyser in horses: reference range and influence of a platelet aggregation inhibitor. *Vet. J.* 170 (1): 108–112.

57 Macieira, S., Rivard, G.-E., Champagne, J. et al. (2007). Glanzmann thrombasthenia in an Oldenbourg filly. *Vet. Clin. Pathol.* 36 (2): 204–208.

58 Christopherson, P.W., van Santen, V.L., Livesey, L., and Boudreaux, M.K. (2007). A 10-base-pair deletion in the gene encoding platelet glycoprotein IIb associated with Glanzmann thrombasthenia in a horse. *J. Vet. Intern. Med.* 21 (1): 196–198.

59 Norris, J.W., Pratt, S.M., Auh, J.-H. et al. (2006). Investigation of a novel, heritable bleeding diathesis of thoroughbred horses and development of a screening assay. *J. Vet. Intern. Med.* 20 (6): 1450–1456.

60 Norris, J.W., Pratt, S.M., Hunter, J.F. et al. (2007). Prevalence of reduced fibrinogen binding to platelets in a population of thoroughbreds. *Am. J. Vet. Res.* 68 (7): 716–721.

61 Norris, J.W., Pombo, M., Shirley, E. et al. (2015). Association of factor V secretion with protein kinase B signaling in platelets from horses with atypical equine thrombasthenia. *J. Vet. Intern. Med.* 29 (5): 1387–1394.

62 Rathgeber, R.A., Brooks, M.B., Bain, F.T., and Byars, T.D. (2001). Clinical vignette. Von Willebrand disease in a thoroughbred mare and foal. *J. Vet. Intern. Med.* 15 (1): 63–66.

63 Mackenzie, C.J., McGowan, C.M., Pinchbeck, G., and Carslake, H.B. (2018). Comparison of two blood sampling techniques for the determination of coagulation parameters in the horse: jugular venipuncture and indwelling intravenous catheter. *Equine Vet. J.* 50 (3): 333–338.

64 Casella, S., Giannetto, C., Fazio, F. et al. (2009). Assessment of prothrombin time, activated partial thromboplastin time, and fibrinogen concentration on equine plasma samples following different storage conditions. *J. Vet. Diagn. Investig.* 21 (5): 674–678.

65 Maunder, C.L., Costa, M., Cue, S.M. et al. (2012). Measurement of prothrombin time and activated partial thromboplastin time in citrated whole blood samples from clinically ill dogs following storage. *J. Small Anim. Pract.* 53 (9): 531–535.

66 Zürcher, M., Sulzer, I., Barizzi, G. et al. (2008). Stability of coagulation assays performed in plasma from citrated whole blood transported at ambient temperature. *Thromb. Hemost.* 99 (2): 416–426.

67 Geor, R.J., Jackson, M.L., Lewis, K.D., and Fretz, P.B. (1990). Prekallikrein deficiency in a family of Belgian horses. *J. Am. Vet. Med. Assoc.* 197 (6): 741–745.

68 Littlewood, J.D., Bevan, S.A., and Corke, M.J. (1991). Hemophilia A (classic hemophilia, factor VIII deficiency) in a thoroughbred colt foal. *Equine Vet. J.* 23 (1): 70–72.

69 Norton, E.M., Wooldridge, A.A., Stewart, A.J. et al. (2016). Abnormal coagulation factor VIII transcript in a tennessee walking horse colt with hemophilia A. *Vet. Clin. Pathol.* 45 (1): 96–102.

70 Hinton, M., Jones, D.R., Lewis, I.M., and Thomson, P.E. (1977). A clotting defect in an Arab colt foal. *Equine Vet. J.* 9 (1): 1–3.

71 Dolente, B.A., Wilkins, P.A., and Boston, R.C. (2002). Clinicopathologic evidence of disseminated intravascular coagulation in horses with acute colitis. *J. Am. Vet. Med. Assoc.* 220 (7): 1034–1038.

72 Topper, M.J. and Prasse, K.W. (1998). Analysis of coagulation proteins as acute-phase reactants in horses with colic. *Am. J. Vet. Res.* 59 (5): 542–545.

73 Topper, M.J. and Prasse, K.W. (1998). Chromogenic assays for equine coagulation factors VII, VIII:C, IX, and X, and C1-esterase inhibitor. *Am. J. Vet. Res.* 59 (5): 538–541.

74 Topper, M.J., Prasse, K.W., Morris, M.J. et al. (1996). Enzyme-linked immunosorbent assay for thrombin-antithrombin III complexes in horses. *Am. J. Vet. Res.* 57 (4): 427–431.

75 Topper, M.J. and Prasse, K.W. (1996). Use of enzyme-linked immunosorbent assay to measure thrombin-antithrombin III complexes in horses with colic. *Am. J. Vet. Res.* 57 (4): 456–462.

76 Johnstone, I.B. and Crane, S. (1986). Hemostatic abnormalities in horses with colic – their prognostic value. *Equine Vet. J.* 18 (4): 271–274.

77 Monreal, L., Anglés, A., Espada, Y. et al. (2000). Hypercoagulation and hypofibrinolysis in horses with colic and DIC. *Equine Vet. J. Suppl.* 32: 19–25.

78 Feige, K., Kästner, S.B.R., Dempfle, C.E., and Balestra, E. (2003). Changes in coagulation and markers of fibrinolysis in horses undergoing colic surgery. *J. Vet. Med. A Physiol. Pathol. Clin. Med.* 50 (1): 30–36.

79 Holland, M., Kelly, A.B., Snyder, J.R. et al. (1986). Antithrombin III activity in horses with large colon torsion. *Am. J. Vet. Res.* 47 (4): 897–900.

80 Dallap Schaer, B.L. and Epstein, K. (2009). Coagulopathy of the critically ill equine patient. *J. Vet. Emerg. Crit. Care* 19 (1): 53–65.

81 Carrier, M., Le Gal, G., Bates, S.M. et al. (2008). D-dimer testing is useful to exclude deep vein thrombosis in elderly outpatients. *J. Thromb. Hemost.* 6 (7): 1072–1076.

82 Nelson, O.L. and Andreasen, C. (2003). The utility of plasma D-dimer to identify thromboembolic disease in dogs. *J. Vet. Intern. Med.* 17 (6): 830–834.

83 Delgado, M.A., Monreal, L., Armengou, L. et al. (2009). Peritoneal D-dimer concentration for assessing peritoneal fibrinolytic activity in horses with colic. *J. Vet. Intern. Med.* 23 (4): 882–889.

84 Epstein, K.L., Brainard, B.M., Giguère, S. et al. (2013). Serial viscoelastic and traditional coagulation testing in horses with gastrointestinal disease. *J. Vet. Emerg. Crit. Care* 23 (5): 504–516.

85 Mendez-Angulo, J.L., Mudge, M.C., and Couto, C.G. (2012). Thromboelastography in equine medicine: technique and use in clinical research. *Equine Vet. Educ.* 24 (12): 639–649.

86 Epstein, K.L., Brainard, B.M., Lopes, M.A.F. et al. (2009). Thrombelastography in 26 healthy horses with and without activation by recombinant human tissue factor. *J. Vet. Emerg. Crit. Care* 19 (1): 96–101.

87 Epstein, K.L., Brainard, B.M., Gomez-Ibanez, S.E. et al. (2011). Thrombelastography in horses with acute gastrointestinal disease. *J. Vet. Intern. Med.* 25 (2): 307–314.

88 Mendez-Angulo, J.L., Mudge, M.C., Vilar-Saavedra, P. et al. (2010). Thromboelastography in healthy horses and horses with inflammatory gastrointestinal disorders and suspected coagulopathies. *J. Vet. Emerg. Crit. Care* 20 (5): 488–493.

89 Mendez-Angulo, J., Mudge, M., Zaldivar-Lopez, S. et al. (2011). Thromboelastography in healthy, sick non-septic and septic neonatal foals. *Aust. Vet. J.* 89 (12): 500–505.

90 Thane, K., Bedenice, D., and Pacheco, A. (2017). Operator-based variability of equine thromboelastography. *J. Vet. Emerg. Crit. Care* 27 (4): 419–424.

91 Cotovio, M., Monreal, L., Navarro, M. et al. (2007). Detection of fibrin deposits in tissues from horses with severe gastrointestinal disorders. *J. Vet. Intern. Med.* 21 (2): 308–313.

92 Dallap, B.L., Dolente, B., and Veterinary, R.B.J.O. (2003). Coagulation profiles in 27 horses with large colon volvulus. *J. Vet. Emerg. Crit. Care* 13 (4): 215–225.

93 Cotovio, M., Monreal, L., Armengou, L. et al. (2008). Fibrin deposits and organ failure in newborn foals with severe septicemia. *J. Vet. Intern. Med.* 22 (6): 1403–1410.

94 Divers, T.J. (2003). Prevention and treatment of thrombosis, phlebitis, and laminitis in horses with gastrointestinal diseases. *Vet. Clin. North Am. Equine Pract.* 19 (3): 779–790.

95 Dolente, B.A., Beech, J., Lindborg, S., and Smith, G. (2005). Evaluation of risk factors for development of catheter-associated jugular thrombophlebitis in horses: 50 cases (1993–1998). *J. Am. Vet. Med. Assoc.* 227 (7): 1134–1141.

96 Bentz, A.I., Palmer, J.E., Dallap, B.L. et al. (2009). Prospective evaluation of coagulation in critically ill neonatal foals. *J. Vet. Intern. Med.* 23 (1): 161–167.

97 Armengou, L., Monreal, L., Tarancón, I. et al. (2008). Plasma D-dimer concentration in sick newborn foals. *J. Vet. Intern. Med.* 22 (2): 411–417.

98 Prasse, K.W., Topper, M.J., Moore, J.N., and Welles, E.G. (1993). Analysis of hemostasis in horses with colic. *J. Am. Vet. Med. Assoc.* 203 (5): 685–693.

5

The Liver

Dennis J. Meyer[1] and Raquel M. Walton[2]

[1] *Charles River Laboratories, Reno, NV, USA*
[2] *IDEXX Laboratories, Inc., Langhorne, PA, USA*

While the diagnostic and prognostic gold standard for hepatic disease is histological evaluation, biopsy is an invasive procedure. Diagnosis of hepatic disease can be achieved with noninvasive procedures such as evaluation of serum biochemical data in conjunction with clinical findings, history, and ultrasound examination. Clinical signs of hepatic disease in horses can include dullness, anorexia, abdominal pain, encephalopathy, weight loss, jaundice, diarrhea, photosensitization, and coagulopathy [1]. In one study, the diagnostic specificity of clinical signs for the presence of hepatic disease was good (81%) but sensitivity was poor (28%), while the most useful noninvasive prognostic test in mature horses with suspected liver disease was the severity of clinical signs [2, 3]. Certain biochemical tests have better sensitivity than clinical signs in predicting the presence of liver disease when they are abnormal, but normal test results do not preclude the presence of liver disease.

5.1 Liver Enzymes

Liver enzymes are generally categorized as hepatocellular and hepatobiliary for diagnostic purposes. The hepatocellular enzymes are aspartate aminotransferase (AST), sorbitol dehydrogenase (SDH), and glutamate dehydrogenase (GLDH). Alanine aminotransferase (ALT), a hepatocellular enzyme that is identified as "liver specific" in humans, dogs, and cats, has limited activity in the horse liver and therefore no correlative diagnostic utility. Alkaline phosphatase (ALP) and gamma-glutamyltransferase (GGT) constitute the hepatobiliary enzymes. In contrast to the use of ALP in humans, dogs, and cats, GGT is considered the preferable hepatobiliary enzyme in the horse. The location of these enzymes is illustrated in Figure 5.1.

Patterns of enzyme changes are associated with different types of liver pathology. An acute, severe, predominantly hepatocellular injury is initially associated with high activity of hepatocellular enzymes with increased values for GGT gradually developing over days and even persisting after the hepatocellular enzymes have returned within the reference interval after complete recovery. Persistent injury is associated with minimal to mild changes in both hepatocellular and hepatobiliary enzymes and requires other diagnostics to define the causation of their persistent increase. A disorder that causes predominantly cholestasis is associated with increases in GGT with low elevations for the hepatocellular enzymes developing over days to weeks. Sufficiently severe liver pathology, acute or chronic and persistent, is likely to alter one or more tests of liver function.

5.1.1 Hepatocellular Enzymes

The hepatocellular enzymes are preformed and located in high activity within the hepatocyte. Altered membrane permeability, generally some type of injury, permits increased leakage into the circulation; the magnitude of increase generally correlates with the number of affected hepatocytes when the pathology is acute and severe. The time to return to reference values following complete recovery is dependent on their respective plasma half-life; the half-life of SDH is shorter than that of AST and GLDH (Figure 5.2). Incomplete return to reference values after several weeks of repeated testing suggests persistent pathology, referred to as chronic persistent (active) hepatitis.

Equine Hematology, Cytology, and Clinical Chemistry, Second Edition.
Edited by Raquel M. Walton, Rick L. Cowell, and Amy C. Valenciano.

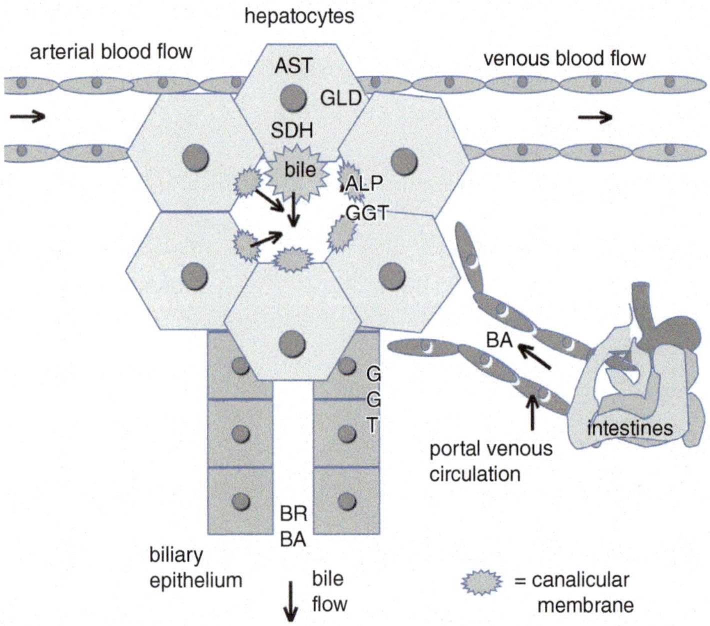

Figure 5.1 The cells and the structures they form along with their constituent enzymes are illustrated. The hepatocellular enzymes, AST, SDH, and GLD, are preformed and located within the hepatocyte. Altered integrity of the hepatocyte membrane, generally due to some type of injury, allows increased "leakage" of these enzymes into the circulation as a reflection of the underlying pathology. The hepatobiliary enzymes, ALP and GGT, are associated with the bile canaliculi and biliary epithelium. Minimal activity is preformed and a stimulus is required to increase their production. An increase in their synthesis and release into the circulation is generally due to impairment of bile flow (cholestasis). Bile acids and bilirubin are eliminated via bile. An increase in their concentrations in the circulation occurs if the cause of the cholestasis is acute and severe (attendant high activities of SDH, GLD, and AST) or chronic and diffuse (high activities of ALP and/or GGT). An increase in bile acids generally precedes an increase in bilirubin. AST, aspartate aminotransferase; GLD, glutamate dehydrogenase; SDH, sorbitol dehydrogenase; ALP, alkaline phosphatase; GGT, gamma-glutamyltransferase; BA, bile acids; BR, total bilirubin. *Source:* Modified from Meyer and Harvey [4].

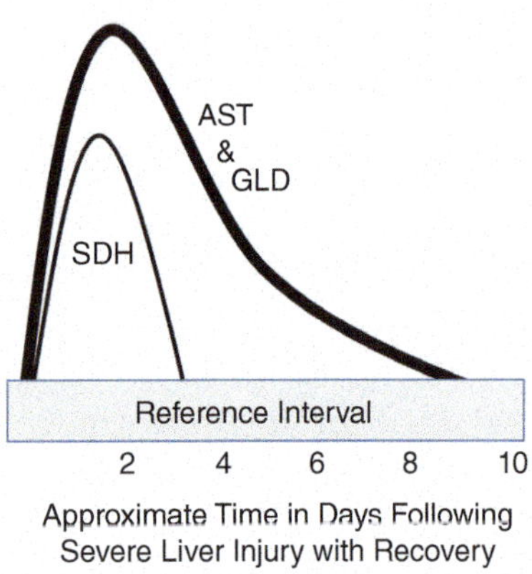

Figure 5.2 The approximate magnitude and duration of SDH, AST, and GLD increases in the circulation following severe hepatic injury with recovery are illustrated. Persistent increases for several weeks in one or more of these enzymes with repeat testing, especially if accompanied by an increase in hepatobiliary enzymes, are suggestive of persistent, progressive (chronic) liver pathology. AST, aspartate aminotransferase; SDH, sorbitol dehydrogenase; GLD, glutamate dehydrogenase. *Source:* Modified from Meyer and Harvey [4].

5.1.1.1 Sorbitol Dehydrogenase

Sorbitol dehydrogenase is considered a liver-specific enzyme, present in high concentrations in the equine liver but in low concentrations in other tissues. The enzyme is free within hepatocyte cytoplasm and is more specific than AST or GLDH in detecting hepatocellular damage. The half-life is less than 12 hours, so serum concentrations can return to reference values within days after a single insult. The *in vitro* stability is much less than other diagnostic enzymes, which can limit the utility of the test; it should be performed on serum within five hours if stored at room temperature, and within 48 hours if frozen [5]. While SDH is very specific for liver disease, its sensitivity is lower than either GLDH or AST for detection of hepatic lipidosis, cirrhosis, and necrosis in horses [6].

5.1.1.2 Glutamate Dehydrogenase

Similar to SDH, GLDH is a liver-specific enzyme present in high concentrations in hepatocytes but in low concentrations in other tissues. It is located primarily in the central lobular region. In contrast to SDH, it is mitochondrial rather than cytosolic, and is therefore typically released only with irreversible cell injury. The half-life of GLDH in the horse is about 14 hours, slightly longer than for SDH but shorter than AST. The *in vitro* stability of enzyme activity is considered greater than SDH. The activity of bovine GLDH is reported to be stable for a month at −20 °C [7].

The sensitivity of GLDH for diagnosis of hepatic disease in mature horses is reported to be 63%, which exceeds the reported sensitivity of SDH [2]. As a liver-specific enzyme with greater stability than SDH, GLDH is a valuable tool for the diagnosis of acute liver injury in horses but the limited availability of the assay in the US restricts its use in practice.

5.1.1.3 Aspartate Aminotransferase

Aspartate aminotransferase is present in high concentrations in hepatocytes and myocytes (see Chapter 10).

Creatine kinase (CK) has high activity in skeletal muscle but is not present in the liver. An enzyme profile of marked increases in AST and CK (without increases in SDH and GLDH) is indicative of primarily skeletal muscle injury. Erythrocytes also contain AST so the presence of hemolysis in samples will increase AST activity. The enzyme is present in both the cytosol and mitochondria of hepatocytes, but in higher concentrations in the mitochondria. In theory, higher magnitude increases in AST would be expected with irreversible than reversible hepatocyte (or myocyte) injury, but this has not been proven. *In vitro* stability at room temperature or refrigerated is days rather than hours, in contrast to SDH or GLDH.

Marked increases in serum AST and SDH or GLDH suggest acute or active hepatocellular injury, whereas marked increases in serum AST with mild to moderate increases in SDH or GLDH suggest chronic hepatic injury or recovery from acute liver injury (Figure 5.2). In one study, the diagnostic sensitivity of AST was determined to be 100% for hepatic lipidosis and 72% for hepatic necrosis in horses [6].

5.1.2 Hepatobiliary Enzymes

The hepatobiliary enzymes require a stimulus for increased production with a resultant increase in the circulation. Retained bile is generally considered the primary stimulant for increased production by the liver, with GGT having relatively greater responsiveness and magnitude of production compared to ALP in the horse. Both GGT and ALP, when increased, have high diagnostic value for the presence of cholestatic liver disease.

5.1.2.1 Alkaline Phosphatase

Alkaline phosphatase is present in multiple tissues, but serum ALP activity does not necessarily correlate with tissue concentrations. ALP is present in relatively low concentrations in liver and yet liver ALP is found in serum, whereas intestinal ALP, present in high tissue concentrations in horses, is not. In hepatocytes, the majority of ALP is bound to bile canalicular surface membranes.

In health, serum ALP originates primarily from liver and bone and is therefore higher in growing horses. In foals, serum ALP may be 100-fold greater than in adults due to bone ALP. In mature horses, roughly 80% of serum ALP is liver ALP and 20% is bone ALP. The ALP isoforms can be distinguished on the basis of differences in heat stability, electrophoretic migration, and wheat germ lectin precipitation. The bone isoform is more susceptible to wheat germ lectin precipitation than the liver, has slower anodal electrophoretic migration, and is more sensitive to heat inhibition. Bone ALP can be directly measured using commercially available antibodies for human bone ALP that have been validated for use in the horse [8]. Often, evaluation of ALP in conjunction with another biliary-specific enzyme such as GGT is sufficient in determining the origin and significance of increased serum ALP concentrations.

The most common cause of increased serum ALP concentrations is cholestasis. Cholestasis induces the synthesis of ALP, which concentrates on the basolateral hepatocyte membrane where it is released into blood or lymphatics [9]. The highest concentrations of serum ALP are associated with cholangitis, biliary cirrhosis, or extrahepatic bile duct obstruction.

5.1.2.2 Gamma-Glutamyltransferase

Gamma-glutamyltransferase (also known as gamma-glutamyltranspeptidase) is a membrane-bound enzyme that is primarily associated with biliary epithelial cells in horses, like other domestic animals. Most serum GGT activity originates from the liver, although it is present in high concentrations in the kidney, intestine, and pancreas. This is attributable to its presence on the luminal surfaces in these organs. Serum half-life of GGT in horses is thought to be around three days, similar to ALP [9].

Increases in GGT are associated with cholestasis and biliary hyperplasia. Serum GGT concentrations are more sensitive than ALP in the diagnosis of cholestatic diseases; in horses with cholestasis, GGT increased ninefold whereas ALP activity only increased twofold [9]. GGT activity is high in colostrum and increased serum GGT concentrations are present in calves and goats during suckling, but not in foals. There is no significant difference in GGT concentrations before and after suckling in foals, but GGT concentrations are higher in foals relative to adults [10].

5.2 Liver Function Tests

5.2.1 Excretory Function Tests

5.2.1.1 Total Bilirubin

Total bilirubin has two forms: unconjugated and conjugated. The primary source of bilirubin is from the degradation of hemoglobin from aged erythrocytes, termed unconjugated (indirect-reacting) bilirubin. Unconjugated bilirubin is transported to the liver via albumin for receptor-mediated uptake by hepatocytes, internalized, and altered to form conjugated (direct-reacting) bilirubin, and actively secreted by the specialized portion of the hepatocyte membrane (canalicular membrane) into bile for delivery to the small intestine (Figure 5.3).

A relatively unique feature of bilirubin removal by the horse occurs at the site of uptake by the hepatocyte. Lack of

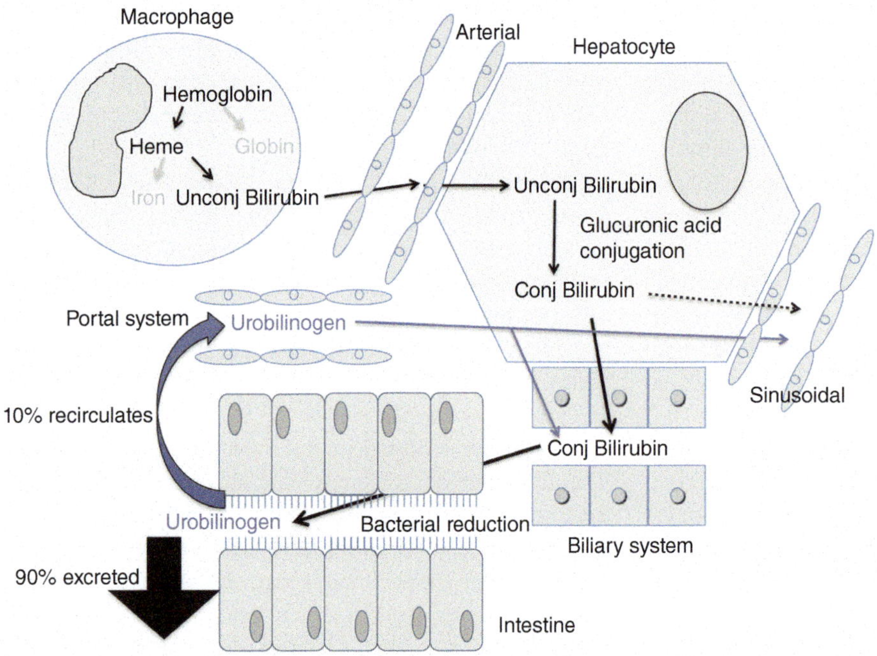

Figure 5.3 Bilirubin metabolism. Unconjugated bilirubin is released into the plasma from macrophages after the breakdown of hemoglobin to heme, which is further degraded into iron and bilirubin. Unconjugated bilirubin is bound by albumin and transported to the liver where it is conjugated to glucuronic acid. Conjugated bilirubin is excreted into bile via biliary canaliculi and then into the intestinal tract, where it is reduced to urobilinogen or stercobilinogen by the action of bacteria. About 10% of urobilinogen returns to the liver via the portal system and the majority is excreted into bile; a small proportion (1–5%) enters the circulation to be excreted via the kidneys. In cases of biliary obstruction or impaired bilirubin excretion due to hepatocellular dysfunction, conjugated bilirubin will efflux into the plasma (*dotted line*).

food intake is commonly associated with moderate to marked increases in total bilirubin due to increases in the unconjugated form. It is likely that free fatty acids and other metabolic constituents that are increased in the fasted state compete for uptake of unconjugated bilirubin; it decreases once appetite returns.

Another cause of increased unconjugated bilirubin is acute, severe hemolysis. Concomitant moderate to marked decreases in circulating red cell mass as measured by the hematocrit are supportive of a hemolytic process. Intrahepatic diseases and extrahepatic obstruction can both cause increases in total bilirubin, with conjugated bilirubin comprising less than half of the total bilirubin.

5.2.1.2 Bile Acids

The circulating concentrations of bile acids are dependent on an intact enterohepatic circulation. Bile acids are efficiently removed from the intestines into the portal circulation, transported to the liver, efficiently extracted from the blood by receptor-mediated uptake by the hepatocyte, processed by the hepatocyte, and actively excreted by the canalicular membrane into bile for delivery to the intestine where the process is repeated (Figure 5.1). Serum bile acid concentrations in foals are significantly higher than in adult horses in the first six weeks of life and age-specific reference values should be used in interpreting results [11].

Bile acids increase in the circulation before an increase in total bilirubin due to liver disease. In contrast to total bilirubin, serum bile acid concentrations in the horse are not affected by short-term fasting (<3 days) [6, 9]. Postprandial increases are also not observed given the lack of gallbladder in equids. The measurement of bile acids is a diagnostic adjunct when abnormal liver enzyme tests are detected; a concomitant increase in bile acids suggests substantial liver pathology precluding their removal from the sinusoidal blood and supports further diagnostics such as liver biopsy. Congenital abnormalities of the portal circulation, often manifested as encephalopathy, cause bile acids to by-pass the liver, resulting in increases in the circulation [12].

5.2.2 Tests Dependent on Synthetic/Metabolic Functions

5.2.2.1 Albumin

Albumin is produced exclusively by hepatocytes. The formation of albumin is relatively well preserved and decreases are not significant until there is substantial loss of hepatocellular mass due to disease (>60–80% of functional mass). Moreover, the half-life of albumin in horses is longer than in other species (19.4 days). Hypoalbuminemia is an infrequent finding with severe acute or chronic liver disease, occurring in only 13–16% of cases in two studies [13, 14]. Hypoalbuminemia occurred more frequently in chronic than acute liver disease.

When there are no liver test abnormalities to suggest liver disease, other causes should be considered. These primarily include losses of albumin due to diseases involving the intestines and kidney. Mild decreases in albumin production can occur when globulins are increased in association with chronic inflammation, and with acute inflammation as albumin is a negative acute-phase protein (see Chapter 8).

5.2.2.2 Ammonia

Ammonia is formed in the intestines and carried to the liver by the portal circulation where it is metabolized in hepatocytes via the Krebs–Henseleit urea cycle with urea nitrogen as one by-product. Loss of hepatocellular mass due to severe disease and congenital portosystemic shunts permits high concentrations to enter the circulation where it can cause cerebral dysfunction (hepatic encephalopathy). A concomitant decrease in blood urea nitrogen (BUN) may be noted although this is not a consistent finding [13, 15]. While ammonia has neurotoxic effects, the etiopathogenesis of hepatic encephalopathy is multifactorial and it is not attributable solely to hyperammonemia as signs cannot be experimentally induced by injection of ammonia in similar concentrations to those associated with encephalopathy [16]. Moreover, while hyperammonemia is common in horses with hepatic encephalopathy, in some cases ammonia concentration remains within reference limits. The measurement of bile acids is a more dependable liver function test for the differential diagnosis of hepatic encephalopathy; moreover, ammonia is labile in blood samples, which limits its diagnostic utility.

Hyperammonemia with encephalopathy in the absence of detectable hepatic disease has been reported in adult horses [17–19]. These cases are associated with gastrointestinal disease and referred to as intestinal hyperammonemia or primary enteric hyperammonemia syndrome resulting. The pathogenesis is attributed to increased ammonia production by gastrointestinal bacteria in conjunction with increased gut permeability [19]. In cases of intestinal hyperammonemia, bile acids concentration and hepatic enzyme activities are reported to be within reference limits.

Hyperammonemia with clinical signs of encephalopathy has also been described in the absence of hepatic disease in related young Morgan horses as a presumptive inherited hyperornithinemia, hyperammonemia, and homocitrullinuria syndrome due to a urea cycle defect [20].

5.2.2.3 Globulins

In one study, nearly half of horses with severe liver disease showed hyperproteinemia attributable to hyperglobulinemia [14]. Hyperglobulinemia has high diagnostic value for the presence of liver disease, with intermediate sensitivity (56%) and good specificity (80%) [3]. Hyperglobulinemia is a result of increased synthesis of alpha-, beta-, and/or gamma-globulins [14].

Beta-gamma bridging, an electrophoretic pattern observed when there is poor demarcation between the beta- and gamma-globulin peaks, in conjunction with a decreased albumin to globulin ratio, has been reported in many veterinary textbooks to be pathognomonic for chronic active hepatitis or hepatic cirrhosis. Recent data show that beta-gamma bridging in horses does not have a strong predictive value for hepatic disease; of three horses with beta-gamma bridging, two had liver disease and one had pulmonary carcinoma with no liver involvement [21].

5.2.2.4 Glucose

Glucose is dependent on the liver as one of several organs for maintenance of normal concentrations in the circulation. However, liver-related decreases in glucose are uncommon and develop only after severe loss of hepatocellular mass due to disease. In a study of primary hepatic disease in adult horses, of the 28 cases for which glucose concentrations were available, none were hypoglycemic [13]. However, in foals with hepatic disease hypoglycemia is reported, likely as a result of decreased hepatic gluconeogenesis capacity relative to adults [22, 23].

5.2.2.5 Coagulation Factors

Coagulation factors (except FXIII) are formed by the liver. Acute, severe, or chronic loss of hepatocellular mass can result in sufficient deficiency of one or more coagulation factors, resulting in prolongation of the prothrombin time and/or activated partial thromboplastin time. It is important to note that with liver disease, no biopsy procedure should be considered until coagulation testing is conducted.

5.2.3 Other Tests

Increases in liver enzyme tests are often the initial indication that liver disease may be present and the cause of clinical signs. Liver function tests can further support the presence of liver disease and define the extent of the liver pathology. Repeated testing is helpful to determine if the liver disease is recovering or persistent. Further assessment of the cause of abnormal liver tests includes ultrasound evaluation and microscopic examination of a cytology aspirate or biopsy.

5.2.3.1 Biopsy

Hepatic biopsy with histological evaluation is considered the gold standard for diagnosis and prognosis of hepatic disease, but is an invasive procedure. Depending upon the distribution of lesions, biopsy, especially single biopsy, may not detect liver disease. While ultrasound guidance may increase the chances of sampling a diseased area, histological lesions can be present in ultrasonographically normal liver.

Histological evaluation of the liver succeeds most often in establishing presence of disease, but may fail in identifying a specific etiology. One study evaluating the prognostic use of hepatic biopsy for equine liver disease showed that the most useful negative prognostic indicators were hepatic fibrosis and biliary hyperplasia [24]. Previous findings support fibrosis as a negative prognostic factor [25]. Common hepatopathies and their associated lesions are listed in Tables 5.1 and 5.2, respectively.

5.3 Hepatic Diseases

5.3.1 Toxins

Toxic hepatopathies are relatively common in equids as a result of grazing behavior. The distribution of lesions is often similar with most hepatotoxins, but unique histological

Table 5.1 Etiologies of liver disease in horses.

Toxic	Parasitic	Infectious	Miscellaneous	Primary neoplasms
Pyrrolizidine alkaloid	*Fasciola hepatica*	*Clostridium piliforme*	Cholelithiasis	Hepatoblastoma
Panicum grasses	*Heterobilharzia americana*	Cholangiohepatitis[a]	Lipidosis	Hepatocellular carcinoma
Xanthium (cocklebur)	*Parascaris equorum*	*Salmonella* spp.		Cholangiocellular carcinoma
Mycotoxins	Strongyle larvae	*E. coli*		
Alsike clover		*Pseudomonas* spp.		
Iron		*Actinobacillus equuli*		
		Equine parvovirus-hepatitis[b]		
		Equine hepacivirus		

[a] Ascending bacterial infections.
[b] Possible etiology of Theiler disease.

Table 5.2 Lesions associated with various etiologies of liver disease.

Etiology	Lesions
Pyrrolizidine alkaloid	Megalocytosis, periacinar necrosis, biliary hyperplasia, periportal fibrosis
Panicum grasses	Biliary fibrosis, periacinar necrosis, crystalline material in bile ducts
Alsike clover	Portal fibrosis, biliary hyperplasia
Mycotoxins	Centrilobular necrosis, biliary hyperplasia, megalocytosis
Cocklebur (*Xanthium* spp.)	Periacinar necrosis
Iron	Portal necrosis, increased iron stores
Clostridium piliforme	Liver necrosis with neutrophilic infiltrate, intrahepatocellular filamentous bacteria
Salmonella spp., *Pseudomonas* spp., *Actinobacillus equuli*, *Escherichia coli*	Cholangiohepatitis: biliary hyperplasia, periductular inflammation, periportal fibrosis
Parasitic (*Heterobilharzia americana*, *Fasciola hepatica*)	Multifocal granulomas with eosinophilic and lymphocytic inflammation
Theiler disease, equine parvovirus-hepatitis	Acute hepatitis: centrilobular to massive necrosis, inflammatory cell infiltrates

features are noted with some toxins (e.g., megalocytes with pyrrols and mycotoxins). The type (acute necrosis or chronic disease) and distribution of hepatocellular damage will influence the pattern of enzyme increases.

5.3.1.1 Pyrrolizidine Alkaloids

Pyrrolizidine alkaloids (PA) are found in several species of plants, including *Senecio*, *Crotalaria*, *Amsinkia*, *Heliotropium*, and *Cynoglossum*. The toxic principle is the pyrrols, which are broken down from the alkaloids in the liver and cross-link with DNA. Liver enzymes typically are elevated before clinical signs appear and the dehydrogenases (SDH, GLDH) may be within reference limits by the time the animal presents with signs of disease. Serum GGT, ALP, and bile acids are more sensitive indicators of PA toxicity because the disease is typically chronic. In one study, serum GGT was shown to be relatively sensitive (75%) and specific (90%) as a screening test for subclinical PA toxicosis, defined by histological evidence of PA toxicity in the absence of clinical signs [26]. In this same study, ALP was shown to have lower sensitivity (58%) and higher specificity (100%) as a screening test.

5.3.1.2 Mycotoxins

There are a number of mycotoxins that are hepatotoxic. Some of the more common ones include aflatoxins and fumonisin. Like pyrrolizidine alkaloids, mycotoxins can cause megalocytosis. In addition to megalocytosis, histological changes seen with mycotoxins include hepatocellular necrosis, depletion of centrilobular hepatocytes, lobular disarray, and biliary hyperplasia.

5.3.1.3 Alsike Clover, Cocklebur, and *Panicum* Grasses

It is thought that the toxic principles associated with alsike clover (*Trifolium hybridum*) and *Panicum* grasses are mycotoxins or plant metabolites because the hepatotoxicity is sporadic and often weather related [1]. Deposition of crystalline substances in bile ducts that are plant saponin derivatives has been reported with *Panicum coloratum*. In one report of *Panicum* toxicosis, increases in SDH, AST, GGT, and ALP were documented along with hepatic necrosis [27]. The toxic principle in cocklebur (*Xanthium*) inhibits the exchange of ATP for ADP in the mitochondria and cytosol, respectively, resulting in hepatic necrosis with a periacinar distribution. Serum chemistry changes characterized by marked increases in serum AST and SDH or GLDH reflect the acute hepatocellular necrosis.

5.3.1.4 Iron

Iron toxicosis causes acute hepatotoxicity with massive periacinar necrosis and deposition of iron in Kupffer cells. Toxicosis is typically the result of administration of ferrous fumarate or sulfate containing vitamin supplements and has been reported in foals and adult horses, although foals are much more susceptible to iron toxicosis than adults [28, 29]. Iron hepatotoxicity was reported as a result of administration of 16 mg/kg ferrous fumarate to neonatal Shetland ponies, whereas administration of 50 mg/kg of ferrous sulfate for eight weeks was not sufficient to induce hepatotoxicity in adult ponies [30]. Although in one of the reported cases of adult iron toxicity a dose of approximately 390 mg iron/kg (ferrous fumarate) over a period of five days was reported, concomitant selenium/vitamin E deficiency with iron excess may have been a contributing factor in other cases of adult iron toxicosis [28].

While adult equids appear to be resistant to iron toxicosis associated with short-term increases in dietary iron intake, hepatotoxicity has been documented in 21 adult horses and a donkey exposed to chronic (>9 years) excessive iron intake in contaminated drinking water [31]. The most common serum chemistry abnormalities included increased GLDH, AST, ALP, and GGT. Bile acids were abnormally high in 10 of 18 horses tested. Histological evaluation of the liver ($n = 12$) showed moderate to severe hemosiderosis in macrophages and hepatocytes with varying degrees of inflammation and fibrosis.

Cases of hemochromatosis in adult horses characterized by hepatic cirrhosis with marked increases in iron storage in hepatocytes, Kupffer cells, and portal macrophages have been described [13, 32, 33]. Whether these cases represent hepatotoxicity secondary to iron overload or a primary hepatopathy with secondary iron overload is uncertain. Iron intake was not excessive in any of the horses for which it was evaluated.

5.3.1.5 Equine Dysautonomia (Grass Sickness)

Equine dysautonomia (see Chapter 10) is a neurodegenerative disease of unknown etiology affecting grazing equids. There is evidence to suggest that *Clostridium botulinum* type C and *Clostridium perfringens* (particularly type A) may play a role in the etiopathogenesis [34, 35]. Histological and biochemical evidence of hepatocellular and hepatobiliary disease has been reported in some cases of grass sickness in horses [36]. Biochemical changes are noted most often in acute and subacute cases (<7 days of illness) and are characterized by significant increases in GLDH, AST, and unconjugated and conjugated bilirubin. Histopathological abnormalities include enlarged hepatocytes/hepatocyte nuclei, lipid accumulation (fatty change), and periportal infiltration of lymphocytes (sometimes with neutrophils). Although these changes may be attributable to direct damage from a putative toxin, it is also possible

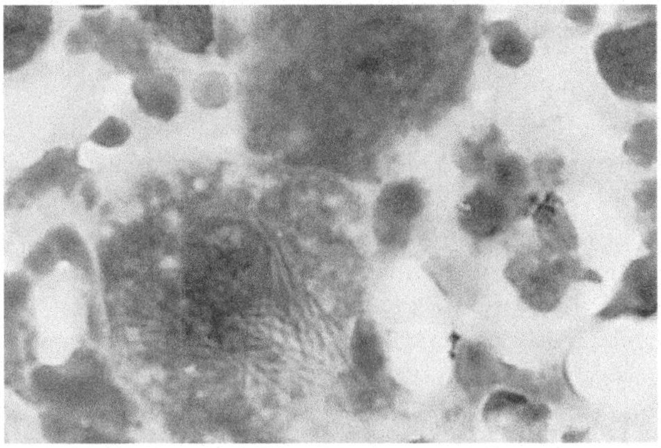

Figure 5.4 Liver impression smear showing a hepatocyte containing *Clostridium piliforme*, the etiologic agent for Tyzzer disease. The linear blue-black organisms are visible within the cytoplasm of the lower hepatocyte. (Wright's stain, original magnification 250×.) *Source:* Courtesy of Oklahoma State University, Stillwater.

that the hepatopathology is secondary to autonomic nervous system injury that is the hallmark of the disease.

5.3.2 Infections

5.3.2.1 *Clostridium piliforme* (Tyzzer Disease)

Infection by *C. piliforme* (formerly *Bacillus piliformis*) usually occurs in foals 1–6 weeks old and causes acute or peracute hepatitis that usually results in death within hours to days. The infection is characterized by multifocal to confluent central coagulation necrosis with inflammatory cells and degenerate hepatocytes at the periphery. A definitive diagnosis is made by identifying filamentous bacteria within hepatocytes at the periphery of the necrotic areas; this may be accomplished via cytology or histology (Figure 5.4). Use of silver stains such as Warthin–Starry facilitates visualization of the organisms on histological sections. There is a marked increase in SDH concentration due to the severe necrosis with moderate to marked hyperbilirubinemia and mild to moderate increases in GGT concentration; ALP is not increased [22].

5.3.2.2 Ascending Cholangiohepatitis

Ascending infection from the intestinal tract with *Salmonella* sp., *Escherichia coli*, *Pseudomonas* sp., *Actinobacillus equuli*, and (less commonly) *Pasteurella* sp., *Streptococcus* sp., or *Clostridium* sp. is associated with inflammation of the biliary tracts and adjacent liver. Histologically, there is biliary hyperplasia, periductular inflammation, and periportal fibrosis. Cholangiocellular enzymes GGT and ALP may be disproportionately high relative to SDH or GLDH, but this depends upon the amount of hepatocellular involvement. Hyperglobulinemia can be seen with chronic (>3 weeks) conditions. Cholelithiasis is frequently encountered with cholangiohepatitis, possibly as a result of decreased biliary flow [37].

5.3.2.3 Theiler Disease

In horses, acute central lobular necrosis has been associated with administration of tetanus antitoxin, antiserum for various diseases (influenza, equine encephalomyelitis, strangles), vaccines prepared from equine foetal tissues, and commercial plasma [38, 39]. The disease was originally described in 1918 by Sir Arnold Theiler and was subsequently dubbed Theiler disease or serum hepatitis.

Clinical presentation is acute and increases in both hepatocellular and hepatobiliary enzymes are seen, although hepatocellular enzyme increases are typically of greater magnitude. There is a seasonal incidence of Theiler disease and horses in contact with serum hepatitis cases have developed disease. These findings, in conjunction with its association with the use of equine serum and plasma products, suggested a possible infectious etiology. With the development of unbiased deep sequencing techniques, four viruses have been identified in hepatitis cases and/or equine plasma products to date: Theiler-disease associated virus (TDAV), equine parvovirus-hepatitis (EqPV-H), equine hepacivirus, and equine pegivirus [40–43]. Subsequent experimental and clinical investigations currently support EqPV-H as the prime etiologic agent in Theiler disease [41, 44–46]. Equine hepacivirus has been shown to cause mild liver disease, but its ability to cause clinical hepatitis or liver failure is currently under investigation. TDAV and equine pegivirus are not hepatotropic and current consensus is that they likely do not cause clinical disease.

5.3.2.4 Parasites

Parascaris equorum and strongyle larvae migrate through the liver and can cause hemorrhagic tracts with necrosis, inflammatory cells (especially eosinophils), and fibrosis. Histopathological findings with liver flukes (*Fasciola hepatica*) include multifocal granulomas with eosinophilic and lymphocytic inflammation. Experimental infection with *F. hepatica* resulted in increases in GLDH and GGT 3–5 months post infection [47]. These findings were similar to natural infection in horses in the United Kingdom in which 39% and 71% of cases had increased GLDH and GGT, respectively [48]. Some infected horses did not have any clinical or biochemical abnormalities; the presence or absence of abnormalities likely reflects the stage and intensity of infection and thus is more useful in prognosis than diagnosis. A *F. hepatica* excretory-secretory antibody detection ELISA validated for horses has good reported diagnostic specificity of 96–97% but varying results for sensitivity, with one study citing a sensitivity of 71% [48] and another reporting 42% sensitivity [49]. The differences may reflect the finding that some horses, unlike cattle, fail to mount a detectable antibody response to excretory-secretory antigen. Fecal egg detection for *F. hepatica* using sedimentation or zinc sulfate flotation techniques can have a sensitivity as low as 16%, however.

The schistosome *Heterobilharzia americana* has been recognized as a cause of multifocal fibrosing eosinophilic and lymphocytic granulomas in the liver of horses in the southern US [50]. These disseminated granulomas present grossly as a starry-sky appearance to the liver. *H. americana*, similar to other schistosomal species, can infect the liver from the intestinal tract via the portal circulation. In many of the reported cases, the granulomas were incidental findings unrelated to a primary disease for which the horse was presented.

5.3.3 Hepatic Lipidosis

Hepatic lipidosis in equids is associated with hyperlipemia, a disorder of lipid metabolism that is discussed in depth in Chapter 9. Hyperlipemia frequently occurs secondary to primary disease processes such as enterocolitis/colitis and colic that produce a negative energy balance and affect insulin sensitivity. Ponies and donkeys can present with primary hyperlipemia; stress and obesity are predisposing factors. Both stress and obesity induce decreases in insulin sensitivity, which is considered the primary predisposing factor (see Chapter 9). There appears to be a genetic predisposition to hyperlipemia in the case of Shetland ponies.

Stimulation of hormone-sensitive lipase in adipocytes by glucagon, corticosteroids, adrenocorticotropic hormone (ACTH), or epinephrine (hormones associated with illness) catalyzes the hydrolysis of stored triglycerides and releases nonesterified fatty acids (NEFA). When there is increased release of fatty acids from adipocytes, the NEFA not utilized by peripheral tissues are taken up by hepatocytes to be oxidized for energy, converted into ketones, or used to synthesize triglycerides that are either stored or released as very low-density lipoproteins (VLDL). Equids have a limited ability to form ketones, thus increases in circulating fatty acids contribute to hepatic triglyceride storage and hypertriglyceridemia via hepatic VLDL synthesis.

5.3.4 Hepatocellular Neoplasia

Primary liver neoplasms are rare in the horse and comprise hepatoblastoma, hepatocellular carcinoma, and cholangiocarcinoma [51]. Hepatoblastomas are reported in neonates and juveniles up to 4 years of age. Hepatocellular carcinomas occur in juveniles and mature horses, whereas reports of cholangiocarcinomas are rare in mature horses. A single case report of a biliary cystadenoma morphologic variant (biliary adenofibroma) has been described as an incidental finding in a mature horse [52].

References

1 Bergero, D. and Nery, J. (2008). Hepatic diseases in horses. *J. Anim. Physiol. Anim. Nutr.* 92: 345–355.

2 Durham, A.E., Newton, J.R., Smith, K.C. et al. (2003). Retrospective analysis of historical, clinical, ultrasonographic, serum biochemical and haematological data in prognostic evaluation of equine liver disease. *Equine Vet. J.* 35: 542–547.

3 Durham, A.E., Smith, K.C., and Newton, J.R. (2003). An evaluation of diagnostic data in comparison to the results of liver biopsies in mature horses. *Equine Vet. J.* 35: 554–559.

4 Meyer, D.J. and Harvey, J.W. (2004). *Veterinary Laboratory Medicine-Interpretation and Diagnosis*, 3e. St Louis: Elsevier, Inc.

5 Horney, B.S., Honor, D.J., MacKenzie, A., and Burton, S. (1993). Stability of sorbitol dehydrogenase activity in bovine and equine sera. *Vet. Clin. Pathol.* 22: 5–9.

6 West, H.J. (1989). Evaluation of total plasma bile acid concentrations for the diagnosis of hepatobiliary disease in horses. *Res. Vet. Sci.* 46: 264–270.

7 West, H.J. (1991). Evaluation of total serum bile acid concentrations for the diagnosis of hepatobiliary disease in cattle. *Res. Vet. Sci.* 51: 133–140.

8 Jackson, B., Eastell, R., Russell, R.G.G. et al. (1996). Measurement of bone specific alkaline phosphatase in the horse: a comparison of two techniques. *Res. Vet. Sci.* 61: 160–164.

9 Hoffmann, W.E., Baker, G., Rieser, S., and Dorner, J.L. (1987). Alterations in selected serum biochemical constituents in equids after induced hepatic disease. *Am. J. Vet. Res.* 48: 1343–1347.

10 Patterson, W.H. and Brown, C.M. (1986). Increase of serum gamma-glutamyltransferase in neonatal Standardbred foals. *Am. J. Vet. Res.* 47: 2461–2463.

11 Barton, M.H. and LeRoy, B.E. (2007). Serum bile acids concentrations in healthy and clinically III neonatal foals. *J. Vet. Intern. Med.* 21: 508–513.

12 Buonanno, A.M., Carlson, G.P., and Kantrowitz, B. (1988). Clinical and diagnostic features of portosystemic shunt in a foal. *J. Am. Vet. Med. Assoc.* 192: 387–389.

13 McGorum, B.C., Murphy, D., Love, S., and Milne, E.M. (1999). Clinicopathological features of equine primary hepatic disease: a review of 50 cases. *Vet. Rec.* 145: 134–139.

14 Parraga, M.E., Carlson, G.P., and Thurmond, M. (1995). Serum protein concentrations in horses with severe liver disease: a retrospective study and review of the literature. *J. Vet. Intern. Med.* 9: 154–161.

15 West, H.J. (1996). Clinical and pathological studies in horses with hepatic disease. *Equine Vet. J.* 28: 146–156.

16 Maddison, J.E. (1992). Hepatic encephalopathy. Current concepts of the pathogenesis. *J. Vet. Intern. Med.* 6: 341–353.

17 Dunkel, B., Chaney, K.P., Dallap Schaer, B.L. et al. (2011). Putative intestinal hyperammonaemia in horses: 36 cases. *Equine Vet. J.* 43: 133–140.

18 Peek, S.F., Divers, T.J., and Jackson, C.J. (1997). Hyperammonaemia associated with encephalopathy and abdominal pain without evidence of liver disease in four mature horses. *Equine Vet. J.* 29: 70–74.

19 Sharkey, L.C., DeWitt, S., and Stockman, C. (2006). Neurologic signs and hyperammonemia in a horse with colic. *Vet. Clin. Pathol.* 35: 254–258.

20 McCornico, R.S., Duckett, W.M., and Wood, P.A. (1997). Persistent hyperammonemia in two related Morgan weanlings. *J. Vet. Intern. Med.* 11: 264–266.

21 Camus, M.S., Krimer, P.M., Leroy, B.E., and Almy, F.S. (2010). Evaluation of the positive predictive value of serum protein electrophoresis beta-gamma bridging for hepatic disease in three domestic animal species. *Vet. Pathol.* 47: 1064–1070.

22 Borchers, A., Magdesian, K.G., Halland, S. et al. (2006). Successful treatment and polymerase chain reaction (PCR) confirmation of Tyzzer's disease in a foal and clinical and pathologic characteristics of 6 additional foals (1986–2005). *J. Vet. Intern. Med.* 20: 1212–1218.

23 Humber, K.A., Sweeney, R.W., Saik, J.E. et al. (1988). Clinical and clinicopathologic findings in two foals infected with *Bacillus piliformis*. *J. Am. Vet. Med. Assoc.* 193: 1425–1428.

24 Durham, A.E., Smitht, K.C., Newton, J.R. et al. (2003). Development and application of a scoring system for prognostic evaluation of equine liver biopsies. *Equine Vet. J.* 35: 534–540.

25 Johnston, J.K., Divers, T.J., Reef, V.B., and Acland, H. (1989). Cholelithiasis in horses: ten cases (1982–1986). *J. Am. Vet. Med. Assoc.* 194: 405–409.

26 Curran, J.M., Sutherland, R.J., and Peet, R.L. (1996). A screening test for subclinical liver disease in horses affected by pyrrolizidine alkaloid toxicosis. *Aust. Vet. J.* 74: 236–240.

27 Johnson, A.L., Divers, T.J., Freckleton, M.L. et al. (2006). Fall panicum (*Panicum dichotomiflorum*) hepatotoxicosis in horses and sheep. *J. Vet. Intern. Med.* 20: 1414–1421.

28 Ambjerg, J. (1981). Poisoning in animals due to oral application of iron. *Nord. Vet. Med.* 33: 71–76.

29 Mullaney, T.P. and Brown, C.M. (1988). Iron toxicity in neonatal foals. *Equine Vet. J.* 20: 119–124.

30 Pearson, E.G. and Andreasen, C.B. (2001). Effect of oral administration of excessive iron in adult ponies. *J. Am. Vet. Med. Assoc.* 218: 400–404.

31 Theelen, M.J.P., Beukers, M., GCM, G., and Sloet van Oldruitenborgh-Oosterbaan, M.M. (2019). Chronic iron overload causing haemochromatosis and hepatopathy in 21 horses and one donkey. *Equine Vet. J.* 51: 304–309.

32 Lavoie, J.P. and Teuscher, E. (1993). Massive iron overload and liver fibrosis resembling haemochromatosis in a racing pony. *Equine Vet. J.* 25: 552–554.

33 Pearson, E.G., Hedstrom, O.R., and Poppenga, R.H. (1994). Hepatic cirrhosis and hemochromatosis in three horses. *J. Am. Vet. Med. Assoc.* 204: 1053–1056.

34 McCarthy, H.E., French, N.P., Edwards, G.B. et al. (2004). Equine grass sickness is associated with low antibody levels to *Clostridium botulinum*: a matched case-control study. *Equine Vet. J.* 36: 123–129.

35 Girling, S.J., Fraser, M.A., Richardson, D. et al. (2017). An acute outbreak of equine dysautonomia (equine grass sickness) in a group of eight Przewalski's horses (*Equus ferus [caballus] przewalskii*). *Equine Vet. Educ.* 29: 358–361.

36 Marrs, J., Small, J., Milne, E.M., and John, H.A. (2001). Liver and biliary system pathology in equine dysautonomia (grass sickness). *J. Vet. Med. A Physiol. Pathol. Clin. Med.* 48: 243–255.

37 Peek, S.F. (2004). Cholangiohepatitis in the mature horse. *Equine Vet. Educ.* 16: 72–75.

38 Aleman, M., Nieto, J.E., Carr, E.A., and Carlson, G.P. (2005). Serum hepatitis associated with commercial plasma transfusion in horses. *J. Vet. Intern. Med.* 19: 120–122.

39 Messer, N.T. and Johnson, P.J. (1994). Idiopathic acute hepatic disease in horses: 12 cases (1982–1992). *J. Am. Vet. Med. Assoc.* 204: 1934–1937.

40 Chandriani, S., Skewes-Cox, P., Zhong, W. et al. (2013). Identification of a previously undescribed divergent virus from the Flaviviridae family in an outbreak of equine serum hepatitis. *Proc. Natl. Acad. Sci. USA* 110: E1407–E1415.

41 Divers, T.J., Tennant, B.C., Kumar, A. et al. (2018). New parvovirus associated with serum hepatitis in horses after inoculation of common biological product. *Emerg. Infect. Dis.* 24: 303–310.

42 Kapoor, A., Simmonds, P., Cullen, J.M. et al. (2013). Identification of a pegivirus (GB virus-like virus) that infects horses. *J. Virol.* 87: 7185–7190.

43 Ramsay, J.D., Evanoff, R., Wilkinson, T.E. et al. (2015). Experimental transmission of equine hepacivirus in horses as a model for hepatitis C virus. *Hepatology* 61: 1533–1546.

44 Tomlinson, J.E., Kapoor, A., Kumar, A. et al. (2019). Viral testing of 18 consecutive cases of equine serum hepatitis: a prospective study (2014–2018). *J. Vet. Intern. Med.* 33: 251–257.

45 Tomlinson, J.E., Tennant, B.C., Struzyna, A. et al. (2019). Viral testing of 10 cases of Theiler's disease and 37 in-contact horses in the absence of equine biologic product administration: a prospective study (2014–2018). *J. Vet. Intern. Med.* 33: 258–265.

46 Tomlinson, J.E., van de Walle, G.R., and Divers, T.J. (2019). What do we know about hepatitis viruses in horses? *Vet. Clin. North Am. Equine Pract.* 35: 351–362.

47 Soulé, C., Boulard, C., Levieux, D. et al. (1989). Experimental equine fascioliasis: evolution of serologic, enzymatic and parasitic parameters. *Ann. Rech. Vet.* 20: 295–307.

48 Howell, A.K., Malalana, F., Beesley, N.J. et al. (2019). *Fasciola hepatica* in UK horses. *Equine Vet. J.* 55: 157–162.

49 Quigley, A., Sekiya, M., Egan, S. et al. (2017). Prevalence of liver fluke infection in Irish horses and assessment of a serological test for diagnosis of equine fasciolosis. *Equine Vet. J.* 49: 183–188.

50 Corapi, W.V., Birch, S.M., Carlson, K.L. et al. (2011). *Heterobilharzia americana* infection as a cause of hepatic parasitic granulomas in a horse. *J. Am. Vet. Med. Assoc.* 239: 1117–1122.

51 Beeler-Marfisi, J., Arroyo, L., Caswell, J.L. et al. (2010). Equine primary liver tumors: a case series and review of the literature. *J. Vet. Diagn. Invest.* 22: 174–183.

52 Salvaggio, A., Caracappa, S., Gurrera, A., and Magro, G. (2003). Hepatic biliary adenofibroma: a hitherto unrecognized tumor in equines. Report of a case. *Vet. Pathol.* 40: 114–116.

6

The Kidney

Andrea A. Bohn[1] and Raquel M. Walton[2]

[1] *Department of Microbiology, Immunology, and Pathology, College of Veterinary Medicine and Biomedical Sciences, Colorado State University, Fort Collins, CO, USA*
[2] *IDEXX Laboratories, Inc., Langhorne, PA, USA*

Abnormalities in laboratory values can help determine the presence and severity of urinary tract disease. Many different disorders of the equine urinary tract have been described and include prerenal, intrarenal, and postrenal processes. Routine laboratory data are used to assess glomerular filtration rate (GFR) as well as other functions of the kidney. The kidney is very important in filtering wastes from the blood as well as maintaining electrolyte, water, and acid–base balances. The kidney also plays an important role in erythropoiesis and vitamin D activation.

Comprehensive evaluation of the equine renal system requires a complete blood count (CBC), serum biochemical panel, and full urinalysis. The CBC can help detect inflammatory conditions and the presence of anemia. Serum biochemical analysis will detect increases in nitrogenous waste products normally excreted by the kidneys, reveal electrolyte and protein abnormalities, and provide information regarding acid–base status. Urinalysis is essential in differentiating causes of azotemia as well as providing clues as to the presence, location, and cause of urinary tract disorders (Table 6.1).

6.1 Laboratory Assessment of the Kidney

In examining laboratory data for evaluation of the urinary tract, the functions of the kidney can essentially be broken down into three main actions (Figure 6.1). The first is the filtering of blood through the glomerulus; total plasma volume is filtered approximately 60–70 times every day [1]. While this is essential for removal of waste substances, essential blood solutes are also filtered during this process. Therefore, the second major action of the kidney is to reabsorb those solutes so that appropriate plasma concentrations are maintained. The third major action is the maintenance of blood volume or body water. This is predominantly regulated in the collecting ducts under the influence of vasopressin.

6.1.1 Glomerular Filtration Rate

6.1.1.1 Creatinine and Serum Urea

The ability of the kidneys to filter blood can be evaluated by determining the GFR. While there are more complicated methods to precisely determine GFR, serum urea and creatinine provide a readily available estimation of GFR. If there is an elevation of these nitrogenous waste products in serum, termed azotemia, it indicates that GFR is decreased. Creatinine has been considered an insensitive method of detecting a decrease in renal functional capacity, as three-fourths of nephron mass is typically lost before azotemia is seen. However, the loss of 75% renal mass translates to a lower functional loss due to compensatory renal hypertrophy, so the actual sensitivity of serum creatinine for detecting decreased renal function is higher than historically assumed [2]. For example, in dogs, creatinine was shown to increase after GFR decreases of 48% on average [3].

Decreases in GFR can be due to prerenal, renal, or postrenal factors or a combination of these processes. If the rate of glomerular filtration decreases, serum urea and creatinine concentrations will increase. Urea concentrations can rise faster than creatinine because of the tubules' ability to reabsorb urea, particularly with a prerenal cause of decreased GFR. Other values that increase with a decrease in GFR are serum phosphorus and total magnesium concentrations.

If the cause of a decrease in GFR is purely prerenal and there are no extenuating circumstances, a horse should

Equine Hematology, Cytology, and Clinical Chemistry, Second Edition.
Edited by Raquel M. Walton, Rick L. Cowell, and Amy C. Valenciano.

Table 6.1 Common laboratory findings associated with different renal diseases.

	CRF	ARF	Early disease	Glomerular disease	Bladder rupture	Strenuous exercise	Dehydration
Azotemia	+	+	−	±	±	±	+
Urea/Creat	>1:10	<1:10					
USG	1.008–1.012	1.008–1.012	Variable	Variable	Variable	>1.025	>1.035
Proteinuria	+	+	±	+++	−	+	−
Other potential findings	Nonregenerative anemia HyperMg Hyperlipidemia Hypoalbuminemia Metabolic acidosis	Glycosuria High FE HyperMg Enzymuria Urine casts and WBCs Metabolic acidosis	Glycosuria High FE Enzymuria	Red cell casts		Hematuria Hemoglobinuria Myoglobinuria	
Serum electrolytes							
Na/Cl	N-L	N-L	N	N	L	L-N-H	N-H
K	N-H	L-N-H	N	N	N-H	N	N
Ca	N-H	L-N-H	N	N-L	N	N-L	N
Phosphorus	N-L	H	N	N-H	N	N	N-H
Additional testing			FE Enzymuria USG Water deprivation test	UPC ratio	Ratio of abdominal fluid creat to serum creat	Retest later	

ARF, acute renal failure; CRF, chronic renal failure; Creat, creatinine; FE, fractional excretion; Mg, magnesium; L, low; N, normal; H, high; UPC, urine protein creatinine ratio; USG, urine specific gravity; WBC, white blood cell.

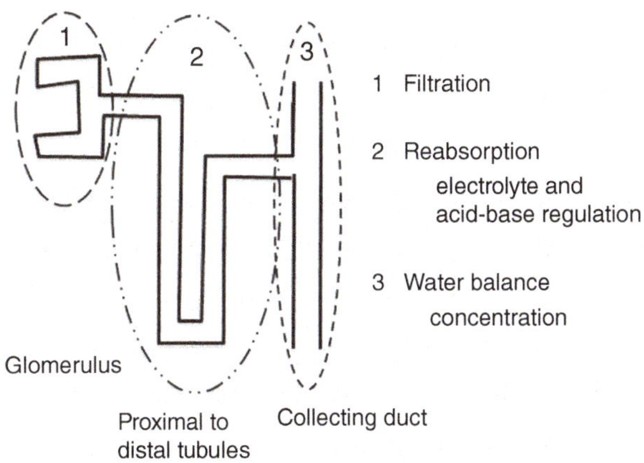

Figure 6.1 Simplified illustration of the three major functions of the kidney that can be assessed by laboratory methods.

have a urine specific gravity >1.025 in the face of azotemia. If a horse is not able to concentrate its urine in the face of azotemia (and the animal has not been treated with fluids), the kidney is not functioning properly and one of the most common causes is renal disease. There are, however, other reasons for the kidneys not being able to concentrate urine, as discussed below. These factors need to be considered before a definitive diagnosis of renal failure is made. With postrenal azotemia, urine specific gravity can be variable and is often isosthenuric in the postobstructive phase. The diagnosis of most postrenal urinary tract disorders is usually predominantly based on history and clinical signs.

Both urea and creatinine concentrations can be elevated for reasons other than decreased GFR. Urea is a by-product of protein metabolism so urea concentration can increase with a high protein diet or urea supplementation. Mild increases in urea may be seen with protein catabolism associated with fasting or prolonged exercise [1]. Interestingly, while urea concentration may increase with fasting in horses, it tends to decrease in ponies [1]. Decreases in urea can also occur with protein-poor diets or liver failure.

Creatinine is a by-product of muscle metabolism and therefore is correlated with total muscle mass. Heavily muscled animals may have creatinine concentrations that are normally slightly above reported reference intervals. Release of creatinine from muscle during exercise, fasting, muscle wasting, or rhabdomyolysis can influence creatinine concentration. In addition, if the Jaffe colorimetric method is used to measure creatinine, the concentration of creatinine may be artefactually increased in the presence of non-creatinine chromagens; this may actually be the main reason for the increase in creatinine associated with fasting. Spurious increases in creatinine have also been associated with various metabolic disorders and administration of cephalosporin antibiotics [4]. Hyperbilirubinemia can interfere with the measurement of creatinine, resulting in falsely low values. During the first few days of a foal's life, creatinine concentration can be quite high relative to adult reference values, but should decrease to adult reference values by 3–5 days if the kidneys are healthy [1, 5].

The blood urea nitrogen (BUN):creatinine ratio is not very useful in determining whether azotemia is prerenal, renal, or postrenal, but it has been used to help differentiate between acute and chronic renal disease. In many (but not all) cases, the ratio will be <10:1 in acute renal failure (ARF) and >10:1 in chronic renal failure (CRF) [4]. If the ratio becomes >15:1 with CRF, this may be an indication of excess protein in the diet [6].

6.1.1.2 Symmetric Dimethylarginine (SDMA)

Symmetric dimethylarginine is an amino acid released from cells during protein degradation that is primarily eliminated by renal excretion; the concentration has been shown to be correlated with GFR in animals and humans. Some reports show SDMA to be an earlier indicator of kidney dysfunction than serum creatinine concentration in dogs and cats with chronic kidney disease [3, 7]. SDMA is not influenced by muscle mass, the major nonrenal influence on serum creatinine concentration [2]. Currently, very little information is available on the use of SDMA for detection of kidney dysfunction in horses. Preliminary evaluations of SDMA in healthy draught-breed horses ($n = 165$) showed correlation with serum creatinine ($R = 0.59$, $P<0.001$) and no significant differences in SDMA between sexes. SDMA concentrations in all healthy draught-breed horses (Belgian, Percheron, and Clydesdale) were <14 μg/dL, similar to the reported reference limit in cats and dogs [8].

6.1.2 Reabsorption and Electrolyte Regulation

For many of the solutes that are filtered through glomeruli, reabsorption predominantly occurs in the proximal tubules, whereas additional regulation may occur further along the nephron. Because all glucose is normally absorbed in the proximal tubules unless the serum concentration exceeds the renal threshold, the presence of glycosuria without hyperglycemia is an indication of proximal tubule dysfunction. Glycosuria is more commonly seen with ARF than CRF.

Serum electrolyte abnormalities can also be seen with tubular dysfunction, including hyponatremia, hypochloremia, hyper- or hypocalcemia, hypophosphatemia, hyper- or hypokalemia, and increased or decreased bicarbonate levels. Horses normally excrete a large amount of calcium and serum calcium concentrations are often abnormal with equine renal failure. Hypercalcemia is commonly seen with CRF whereas hypocalcemia is more commonly associated with ARF.

A relatively easy way to assess whether there is decreased reabsorption of electrolytes by the kidney is to determine their fractional excretion (FE). The FE of sodium is most commonly determined; the second most common electrolyte used is phosphorus. FE is calculated using the concentrations of the electrolyte and creatinine in both serum and urine and plugging those numbers into the following equation:

$$\frac{\text{Serum creatinine}}{\text{Urine creatinine}} \times \frac{\text{Urine sodium}}{\text{Serum sodium}} \times 100 \tag{6.1}$$

The FE of sodium and phosphorus is normally <1%. Values greater than 1% (0.8%) imply tubular dysfunction, unless the animal is receiving a diet very high in sodium or phosphorus, has been administered polyionic intravenous fluids or certain medications (furosemide), recently performed low-intensity exercise, or there is aldosterone or parathormone deficiency [9].

6.1.3 Water Conservation and Blood Volume Regulation

Greater than 99% of what is filtered through the glomerulus is reabsorbed by the renal tubules. Water is largely reabsorbed in the proximal tubules and additional water is reabsorbed as the tubular fluid travels through the descending limb of the loop of Henle. The final concentration of urine is determined by processes within the collecting ducts. Glomerular filtrate, as it enters proximal tubules, has a specific gravity of 1.008–1.014. Therefore, if urine leaving the bladder has a similar specific gravity, it is considered isosthenuric. The specific gravity becomes more concentrated (hypersthenuric) as the tubular fluid travels through the descending limb of the loop of Henle, but then becomes less concentrated (hyposthenuric) as electrolytes are actively reabsorbed in the ascending limb which is relatively impermeable to water. Hyposthenuric urine, therefore, requires energy and functioning tubules. As the tubular fluid travels through collecting ducts, final water regulation occurs under the influence of vasopressin. Vasopressin causes the collecting ducts to become permeable to water so that water can flow from the less concentrated tubular fluid to the highly osmotic medullary interstitium. Hypertonicity of the medulla is necessary for this water movement and is reliant on adequate urea and sodium concentrations in maintaining an osmotic gradient.

If an animal becomes dehydrated, the urine should become concentrated before azotemia occurs. Therefore, if an animal is azotemic with a urine specific gravity <1.025, the kidneys are not able to concentrate appropriately. This is most often due to renal disease, which should be a differential whenever one sees azotemia with lack of urine concentration, but it is possible that the kidneys are not concentrating urine for other reasons. Marked hyponatremia can lead to medullary washout (the lack of a hypertonic medullary interstitium) so that water is not drawn through the pores of the collecting ducts. Osmotic diuresis, as can occur with diabetes mellitus, decreases the concentration difference between the tubular fluid and medullary interstitium as well as increasing the rate of flow through the tubules, resulting in lack of urine concentration. If vasopressin is lacking (central diabetes insipidus), water cannot be reabsorbed across the collecting ducts. Likewise, the kidneys can be resistant to the action of vasopressin, which is thought to contribute to the lack of urine concentrating ability associated with hyperadrenocorticism, endotoxemia, and hypercalcemia.

6.1.4 Other Renal Functions

Glomeruli, whilst allowing many solutes to enter the nephron, are also designed to prevent many blood products from being filtered into the urinary space. Substances about the size of albumin and above do not readily make their way into the glomerular filtrate. In addition to size, the negative charge of the glomerular basement membrane helps maintain the filtration barrier [10]. If this barrier is damaged, substances that normally do not freely filter across, such as albumin, can be lost into the urine, resulting in proteinuria and, eventually, hypoalbuminemia.

An additional function of the kidney is the production of erythropoietin to maintain erythrocyte numbers. Nonregenerative anemia can occur with chronic renal disease due to decreased erythropoietin production.

6.2 Urinalysis

6.2.1 Gross Evaluation

A full urinalysis is important in the evaluation of the urinary tract. The gross appearance of the urine should be documented, as well as any changes in character of the urine observed during micturition. Evidence of hemorrhage seen only in the early phase of micturition is indicative of urethral hemorrhage, while consistent bloodiness is suggestive of hemorrhage in the bladder or above. Urine often contains more particulates during the end of micturition, as settled sludge within the bladder is often expelled then [11]. Equine urine can normally appear light yellow to dark amber or light brown and is often cloudy, containing

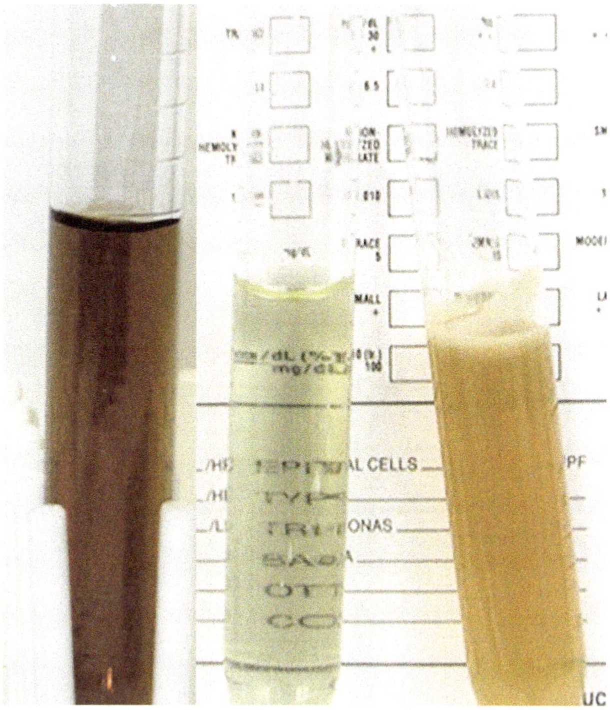

Figure 6.2 Gross evaluation of urine. Equine urine is frequently cloudy as seen in the right tube. The middle tube contains pale, clear urine, as often seen with polyuria. The reddish brown color of the urine on the left is due to myoglobinuria.

crystalline material and mucus (Figure 6.2). Pale, clear urine is associated with polyuria. Urine can appear pink to red with hematuria or hemoglobinuria, red to dark-brown with myoglobinuria or methemoglobinuria, and yellow-brown with bilirubinuria. Normal urine can become darker or even reddish in color over time due to oxidation products [12]. Ideally, urinalysis should be performed within one hour of collection as objects such as casts can dissolve quickly.

6.2.2 Urine Specific Gravity

It is recommended that urine specific gravity be measured with a refractometer rather than relying on a dipstick reading. Healthy horses typically maintain a urine specific gravity >1.020. The isosthenuric range of horse urine is 1.008–1.014, indicating that the urine coming out of the bladder has a similar concentration to the glomerular filtrate from the blood, without any significant concentration or dilution. If urine specific gravity is greater than 1.025 or less than 1.008, it can be presumed that at least 33% of kidney mass is functioning since dilution of urine, as well as concentration, requires functional tubules.

Prerenal azotemia is usually due to dehydration and properly functioning kidneys will conserve water, resulting in concentrated urine, before an animal will become azotemic. Therefore, isosthenuric urine in the face of azotemia is always abnormal. Isosthenuria without azotemia could indicate a lack of ability to concentrate urine, but this would have to be confirmed by some other means.

Concentrating ability is tested by a water deprivation test. This needs to be done carefully, so that the animal will not become dangerously dehydrated if they are not able to concentrate their urine. The animal may also need time to reestablish hyperosmolarity of the medullary interstitium if there has been medullary washout. If urine concentration occurs only after administration of vasopressin, this confirms that a deficit of endogenous vasopressin is the reason for the lack of concentration and not renal disease.

Hyposthenuric urine typically implies interference with or lack of vasopressin or, possibly, water overload. Nursing foals frequently have dilute urine because of their diet, but they normally have the ability to concentrate urine >1.030 from the time of birth [13].

6.2.3 Reagent Test Strips

The pH of urine from healthy adult horses is alkaline, usually between 7.5 and 8.5, largely as a result of an herbivorous diet. Bacteriuria, high-grain diets, intravenous fluids, strenuous exercise, and starvation can result in acid urine. Healthy suckling foals have acidic urine due to their milk diet. Metabolic acidosis is a common cause of acid urine in adult horses and paradoxical aciduria can also be seen with metabolic alkalosis, especially when combined with hypokalemia (Figure 6.3).

Equine urine does not normally contain glucose, ketones, or bilirubin. It is thought that the renal threshold for serum glucose is around 150 mg/dL. If glucosuria is present and the serum glucose concentration is less than 150 mg/dL, this is an indication of renal tubular dysfunction. Ketonuria is uncommon as horses are poorly ketogenic. The presence of bilirubinuria should be correlated with the serum chemistry panel and CBC for detection of liver disease, posthepatic biliary obstruction or hemolytic anemia.

Equine urine should contain very little protein. In concentrated urine (>1.035), normal protein concentrations may produce a trace to 1+ reaction on the dipstick. False elevations in protein concentration can be expected in horses since alkaline urine may cause false positives on reagent pads. Any increase in urine protein as indicated by a dipstick should be verified; this is often done using the semiquantitative sulfosalicylic acid precipitation test.

Glomerular diseases are often associated with marked proteinuria, while tubular lesions can result in milder proteinuria. Hemorrhage into the urinary tract and inflammation can also result in high urine protein concentrations.

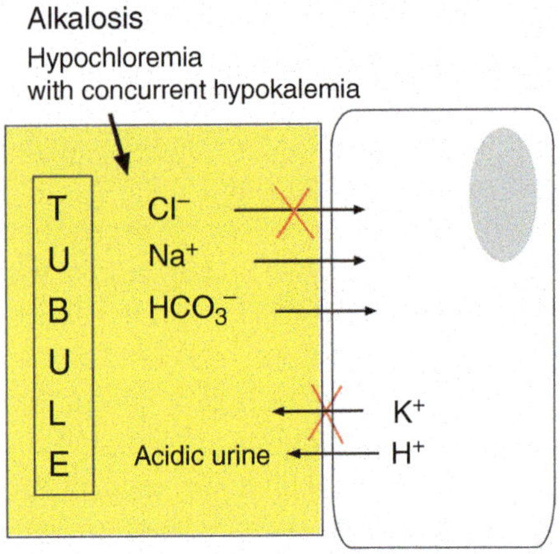

Figure 6.3 Paradoxical aciduria. In horses with metabolic alkalosis, chloride is less available for reabsorption with sodium into proximal tubular epithelial cells so there is decreased sodium resorption in the proximal tubule. Depletion of chloride results in reabsorption of bicarbonate with sodium, exacerbating the alkalosis. If there is a metabolic alkalosis with concurrent volume depletion, sodium resorption is increased in the distal tubule via aldosterone by exchange with a cation, usually hydrogen, but also potassium. With concurrent hypokalemia, potassium is conserved and increased hydrogen is excreted in its place, resulting in aciduria and an exacerbated alkalosis.

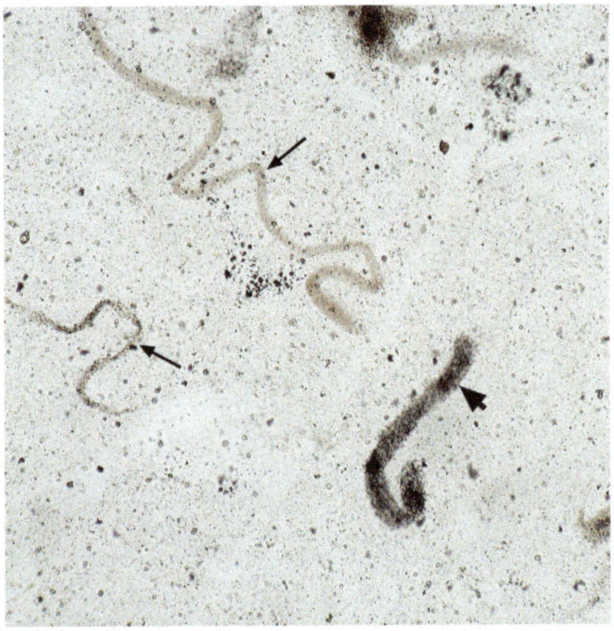

Figure 6.4 Sedimented urine from a horse with rhabdomyolysis. Granular casts indicate renal tubular damage (*large arrowhead*). Mucus strands are common in equine urine and should not be confused with casts (*small arrows*). Unstained wet mount, 10× objective.

Urine protein to creatinine (UPC) ratios can be used to more accurately assess the amount of protein in the urine. The UPC ratio should be <1.0 in a normal horse [14]. UPC ratios are not indicated if there is evidence of inflammation or hemorrhage in the urinary tract since protein associated with these processes cannot be differentiated from proteins that may be present due to glomerular or tubular disease. Proteinuria can be transient and not indicative of renal disease, such as can occur after exercise in horses [4, 11]. It is therefore important to establish if proteinuria is persistent before further work-up.

The reagent pad for blood measures myoglobin as well as hemoglobin. Therefore, a positive reaction can be due to free hemoglobin from lyzed erythrocytes, whole red blood cells, or myoglobin. Some pads help distinguish whole erythrocytes from free hemoglobin. Hemoglobin from intravascular hemolysis may be differentiated from myoglobinuria by examining the color of plasma or serum since hemoglobin can often be visualized while myoglobin will not be. Measuring serum creatine kinase concentration to assess muscle injury and performing a CBC to look for anemia can also be useful in differentiating the cause of a positive blood pad. Most positive blood reactions are due to hemorrhage within the urinary tract. This can be due to trauma, uroliths, inflammation, neoplasia, vascular defects, or coagulopathy.

6.2.4 Urine Sediment Exam

The sediment exam is performed by centrifuging 5–10 mL of urine at 1000–1500 rpm for five minutes and removing the supernatant. After resuspending the sedimented material in the small amount of fluid left over, a drop is placed on a slide and coverslipped. The microscope should be adjusted for high contrast; a sediment stain can also be used to enhance visualization.

At low power (10× objective), casts can be detected and counted and an overall view of the sample obtained. In horses, it is important not to mistake strands of mucus for casts (Figure 6.4). The sample should then be examined at high magnification (40× objective) for erythrocytes, leukocytes, epithelial cells, bacteria, crystals, or any unusual findings. If high numbers of calcium carbonate crystals are obscuring other objects within the sediment, 10% acidic acid can be added to the sediment to dissolve the crystals. If there is uncertainty about what is visualized in a wet mount, the coverslip can be carefully removed (or a new slide made from the sediment), air dried, and then stained for cytological evaluation.

Casts are formed from material within and take the shape of renal tubule lumens. The foundation of all casts is Tamm–Horsfall glycoprotein, which is a normal secretion of renal tubular cells. Hyaline casts contain mostly protein and their number can be increased with renal disease,

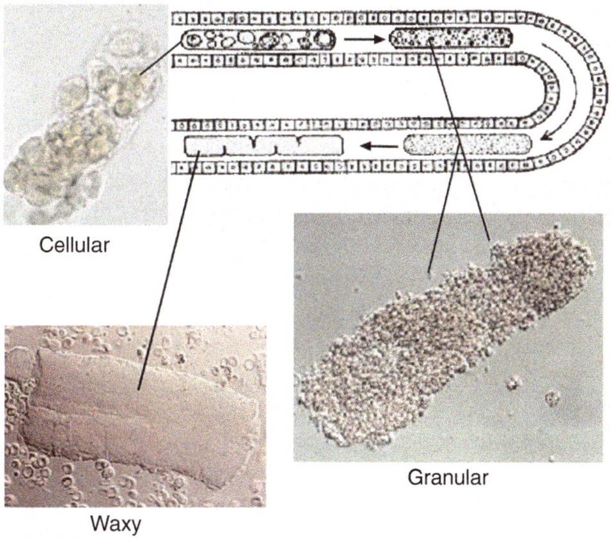

Figure 6.5 Cast formation in the renal tubules. Tubular epithelial cells, leukocytes, and/or erythrocytes sloughed into the tubular lumen form a cast of the tubule. Cellular casts have been immediately flushed from the lumen into urine. In contrast, granular and waxy casts have been retained in the lumen, where they degrade from a cellular to granular then waxy appearance. Thus, cellular, granular, and waxy casts imply a single process.

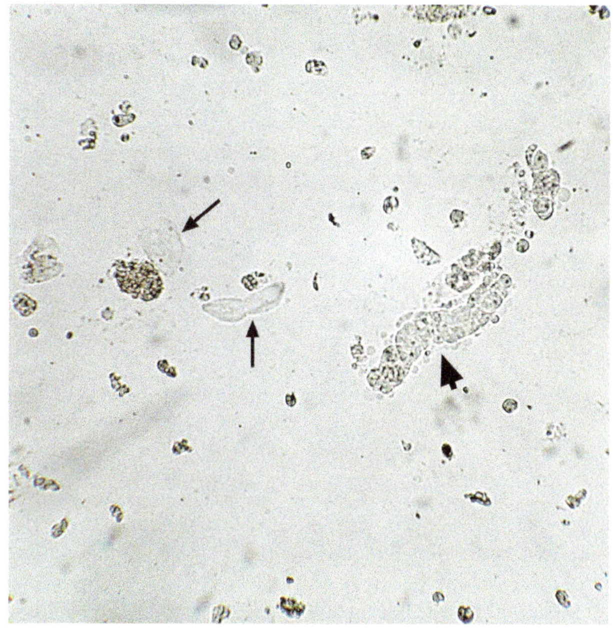

Figure 6.6 Sedimented urine from a severely dehydrated animal. Cellular casts are present, indicating sloughing of renal tubular cells (*large arrowhead*). A few squamous epithelial cells can be seen in free-catch urine samples (*small arrows*). Unstained wet mount, 40× objective.

severe dehydration, and protein-losing nephropathy. Other casts are characterized by the type of cells trapped within the protein framework (erythrocytes, leukocytes, epithelial cells), as granular casts if cellular features have degraded so that cells cannot be recognized, or as waxy casts if cellular products are extremely broken down (Figure 6.5). Erythrocytes and leukocytes indicate hemorrhage or inflammation within the nephron, respectively. Epithelial cell casts indicate a tubular insult that has caused cell sloughing (Figure 6.6). A few hyaline and rare granular casts may be seen in normal urine but if increased numbers of casts are present, this is an indication of renal insult.

Urine should contain very few cells. A sediment preparation made from 10 mL of urine should contain <5–8 erythrocytes or leukocytes per high magnification (40× objective) field [12]. Few epithelial cells should also be present. Squamous epithelial cells may be present within voided samples (Figure 6.6). Increased numbers of transitional epithelial cells may be seen with inflammation, neoplasia, or trauma. Dysplastic changes occur within transitional epithelial cells associated with inflammation, therefore a few irregular clusters of epithelial cells should not raise immediate concern for neoplasia if associated with an inflammatory process.

Inflammation is present with >8 neutrophils per high-power field (40× objective). Bacterial infection may be present even if bacteria are not seen. For culture, urine should be collected by catheterization; foals also can be collected by cystocentesis. Greater than eight erythrocytes per high dry field indicates hemorrhage within the urinary tract. This could be due to trauma, uroliths, inflammation, neoplasia, vascular defects, or coagulopathy. Mild hematuria can be seen post exercise [12, 15].

Crystals are very common in horse urine, particularly calcium carbonate crystals (Figure 6.7). Calcium phosphate, triple phosphate, and low numbers of calcium oxalate crystals can also be seen. If urine is carefully collected, it should contain very few or no bacteria. Other substances that may be seen in urine include sperm from stallions, plant or other particulate matter in a voided sample, parasite eggs, or lymphoma cells.

6.3 Laboratory Abnormalities Associated with Different Disease States

6.3.1 Acute Renal Failure

In ARF, the horse will be azotemic with isosthenuria. BUN to creatinine ratios are typically <10:1. Hypermagnesemia is often associated with the decrease in GFR. Hyponatremia and hypochloremia are often present and the FE of sodium is >1.0. Serum calcium and phosphorus concentrations can be variable, from low, normal, to high. Phosphaturia is

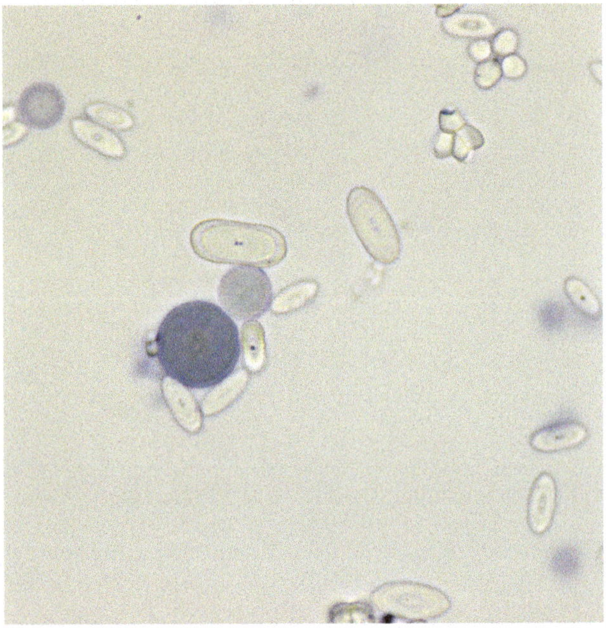

Figure 6.7 Calcium carbonate crystals. Note the concentric lamellar structure and the range of possible shapes of the crystals. Wright–Giemsa stain, 100× objective.

typically present early in the disease process. Enzymuria and glycosuria are also often present.

There is typically a mild to moderate proteinuria associated with ARF. Results of the urine sediment examination may vary with disease process. With acute interstitial nephritis, there may be pyuria, white blood cell casts, eosinophiluria and eosinophilia, and/or hematuria. With acute tubular necrosis, associated with either ischemia or nephrotoxins, granular casts are often present but hematuria is less common.

6.3.2 Chronic Renal Failure

Horses with CRF will be azotemic and have a urine specific gravity <1.020. BUN to creatinine ratios are often >10:1, likely due to variable distribution of these nitrogenous compounds within body fluids. It is also thought that urinary excretion of creatinine occurs in CRF. Serum creatinine concentration can be used as a rough guide to the prognosis of CRF, keeping in mind that there are other factors that also influence creatinine levels. In general, a doubling of creatinine roughly equals a 50% decline in GFR [6]. Horses with creatinine concentrations below 5 mg/dL can do fairly well, at least in the short term and possibly long term, with management, whilst creatinine concentrations between 5 and 10 mg/dL are associated with declining renal function. Creatinine concentrations >15 mg/dL indicate a grave prognosis [6]. Monitoring creatinine concentrations over time can be useful in monitoring disease progression.

Hypercalcemia and hypophosphatemia are common in equine CFR. The degree of hypercalcemia is related to the amount of calcium in the diet as the kidney normally plays a large role in excreting excess calcium [16]. Mild hyponatremia and hypochloremia may be present due to decreased tubular reabsorption, although FE values may not be abnormal. Most horses with CRF have a normal acid–base status or may be slightly alkalotic. Metabolic acidosis typically occurs in the terminal stages of CRF. Horses with CRF may also be hyperkalemic due to decreased excretion or metabolic acidosis. Because of decreased erythropoietin production associated with CRF and, possibly, decreased erythrocyte life span with exposure to uremic toxins, a mild nonregenerative anemia is often associated with CRF. Horses with CRF can also develop hypercholesterolemia and hypertriglyceridemia, occasionally severe enough to be seen as lipemia [6]. Glycosuria and enzymuria are less common in CRF than in ARF, as are elevated FEs, despite urinary electrolyte losses [6].

There is typically a degree of proteinuria associated with CRF and horses are commonly mildly hypoalbuminemic. UPC ratios can be used to more quantitatively assess protein loss. Because urine is isosthenuric and the animals are polyuric, urine sediment is typically devoid of crystals and mucus. Pyuria may also be nonexistent even with infection of the urinary tract. Occasionally, erythrocytes or leukocytes may be seen in urine, depending on the underlying disease process.

6.3.3 Urinary Tract Rupture

Uroperitoneum secondary to rupture of the urinary bladder is not always easy to diagnose based on serum biochemical changes. The presence of azotemia is variable. The most consistent serum biochemical finding is hyponatremia. Hyperkalemia and hypochloremia are the next most common serum biochemical abnormalities, although all these changes are less likely if there has been prior fluid administration [9, 17–19]. Since other disease processes can manifest similarly, collection of abdominal fluid and comparing the concentration of creatinine in the fluid to the serum creatinine concentration is a valuable diagnostic tool. A fluid creatinine concentration >2 times the serum concentration confirms uroperitoneum [19]. Presence of calcium carbonate crystals in the peritoneal fluid cytology is also diagnostic for uroperitoneum (see Chapter 18).

6.3.4 "Early" Renal Disease

Horses are considered to be in renal failure when there is azotemia and isosthenuria, but these are relatively insensitive markers for renal disease. In general, approximately 50% of renal function is lost by the time an animal becomes azotemic [2] and approximately 67% function is lost before urine can no longer be concentrated. Ideally, it would be advantageous to be able to diagnose renal disease before 50–67% of the functional kidney is lost so that appropriate therapies or preventive measures can be taken in a timely manner.

Direct measurement of GFR is a good way to detect renal dysfunction early in the disease course, but this is not routinely performed and readers are encouraged to look elsewhere for information on this technique [4, 11]. Because the relatively low sensitivity of creatinine partly stems from reference intervals that are overly wide for patients with a low baseline concentration, sensitivity could be improved by establishing age-, breed-, and sex-specific reference intervals. Creatinine is an analyte with variability that is higher between individuals than within an individual animal [2]. Thus, creatinine is best evaluated with individual rather than population-based reference values [20]; comparing the patient's own historical values over time may lead to much earlier detection of kidney disease than comparison to the laboratory's population-based reference limits.

If a horse presents with isosthenuria without azotemia, it should be determined whether this is because of intrinsic renal disease or due to some other reason. In this scenario, if a cause for the isosthenuric urine is not evident on the CBC, biochemical panel, or urinalysis, one may wish to first determine if the horse can concentrate its urine by rechecking at a later date. If the horse is persistently isosthenuric, one should consider performing a water deprivation test.

Other tests of renal functional ability or injury include FE of sodium and assessment of enzymuria. Elevations in FE indicate that the renal tubules are not functioning properly and the presence of enzymuria indicates damage to the renal tubular cells. Serial assessments may be more useful than a one-time test and negative findings do not necessarily rule out intrinsic renal diseases.

The urine enzymes that have shown some utility in assessing equine renal insult are gamma-glutamyltransferase (GGT), N-acetyl-beta-glucoaminidase (NAG), alkaline phosphatase (ALP) (all proximal tubular), and lactate dehydrogenase (LDH) (distal tubular) [4]. Enzyme activity is typically compared to creatinine concentrations and reported as a ratio. Activities for these enzymes in healthy horse urine are reported to be <36.54 IU GGT/g creatinine (<1.85 IU GGT/mmol creatinine), <1 IU NAG/g creatinine, 0–28 IU ALP/g creatinine, and 0–12 IU LDH/g creatinine [2, 4]. Clinically significant thresholds of increased enzymatic activity have not been defined so caution must be used in the interpretation of results. For GGT, a ratio >100 IU/g is likely clinically significant [4, 11]. Many conditions can affect enzymatic activity so measurements should be assessed within 72 hours of collection and the sample should be refrigerated but not frozen if not immediately analyzed [4]. NAG activity is affected by alkaline urine and is most useful when urine pH is acidic to neutral. Currently, the usefulness of these markers in predicting clinically significant tubular damage is unknown as studies have yielded inconsistent results with respect to the magnitude of enzymuria, whether histological changes are observed, and whether or not azotemia develops following the insult.

6.3.5 Glomerular Disease

Renal amyloidosis is rare in horses, but diseases of renal glomeruli are typically characterized by moderate to marked proteinuria. With glomerular disease, animals may become azotemic, but can still concentrate urine if the distal tubules are not involved in the disease process. With acute glomerulonephritis, red cell casts may be seen on urinalysis.

6.3.6 Strenuous Exercise

Exercise has been associated with transient proteinuria, hematuria, hemoglobinuria, and myoglobinuria [4, 11, 12]. It is important to keep in mind the timing of urine collection with respect to exercise or to confirm persistence of abnormal findings at a later date.

References

1 Schott, H.C. II (2004). Renal physiology. In: *Equine Internal Medicine*, 2e (eds. S.M. Reed, W.M. Bayly and D.C. Sellon), 1184–1199. St Louis: Saunders.

2 Hokamp, J.A. and Nabity, M.B. (2016). Renal biomarkers in domestic species. *Vet. Clin. Pathol.* 45 (1): 28–56.

3 Nabity, M.B., Lees, G.E., Boggess, M.M. et al. (2015). Symmetric dimethylarginine assay validation, stability, and evaluation as a marker for the early detection of chronic kidney disease in dogs. *J. Vet. Intern. Med.* 29 (4): 1036–1044.

4 Schott, H.C. II (2004). Examination of the urinary system. In: *Equine Internal Medicine*, 2e (eds. S.M. Reed, W.M. Bayly and D.C. Sellon), 1200–1220. St Louis: Saunders.

5 Chaney, K.P., Holcombe, S.J., Schott, H.C., and Barr, B.S. (2010). Spurious hypercreatininemia: 28 neonatal foals (2000–2008). *J. Vet. Emerg. Crit. Care* 20 (2): 244–249.

6 Schott, H.C. II (2004). Chronic renal failure. In: *Equine Internal Medicine*, 2e (eds. S.M. Reed, W.M. Bayly and D.C. Sellon), 1231–1253. St Louis: Saunders.

7 Hall, J.A., Obare, E., Yerramilli, M., and Jewell, D.E. (2014). Comparison of serum concentrations of symmetric dimethylarginine and creatinine as kidney function biomarkers in cats with chronic kidney disease. *J. Vet. Intern. Med.* 28 (6): 1676–1683.

8 Schott, H.C. II, Gallant, L., Coyne, M. et al. (2018). *Symmetric dimethylarginine and creatinine concentrations in draft breed horses.* Abstract presented at 11th Annual European College of Equine Internal Medicine Congress; Belgium (November 9–10).

9 Higuchi, T., Nanao, Y., and Senba, H. (2002). Repair of urinary bladder rupture through a urethrotomy and urethral sphincterotomy in four postpartum mares. *Vet. Surg.* 31 (4): 344–348.

10 Toribio, R.E. (2007). Essentials of equine renal and urinary tract physiology. *Vet. Clin. North Am. Equine Pract.* 23 (3): 533–561.

11 Savage, C.J. (2008). Urinary clinical pathologic findings and glomerular filtration rate in the horse. *Vet. Clin. North Am. Equine Pract.* 24 (2): 387–404.

12 Schumacher, J. (2007). Hematuria and pigmenturia of horses. *Vet. Clin. North Am. Equine Pract.* 23 (3): 655–675.

13 Axon, J.E. and Palmer, J.E. (2008). Clinical pathology of the foal. *Vet. Clin. North Am. Equine Pract.* 24 (2): 357–385.

14 Uberti, B., Eberle, D.B., Pressler, B.M. et al. (2009). Determination of and correlation between urine protein excretion and urine protein-to-creatinine ratio values during a 24-hour period in healthy horses and ponies. *Am. J. Vet. Res.* 70 (12): 1551–1556.

15 Schott, H.C. II (2004). Hematuria. In: *Equine Internal Medicine*, 2e (eds. S.M. Reed, W.M. Bayly and D.C. Sellon), 1270–1276. St Louis: Saunders.

16 LeRoy, B., Woolums, A., Wass, J. et al. (2011). The relationship between serum calcium concentration and outcome in horses with renal failure presented to referral hospitals. *J. Vet. Intern. Med.* 25 (6): 1426–1430.

17 Behr, M.J., Hackett, R.P., Bentinck-Smith, J. et al. (1981). Metabolic abnormalities associated with rupture of the urinary bladder in neonatal foals. *J. Am. Vet. Med. Assoc.* 178 (3): 263–266.

18 Dunkel, B., Palmer, J.E., Olson, K.N. et al. (2005). Uroperitoneum in 32 foals: influence of intravenous fluid therapy, infection, and sepsis. *J. Vet. Intern. Med.* 19 (6): 889–893.

19 Richardson, D.W. and Kohn, C.W. (1983). Uroperitoneum in the foal. *J. Am. Vet. Med. Assoc.* 182 (3): 267–271.

20 Walton, R.M. (2012). Subject-based reference values: biological variation, individuality, and reference change values. *Vet. Clin. Pathol.* 41 (2): 175–181.

7

Acid–Base and Electrolytes

Andrea A. Bohn

Department of Microbiology, Immunology, and Pathology, College of Veterinary Medicine and Biomedical Sciences, Colorado State University, Fort Collins, CO, USA

Evaluation of electrolyte concentrations and acid–base balance is typically used more to assess severity of disease and to guide treatment rather than as a diagnostic tool, although certain changes can aid in the diagnosis of some disorders. Abnormalities in electrolyte concentrations and acid–base balance are often associated with diarrhea, colic, rhabdomyolysis, prolonged exercise and sweating, renal disease, and endocrine abnormalities. This chapter will focus on acid–base and electrolyte changes commonly seen in horses and their causes.

7.1 Acid–Base

Maintaining the proper pH of blood and tissues is important for optimal enzymatic and cellular function. The normal pH range for horse blood is approximately 7.38–7.44. Below this range, the blood is acidemic and above the range it is alkalemic. Various processes are in place to help maintain normal pH. These involve the respiratory system, in which carbon dioxide (CO_2) is exhaled, the kidneys, where excess acids or bases can be excreted, and buffer systems, the most important of which for our purposes of evaluation is bicarbonate (HCO_3). An abnormality in acid–base balance is not a disease but a reflection of many possible disease processes. Evaluation of the acid–base status can give an indication that a serious problem exists.

Acid–base abnormalities are traditionally described as being either a respiratory acidosis or alkalosis or a metabolic acidosis or alkalosis. A primary disorder within one of these systems typically results in a compensatory response in the other. Since the respiratory system is concerned with CO_2 which is weakly acidic, and the metabolic system handles HCO_3, which is a weak base, the movement of the compensatory response should be in the same direction (up or down) as the primary disorder. To determine which is the primary disorder, one must look at the blood pH. If the blood is acidemic, the system that is moving in the acidic direction is the source of the primary disorder. If the blood is alkalemic, the system that is moving in the alkaline direction has the primary disorder. If both branches are moving in an alkaline or acidic direction, there is a mixed acid–base disorder. Likewise, if the compensatory side has shifted more than expected for a compensatory response, there is likely a mixed acid–base disorder. In those cases, the pH may be normal, even with marked acid–base abnormalities.

7.1.1 Steps to Evaluating Acid–Base Status

The following six-point approach to acid–base status is very useful for a complete characterization.

1) What is the blood pH? Is there an acidemia (<7.38 pH) or alkalemia (>7.44 pH)?
2) Is pCO_2 high (acidic) or low (alkalotic)?
   Is this contributing to the pH change?
   Is this a compensatory response?
3) Is HCO_3 low (acidic) or high (alkalotic)?
   Is this contributing to the pH change?
   Is this a compensatory response?
4) What is the anion gap (AG)?
5) What is the corrected chloride concentration?
6) What is the albumin concentration?

Bicarbonate and chloride (Cl) concentrations as well as AG are routinely provided within a serum biochemistry panel, which provides important information on the acid–base status of a horse. However, a complete characterization of acid–base status requires a full blood gas panel (preferably on arterial blood). AG, when increased, is

Equine Hematology, Cytology, and Clinical Chemistry, Second Edition.
Edited by Raquel M. Walton, Rick L. Cowell, and Amy C. Valenciano.

always an indication of metabolic acidosis. Bicarbonate and Cl concentrations also reflect acid–base status, but whether abnormalities in these substances are due to primary metabolic derangements, compensatory mechanisms in response to respiratory acid–base imbalances, or there is a mixed acid–base disturbance often cannot be determined without also knowing the pH and pCO_2 of the blood. Table 7.1 describes expected results for uncomplicated acid–base abnormalities.

7.1.2 Bicarbonate

Bicarbonate is an important buffer in the blood and its concentration therefore reflects the acid–base status of an animal. Changes in HCO_3 concentration can be due to metabolic derangements or compensation for respiratory acidosis or alkalosis. Bicarbonate concentration is typically reported either as total CO_2 (TCO_2), which is normally about 5% higher than HCO_3, or as HCO_3 concentration. In this chapter, bicarbonate will be designated as HCO_3.

Exposure of blood or serum to air can result in CO_2 release, which causes underestimation of HCO_3. In contrast, allowing blood to stand without exposure to air may result in overestimation of HCO_3 due to metabolic processes. Therefore, appropriate handling of blood samples is an important step in laboratory analysis.

7.1.3 Metabolic Acidosis and Alkalosis

7.1.3.1 Chloride-Associated Acid–Base Abnormalities

With primary metabolic acid–base abnormalities, when AG is normal (no increase in organic acids) changes in HCO_3 concentration are associated with a converse shift in Cl concentration. In this instance, the pH should reflect the HCO_3 and Cl concentrations and if there is respiratory compensation, the pCO_2 will have moved in the same direction (increased or decreased) as HCO_3. To determine that there is a primary metabolic acidosis or alkalosis with respiratory compensation or vice versa, it is again necessary to evaluate the pH and pCO_2. Hypochloremic metabolic alkalosis occurs when HCO_3 is retained in the blood as Cl is lost from or sequestered within the upper gastrointestinal (GI) tract or lost from excessive sweating. Hyperchloremic metabolic acidosis occurs when Cl is retained in response to HCO_3 loss from the intestinal tract or the kidneys (renal tubular acidosis).

7.1.3.2 Anion Gap

Bicarbonate is a very important buffer for endogenous and exogenous acids. Endogenous acids include lactic acid and uremic acids; ketoacids are common in other species but horses are poorly ketogenic. Exogenous acids include metabolites of ethylene glycol and salicylate. An increase in any of these acids results in a decrease in HCO_3 concentration as it buffers the hydrogen ion.

While there are methods to measure many of the acids that cause a metabolic acidosis, an easy way to determine their presence is by calculating the AG. The AG is based on the fact that the numbers of negative and positive charges in plasma are equal. We do not routinely measure all substances in the blood and there are therefore many unmeasured anions and cations present. The commonly measured cations are sodium (Na) and potassium (K) and the commonly measured anions are Cl and HCO_3. Because the sum of unmeasured and measured cations must equal the sum of unmeasured and measured anions in blood, we can determine the difference between the unmeasured components (AG) by calculating the difference between the measured components. And since the number of unmeasured

Table 7.1 Uncomplicated acid–base abnormalities and their expected changes.

Acid–base abnormality	pH	pCO_2	HCO_3	Cl	AG
High anion gap metabolic acidosis with respiratory compensation	L	L	L	N	H
Hyperchloremic metabolic acidosis with respiratory compensation	L	L	L	H	N
Hypochloremic metabolic alkalosis with respiratory compensation	H	H	H	L	N
Respiratory acidosis with metabolic compensation	L	H	H	L	N
Respiratory alkalosis with metabolic compensation	H	L	L	H	N

H, high; L, low; N, normal; AG, anion gap.

cations usually does not change significantly, any abnormality in AG is related to the number of anions.

A decrease in AG is associated with hypoalbuminemia since the predominant unmeasured anion in health is albumin. An increased AG indicates the presence of additional unmeasured anions in the blood; after HCO_3 buffers the hydrogen ion from excess endogenous or exogenous acids, the corresponding anion is left in circulation. Chloride concentration does not change with high AG metabolic acidosis since the decrease in negative charge from HCO_3 buffering is offset by the negative charge of the unmeasured anion present. Hypoalbuminemia can offset and mask the presence of other unmeasured anions when determined by AG.

7.1.4 Respiratory Acidosis and Alkalosis

Respiratory acidosis typically occurs with respiratory depression or pulmonary disease and the resulting decrease in the amount of CO_2 exhaled. Respiratory alkalosis occurs with hyperventilation (due to pain, anxiety, or iatrogenic means) as the result of increased amounts of CO_2 being exhaled.

The evaluation of the respiratory components of acid–base balance requires knowledge of blood pH and pCO_2. Since pCO_2 is acidic and HCO_3 is basic, a primary increase in pCO_2 is compensated by an increase in HCO_3 and a primary decrease in pCO_2 is compensated by a decrease in HCO_3. When there is a primary respiratory acidosis (increased pCO_2), HCO_3 is retained by the kidneys to compensate for the acidemia. When there is a primary respiratory alkalosis (decreased pCO_2), the kidneys increase HCO_3 excretion in compensation. As HCO_3 concentrations shift to compensate for respiratory acid–base imbalances, Cl concentrations shift in the opposite direction to maintain electrical neutrality.

7.1.5 Compensatory Mechanisms

If there are abnormalities in the acid–base balance from metabolic processes, the respiratory system can act quickly to blow off either more or less CO_2 to help maintain blood pH. This compensation can take place within minutes to hours. In general, for every 1 mEq of HCO_3 abnormality, the respiratory system is able to adjust by about 0.7 mmHg CO_2. The lungs blow off extra CO_2 to compensate for metabolic acidosis and they retain CO_2 to compensate for metabolic alkalosis.

Several hours to days are needed for the kidneys to respond to respiratory acidosis or alkalosis. The kidneys eventually excrete an increased amount of HCO_3 to compensate for respiratory alkalosis or retain an increased amount for respiratory acidosis. In respiratory acidosis, for every 10 mmHg increase in PCO_2, the HCO_3 concentration is expected to increase by 1–2 mEq in the acute phase and by 3–4 mEq if chronic. In respiratory alkalosis, for every 10 mmHg decrease in PCO_2, the HCO_3 concentration is expected to decrease by 2–3 mEq in the acute phase and by 4–6 mEq if chronic.

7.1.6 Base Excess

Other buffers in the blood besides HCO_3 include sulfates, phosphates, and hemoglobin, so the concentration of HCO_3 does not always reflect the total buffering capacity of the blood. Base excess (BE) is a reported value that indicates how far off from the normal total buffering capacity an animal is. Another way to think of it is that BE indicates how much acid needs to be added in order to bring the pH back to normal. In health, the reference interval of BE is about −4 to +4. Numbers less than −4 indicate a deficiency in anionic buffers (a negative BE) and therefore an acidosis, while numbers greater than +4 indicate an excess of anionic buffers and the presence of an alkalosis that may require addition of acid to bring the pH back to normal.

7.2 Electrolytes

7.2.1 Sodium

Sodium concentration and water balance are dependent on each other so when considering reasons for abnormalities in serum Na concentrations, one must also take into consideration water balance. Hydration status is typically determined by a combination of physical examination and laboratory assessments. Decreased skin turgor, increased capillary refill time, and tacky mucous membranes are subjective assessments of dehydration. Hemoconcentration is a result of dehydration that may be evidenced by detecting an increase in packed cell volume (PCV) and plasma protein concentration. Overhydration in horses is rare and typically does not occur unless there is decreased water excretion from the kidneys, which can be associated with renal, cardiac, or liver disorders. Psychogenic polydypsia can potentially lead to overhydration, but the renal system can usually handle increased water intake.

7.2.1.1 Hypernatremia

Hypernatremia occurs if there is excess Na (rare) or decreased water content (Table 7.2). The potential for excess Na exists if animals have access to and ingest salt without having access to fresh water. Inappropriate administration of hypertonic fluids can also lead to Na excess.

Table 7.2 Common causes of sodium and chloride abnormalities in horses.

Sodium
Hypernatremia
Dehydration
Insensible water loss
Diabetes insipidus (central or nephrogenic)
Hyponatremia
Hypertonic fluid loss or isotonic loss with water repletion
Gastrointestinal disease
Renal disease
Sweat loss
Electrolyte and fluid shifts due to third-spacing of fluids
Uroperitoneum
Severe hypoalbuminemia
Severe hepatic disease
Severe cardiac disease
Chloride
Hyperchloremia
See hypernatremia
Metabolic acidosis
HCO_3 loss or sequestration
Intestinal disease
Renal loss
Metabolic compensation for respiratory alkalosis
Hypochloremia
See hyponatremia
Metabolic alkalosis
HCO_3 retention with Cl loss/sequestration
Upper gastrointestinal obstruction
Sweat loss
Metabolic compensation for respiratory acidosis

Most causes of hypernatremia include either pure water loss or loss of hypotonic fluids where water loss is greater than electrolyte loss.

Pure water loss occurs with insensible water loss associated with evaporation from lungs and skin as well as fecal and urine water excretion. If insensible water losses are greater than water intake, serum Na concentration will increase. Increased water loss can occur with strenuous exercise, resulting in hypernatremia immediately post exercise. Decreased water intake can be due to an animal not having access to water or to a defective thirst response, as has been seen in horses with debilitating brain disease [1]. It must be remembered that serum Na concentration is related to the ratio of Na to water within vascular plasma and does not necessarily reflect the body's Na content. Hypernatremia may be present when there is decreased water intake and/or increased water loss even though total body Na concentrations may be depleted from excessive loss during sweating [2–4].

With renal disease, there is often loss of electrolytes along with decreased urine concentrating ability, but when there is a defect primarily associated with concentration, as with either central or nephrogenic diabetes insipidus (lack of antidiuretic hormone [ADH] activity), hypotonic fluid loss and hypernatremia can occur.

7.2.1.2 Hyponatremia

Hyponatremia most commonly occurs with loss of isotonic fluid and subsequent water repletion or, possibly, with loss of hypertonic fluid (more Na lost than water; see Table 7.2). Loss of isotonic fluid can result in hypovolemia, which stimulates renal water retention and thirst. Common sites of isotonic fluid loss include body cavities, intestinal tract, kidneys, and skin (sweating).

Many different digestive system disorders cause isotonic fluid loss, including diarrhea, sequestration of fluid in the GI tract with ileus or obstruction, gastric reflux, or esophageal obstruction and loss of saliva. Renal failure or diuresis can lead to sodium wasting into the urine. Hyponatremia is also often seen with uroperitoneum since the urine leaking into the abdominal cavity is of low Na concentration, which rapidly equilibrates with plasma Na [5]. Third-space fluid accumulation can lead to hyponatremia because of electrolyte and fluid shifts; hyponatremia can become pronounced with repeated removal of isotonic fluid from body cavities. If there is increased water intake and an ADH response, dilutional hyponatremia may ensue. Severe hypoalbuminemia, liver disease, or cardiac disease leading to third-spacing of fluids (edema) may result in mild hyponatremia due to water retention in excess of Na retention, especially if total body Na stores are decreased. Equine sweat contains a Na concentration that is equal to or slightly higher than that of blood [6] so sweat can be a source of significant Na loss, particularly with exercise. At high ambient temperatures, horses at rest are typically able to maintain normal Na levels but after an endurance race, plasma sodium concentrations were shown to drop [7].

Less common reasons for hyponatremia include iatrogenic hypoadrenocorticism, excess administration of Na-poor fluids, excessive water consumption, syndrome of inappropriate ADH secretion, and pseudohyponatremia. Pseudohyponatremia can occur if there are other substances causing hyperosmolality and drawing water into the vascular space, such as marked hyperglycemia or mannitol. Marked hyperlipidemia or hyperproteinemia can also result in pseudohyponatremia on some chemistry analyzers by taking up space within the plasma volume; using an ion-specific electrode to measure serum Na concentration will avoid this problem since it is not affected by protein or lipid content.

7.2.2 Chloride

7.2.2.1 Hyperchloremia and Hypochloremia with Water Imbalance

To maintain electrical neutrality, Cl typically moves either with Na or opposite to HCO_3. The factors that lead to hypernatremia and hyponatremia similarly affect Cl levels. To determine if the cause of hypochloremia or hyperchloremia is due to the same process affecting Na concentration, one can perform an easy calculation to "correct" Cl for the concentration of Na. This is done by dividing "normal" Na (typically a value from the middle of the reference interval) by the actual Na concentration and multiplying this result by the actual Cl concentration:

$$\frac{Na_{Reference}}{Na_{Measured}} \times Cl_{Measured} \tag{7.1}$$

This corrects for any water imbalance that is similarly affecting Na concentration. The corrected Cl is then interpreted in the context of the Cl reference interval. If Cl concentration does not correct into the reference interval (or if Na and Cl abnormalities are obviously disproportional), this suggests that there is an acid–base imbalance that should be reflected by a HCO_3 concentration that is inversely related to the Cl concentration.

7.2.2.2 Hyperchloremia Associated with Acid–Base Abnormalities

Hyperchloremia may be associated with metabolic acidosis or with metabolic compensation for respiratory alkalosis (see Table 7.2). Hyperchloremic metabolic acidosis is seen when there is HCO_3 loss from the intestinal tract or kidneys or sequestration of HCO_3 in the gut. Bicarbonate loss from the kidneys occurs in renal tubular acidosis, which is a rare condition in horses, in which there is decreased reabsorption of HCO_3 by renal tubules [8].

7.2.2.3 Hypochloremia with Acid–Base Abnormalities

Hypochloremia may be associated with metabolic alkalosis or metabolic compensation for respiratory acidosis (see Table 7.2). Metabolic alkalosis is often due to loss or sequestration of stomach contents. Since horses cannot vomit, hypochloremia with hyperbicarbonatemia should alert one to a possible upper GI obstruction, either physical or functional. Equine sweat contains up to twice as much Cl as in plasma and more Cl than Na [6]. Therefore, hypochloremia can become more severe than hyponatremia from sweat loss, leading to a metabolic alkalosis. Chloride losses are also greater than Na losses with furosemide diuresis [9].

7.2.3 Potassium

Potassium (K) is an important intracellular ion and less than 2% of total body K is free within plasma. Therefore, plasma concentrations of K are often not an accurate reflection of the whole-body content of K. Normally, the horse's diet is high in K and the kidneys are very efficient in excreting the excess [9]. Some K is also lost from the GI tract and in sweat. In addition, K can shift between the intracellular and extracellular compartments, resulting in higher or lower serum concentrations. Because equine erythrocytes contain a high concentration of K, serum concentrations of K may be erroneously high with hemolysis; this pseudohyperkalemia should be considered before other causes of hyperkalemia.

7.2.3.1 Hyperkalemia

Hyperkalemia is usually due to either the shifting of K from the intracellular to extracellular compartments or decreased excretion from the urinary system (Table 7.3). Decreased excretion is most commonly associated with anuric or oliguric renal failure or uroperitoneum. The extracellular movement of K is often a result of metabolic acidosis. Potassium is also released from muscle cells during exercise and hyperkalemia may be seen during and

Table 7.3 Common causes of potassium abnormalities in horses.

Potassium
Hyperkalemia
Decreased renal excretion
Metabolic acidosis
Release from muscle cells
Exercise
Rhabdomyolysis
HYPP attack
Hypokalemia
Dietary insufficiency
Loss
Gastrointestinal disease
Renal disease
Sweat loss

shortly after strenuous exercise [10–12]. Severe rhabdomyolysis can result in hyperkalemia because of release from damaged cells [13].

Hyperkalemic periodic paralysis (HYPP) is a genetic disease in which there is a mutation in a sodium channel, seen in quarter horses and some horses with quarter horse blood. HYPP attacks are associated with high serum K levels [14].

7.2.3.2 Hypokalemia

Hypokalemia can result from decreased intake as well as increased loss of K (see Table 7.3). Decreased intake may be due to a number of different causes associated with the quality or amount of food ingested. Loss of K occurs from the kidneys, GI tract, or sweat.

Alkalosis and insulin (often associated with IV administration of glucose-containing fluids) cause the intracellular movement of K and may result in hypokalemia regardless of whole-body potassium content.

7.2.4 Calcium

Calcium (Ca) is a very important electrolyte that is under tight hormonal control. Calcitonin, vitamin D, and parathyroid hormone (PTH) all act to maintain a narrow plasma Ca concentration from what is ingested, absorbed, and excreted by the GI tract, reabsorbed and excreted by the kidneys, and stored within the skeletal system.

Calcium concentration can be measured as total Ca (tCa) or as the ionized form (iCa). The concentration of Ca in its ionized form is what is physiologically relevant and under hormonal control. It is therefore preferable to measure the ionized form, which has become more available with point-of-care analyzers. The remaining Ca in circulation is either bound to albumin or complexed with anions and therefore the concentration of tCa can fluctuate depending on the amount of these other substances. Abnormalities in iCa concentration are typically related to dysregulation of hormonal control or excretion. The amount of iCa in circulation is also pH dependent since the pH determines how much Ca binds to proteins. Acidosis results in higher and alkalosis results in lower iCa concentrations.

7.2.4.1 Hypercalcemia

Hypercalcemia (Table 7.4) is common in horses with chronic renal failure and is thought to be associated with the high Ca content of the equine diet. The kidneys normally excrete a large amount of Ca and tCa concentration was higher in chronic renal failure (CRF) horses fed an alfalfa diet [15]. Reports of iCa in horses with CRF are limited, but in one study three out of three horses with CRF had high concentrations of iCa and low PTH [16].

Table 7.4 Common causes of calcium, magnesium, and phosphorus abnormalities.

Calcium
Hypercalcemia
Chronic renal failure
Humoral hypercalcemia of malignancy
Hypocalcemia
Hypoalbuminemia (only total Ca, not ionized Ca)
Lactation or transport tetany
Inflammatory mediators
Colic
Sepsis
Heavy exercise
Canthardin toxicity
Acute renal failure
Magnesium
Hypermagnesemia
Renal failure
Iatrogenic overdose
Hypomagnesemia
See hypocalcemia
Long-term parenteral or enteral support with low Mg
Phosphorus
Hyperphosphatemia
Acute renal failure
Release from damaged cells
Phosphate-containing enema
Dietary excess
Hypophosphatemia
Chronic renal failure
Humoral hypercalcemia of malignancy
Intracellular shifts

Hypercalcemia associated with neoplastic processes occurs in horses, as in other species, and has been reported with a variety of tumors, including lymphoma, multiple myeloma, and some carcinomas [17–25]. Humoral hypercalcemia of malignancy is often associated with PTHrP, a protein with PTH-like activity. Neoplasms that cause bony lysis can also result in hypercalcemia.

Less common causes of hypercalcemia include the ingestion of calcinogenic plants (*Cestrum diurnum*) or other means of vitamin D toxicosis, granulomatous disease, and primary hyperparathyroidism [26–28]. Primary hyperparathyroidism is associated with increased levels of PTH from a parathyroid adenoma or parathyroid hyperplasia, which results in hypercalcemia from increased absorption and hypophosphatemia due to a strong phosphaturic effect. Primary hyperparathyroidism has been reported in horses, ponies, and a mule [29–31].

7.2.4.2 Hypocalcemia

Hypocalcemia (see Table 7.4) is only relevant physiologically if pertaining to iCa. One of the more common causes of hypocalcemia is hypoalbuminemia, but this only affects tCa concentration; iCa concentration is unaffected. Clinical hypocalcemia, when acute, can be associated with synchronous diaphragmatic flutter, tetany, or ileus. Chronic hypocalcemia can lead to skeletal abnormalities. Hypocalcemia causing metabolic tetany most often occurs in horses that are lactating [32]. Metabolic tetany also can occur in horses that have been transported long distances [32]. In these horses, it is usually a combination of decreased feed intake and associated stress, as corticosteroids decrease activity of vitamin D and decrease Ca absorption.

Horses with colic are often hypocalcemic [32]. The pathogenesis is likely associated with endotoxemia and activation of inflammatory mediators that impair parathyroid gland function. Sepsis is also commonly associated with hypocalcemia, most often seen in foals [32]. The mechanism of hypocalcemia with sepsis includes parathyroid gland dysfunction, but is likely multifactorial.

Heavily exercised horses can become hypocalcemic via an unknown mechanism. Sweat contains Ca, so excessive sweating may be a factor [33]. In addition, metabolic alkalosis associated with exercise and sweating can result in lower concentrations of iCa due to increased binding to albumin and other anions. It has also been hypothesized that parathyroid gland dysfunction may play a role in exercise-induced hypocalcemia, although most horses participating in endurance rides had elevated levels of PTH in conjunction with low iCa concentrations [34].

Canthardin (blister beetle) toxicity is associated with severe hypocalcemia [35, 36]. While the underlying mechanism is not known, it is likely related to toxin-induced damage to mucosal surfaces of the GI and urinary systems [32]. Tissue damage associated with severe rhabdomyolysis may also cause hypocalcemia [13]. Although rare in horses, pancreatitis may cause hypocalcemia, likely due to saponification of peripancreatic fat [37, 38]. Oxalate toxicity can cause chronic hypocalcemia by decreasing the absorption of calcium from the GI tract through binding to oxalates [39]. Oxalate binding of dietary calcium is one potential cause of nutritional secondary hyperparathyroidism, resulting in dietary phosphate in excess of calcium [40].

Primary hypoparathyroidism is rare but has been described in foals and horses [41, 42]. Failure of the parathyroid gland to secrete adequate PTH results in hypocalcemia and hyperphosphatemia. Functional or acquired hypoparathyroidism is also associated with decreased excretion of PTH, but as a result of inflammatory mediators or magnesium deficiency and not a problem with the gland itself.

Iatrogenic hypocalcemia can occur with administration of furosemide or tetracyclines [32]. Loop diuretics result in calcium wasting in urine. Tetracyclines chelate Ca and can result in a transient hypocalcemia.

7.2.5 Magnesium

Magnesium (Mg) is a cation with a charge similar to calcium and is also present in the plasma as ionized, protein-bound, or complexed forms. Similar to Ca, the ionized form is the physiologically relevant form, the concentration of total Mg is influenced by the amount of albumin and complexing anions in circulation, and the concentration of the ionized form is pH dependent. Most Mg is intracellular with less than 1% of total body Mg in the extracellular fluid, so total Mg concentration may not reflect body content. Hemolysis can erroneously increase measured concentrations due to high intracellular Mg concentration.

Magnesium is absorbed from the GI tract. The kidneys are primarily responsible for excretion but there is also some excretion from the GI tract and mammary gland, as well as small amounts in sweat and the growing fetus. Magnesium is important in maintaining electrochemical gradients within excitable tissues and is used in hundreds of enzymatic reactions, including those involving ATP. Hypomagnesemia affects PTH production and secretion and can lead to hypocalcemia. Hypokalemia is also associated with hypomagnesemia as Mg is important in the action of the Na+/K+ ATPase pump [43].

7.2.5.1 Hypomagnesemia

Causes of hypomagnesemia are similar to those of hypocalcemia (see Table 7.4): lactation and transport over long distances (especially with decreased intake), excessive sweating, endotoxemia, sepsis, canthardin toxicity, and GI disorders. Long-term parenteral or enteral support that is deficient in Mg can also result in hypomagnesemia.

7.2.5.2 Hypermagnesemia

Hypermagnesemia most commonly occurs with either iatrogenic overdose, including with Epsom salts, or with renal failure (see Table 7.4) [43]. Given the high intracellular concentration of Mg, severe tissue damage associated with rhabdomyolysis or acute tumor lysis syndrome can result in hypermagnesemia, along with hyperkalemia and hyperphosphatemia.

7.2.6 Phosphate

The concentration of inorganic phosphorus (Pi) is traditionally interpreted along with Ca although it does not maintain as narrow a plasma concentration as Ca does. Serum Pi concentration is normally regulated by GI absorption and renal reabsorption. Vitamin D increases the intestinal and renal absorption of both Ca and Pi while PTH acts on the kidney to reabsorb Ca but increase the renal excretion of Pi. In addition, phosphatonin release from the intestine is dependent on the concentration of phosphates within the intestinal lumen and influences the rate of Pi excretion by the kidney. Phosphatonins (e.g., fibroblast growth factor 23 and secreted frizzled related protein 4) are a group of compounds that may act on multiple organs to regulate phosphate metabolism [44].

Phosphorus is the predominant intracellular anion and there can be rapid translocation between intracellular and extracellular pools. Therefore, in contrast to Ca, serum fluctuations in Pi concentrations are often associated with diet, age (higher in foals), physiological state, insulin/glucose status, energy utilization, and sample handling [45].

7.2.6.1 Hyperphosphatemia

Causes of hyperphosphatemia include acute renal failure, vitamin D toxicosis, and primary hypoparathyroidism (see Table 7.4). Massive tissue damage associated with rhabdomyolysis, acute tumor lysis, devitalized intestine, or hemolysis may result in hyperphosphatemia from release of intracellular Pi. Foals receiving phosphate-containing enemas can become hyperphosphatemic. Excess Pi in the diet or high Pi to Ca ratios can result in nutritional secondary hyperparathyroidism with hyperphosphatemia as the body attempts to maintain normal Ca levels.

7.2.6.2 Hypophosphatemia

While acute renal failure is more commonly associated with hyperphosphatemia, hypophosphatemia frequently occurs with chronic renal failure and hypercalcemia (see Table 7.4). Because of its phosphaturic action, primary hyperparathyroidism or PTHrP-associated hypercalcemia of malignancy results in hypophosphatemia.

Many causes of hypophosphatemia are due to shifting of the extracellular Pi to the intracellular space. This can occur with sepsis, refeeding syndrome, alkalosis, and hyperinsulinism, which is thought to be the mechanism associated with parenteral nutrition and hyperglycemia-induced hypophosphatemia [45].

References

1 Heath, S.E., Peter, A.T., Janovitz, E.B. et al. (1995). Ependymoma of the neurohypophysis and hypernatremia in a horse. *J. Am. Vet. Med. Assoc.* 207 (6): 738–741.

2 Flaminio, M.J. and Rush, B.R. (1998). Fluid and electrolyte balance in endurance horses. *Vet. Clin. North Am. Equine Pract.* 14 (1): 147–158.

3 Hyyppä, S. and Pösö, A.R. (1998). Fluid, electrolyte, and acid–base responses to exercise in racehorses. *Vet. Clin. North Am. Equine Pract.* 14 (1): 121–136.

4 Kingston, J.K. and Bayly, W.M. (1998). Effect of exercise on acid-base status of horses. *Vet. Clin. North Am. Equine Pract.* 14 (1): 61–73.

5 Dunkel, B., Palmer, J.E., Olson, K.N. et al. (2005). Uroperitoneum in 32 foals: influence of intravenous fluid therapy, infection, and sepsis. *J. Vet. Intern. Med.* 19 (6): 889–893.

6 McEwan Jenkinson, D., Elder, H.Y., and Bovell, D.L. (2006). Equine sweating and anhidrosis part 1 – equine sweating. *Vet. Dermatol.* 17 (6): 361–392.

7 Schott, H.C., Marlin, D.J., Geor, R.J. et al. (2006). Changes in selected physiological and laboratory measurements in elite horses competing in a 160 km endurance ride. *Equine Vet. J. Suppl.* 38 (36): 37–42.

8 Arroyo, L.G. and Stämpfli, H.R. (2007). Equine renal tubular disorders. *Vet. Clin. North Am. Equine Pract.* 23 (3): 631–639.

9 Johnson, P.J. (1995). Electrolyte and acid–base disturbances in the horse. *Vet. Clin. North Am. Equine Pract.* 11 (3): 491–514.

10 Harris, P. and Snow, D.H. (1988). The effects of high intensity exercise on the plasma concentration of lactate, potassium and other electrolytes. *Equine Vet. J.* 20 (2): 109–113.

11 Harris, P. and Snow, D.H. (1992). Plasma potassium and lactate concentrations in thoroughbred horses during exercise of varying intensity. *Equine Vet. J.* 24 (3): 220–225.

12 Nostell, K., Funkquist, P., Nyman, G. et al. (2006). The physiological responses to simulated race tests on a track and on a treadmill in standardbred trotters. *Equine Vet. J. Suppl.* 38 (36): 123–127.

13 Perkins, G., Valberg, S.J., Madigan, J.M. et al. (1998). Electrolyte disturbances in foals with severe rhabdomyolysis. *J. Vet. Intern. Med.* 12 (3): 173–177.

14 Aleman, M. (2008). A review of equine muscle disorders. *Neuromuscul. Disord.* 18 (4): 277–287.

15 LeRoy, B., Woolums, A., Wass, J. et al. (2011). The relationship between serum calcium concentration and outcome in horses with renal failure presented to referral hospitals. *J. Vet. Intern. Med.* 25 (6): 1426–1430.

16 Estepa, J.C., Garfia, B., Gao, P.R. et al. (2003). Validation and clinical utility of a novel immunoradiometric assay exclusively for biologically active whole parathyroid hormone in the horse. *Equine Vet. J.* 35 (3): 291–295.

17 Barton, M.H., Sharma, P., LeRoy, B.E., and Howerth, E.W. (2004). Hypercalcemia and high serum parathyroid hormone-related protein concentration in a horse with multiple myeloma. *J. Am. Vet. Med. Assoc.* 225 (3): 409–413.

18 Cook, G., Divers, T.J., and Rowland, P.H. (1995). Hypercalcaemia and erythrocytosis in a mare associated with a metastatic carcinoma. *Equine Vet. J.* 27 (4): 316–318.

19 Esplin, D.G. and Taylor, J.L. (1977). Hypercalcemia in a horse with lymphosarcoma. *J. Am. Vet. Med. Assoc.* 170 (2): 180–182.

20 Finley, M.R., Rebhun, W.C., Dee, A., and Langsetmo, I. (1998). Paraneoplastic pruritus and alopecia in a horse with diffuse lymphoma. *J. Am. Vet. Med. Assoc.* 213 (1): 102–104.

21 Fix, A.S. and Miller, L.D. (1987). Equine adrenocortical carcinoma with hypercalcemia. *Vet. Pathol.* 24 (2): 190–192.

22 Karcher, L.F., Le Net, J.L., Turner, B.F. et al. (1990). Pseudohyperparathyroidism in a mare associated with squamous cell carcinoma of the vulva. *Cornell Vet.* 80 (2): 153–162.

23 Mair, T.S., Yeo, S.P., and Lucke, V.M. (1990). Hypercalcaemia and soft tissue mineralisation associated with lymphosarcoma in two horses. *Vet. Rec.* 126 (5): 99–101.

24 Meuten, D.J., Price, S.M., Seiler, R.M., and Krook, L. (1978). Gastrict carcinoma with pseudohyperparathyroidism in a horse. *Cornell Vet.* 68 (2): 179–195.

25 Rosol, T.J., Nagode, L.A., Robertson, J.T. et al. (1994). Humoral hypercalcemia of malignancy associated with ameloblastoma in a horse. *J. Am. Vet. Med. Assoc.* 204 (12): 1930–1939.

26 Krook, L., Wasserman, R.H., Shively, J.N. et al. (1975). Hypercalcemia and calcinosis in Florida horses: implication of the shrub, Cestrum diurnum, as the causative agent. *Cornell Vet.* 65 (1): 26–56.

27 Muylle, E., Oyaert, W., de Roose, P., and van den Hende, C. (1974). Hypercalcaemia and mineralisation of non-osseous tissues in horses due to vitamin-D toxicity. *Zentralbl. Veterinarmed. A* 21 (8): 638–643.

28 Sellers, R.S., Toribio, R.E., and Blomme, E.A. (2001). Idiopathic systemic granulomatous disease and macrophage expression of PTHrP in a miniature pony. *J. Comp. Pathol.* 125 (2–3): 214–218.

29 Frank, N., Hawkins, J.F., Couëtil, L.L., and Raymond, J.T. (1998). Primary hyperparathyroidism with osteodystrophia fibrosa of the facial bones in a pony. *J. Am. Vet. Med. Assoc.* 212 (1): 84–86.

30 Peauroi, J.R., Fisher, D.J., Mohr, F.C., and Vivrette, S.L. (1998). Primary hyperparathyroidism caused by a functional parathyroid adenoma in a horse. *J. Am. Vet. Med. Assoc.* 212 (12): 1915–1918.

31 Wong, D., Sponseller, B., Miles, K. et al. (2004). Failure of technetium Tc 99m sestamibi scanning to detect abnormal parathyroid tissue in a horse and a mule with primary hyperparathyroidism. *J. Vet. Intern. Med.* 18 (4): 589–593.

32 Toribio, R.E. (2004). Calcium disorders. In: *Equine Internal Medicine*, 2e (eds. S.M. Reed, W.M. Bayly and D.C. Sellon), 1295–1326. St Louis.

33 Kerr, M.G. and Snow, D.H. (1983). Composition of sweat of the horse during prolonged epinephrine (adrenaline) infusion, heat exposure, and exercise. *Am. J. Vet. Res.* 44 (8): 1571–1577.

34 Aguilera-Tejero, E., Estepa, J.C., Lopez, I. et al. (2001). Plasma ionized calcium and parathyroid hormone concentrations in horses after endurance rides. *J. Am. Vet. Med. Assoc.* 219 (4): 488–490.

35 Helman, R.G. and Edwards, W.C. (1997). Clinical features of blister beetle poisoning in equids: 70 cases (1983–1996). *J. Am. Vet. Med. Assoc.* 211 (8): 1018–1021.

36 Schmitz, D.G. (1989). Cantharidin toxicosis in horses. *J. Vet. Intern. Med.* 3 (4): 208–215.

37 Bakos, Z., Krajcsovics, L., and Tóth, J. (2008). Successful medical treatment of acute pancreatitis in a horse. *Vet. Rec.* 162 (3): 95–96.

38 Ollivett, T.L., Divers, T.J., Cushing, T. et al. (2012). Acute pancreatitis in two five-day-old appaloosa foals. *Equine Vet. J. Suppl.* 44 (41): 96–99.

39 Laan, T.T., Spoorenberg, J.F., and van der Kolk, J.H. (2000). Hypocalcemia in a four-week-old foal. *Tijdschr. Diergeneeskd.* 125 (6): 185–187.

40 Estepa, J.C., Aguilera-Tejero, E., Zafra, R. et al. (2006). An unusual case of generalized soft-tissue mineralization in a suckling foal. *Vet. Pathol.* 43 (1): 64–67.

41 Durie, I., van Loon, G., Hesta, M. et al. (2010). Hypocalcemia caused by primary hypoparathyroidism in a 3-month-old filly. *J. Vet. Intern. Med.* 24 (2): 439–442.

42 Hudson, N.P., Church, D.B., Trevena, J. et al. (1999). Primary hypoparathyroidism in two horses. *Aust. Vet. J.* 77 (8): 504–508.

43 Stewart, A.J. (2011). Magnesium disorders in horses. *Vet. Clin. North Am. Equine Pract.* 27 (1): 149–163.

44 Shaikh, A., Berndt, T., and Kumar, R. (2008). Regulation of phosphate homeostasis by the phosphatonins and other novel mediators. *Pediatr. Nephrol.* 23 (8): 1203–1210.

45 Toribio, R.E. (2011). Disorders of calcium and phosphate metabolism in horses. *Vet. Clin. North Am. Equine Pract.* 27 (1): 129–147.

8

Proteins

Koranda A. Walsh

Department of Pathobiology, School of Veterinary Medicine, University of Pennsylvania, Philadelphia, PA, USA

Proteins are a vast array of molecules essential for an abundant variety of biological functions, which include serving as enzymes, antibodies, hormones, and carriers. Proteins are often combined with other substances including triglycerides or polysaccharides. The most clinically relevant plasma and serum proteins in the biochemistry of domestic animals include albumin, globulin, clotting factors, and acute-phase proteins (APPs) such as serum amyloid A (SAA) and fibrinogen. In contrast to plasma, serum does not contain clotting factors or fibrinogen.

Major plasma proteins are produced predominantly in the liver with some contribution from B-cells (immunoglobulins) [1]. B-cells produce immunoglobulins after appropriate stimulation in the presence of pathogens. Hepatocytes produce other proteins under the influence of various regulatory factors such as cytokines produced during inflammation. Other tissues (intestine, lung, adipose tissue, mammary gland, pituitary) are also capable of protein production under certain conditions [2, 3]. This chapter will discuss proteins, including APPs, and how they relate to the horse.

8.1 Acute-Phase Proteins

Aucte-phase proteins are defined as proteins whose plasma concentrations increase or decrease by at least 25% after an inflammatory stimulus [4]. They are a key component of an acute-phase response (APR) which is a highly complex response to multiple stimuli including inflammation, infection, trauma, stress, and/or neoplasia [1]. It acts as a component of the innate immune system serving to minimize tissue damage while enhancing healing and restoring homeostasis (Figure 8.1) [5–7].

Acute-phase proteins are generally classified as positive proteins (major, moderate, or minor) and negative proteins depending on whether values increase or decrease in response to a challenge. Positive major proteins have the following characteristics: low to undetectable concentrations in plasma during health; rapid plasma increases (>10-fold in concentration) after an APR; a large dynamic range; rapid decreases in concentration once disease has resolved; and increases following secondary infection or disease relapse. Positive moderate APPs are always present in the plasma of healthy horses and have the following characteristics: 5–10-fold increases in concentration in an APR and slower response (days to weeks) to an APR with a later increase, peak, and return to baseline [1, 8, 9]. Minor proteins increase slowly and to a small extent (less than 2-fold). The quantification of APP may provide valuable diagnostic and prognostic information. Negative APPs decrease during the APR (see albumin below).

The most commonly measured positive APPs in equine medicine include SAA (major APP), fibrinogen (moderate APP), and haptoglobin (Hp; moderate APP). Other relevant APPs include alpha-1-acid glycoprotein (AGP; minor APP) and C-reactive protein (CRP; minor APP) [9]. The most commonly measured negative APP is albumin (Table 8.1).

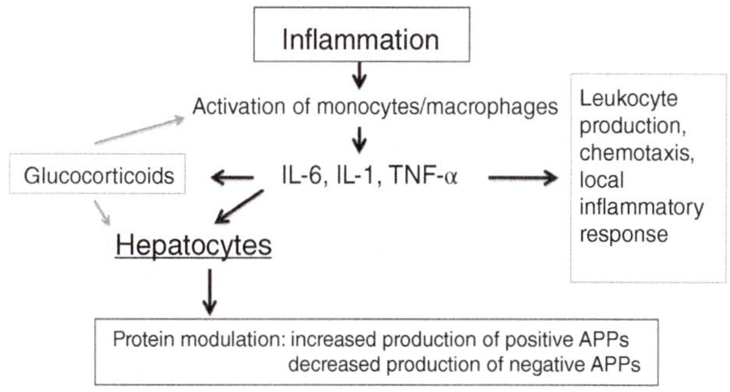

Figure 8.1 Schema depicting the acute-phase response.

Equine Hematology, Cytology, and Clinical Chemistry, Second Edition.
Edited by Raquel M. Walton, Rick L. Cowell, and Amy C. Valenciano.

Table 8.1 Common acute-phase proteins in the horse.

Positive APP			Negative APP
Major	**Moderate**	**Minor**	
SAA	Fibrinogen Haptoglobin	Alpha-1-acid glycoprotein C-reactive protein	Albumin

SAA, serum amyloid A; APP, acute-phase protein.

8.2 Albumin

Albumin, a water-soluble protein synthesized by the liver, makes up the vast majority of plasma proteins (35–50%) [1]. It plays a central role in the generation of colloid osmotic pressure and acts as a carrier for hormones, fatty acid, metal ions, and pharmaceutical products [10]. Its production is regulated by colloid osmotic pressure, as well as hormones such as insulin, thyroxine, and cortisol. In an APR, albumin is considered a negative APP. Hepatic production of albumin is thought to be downregulated in the APR due to amino acid demand to produce other APPs [11]. The half-life of albumin varies by species and is reported as 19.4 days in the horse [12].

There are several dye-binding assays available for the measurement of albumin. The most widely used dyes include bromocresol green (BCG) and bromocresol purple (BCP). The dye binds to albumin, thereby altering its absorbance and making it measureable via spectrophotometry. Dye-binding methods are considered accurate when albumin is within the reference interval, but the accuracy decreases when albumin is very low or high [1]. Interpretation of albumin is often combined with assessment of globulin (see below for interpretation of albumin and globulin).

8.3 Globulin

Globulins comprise a variety of proteins that can be separated, via protein electrophoresis, into several fractions: alpha-1, alpha-2, beta-1, beta-2, and gamma. Alpha- and beta-globulins are predominantly synthesized by the liver and include APPs as well as select immunoglobulins (i.e., IgM and IgA), which may extend away from the gamma-globulin fraction. The gamma-globulin fraction consists predominantly of immunoglobulins, which are produced by B-lymphocytes and plasma cells.

The simplest way to estimate the globulin fraction is to measure the total protein content of serum and subtract the albumin concentration. The globulin fraction can then be subdivided and the percentage of each fraction can be determined via electrophoretic methods. The most utilized method is serum protein electrophoresis (SPE) which is commonly performed using cellulose acetate or agarose gel. To decrease the complexity of interpretation, serum is used rather than plasma to exclude fibrinogen measurement.

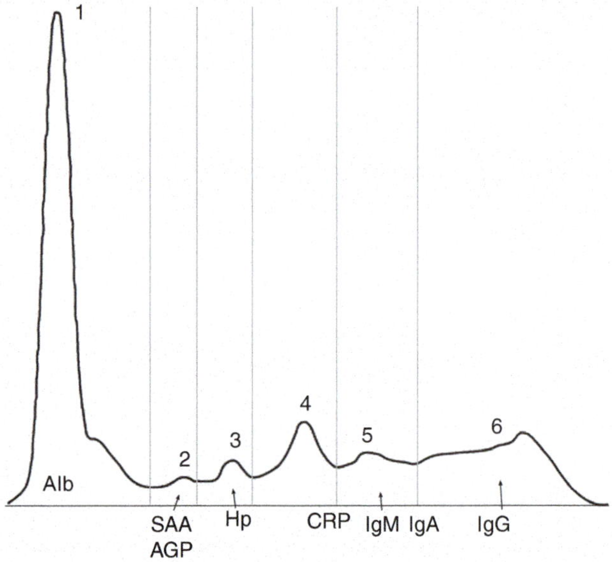

Figure 8.2 Serum electrophoretogram densitometer tracing from a healthy horse. 1. Albumin fraction. 2. Alpha-1-globulin fraction. 3. Alpha-2-globulin fraction. 4. Beta-1-globulin fraction. 5. Beta-2-globulin fraction. 6. Gamma-globulin fraction. Alb, albumin; AGP, alpha-1-acid glycoprotein; CRP, C-reactive protein; Hp, haptoglobin; SAA, serum amyloid A.

Principles of electrophoresis are discussed in detail in other major texts and will only be briefly addressed here. Electrophoresis is based on the movement of charged proteins within an electrical field. Proteins separate depending upon their size, shape, and charge, and the strength of the electric field. Negatively charged proteins move towards the positively charged electrode and away from the negative electrode. Once proteins are separated, they are stained and the proportion of each protein is estimated by densitometry. Computer software converts absorbance readings from the densitometer to a graphical representation and calculates the percentage of protein per fraction, leading to the depiction of peaks for each fraction. Albumin is represented by a large peak on the left (nearest the positive electrode) and is followed by alpha-1, alpha-2, beta-1, beta-2, and gamma fractions (Figure 8.2). Typically, agarose gel matrix electrophoresis results in these six protein fractions in horses, although in the literature the number of fractions ranges from four to nine depending on the interpretation of peaks [13].

8.4 Interpreting Albumin and Globulin Relative to Each Other

Albumin and globulin are often interpreted according to how they change relative to each other. Interpretation of altered protein concentrations depends on determining which fraction of proteins, albumin, or globulins, is altered. Causes for alterations in protein concentrations in the horse are summarized below.

8.4.1 Hypoalbuminemia with Hypoglobulinemia

Concurrent decreases in both albumin and globulin can be the result of proportional loss of both constituents, or less commonly result from dilution (e.g., excess antidiuretic hormone [ADH] secretion) [14]. Examples where both are lost proportionally include blood loss, protein-losing enteropathy, exudative skin disease, and plasma loss (e.g., vasculitis). In blood loss, albumin and globulins are lost proportionately and then diluted as fluid shifts from the extracellular space to the intracellular space in response to hypovolemia. Protein loss via the intestines results from a variety of intestinal lesions including ulceration, parasitism, bacterial infection (e.g., *Salmonella*, *Lawsonia*) [15], neoplasia, and inflammatory infiltrates. In these cases, both albumin and globulin leak into the intestinal tract and are lost in the feces or are degraded. Severe exudative skin disease, for example with burns, causes increased vascular permeability and loss of proteins. However, in severe cases, globulins may increase due to severe inflammation. In effusive disease (peritonitis, pleuritis, vasculitis), protein-rich fluids may accumulate in body cavities, resulting in decreases in albumin and globulin concentrations.

8.4.2 Hypoalbuminemia with Normal or Increased Globulins

Conditions that result in hypoalbuminemia with normal or increased globulins are due to either selective albumin loss or decreased albumin production. One cause of selective albumin loss is glomerular disease. Glomerulonephritis in the horse has been reported as mesangioproliferative, non-proliferative (membranous), or as membranoproliferative lesions [16–18]. The disease can be subclinical or clinical. Biochemical changes can include proteinuria, hematuria, hypoalbuminemia, and hypercholesterolemia.

Decreased albumin production from the liver can be the result of a negative APR whereby albumin is down-regulated [11]. Decreased production due to negative APP responses are mild [9]. Albumin production can also be decreased due to hepatic failure but typically not until 80% of functional liver mass is compromised [14] (see Chapter 5). This finding is often supported by other biochemical changes in liver function values such as hypocholesterolemia, low blood urea nitrogen (BUN), hyperbilirubinemia, and/or hypoglycemia. Because of the aforementioned half-life of albumin (approximately 19 days), low albumin is often uncommon unless the disease is a chronic process [19]. This can be true even when other functional parameters are affected. Starvation and/or malabsorption can lead to deficiencies in amino acids severe enough to compromise albumin production. Chronic gastrointestinal signs usually accompany malabsorption.

8.4.3 Hypoglobulinemia with Normal to Increased Albumin

The pattern of decreased globulin and normal to increased albumin is highly associated with decreases in the beta- or gamma-globulin fractions, typically due to decreased immunoglobulins. This can occur with failure of passive transfer (FPT) or immunodeficiencies. Passive transfer occurs when immunoglobulins (predominantly IgG) are transferred from the mare's colostrum through the semipermeable intestinal tract of the neonate. Failure to ingest or absorb sufficient colostrum results in FPT. FPT may be masked by concurrent inflammation or dehydration that can increase globulin levels. There are several tests for FPT, but the gold standard is considered to be the radial immunodiffusion assay (RID) for IgG. The majority of neonatal foals have serum IgG concentrations >800 mg/dL after absorption of sufficient colostrum; foals with concentrations <400 mg/dL are classified as having FPT and those between 800 and 400 mg/dL have partial FPT [20, 21].

Inherited or acquired immunodeficiency syndromes can result in low concentrations of immunoglobulins and in some cases low globulins. Diseases reported in foals include severe combined immunodeficiency (SCID), Fell pony syndrome, selective IgM deficiencies, and agammaglobulinemia [22].

8.4.4 Hyperalbuminemia

Hyperalbuminemia is primarily and most commonly caused by dehydration. Pseudohyperalbuminemia, however, can result from concentrations determined by BCG dye methods. While BCG preferentially binds to albumin, it can also bind some alpha- and beta-globulins. Additionally, it can bind fibrinogen in heparinized plasma samples (similar to canine data) [23].

8.4.5 Hyperalbuminemia and Hyperglobulinemia

The combination of both hyperalbuminemia and hyperglobulinemia is generally a result of dehydration; water loss causes relative increases in both constituents. Other considerations for selective hyperglobulinemia should be considered (see below). In the face of dehydration, concurrent increased or high normal red blood cell volumes should be expected (unless there is a concomitant anemia).

8.4.6 Hyperglobulinemia

The significance of hyperglobulinemia depends on which fraction is increased. The alpha-globulins include many of the APPs. AGP and alpha-1-antitrypsin migrate in the alpha-1 fraction while Hp, ceruloplasmin, alpha-2-lipoproteins (VLDL), and alpha-2-macroglobulin migrate in the alpha-2 fraction. Therefore, increases in the alpha-1 and alpha-2 fractions may be associated with acute inflammatory disease. Increases in the alpha-2 fraction can also be associated with nephrotic syndrome given that VLDLs can increase with this disease process.

Beta-globulins include beta-2 lipoproteins (LDL), IgM, IgA, and complement and are rarely increased independently of other fractions [7, 14]. Antigenic responses may increase complement and IgM in the beta fraction. Although most increases are polyclonal, occasionally there are monoclonal spikes, for example with multiple myeloma or lymphoma [24–27]. However, monoclonal gammopathies have also been noted in horses infected with intestinal parasites (*Strongylus vulgaris*, *Strongyloides westeri*) due to an increase in an equine-specific immunoglobulin, IgG(T) (a subclass of IgG found in the horse), found in the beta fraction [28]; IgG(T) can also migrate in the alpha-2 fraction on SPE [29].

Beta-gamma bridging is the phenomenon whereby there is no clear separation between beta and gamma fractions in conjunction with a decreased albumin to globulin ratio. Although historically beta-gamma bridging was thought to be pathognomonic for hepatic disease, a study evaluating the prevalence of hepatic disease in animals with beta-gamma bridging showed the finding is not specific for hepatic disease, and is found just as frequently with infectious disease [30].

Gamma-globulins include immunoglobulins of all types (though some immunoglobulins exhibit beta and alpha electrophoretic mobility) and CRP [14, 31]. Increased gamma-globulins with broad peaks are regarded as polyclonal gammopathies while those with sharp peaks are considered monoclonal gammopathies. The sharpness of a peak can be visually identified by comparing the width of the peak in question with the width of the albumin peak. Polyclonal gammopathies are a result of a heterogeneous group of plasma cells producing a mixture of immunoglobulins. Causes of polyclonal gammopathies include infectious disease and chronic inflammatory disease. Monoclonal spikes are the result of proliferation of a single clone of the B-lymphocyte lineage producing a homogeneous population of immunoglobulin, or its fragment, which migrate together [32]. The immunologically homogeneous protein is often called a paraprotein or M-protein, "M" for monoclonal. This type of gammopathy can be produced by neoplastic proliferations of B-cells or plasma cells (e.g., multiple myeloma, lymphoma, lymphocytic leukemia), some infectious diseases, and idiopathic conditions [24, 29, 33].

8.4.6.1 Serum Amyloid A

Serum amyloid A, a small hydrophobic protein produced predominantly by the liver, is found complexed with lipoproteins and comprises several different isoforms [34]. In the horse, the major isoform is SAA3, which can also be produced by mammary tissue [35, 36]. The physiological role of SAA is not completely understood, but it is highly conserved amongst mammals and may serve basic and essential roles in innate immunity [8]. SAA binds and opsonizes gram-negative bacteria, participates in leukocyte chemotaxis, inhibits oxidative burst, and may modulate connective tissue remodeling and repair [37–39]. SAA is the precursor of amyloid A and is implicated in the pathogenesis of amyloidosis, atherosclerosis, and rheumatoid arthritis in humans [39].

Multiple methods have been used to measure equine SAA, including ELISA, slide-reversed passive latex agglutination test, single radial immunodiffusion, latex agglutination immunoturbidimetric assays, and electroimmunoassays [35, 40–44]. A turbidimetric immunoassay for human SAA was noted to have excellent reactivity in horses [45]. The assay is based on binding of SAA to a latex conjugated mixture of rabbit polyclonal and mouse monoclonal antihuman SAA antibodies. The mixture causes a precipitate that can be measured turbidimetrically. Automated assays are available and are based on an automated latex agglutination turbidimetric immunoassay using monoclonal antihuman SAA antibodies [46]. A new stall-side test is also available from Stablelab which uses a proprietary, lateral-flow, membrane-based immunoassay [47]. The test is reported to have acceptable accuracy and precision in equine serum and plasma for SAA concentrations of up to at least 1000 mg/mL.

In healthy horses, a commonly accepted reference interval for SAA has been reported as 0–20 mg/L with no differences based on sex, but reported differences with age [48]. SAA is considered a sensitive indicator of the APR in horses and has a short half-life and a large dynamic range between resting levels in healthy patients versus those with infection or inflammation [35, 38, 43, 48–50]. SAA concentrations increase in as little as six hours after an inflammatory stimulus and decrease within 12 hours of resolution of the stimulus [45, 48]. It is considered to be a more sensitive indicator of inflammation than white blood cell (WBC) counts and fibrinogen [51]. Most commonly, immunoturbidometric and ELISA tests are used and it is recommended to compare SAA levels obtained during health with those obtained during disease. SAA can be helpful in detection of early disease but it is still a nonspecific parameter and should always be considered in the context of the clinical picture including history, physical exam, blood work, and any additional testing modalities.

Increases in SAA have been used in evaluating and monitoring a multitude of physiological states and disease processes including reproductive health and disease, respiratory diseases, orthopedic disease, gastrointestinal disease, neonatal sepsis, neurological disease [52], and changes due to exercise. A review of all uses for SAA is not provided here and the reader is referred instead to Witkowska-Piłaszewicz et al. [48] and Nolen-Walston [53].

8.4.6.2 Fibrinogen

Fibrinogen, a soluble plasma glycoprotein synthesized by the liver, is a large protein composed of a glycoprotein and two sets of three polypeptide chains joined by disulfide bridges [54]. It is converted to fibrin in the presence of thrombin and is essential for clotting. In addition to its role in clotting, it also binds to cell surface integrins (CD11/CD18) found on phagocytic cells, which initiates cell functions such as phagocytosis, degranulation, and antibody-dependent cytotoxicity [7].

In healthy horses, a reported reference interval is 200–400 mg/dL [9]. Concentrations of this moderate APP increase 1-10-fold over 24–72 hours during an APR and are reported to peak 72–144 hours after a stimulation of the APR [9]. Fibrinogen represents the largest proportion of plasma protein synthesized during an APR. It is considered a fairly insensitive indicator of inflammation, but the presence of increased values tends to be specific for inflammation [51].

There are several assays for fibrinogen, including quick estimation methods such as refractometry readings before and after heat precipitation, as well as ELISA-based methods. More precise methods include the Ratnoff–Menzies assay, clot weight measurement, and antifibrinogen antiserum with immunoprecipitate quantification and thrombin time [7].

8.4.6.2.1 Hyperfibrinogenemia The two main differentials for increased fibrinogen concentrations are dehydration and inflammation. The calculation of a plasma protein to fibrinogen ratio can be helpful in distinguishing between the two by eliminating the effect of hydration status. The ratio is simply performed by dividing the plasma protein value by the fibrinogen value once its units have been converted to g/dL. For the horse, a ratio ≥15 suggests dehydration and a ratio <15 is consistent with a true increase in fibrinogen secondary to inflammation. Concurrent dehydration and inflammation will obscure the clarity of the ratio. The ratio should not be performed on neonatal animals or those with concurrent hypoproteinemia.

While renal disease, especially glomerular disease, has been implicated in increased fibrinogen levels in cattle and dogs, it is not generally thought to be a cause of hyperfibrinogenemia in the horse. Neoplasia has been associated with increases in fibrinogen. Although data are lacking on this point, one study of clinical data associated with equine lymphoma reported that hyperfibrinogenemia was one of the most commonly noted abnormalities [27].

8.4.6.3 Haptoglobin

Haptoglobin, a glycoprotein produced primarily by hepatocytes, is composed of two alpha and two beta subunits [8]. The physiological role of Hp is to bind free hemoglobin (Hp–hemoglobin complex), which is then phagocytized by macrophages via the CD163 receptor, ultimately preventing iron loss [6]. Hemoglobin binding reduces the availability of iron and heme groups for bacterial use, contributing to Hp's indirect antibacterial activity [55]. Production of Hp is stimulated by free hemoglobin in the blood [56].

Equine Hp is laborious to assess and is generally assayed in research laboratories. Automated assays using cyanmethemoglobin are available and are based on Hp's strong affinity for hemoglobin [57]. Other assays, based on human Hp immunoturbidimetric assays, have been validated for use in horses [58]. Recently, a two-site heterogeneous immunoassay test kit has become available from LifeAssays® (Lund, Sweden). It is important to note that because Hp functions in binding hemoglobin, it may be consumed in cases of hemolysis.

Haptoglobin is considered a moderate APP in the horse which peaks 72–120 hours after a stimulus [9]. Hp increases in horses were noted after surgery, noninfectious arthritis, and carbohydrate-induced laminitis [35, 59, 60]. Hp was not shown to distinguish inflammatory airway disease (IAD) from other causes of exercise intolerance [61], and was shown to be a marker of both acute and chronic systemic inflammation in horses with heaves [62].

8.4.6.4 Alpha-1 Acid Glycoprotein

Alpha-1 AGP, one of the most heavily glycosylated proteins in serum, is produced by hepatocytes [63]. It is considered a moderate APP in most species due to its slow increase and prolonged elevation compared with major APPs and is associated with chronic rather than acute inflammation [1].

Acid glycoprotein has the ability to bind many endogenous metabolites including heparin, histamine, serotonin, steroids, and catecholamines [64]. AGP is involved in modulating the immune system reaction by inhibiting phagocytosis, neutrophil activation, and platelet aggregation and may have some role in T- and B-lymphocyte maturation [1]. Quantitative measurement is performed via single radial immunodiffusion with serum. In horses, AGP shows a peak value 2–3 days after castration or jejunostomy with return to baseline by 14–28 days post surgery [65].

8.4.6.5 C-reactive Protein

C-reactive protein, composed of five subunits, is a well-documented APP in dogs and, to a lesser extent, horses [7, 66]. It functions as an activator of the classic complement pathway, an inducer of pro- and antiinflammatory cytokines, and modulator of phagocytosis. Both an antibody-based ELISA test and a nonspecies-dependent assay based on a soybean oil–phosphocholine interaction have been validated in horses and verify that CRP is an APP in this species [67, 68].

Increases in equine CRP have been reported in arthritis, pneumonia, enteritis, and post castration [67]. In heaves, CRP was not shown to be a good marker of acute or chronic systemic inflammation [62].

References

1 Eckersall, P.D. (2008). Proteins, proteomics, and the dysproteinemias. In: *Clinical Biochemistry of Domestic Animals*, 6e (eds. J.J. Kaneko, J.W. Harvey and M.L. Bruss), 117–155. San Diego: Academic Press.

2 Eckersall, P.D., Young, F.J., McComb, C. et al. (2001). Acute phase proteins in serum and milk from dairy cows with clinical mastitis. *Vet. Rec.* 148 (2): 35–41.

3 Jacobsen, S., Niewold, T.A., Kornalijnslijper, E. et al. (2005). Kinetics of local and systemic isoforms of serum amyloid A in bovine mastitic milk. *Vet. Immunol. Immunopathol.* 104 (1–2): 21–31.

4 Gabay, C. and Kushner, I. (1999). Acute-phase proteins and other systemic responses to inflammation. *N. Engl. J. Med.* 340 (6): 448–454.

5 Beutler, B. (2004). Innate immunity: an overview. *Mol. Immunol.* 40 (12): 845–859.

6 Cray, C., Zaias, J., and Altman, N.H. (2009). Acute phase response in animals: a review. *Comp. Med.* 59 (6): 517–526.

7 Crisman, M.V., Scarratt, W.K., and Zimmerman, K.L. (2008). Blood proteins and inflammation in the horse. *Vet. Clin. North Am. Equine Pract.* 24 (2): 285–297.

8 Cray, C. (2012). Acute phase proteins in animals. *Prog. Mol. Biol. Transl. Sci.* 105: 113–150.

9 Jacobsen, S. (2007). Review of equine acute-phase proteins. *Proc. Am. Assoc. Equine Pract.* 53: 230–235.

10 Evans, T.W. (2002). Review article: albumin as a drug – biological effects of albumin unrelated to oncotic pressure. *Aliment. Pharmacol. Ther.* 16 (s5): 6–11.

11 Aldred, A. and Schreiber, G. (1993). The negative acute phase proteins. In: *Acute Phase Proteins: Molecular Biology, Biochemistry, and Clinical Applications* (eds. A. Mackiewicz, I. Kushner and H. Baumann), 686. Boca Raton: CRC Press.

12 Matteeuws, D.R., Kaneko, J.J., Loy, R.G. et al. (1966). Compartmentalization and turnover of 131-I-labeled albumin and gamma globulin in horses. *Am. J. Vet. Res.* 27 (118): 699–705.

13 Riond, B., Wenger-Riggenbach, B., Hofmann-Lehmann, R., and Lutz, H. (2009). Serum protein concentrations from clinically healthy horses determined by agarose gel electrophoresis. *Vet. Clin. Pathol.* 38 (1): 73–77.

14 Stockham, S.L. and Scott, M.A. (eds.) (2008). Proteins. In: *Fundamentals of Veterinary Clinical Pathology*, 2e, 370–413. Ames: Blackwell.

15 Bihr, T.P. (2003). Protein-losing enteropathy caused by *Lawsonia intracellularis* in a weanling foal. *Can. Vet. J.* 44 (1): 65–66.

16 Banks, K.L. and Henson, J.B. (1972). Immunologically mediated glomerulitis of horses. II. Antiglomerular basement membrane antibody and other mechanisms in spontaneous disease. *Lab. Invest.* 26 (6): 708–715.

17 Felippe, M. (ed.) (2016). Glomerulonephritis. In: *Equine Clinical Immunology*, 87–90. Ames: Wiley.

18 Waldvogel, A., Wild, P., and Wegmann, C. (1983). Membranoproliferative glomerulonephritis in a horse. *Vet. Pathol.* 20 (4): 500–503.

19 Parraga, M.E., Carlson, G.P., and Thurmond, M. (1995). Serum protein concentrations in horses with severe liver disease: a retrospective study and review of the literature. *J. Vet. Intern. Med.* 9 (3): 154–161.

20 Davis, R. and Siguère, S. (2005). Evaluation of five commercially available assays and measurement of serum total protein concentration via refractometry for

the diagnosis of failure of passive transfer of immunity in foals. *J. Am. Vet. Med. Assoc.* 227 (10): 1640–1645.

21 McClure, J.T., Miller, J., and DeLuca, J.L. (2003). Comparison of two ELISA screening tests and a non-commercial glutaraldehyde coagulation screening test for the detection of failure of passive transfer in neonatal foals. *Proc. Am. Assoc. Equine Pract.* 2003: 301–305.

22 Crisman, M.V. and Scarratt, W.K. (2008). Immunodeficiency disorders in horses. *Vet. Clin. North Am. Equine Pract.* 24 (2): 299–310.

23 Stokol, T., Tarrant, J.M., and Scarlett, J.M. (2001). Overestimation of canine albumin concentration with the bromcresol green method in heparinized plasma samples. *Vet. Clin. Pathol.* 30 (4): 170–176.

24 Edwards, D.F., Parker, J.W., Wilkinson, J.E., and Helman, R.G. (1993). Plasma cell myeloma in the horse. A case report and literature review. *J. Vet. Intern. Med.* 7 (3): 169–176.

25 Henry, M., Prasse, K., and White, S. (1989). Hemorrhagic diathesis caused by multiple myeloma in a three-month-old foal. *J. Am. Vet. Med. Assoc.* 194 (3): 392–394.

26 Meichner, K., Kraszeski, B.H., Durrant, J.R. et al. (2017). Extreme lymphocytosis with myelomonocytic morphology in a horse with diffuse large B-cell lymphoma. *Vet. Clin. Pathol.* 46 (1): 64–71.

27 Meyer, J., Delay, J., and Bienzle, D. (2006). Clinical, laboratory, and histopathologic features of equine lymphoma. *Vet. Pathol.* 43 (6): 914–924.

28 Mair, T.S., Cripps, P.J., and Ricketts, S.W. (1993). Diagnostic and prognostic value of serum protein electrophoresis in horses with chronic diarrhoea. *Equine Vet. J.* 25 (4): 324–326.

29 Kent, J.E. and Roberts, C.A. (1990). Serum protein changes in four horses with monoclonal gammopathy. *Equine Vet. J.* 22 (5): 373–376.

30 Camus, M.S., Krimer, P.M., Leroy, B.E., and Almy, F.S. (2010). Evaluation of the positive predictive value of serum protein electrophoresis beta-gamma bridging for hepatic disease in three domestic animal species. *Vet. Pathol.* 47 (6): 1064–1070.

31 Allison, R.W. (2012). Laboratory evaluation of plasma and serum proteins. In: *Veterinary Hematology and Clinical Chemistry*, 2e (eds. M.A. Thrall, M.G. Weiser, R.W. Allison and T.W. Campbell), 460–475. Ames: Wiley Blackwell.

32 Glavey, S.V. and Leung, N. (2016). Monoclonal gammopathy: the good, the bad and the ugly. *Blood Rev.* 30 (3): 223–231.

33 Traub-Dargatz, J., Bertone, A., Bennett, D. et al. (1985). Monoclonal aggregating immunoglobulin cryoglobulinaemia in a horse with malignant lymphoma. *Equine Vet. J.* 17 (6): 470–473.

34 Hultén, C., Sletten, K., Foyn Bruun, C., and Marhaug, G. (1997). The acute phase serum amyloid A protein (SAA) in the horse: isolation and characterization of three isoforms. *Vet. Immunol. Immunopathol.* 57 (3–4): 215–227.

35 Hultén, C., Grönlund, U., Hirvonen, J. et al. (2002). Dynamics in serum of the inflammatory markers serum amyloid A (SAA), haptoglobin, fibrinogen and alpha2-globulins during induced noninfectious arthritis in the horse. *Equine Vet. J.* 34 (7): 699–704.

36 McDonald, T.L., Larson, M.A., Mack, D.R., and Weber, A. (2001). Elevated extrahepatic expression and secretion of mammary-associated serum amyloid A 3 (M-SAA3) into colostrum. *Vet. Immunol. Immunopathol.* 83 (3–4): 203–211.

37 Hari-Dass, R., Shah, C., Meyer, D.J., and Raynes, J.G. (2005). Serum amyloid A protein binds to outer membrane protein A of gram-negative bacteria. *J. Biol. Chem.* 280 (19): 18562–18567.

38 Petersen, H.H., Nielsen, J.P., and Heegaard, P.M.H. (2004). Application of acute phase protein measurements in veterinary clinical chemistry. *Vet. Res.* 35 (2): 163–187.

39 Uhlar, C.M. and Whitehead, A.S. (1999). Serum amyloid A, the major vertebrate acute-phase reactant. *Eur. J. Biochem.* 265 (2): 501–523.

40 Chavatte, P.M., Pepys, M.B., Roberts, B. et al. (1991). Measurement of serum amyloid A protein (SAA) as an aid to differential diagnosis of infection in newborn foals. Private publication. Newmarket: R &W Publications, pp. 33–38.

41 Nunokawa, Y., Fujinaga, T., Taira, T. et al. (1993). Evaluation of serum amyloid A protein as an acute-phase reactive protein in horses. *J. Vet. Med. Sci.* 55 (6): 1011–1016.

42 Pepys, M.B., Baltz, M.L., Tennent, G.A. et al. (1989). Serum amyloid A protein (SAA) in horses: objective measurement of the acute phase response. *Equine Vet. J.* 21 (2): 106–109.

43 Stoneham, S.J., Palmer, L., Cash, R., and Rossdale, P.D. (2001). Measurement of serum amyloid A in the neonatal foal using a latex agglutination immunoturbidimetric assay: determination of the normal range, variation with age and response to disease. *Equine Vet. J.* 33 (6): 599–603.

44 Wakimoto, Y. (1996). Slide reversed passive latex agglutination test. A simple, rapid and practical method for equine serum amyloid A (SAA) protein determination. *Jpn. J. Vet. Res.* 44: 43.

45 Jacobsen, S., Kjelgaard-Hansen, M., Hagbard Petersen, H., and Jensen, A.L. (2006). Evaluation of a commercially available human serum amyloid A (SAA) turbidometric immunoassay for determination of equine SAA concentrations. *Vet. J.* 172 (2): 315–319.

46 Christensen, M., Jacobsen, S., Ichiyanagi, T., and Kjelgaard-Hansen, M. (2012). Evaluation of an automated assay based on monoclonal anti-human serum amyloid A (SAA) antibodies for measurement of canine, feline, and equine SAA. *Vet. J.* 194 (3): 332–337.

47 Schwartz, D., Pusterla, N., Jacobsen, S., and Christopher, M.M. (2018). Analytical validation of a new point-of-care assay for serum amyloid A in horses. *Equine Vet. J.* 50 (5): 678–683.

48 Witkowska-Piłaszewicz, O.D., Żmigrodzka, M., Winnicka, A. et al. (2019). Serum amyloid A in equine health and disease. *Equine Vet. J.* 51 (3): 293–298.

49 Belgrave, R.L., Dickey, M.M., Arheart, K.L., and Cray, C. (2013). Assessment of serum amyloid A testing of horses and its clinical application in a specialized equine practice. *J. Am. Vet. Med. Assoc.* 243 (1): 113–119.

50 Jacobsen, S. and Andersen, P.H. (2007). The acute phase protein serum amyloid A (SAA) as a marker of inflammation in horses. *Equine Vet. Educ.* 19 (1): 38–46.

51 Hooijberg, E.H., van den Hoven, R., Tichy, A., and Schwendenwein, I. (2014). Diagnostic and predictive capability of routine laboratory tests for the diagnosis and staging of equine inflammatory disease. *J. Vet. Intern. Med.* 28 (5): 1587–1593.

52 Mittelman, N.S., Stefanovski, D., and Johnson, A.L. (2018). Utility of C-reactive protein and serum amyloid A in the diagnosis of equine protozoal myeloencephalitis. *J. Vet. Intern. Med.* 32 (5): 1726–1730.

53 Nolen-Walston, R. (2015). How to interpret serum amyloid A concentrations. *Proc. Am. Assoc. Equine Pract.* 61: 130–137.

54 Mosesson, M.W. (2005). Fibrinogen and fibrin structure and functions. *J. Thromb. Haemost.* 3 (8): 1894–1904.

55 Theilgaard-Mönch, K., Jacobsen, L.C., Nielsen, M.J. et al. (2006). Haptoglobin is synthesized during granulocyte differentiation, stored in specific granules, and released by neutrophils in response to activation. *Blood* 108 (1): 353–361.

56 Levy, A.P., Asleh, R., Blum, S. et al. (2010). Haptoglobin: basic and clinical aspects. *Antioxid. Redox Signal.* 12 (2): 293–304.

57 Skinner, J.G. and Roberts, L. (1994). Haptoglobin as an indicator of infection in sheep. *Vet. Rec.* 134 (2): 33–36.

58 Wiedmeyer, C.E. and Solter, P.F. (1996). Validation of human haptoglobin immunoturbidimetric assay for detection of haptoglobin in equine and canine serum and plasma. *Vet. Clin. Pathol.* 25 (4): 141–146.

59 Fagliari, J.J., McClenahan, D., Evanson, O.A., and Weiss, D.J. (1998). Changes in plasma protein concentrations in ponies with experimentally induced alimentary laminitis. *Am. J. Vet. Res.* 59 (10): 1234–1237.

60 Kent, J.E. and Goodall, J. (1991). Assessment of an immunoturbidimetric method for measuring equine serum haptoglobin concentrations. *Equine Vet. J.* 23 (1): 59–66.

61 Leclere, M., Lavoie-Lamoureux, A., and Lavoie, J.P. (2015). Acute phase proteins in racehorses with inflammatory airway disease. *J. Vet. Intern. Med.* 29 (3): 940–945.

62 Lavoie-Lamoureux, A., Leclere, M., Lemos, K. et al. (2012). Markers of systemic inflammation in horses with heaves. *J. Vet. Intern. Med.* 26 (6): 1419–1426.

63 Fournier, T., Medjoubi-N, N., and Porquet, D. (2000). Alpha-1-acid glycoprotein. *Biochim. Biophys. Acta* 1482 (1–2): 157–171.

64 Israili, Z.H. and Dayton, P.G. (2001). Human alpha-1-glycoprotein and its interactions with drugs. *Drug Metab. Rev.* 33 (2): 161–235.

65 Taira, T., Fujinaga, T., Tamura, K. et al. (1992). Isolation and characterization of alpha 1-acid glycoprotein from horses, and its evaluation as an acute-phase reactive protein in horses. *Am. J. Vet. Res.* 53 (6): 961–965.

66 Yamashita, K., Fujinaga, T., Okumura, M. et al. (1991). Serum C-reactive protein (CRP) in horses: the effect of aging, sex, delivery and inflammations on its concentration. *J. Vet. Med. Sci.* 53 (6): 1019–1024.

67 Takiguchi, M., Fujinaga, T., Naiki, M. et al. (1990). Isolation, characterization, and quantitative analysis of C-reactive protein from horses. *Am. J. Vet. Res.* 51 (8): 1215–1220.

68 Tugirimana, P.L., de Clercq, D., Holderbeke, A.L. et al. (2011). A functional turbidimetric method to determine C-reactive protein in horses. *J. Vet. Diagn. Investig.* 23 (2): 308–311.

9

Laboratory Assessment of Lipid and Glucose Metabolism

Raquel M. Walton

IDEXX Laboratories, Inc., Langhorne, PA, USA

Acronyms and abbreviations that appear in this chapter include: BCS, body condition score; BM, body mass; DM, diabetes mellitus; GIT, gastrointestinal tract; GLUT, glucose transporter; HDL, high-density lipoprotein; ID, insulin dysregulation; LPL, lipoprotein lipase; LCFA, long chain fatty acids; LDL, low-density lipoprotein; NaF, sodium fluoride; NEFA, nonesterified fatty acids; PPID, pituitary pars intermedia dysfunction; PSSM, polysaccharide storage myopathy; VLDL, very low-density lipoprotein.

9.1 Lipids

Lipids perform a variety of roles in the body, ranging from energy storage to serving as major cell membrane components and polar solvents for fat-soluble vitamin and hormone transport. Of the many lipids present in mammals, only a very few are of clinical and diagnostic relevance. This chapter will discuss the primary lipid abnormalities encountered in equids and the methods for their diagnosis. A preliminary discussion of the types of lipids and their role in metabolism is necessary to adequately understand equine lipid disorders. Hyperlipidemias in horses are largely due to hypertriglyceridemia, so triglyceride metabolism will be emphasized.

9.1.1 Triglyceride Metabolism

Triglycerides are synthesized in intestinal enterocytes from three long chain fatty acids (LCFA) and one glycerol molecule that are absorbed following the digestion of dietary fats by pancreatic lipase (Figure 9.1). Within enterocytes, triglycerides are incorporated into chylomicron particles that are made water soluble by a protein and phospholipid coating. Chylomicrons are released first into lymphatics and then into blood via the thoracic duct. Lipoprotein lipase (LPL), produced by adipocytes and myocytes, translocates to the luminal surface of endothelium where it breaks down plasma triglycerides into LCFA and glycerol, which are extracted into fat and muscle. In nonruminants, glucose is the primary building block for LCFA used in triglyceride synthesis; acetate is used for LCFA synthesis in ruminants [1].

Insulin is involved in lipid metabolism by facilitating glucose uptake into adipocytes and myocytes and increasing LPL activity in endothelial tissue. Glucagon, corticosteroids, adrenocorticotropic hormone (ACTH), and epinephrine stimulate hormone-sensitive lipase in adipocytes to catalyze the hydrolysis of stored triglycerides and release nonesterified fatty acids (NEFA). Hyperinsulinemia promotes triglyceride production and increases adipose tissue, whereas glucagon and corticosteroids counteract these effects. When there is increased release of fatty acids from adipocytes, the NEFA not utilized by peripheral tissues are taken up by hepatocytes to be oxidized for energy, converted into ketones or used to synthesize triglycerides that are either stored or released as very low-density lipoprotein (VLDL). Thus, increases in circulating fatty acids contribute to hepatic triglyceride storage and hypertriglyceridemia via hepatic VLDL synthesis (Figure 9.2).

9.1.2 Laboratory Characterization of Lipid Metabolism

Lipids are a class of compounds that are soluble in organic solvents and insoluble in water. Lipid hydrolysis produces fatty acids or complex alcohols that can combine with fatty acids to form esters [2]. Hyperlipidemia and hyperlipemia are used synonymously to denote increases in serum or plasma lipid concentrations. By convention, lipemia refers to the gross appearance of serum or plasma when hypertriglyceridemia is present.

Equine Hematology, Cytology, and Clinical Chemistry, Second Edition.
Edited by Raquel M. Walton, Rick L. Cowell, and Amy C. Valenciano.

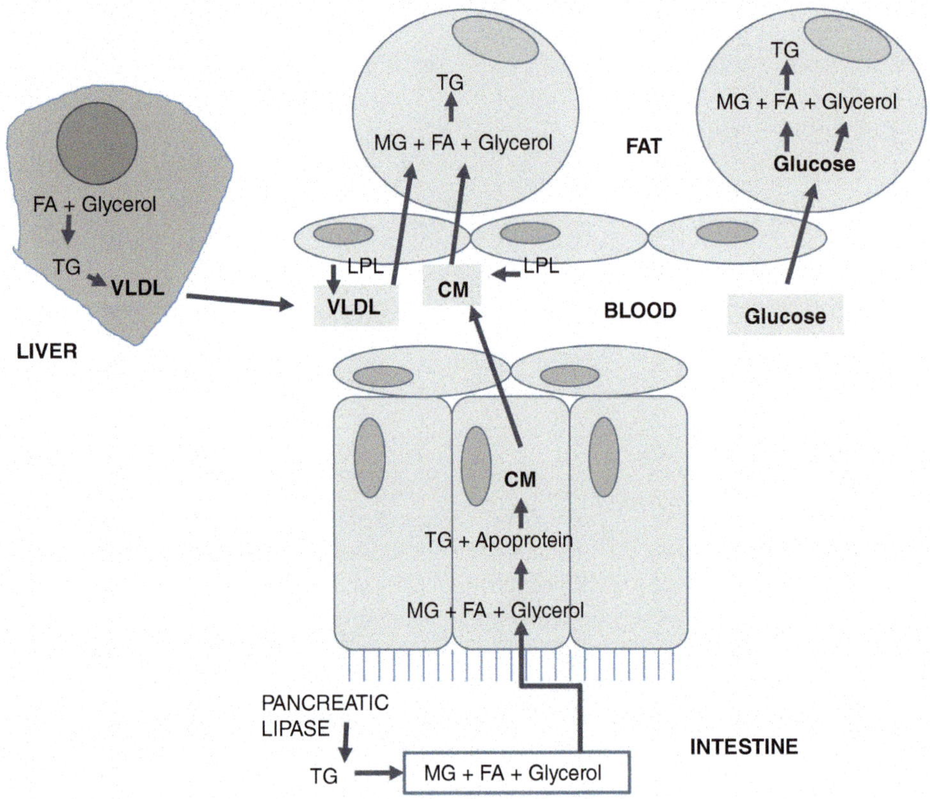

Figure 9.1 Overview of triglyceride (TG) metabolism. TGs are synthesized in enterocytes or in the liver. TGs of dietary origin are synthesized in the intestine from monoglycerides (MG), long chain fatty acids (FA), and glycerol broken down from dietary fats by pancreatic lipase. Within enterocytes, triglycerides are incorporated into chylomicron (CM) particles that are released first into lymphatics and then into blood via the thoracic duct. In the liver, TGs are synthesized and released as very low-density lipoproteins (VLDLs). Lipoprotein lipase (LPL) on the luminal surface of endothelium breaks down plasma triglycerides (in the form of chylomicrons or VLDLs) into FA and glycerol, which are taken up by muscle and fat. In nonruminants, glucose is the primary building block for FAs used in triglyceride synthesis.

9.1.2.1 Lipoproteins

The two principal lipids measured in animals are triglycerides and cholesterol. All triglycerides and the majority of cholesterol are carried within lipoproteins. Lipoproteins are classified according to their relative density, which is dependent upon their composition. The classes of lipoproteins include VLDL, low-density (LDL), and high-density (HDL) lipoproteins. The lipoprotein core is hydrophobic and consists of triglyceride and cholesterol ester molecules surrounded by a hydrophilic membrane composed of proteins (apoproteins), phospholipids, and unesterified cholesterol molecules. Lipoproteins are measured after they are separated using electrophoresis or ultracentrifugation.

The predominant lipoprotein in horses is HDL, comprising 61% of the total plasma lipoprotein mass, with VLDL and LDL comprising 24% and 15%, respectively. Similar to humans, VLDL is triglyceride rich, whereas LDL is cholesterol rich and HDL is protein rich. Normal concentrations of VLDL and total triglyceride are reported to be higher in Shetland ponies than Thoroughbred horses [3]. Although lipoprotein fractions are not typically measured in veterinary medicine, they may be of diagnostic utility in metabolic syndrome (discussed below) [4].

9.1.2.2 Nonesterified Fatty Acids

Glucose is the most important precursor of LCFA in nonruminants, whereas acetate is used in ruminants. As hindgut fermenters, horses absorb short chain fatty acids (acetate, propionate, and butyrate) from insoluble carbohydrates. Horses can readily shift from using glucose-based LCFA synthesis in diets high in soluble carbohydrates to acetate-based synthesis when fed high-roughage diets [5, 6].

Following triglyceride hydrolysis in adipocytes, LCFA are released into circulation as NEFA bound to albumin. Typically, NEFA are produced in response to energy demand, thus increased concentrations are considered an indicator of negative energy balance. Concentrations of NEFA increase with stress, exercise, and low blood glucose as a result of hormonal stimulation of adipocyte lipase (Figure 9.2). Accordingly, care should be taken to

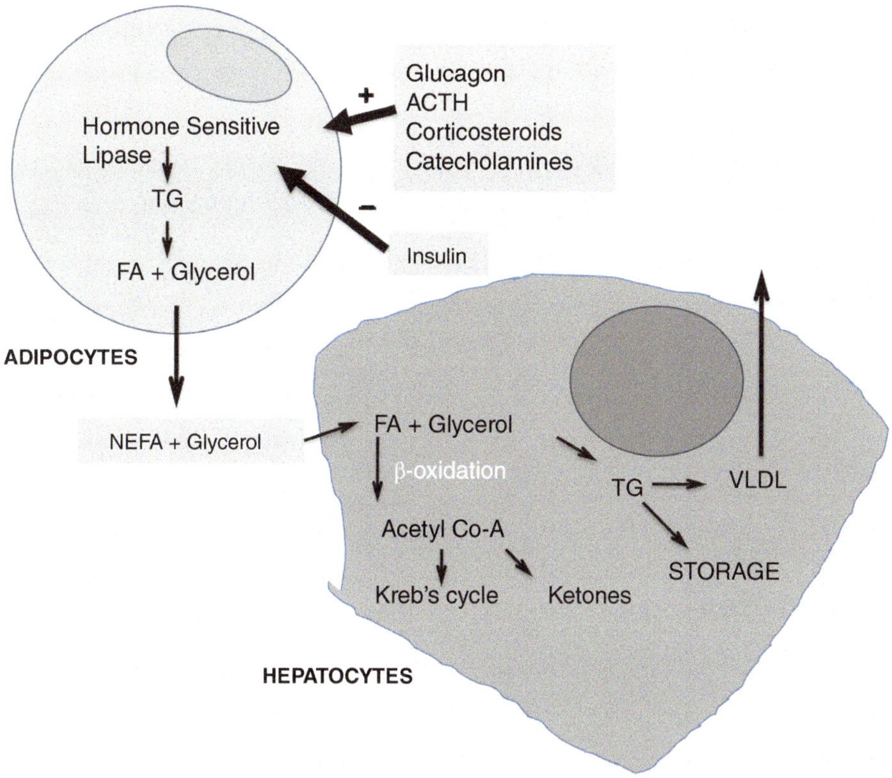

Figure 9.2 Hormone effects on triglyceride (TG) metabolism. Insulin inhibits the breakdown of TGs into nonesterified fatty acids (NEFA) and promotes triglyceride production and increases adipose tissue. Glucocorticoids, ACTH, glucagon, and catecholamines are insulin antagonists that stimulate hormone-sensitive lipase to break down TG into NEFA and glycerol. The increased concentrations of NEFA are taken up by hepatocytes to be oxidized for energy, converted into ketones, or used to synthesize triglycerides that are either stored in the liver or released as VLDL.

minimize excitement and exercise should be restricted in the period immediately before sampling.

Serum or plasma can be used for measurement but heparin anticoagulant should be avoided since it can increase NEFA concentrations during storage. NEFA concentrations are stable in whole blood for 24 hours and in separated serum or plasma for 72 hours as long as the samples are kept at 4 °C; storage at room temperature results in increased NEFA concentrations. Because of the instability of NEFA concentrations, NEFAs are best measured in situations in which the sample can be kept cool and submitted to a diagnostic laboratory relatively quickly.

9.1.2.3 Triglycerides

Circulating triglycerides are present within lipoproteins produced by the liver (VLDL) or intestinal enterocytes (chylomicrons). Triglyceride concentration is preferentially measured in serum and is stable for up to a week at 4 °C, for three months at −20 °C, and for years at −70 °C. Triglycerides are made of three LCFA and a glycerol molecule. Most assays for serum triglycerides use a reaction with a lipase to release glycerol from triglycerides; it is the glycerol that is measured following a coupling reaction with a substance that can be detected spectrophotometrically. Triglycerides should be measured on fasting samples (minimum of 12 hours). Triglycerides are usually reported in mg/dL. To convert into SI units (mmol/L), the concentration in mg/dL is multiplied by a factor of 0.01129.

The gross appearance of lipid in plasma or serum, termed lipemia, is only caused by increased concentrations of triglyceride-rich lipoproteins (chylomicrons and VLDL). Thus, an estimate of triglyceride concentration can be determined visually (Figure 9.3). Serum or plasma that is clear indicates that the triglyceride concentration is <200 mg/dL (2.26 mmol/L); serum with triglyceride concentrations around 300 mg/d: (3.39 mmol/L) appears hazy-turbid, whereas triglycerides >600 mg/dL (6.77 mmol/L) impart an opaque, milky appearance [2]. It is of interest to note that serum triglyceride concentrations exceeding 500 mg/dL (5.65 mmol/L) have been associated with no visible evidence of lipemia in horses [7]. However, the authors may have ignored a hazy-turbid appearance as not consistent with the classic milky appearance associated with lipemia.

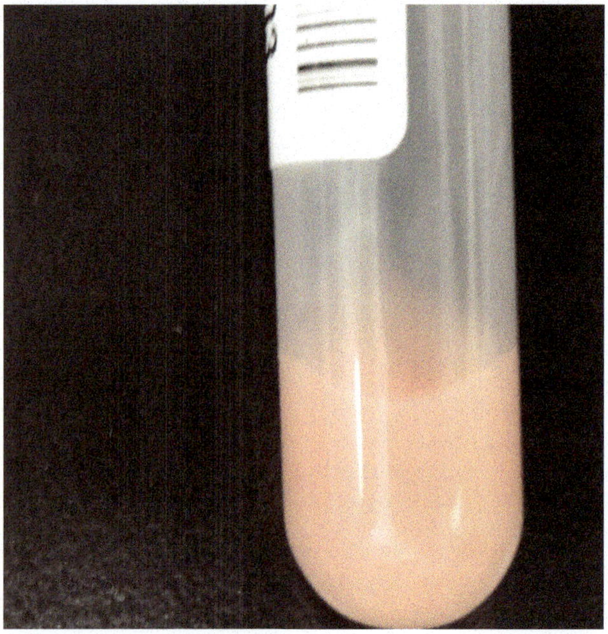

Figure 9.3 Lipemic serum is opaque and white to pink. The pink tinge is commonly due to mild hemolysis that often occurs with lipemic serum.

The presence of chylomicrons is indicated when a creamy, homogeneous layer floating on the surface of plasma or serum appears after refrigeration for several hours. If only chylomicrons are present, the serum below the floating lipid layer is clear. In contrast, lipemia attributable to increases in VLDL produces turbid or milky serum that persists after refrigeration. Fasting lipemia is due to the presence of VLDL, whereas postprandial lipemia is associated with chylomicronemia.

9.1.2.4 Cholesterol

Measurement of cholesterol includes total cholesterol derived mainly from cholesterol-rich lipoproteins LDL and HDL. Like triglycerides, cholesterol can be synthesized in the liver or absorbed from dietary sources in the intestine. Cholesterol concentration is stable for a week at 4 °C, for three months at −20 °C, and for years at −70 °C. Measurement involves hydrolysis of cholesterol esters to produce cholesterol. Added cholesterol oxidase produces hydrogen peroxide, which reacts with an indicator dye for spectrophotometric analysis. Cholesterol can be measured in fasted or nonfasted samples.

9.1.3 Equine Hyperlipidemias

The laboratory definition of hyperlipidemia is an increase in measurable serum lipids, which in horses are usually triglycerides. Diagnosis of hyperlipidemia is dependent upon measurement of serum triglyceride concentration. By convention, equine hyperlipidemias are clinically classified in the following manner: *hyperlipidemia* is characterized by serum triglyceride concentrations from 100 to 500 mg/dL (1.13–5.65 mmol/L) without gross lipemia or clinical signs; *hyperlipemia* is defined as a serum triglyceride concentration more than 500 mg/dL (5.65 mmol/L) with visible lipemia and fatty infiltration of the liver and/or other organs [7, 8]. Hyperlipidemia is usually associated with insufficient food intake and is often unnoticed because it is subclinical.

These categorizations use 100 mg/dL as the cut-off for the lower reference value. Different laboratories and different species under varying conditions will have different cut-off values for hyperlipidemia and hyperlipemia. For example, normal triglyceride concentrations in horses and nonpregnant ponies are often reported as <100 mg/dL, but reference values for ponies during the last trimester of pregnancy concentrations can reach 250 mg/dL (2.83 mmol/L). In one study, concentrations of up to 390 mg/dL (4.4 mmol/L) are reported for healthy donkeys [9]. Thus, hyperlipidemia and hyperlipemia should be defined using the lower end of the reference interval established by the laboratory producing the results.

Hyperlipidemia is typically associated with periods of negative energy balance (e.g., hypophagia, pregnancy, lactation), but is also linked to obesity, stress, sex, and breed. The pathogenesis of equine hyperlipemia lies in disturbances in energy metabolism compounded with insulin resistance. Insulin resistance is the cell's diminished capacity to transport glucose from the blood into peripheral tissues in response to insulin (discussed further in the next section). In the context of insulin resistance, development of a negative energy balance results in excessive and inappropriate mobilization of fatty acids that accumulate in the liver as triglycerides and in the blood as VLDL. The increase in plasma triglyceride and NEFA concentrations can interfere with insulin's inhibition of hormone-sensitive lipase, contributing to increased lipolysis. Catecholamines, cortisol, and ACTH, all of which are increased in illness, also stimulate LPL. The hyperlipemia results in accumulation of fatty acid metabolites in myocytes that can interfere with insulin-mediated glucose transport into cells, enhancing insulin resistance [10]. Concomitant azotemia may inhibit LPL activity, further exacerbating the lipidemia [11]. The ensuing self-perpetuating hyperlipemia results in tissue lipidosis and ultimately organ dysfunction and failure. Many of the biochemical abnormalities present in hyperlipemia (other than the hypertriglyceridemia itself) can be attributed to either a primary disease process that precipitated hyperlipemia and/or to organ dysfunction/failure caused by lipidosis.

9.1.3.1 Hyperlipemia in Ponies, Miniature Horses, and Donkeys

There is a high prevalence of hyperlipemia in pony breeds, especially Shetland ponies, miniature horses, and donkeys. Female ponies show a higher prevalence than males, representing 75% or more of cases [8]. In ponies, hyperlipemia is more prevalent in reproductively active mares, with increased incidence in late pregnancy and early lactation. The increased prevalence of hyperlipemia in female miniature breeds and donkeys applies to both reproductively active and inactive mares [8, 9]. Prevalence reports range from 3–5% up to 11% in the general population and are even higher in hospitalized patients (up to 18%) [9, 12].

Hyperlipemia frequently occurs secondary to primary disease processes such as enterocolitis/colitis and colic that produce a negative energy balance and affect insulin sensitivity (see section on insulin resistance below). In miniature horses, hyperlipemia develops consequent to a primary disease in the vast majority of cases. In contrast, ponies and donkeys can present with primary hyperlipemia; stress and obesity are predisposing factors. Both stress and obesity induce decreases in insulin sensitivity, which is considered the primary predisposing factor. There appears to be a genetic predisposition in the case of Shetland ponies.

9.1.3.2 Horse Hyperlipidemias

Hyperlipidemia (triglyceride concentrations above the reference value limit but without gross lipemia or associated illness) is reported in horses, usually as a result of inadequate food intake. Hyperlipidemia/hypertriglyceridemia due to fasting in horses is reported to range from 100 to 300 mg/dL [7]. In contrast, hyperlipemia, defined as marked increases in serum triglyceride concentrations (e.g., >500 mg/dL) with gross lipemia and clinical illness, is uncommon in large-breed horses compared to ponies, small breeds, and donkeys [13, 14]. A third hyperlipidemic category of marked hypertriglyceridemia (>500 mg/dL) associated with clinical signs but *without* visual evidence of plasma lipemia, has been described [7]. The absence of plasma lipemia distinguishes this disorder from hyperlipemia. It is uncertain why this magnitude of hypertriglyceridemia does not cause visible plasma turbidity or opacity given that triglyceride concentrations >300 gm/dL should cause turbidity and concentrations >600 mg/dL should impart a milky appearance.

Cases of severe hypertriglyceridemia without visible lipemia were associated with systemic inflammatory response syndrome (SIRS), which is defined as presence of two or more of the following abnormalities: fever or hypothermia, tachycardia, tachypnea or hypocapnia, leukocytosis, leukopenia or greater than 10% immature granulocytes (left shift). All horses had one or more primary disease processes and were off feed, and many were azotemic. Thus, most of the factors contributing to the pathogenesis of hyperlipemia were present. A prevalence of 0.6% over the course of a two-year period was reported [7].

9.1.3.3 Equine Metabolic Syndrome

Metabolic syndrome in horses is primarily a disorder of insulin dysregulation (ID) and is discussed in this context in the next section. Equine metabolic syndrome (EMS) is not a disease but rather a combination of factors that imply increased susceptibility to laminitis. The primary components defining the syndrome include obesity (generalized or localized), hyperinsulinemia, and insulin resistance with a predisposition to the development of laminitis. Another main component of EMS is mild hypertriglyceridemia (including increased VLDL concentrations). Hypertriglyceridemia is more commonly seen in ponies than horses with EMS [15]. In humans, hypertriglyceridemia with *decreased* HDL cholesterol concentrations is used as a criterion in the diagnosis of metabolic syndrome. Interestingly, horses with EMS have hypertriglyceridemia (VLDL and VLDL triglycerides) with *increased* HDL cholesterol [4]. A positive correlation between plasma HDL and triglyceride concentrations has also been detected in Shetland ponies [16]. It is postulated that this is a result of the near absence of cholesterol ester transfer protein activity in equine blood. Cholesterol ester transfer protein catalyzes transfer of cholesterol from HDL to VLDL in humans. Thus, in humans, triglyceride carried by VLDLs is exchanged for cholesterol when VLDLs interact with HDL in the blood and, as VLDL concentrations increase, interactions with HDL increase and HDL cholesterol concentrations decrease.

Hypertriglyceridemia has been found to be a significant predictor of laminitis in ponies with cut-off values from 0.64 to 1.06 mmol/L (57–94 mg/dL) [17, 18]. However, triglycerides are correlated with body condition score (BCS); not all obese horses have EMS and cases of EMS in lean horses are reported. Consequently, triglycerides may not be a very specific marker of ID and therefore may not be as valuable in the prediction of laminitis [19].

Obese horses with insulin resistance also have increased blood NEFA concentrations [4]. The NEFA concentration increases with obesity because adipose tissues reach their maximum capacity for fat storage and insulin's inhibitory effects on hormone-sensitive lipase are reduced. As a result, the influx of fatty acids into tissues increases, which causes an accumulation of fatty acid metabolites that interfere with insulin receptor signaling, thereby enhancing insulin resistance. Increased uptake of fatty acids by the liver increases the availability of triglyceride for VLDL synthesis, which is part of the mechanism of hypertriglyceridemia associated with insulin resistance. Increased VLDL production has been associated with feed deprivation and hyperlipemia in horses, which are conditions that develop in response to increased mobilization of NEFA from adipose stores.

9.2 Glucose

In addition to lipids, the other principal component in energy metabolism in mammals is glucose. Glucose is produced in the liver and, to a lesser extent, in the kidney or is absorbed from dietary sources. Production of glucose is accomplished primarily in the liver through gluconeogenesis and glycogenolysis. In nonruminant species, glucose is manufactured using mainly amino acids. The volatile fatty acid propionate, absorbed in the rumen or hindgut, provides the major building block for *de novo* glucose synthesis in ruminants. As a hindgut fermenter, the horse can use either amino acids or propionate in gluconeogenesis [20]. Equids rely heavily on gluconeogenesis to maintain blood glucose concentrations due to limited stores of glycogen. During negative energy balance, protein catabolism increases to provide amino acids for gluconeogenesis.

9.2.1 Glucose Metabolism

There are multiple hormones whose actions result in increases in plasma glucose concentration and one principal hormone that decreases blood glucose. Normoglycemia is the result of the interactions of multiple hormones, but the two primary processes responsible for glucose homeostasis are insulin secretion by pancreatic beta-cells in response to blood glucose concentration and the response of skeletal muscle and adipose tissue to insulin concentrations. Insulin decreases blood glucose concentrations by promoting cellular uptake, utilization, or storage and by inhibiting hepatic gluconeogenesis (Figure 9.4). Glucagon and catecholamines increase blood glucose by stimulating glycogenolysis; glucagon and corticosteroids stimulate gluconeogenesis; and glucagon and corticosteroids inhibit insulin activity at the receptor and postreceptor level. Catecholamines inhibit insulin secretion, stimulate glucagon release, and inhibit insulin activity at the postreceptor level. The effects of these hormones on fat metabolism were described previously (Figure 9.2).

After a meal, insulin is released from pancreatic beta-cells to facilitate glucose uptake by fat and muscle tissue via the GLUT-4 transporter. Insulin is not required for glucose uptake by the hepatic GLUT-2 transporter, but affects hepatic glucose metabolism by stimulating hepatic glycolysis, inhibiting gluconeogenesis, and facilitating glycogen synthesis. When there is a negative energy balance, normoglycemia is maintained in multiple ways. The metabolic rate slows to limit glucose consumption. Glucagon secretion increases and insulin secretion decreases, resulting in gluconeogenesis, glycogenolysis, and peripheral lipolysis. The metabolism shifts from glucose to fatty acids as a primary energy source. Because the liver uses few fatty acids for energy, and the pathway for ketone body formation is not well developed in horses, if the negative energy balance persists, increasing amounts of triglycerides are produced (Figure 9.2) [6]. With time, the hepatocellular triglyceride concentration overwhelms the liver's capacity for synthesizing and exporting VLDL, resulting in increased triglyceride storage and hepatic lipidosis.

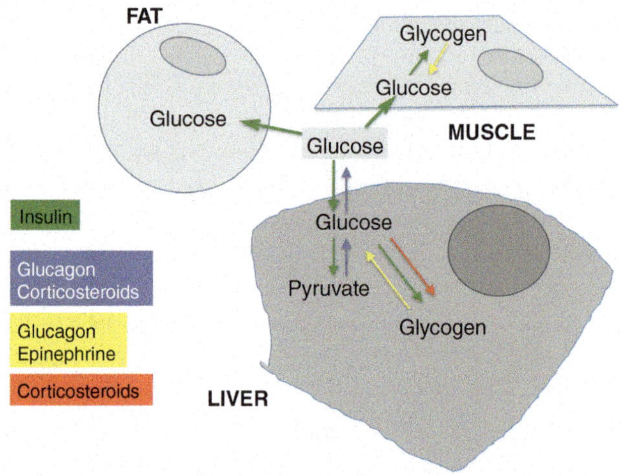

Figure 9.4 The effects of hormones on glucose metabolism. Insulin promotes normoglycemia by increasing glucose uptake, utilization, and storage and inhibiting gluconeogenesis. Glucagon, corticosteroids, and epinephrine cause hyperglycemia through various mechanisms including inhibition of insulin activity and stimulation of gluconeogenesis and glycogenolysis.

9.2.2 Insulin Resistance and Dysregulation

Insulin resistance (IR) is defined as insensitivity to insulin at the cell surface, where glucose entry into the cell is facilitated, or insulin ineffectiveness as a result of the disruption of intracellular glucose metabolism [21]. Insulin dysregulation (ID) comprises states of tissue insulin resistance as well as persistent or intermittent hyperinsulinemia [22]. Hyperinsulinemia was previously thought to occur solely as a response to tissue insulin resistance, but in ponies, transient hyperinsulinemia has also been shown to result from an inappropriate response to ingested carbohydrates in the absence of tissue insulin resistance [23]. Hyperresponsiveness to oral nonstructural carbohydrates without concurrent evidence of insulin resistance is proposed to occur via a functional enteroinsular axis, where alterations in glucose absorption and the secretion of intestinal incretin hormones may account for the difference between healthy and dysregulated ponies.

Glucose and lipid metabolism are intricately linked via insulin, glucagon, and other hormones. Abnormalities in lipid metabolism are therefore associated with dysregulation of glucose metabolism. Increased plasma fatty acid concentrations are associated with several insulin-resistant states in humans through various mechanisms, including inhibition of glucose transport or phosphorylation activity [10]. This appears to be a mechanism of insulin resistance in obesity and type 2 diabetes. Increased concentrations of inflammatory cytokines in humans are reported to be key in the development of obesity-associated insulin resistance. There is evidence that this may also be true in horses [24, 25].

Insulin resistance and dysregulation in equids have been associated with pasture laminitis, hyperlipidemia, obesity, pituitary pars intermedia dysfunction (PPID), type 2 diabetes mellitus (DM), SIRS, and EMS [4, 26–29]. Specific, quantitative methods of measuring insulin sensitivity are available, but are not currently suitable for practical clinical applications [21, 28]. The more commonly used tests are indirect methods of assessing insulin sensitivity and include measurement of resting glucose, insulin, leptin, and adiponectin concentrations, and dynamic tests such as the oral glucose/sugar tolerance test and insulin tolerance test (discussed below).

9.2.3 Laboratory Characterization of Glucose Metabolism

Although there are multiple methods currently in use to assess insulin sensitivity, many are appropriate only in research situations. This section will limit discussion to the nonspecific indicators of insulin resistance that are most applicable to clinical practice rather than specific, quantifiable methods such as the euglycemic hyperinsulinemic clamp, the frequently sampled IV glucose tolerance test with minimal model analysis, and the insulin suppression test [30].

9.2.3.1 Glucose

Blood glucose can be measured in whole blood, serum, or plasma. Because glycolysis continues in blood cells *in vitro*, serum or plasma should be separated as soon as possible from the blood cells, preferably within an hour after collection. If the sample cannot be separated within an hour, glycolysis can be inhibited with special collection tubes containing sodium fluoride (NaF). If NaF is used for collection, glucose assays based on glucose oxidase cannot be used since NaF inhibits glucose oxidase activity. Glycolysis is reported to decrease glucose concentrations by 5–10% per hour at room temperature; greater decreases can occur if there is marked erythrocytosis or leukocytosis.

The most common glucose assays use glucose oxidase for the initial reaction; other assays are based on glucose reduction of copper or ferricyanide. Because these assays are based on color changes, lipemia, hemolysis, and icterus can interfere with results. Nonphotometric assays rely on the use of oxygen or hydrogen peroxide electrodes to measure consumption or production, respectively, in the glucose oxidase reaction.

Glucose concentrations in serum and plasma are roughly equal, but whole-blood glucose concentrations may vary from plasma or serum concentrations. Most commercially available glucometers use whole blood. Many glucometers were designed for human use and therefore assume a constant stable relationship between plasma and whole blood and equilibration between plasma and erythrocyte glucose concentrations. In humans, this relationship holds true: glucose distribution is 50% within erythrocytes and 50% within plasma. This is not the case in many veterinary species. For example, in dogs and cats, glucose distribution is 12.5% and 7% within erythrocytes and 87.5% and 93% within plasma, respectively [31]. Similarly, in foals and horses glucose is largely present in plasma, with little measurable glucose in erythrocytes [32]. Whole-blood glucose measurements in horses using a point-of-care glucometer designed for human use were poorly correlated with the laboratory analyzer. However, when plasma was separated and tested with the glucometer, there was good agreement [33]. Similarly, in neonatal foals, a point-of-care glucometer designed for human use consistently underestimated blood glucose relative to the clinical laboratory analyzer [34]. In contrast, one study using a veterinary glucometer showed good accuracy and precision in horses relative to the laboratory standard [35]. It is important to note that differences in methodology may yield differences in the reference values. Thus, an essential component of test validation is to establish species-specific and instrument-specific reference intervals.

Although point-of-care glucometers use whole blood to measure glucose concentrations, some measure plasma glucose, some measure whole-blood glucose, and others calculate the plasma glucose concentration from a whole-blood glucose measurement [36]. Glucometers that calculate the plasma glucose concentration from the whole-blood glucose concentration may assume a normal hematocrit, which can result in inaccurate results since the erythrocyte concentration can affect the glucose measurement. Few studies have been done on the effects of hematocrit on point-of-care glucometer readings in horses, but one anecdotal report suggests that a high hematocrit does affect accurate glucose measurement by a veterinary glucometer [35].

9.2.3.1.1 Hyperglycemia Hyperglycemia can present either transiently or persistently (Table 9.1). Transient hyperglycemia may be postprandial, physiological, or drug related. Postprandial hyperglycemia, more common with feeds high in simple carbohydrates, can persist for 2–4 hours after feeding. Physiological hyperglycemia is caused by the insulin antagonistic actions of catecholamines, glucocorticoids, growth hormone, and glucagon; drug-associated hyperglycemias are often the result of the drug's stimulation or mimicry of these hormones. Glucose homeostatic dysfunction manifesting as hyperglycemia is reported in up to half of adult horses with acute abdominal disease [37]. The hyperglycemia is likely due to a combination of peripheral insulin resistance and increased gluconeogenesis due to the release of epinephrine, cortisol, tumor necrosis factor, and other mediators. Hyperglycemia has negative prognostic significance in colic patients and prognosis worsens with the severity of hyperglycemia.

Pathological hyperglycemia is associated with glucose metabolic defects associated with relative and/or absolute insulin deficiency. In horses, these are most commonly associated with insulin-resistant (IR) states such as EMS, SIRS, and PPID that have become uncompensated. Type 2 DM is an example of an IR disorder with pancreatic beta-cell dysfunction. Insulin resistance and associated disorders are discussed in more detail later in the chapter.

Table 9.1 Conditions associated with hyperglycemia.

Conditions
Physiological
Postprandial (high simple carbohydrate content)
Glucocorticoids
Stress
Catecholamines
Pain, exertion, excitement
Drugs
Glucocorticoids
Progesterone
Xylazine
Ketamine
Morphine
Pathological
Diabetes mellitus
Pituitary pars intermedia dysfunction[a]
Equine metabolic syndrome[a]
Colic[a]

[a] Hyperglycemia is not present in all cases.

9.2.3.1.2 Hypoglycemia Disorders causing hypoglycemia are attributable to increased glucose utilization by tissues and/or decreased glucose production (Table 9.2). Hypoglycemia is associated with sepsis and/or endotoxemia likely as a result of increased tissue glucose utilization and/or impaired gluconeogenesis and glycogenolysis. Extreme exertion in endurance horses can result in hypoglycemia, presumably as a result of decreased glycogen stores, increased glucose utilization, and/or decreased epinephrine responsiveness. Hypoglycemia due to hepatic failure only occurs after loss of more than 70% of liver function; other clinical signs and laboratory abnormalities will support an interpretation of hypoglycemia due to liver failure (see Chapter 5). Neonatal hypoglycemia may occur with poor nursing due to multiple causes (e.g., diarrhea, hypothermia, or agalactia). Foals have comparatively small glycogen and protein reserves as substrates for gluconeogenesis during times of decreased food intake. Hypoglycemia associated with starvation or malabsorption in adult horses and ponies is uncommon and only occurs with long-term decreased glucose availability.

9.2.3.2 Insulin

Insulin measurement is performed with an immunoassay. Serum or plasma insulin concentration may include proinsulin and is reported in immunoreactive units. Most insulin immunoassays use a commercial radioimmunoassay, but a chemiluminescent immunometric assay (Siemens, Diagnostic Products Corp., Los Angeles, CA) is now available. Equine insulin is stable for 30 days at 6–8 °C and for one year at −20 °C [38]. Serum or heparinized plasma can be used to measure insulin concentration.

Table 9.2 Conditions associated with hypoglycemia.

Conditions
Preanalytic and analytic causes
Delayed serum/plasma separation from blood cells
Marked leukocytosis, erythrocytosis[a]
Assay interference (hemolysis, icterus, lipemia)
Pathological
Sepsis/endotoxemia
Extreme exertion
Hepatic failure
Neonatal hypoglycemia
Starvation, malabsorption[a]
Glycogen storage disease (quarter horse polysaccharide storage myopathy)

[a] Uncommon.

Of the tests that evaluate glucose metabolism, measurement of resting insulin concentration is the most readily available and easy to perform. Resting insulin concentration is a useful screening test for decreased insulin sensitivity because compensatory hyperinsulinemia is a common feature of insulin resistance in horses. However, with mild or early insulin resistance, hyperinsulinemia may not have developed yet or the rise in serum insulin concentration may be too small to be detected using population-based reference values. Moreover, insulin concentration may vary as a result of diurnal variation, stress, or feeding. Prior to testing, acute stress from transportation, environmental factors, or pain should be minimized. Fasting before measuring basal insulin is not recommended as secondary insulin resistance can be induced by fasting. Insulin should also not be evaluated within 4–5 hours of grain feeding as responses are too variable [39].

Basal insulin concentrations of 20 μIU/mL were recommended as cut-off values to distinguish between healthy and insulin-dysregulated horses in the consensus statements of the American College of Veterinary Internal Medicine (ACVIM) [40]. A recent consensus statement by the European College of Equine Internal Medicine recommends that when forage of unknown quality is being fed, increases in basal insulin concentrations of 20–50 μIU/mL with the Immulite 1000 (Siemens) should prompt dynamic testing for ID using an oral glucose or sugar tolerance, and increases in basal insulin concentrations >50 μIU/mL as consistent with ID [39]. The authors of the ACVIM consensus statement specified the 20 μIU/mL cut-off value as being valid for sample analyses generated from the Coat-A-Count insulin radioimmunoassay (Siemens), Immulite insulin solid-phase chemiluminescent assay (Siemens), and DSL-1600 insulin radioimmunoassay (Diagnostic Systems Laboratory Inc., Webster, TX). Use of this cut-off without consideration of the assay method can lead to misdiagnosis due to significant differences in insulin values depending upon the assay method [39, 41]. The specific methodology used for insulin quantification should always be considered when interpreting results, especially when using diagnostic guidelines from published studies.

9.2.3.3 Adipokines (Leptin and Adiponectin)

Adipose tissue functions as a complex endocrine organ, producing adipokines that influence energy metabolism [42]. The use of adipokines as diagnostic tools in investigating ID in equids is increasing; leptin and adiponectin have been most widely studied, although currently only leptin evaluation is available for horses and ponies in some veterinary diagnostic laboratories in the United States.

The hormone leptin is synthesized by adipocytes in greater quantities when the body is in positive energy balance and signals the hypothalamus that adipose stores are replete. Serum leptin concentrations have been positively correlated with BCS in horses, indicating that blood leptin concentrations reflect body fat mass in horses [4, 43]. However, not all obese horses are hyperleptinemic and not all hyperleptinemic horses are obese [44]. Hyperleptinemia has been associated with glucose metabolism disturbances in horses; obese horses with high serum leptin concentrations showed abnormal glucose tolerance test results compared with obese horses that had lower leptin concentrations [44, 45]. These authors speculate that the hyperleptinemic condition is a result of reduced insulin sensitivity causing chronic increases in insulin concentrations with resultant chronic stimulation of adipose tissue output of leptin.

Leptin may decrease as much as 50% with fasting and will rise after feeding up to twofold fasting values [42]. Reference values should clearly state whether they reflect fed or fasting states. Serum and plasma collected in either EDTA or heparin is reported to be acceptable for leptin measurement in horses, but the laboratory offering the test should be consulted before sample submission. In humans, leptin is stable in serum for two months at 4 °C and two years at −20 °C and appears to have similar stability in rodents [42]. Studies in the stability of equine leptin are lacking.

The best characterized effects of adiponectin include enhancement of insulin sensitivity, antiinflammatory properties, and inhibition of the development of atherosclerosis. Unlike leptin, adiponectin levels do not appear to be affected by feeding, exercise, or circadian rhythms [42]. Circulating adiponectin in horses has been shown to be negatively correlated with fat mass, percent body fat, BCS, and leptin levels. Low plasma adiponectin with high basal insulin or insulin post dexamethasone has been reported to be a risk factor for laminitis [19]. Current interpretations for adiponectin espoused by the Equine Endocrinology Group (https://sites.tufts.edu/equineendogroup) cite high molecular weight (HMW) adiponectin concentrations <3.2 μg/mL (ELISA) as "consistent with metabolic derangement and increased risk of laminitis" and total adiponectin concentrations <2.5 μg/mL (radioimmunoassay – RIA) or <24 μg/mL (immunoturbidometric assay) as "consistent with EMS." Equine adiponectin evaluation is not currently offered by veterinary diagnostic laboratories in the United States.

9.2.3.4 Dynamic Testing

9.2.3.4.1 Oral Glucose Tolerance Test Tolerance is typically defined as blood glucose clearance following oral or intravenous glucose administration. Recent work has shown that hyperresponsiveness to glucose in ID individuals may be dependent upon the route of administration. Oral administration stimulates a greater insulin secretion than IV administration in ponies in part as a result of factors that the gastrointestinal tract (GIT) releases that augment glucose-induced pancreatic insulin secretion [23]. The proximal small intestine releases incretin hormones (mainly glucagon-like peptide-1 – GLP-1) that work with glucose to augment pancreatic insulin release. In addition, enhanced glucose bioavailability due to intestinal absorption of glucose (or less metabolism during first pass through the liver) also occurs following oral ingestion of nonstructural carbohydrates in insulin-dysregulated ponies. Because upregulation of the enteroinsular axis is implicated in equine ID, oral administration is now preferred over parenteral administration in tolerance testing.

Oral protocols may have poor compliance due to decreased palatability of the large glucose dose, and test results may be affected by ingestion time, gastric emptying, and intestinal absorption. However, in one study, repeatability of the oral glucose test (OGT) was shown to be satisfactory [46]. OGTs are performed by offering glucose (or dextrose) powder mixed in small, low-glycemic meals. Fasting overnight is recommended before the test to increase compliance with ingesting the test dose and to facilitate gastric glucose transit. Glucose powder 0.5 or 1.0 g/kg body mass (BM) is used; a dose of 0.75 g/kg BM had better acceptance by ponies than 1.0 g/kg BM and test results were satisfactory [46]. Insulin concentrations regarded as indicative of ID, when measured at 120 minutes post feeding, are >68 μIU/mL for 0.5 g/kg BM glucose and >80–90 μIU/mL for 1.0 g/kg BM glucose with Immulite 1000 chemiluminescent analysis [39]. An insulin concentration <65.5 μIU/mL for 1.0 g/kg BM with resting insulin <8.5 μIU/mL using the ADVIA Centaur chemiluminescent assay was not associated with development of laminitis in ponies in another study [47].

9.2.3.4.2 Oral Sugar Test The Equine Endocrinology Group (https://sites.tufts.edu/equineendogroup) currently recommends the oral sugar test (OST) as one of two dynamic screening tests for ID (see Figure 9.6). The OST uses a specific corn syrup (Karo Light Corn Syrup; ACH Food Companies, Inc., Oakbrook Terrace, IL) at a dosage of 0.15 mL/kg BM PO via dosing syringe. It is currently recommended to fast horses for 3–12 hours prior to testing. Blood sampling to measure insulin response is recommended between 60 and 90 minutes after corn syrup administration. Insulin concentrations >60 μIU/mL post dosing were initially used to indicate ID using RIA (Millipore Human RIA), although a lower cut-off of >45 μIU/m) was recommended more recently (https://sites.tufts.edu/equineendogroup). A higher dosage of 0.25 mL/kg BM corn syrup was suggested to improve diagnostic value with a cut-off of >30 μIU/mL between 60 and 90 minutes using Coat-A-Count RIA. An even higher dosage of 0.45 mL/kg BW corn syrup provided higher sensitivity for ID with a value of >110 μIU/mL measured by RIA (Insulin CT, MP Biomedical) at 60 minutes [48]. Proposed high-dose OST cut-off values for insulin concentrations measured with other assays include 40 μIU/mL using the Immulite 1000 and 63 μIU/mL using the Immulite 2000xpi chemiluminescent assays [39].

9.2.3.4.3 Intravenous Glucose Challenge Although intravenous (IV) administration is a more specific assessment of glucose metabolism because it bypasses the GIT, it is less useful in evaluating ID precisely because the GIT is omitted in the test. However, the procedure has historically been of use in both diagnosis and monitoring of EMS and is performed by administering 0.5 g glucose/kg IV. Blood is taken at 0 (baseline), 5, 15, 30, 60, and 90 minutes post infusion and then hourly for 5–6 hours for measurement of glucose and insulin concentrations. Blood glucose concentrations in horses with normal insulin sensitivity should show an immediate rise, a peak at 15 minutes, and a return to baseline within 1–2 hours. The insulin concentration should parallel the glucose response curve, but peak at 30 minutes post infusion. Horses with insulin resistance will show delayed return to reference values (>2 hours) and a higher blood glucose peak (Figure 9.5) [27].

9.2.3.4.4 Combined Glucose–Insulin Test The combined glucose–insulin test requires collection of a baseline blood sample, infusion of 150 mg/kg 50% dextrose solution, and infusion of 0.10 units/kg regular insulin immediately after the dextrose infusion. Blood samples are collected at 1, 5, 15, 25, 35, 45, 60, 75, 90, 105, 120, 135, and 150 minutes post infusion [49]. Other abbreviated protocols end collection at 120 minutes, omitting the last two time points, or measure insulin and glucose at 0, 45, and 75 minutes [39, 50]. With this method, insulin resistance is defined as maintenance of blood glucose concentrations above the baseline value for ≥45 minutes. Insulin concentration should be under 20 μIU/mL both at baseline and at 75 minutes, and remain <100 μIU/mL at 45 minutes when analyzed with the Coat-A-Count RIA [49]. The test can be shortened to 60 minutes when used in the field, but the time taken for the blood concentration to return to baseline is important information that should be recorded for future reference. This allows assessment of the response to diet, exercise, or medication.

Care should be taken to minimize stress, exercise, excitement, or pain before and during the testing because of their effect on glucose concentration. Note that there is a small risk of hypoglycemia when performing this test and signs of

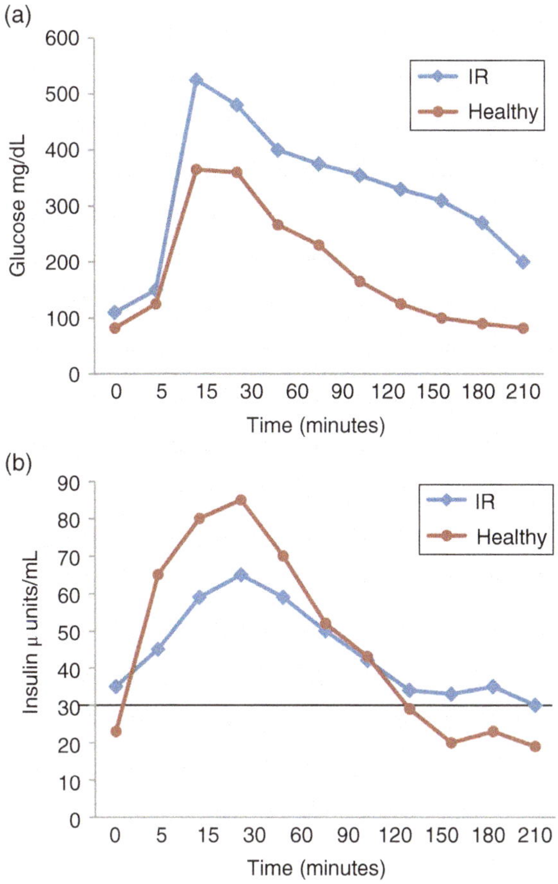

Figure 9.5 Glucose tolerance test. (a) Glucose concentration post administration of intravenous glucose in healthy and insulin-resistant (IR) ponies. The blood glucose concentration in the healthy pony shows an immediate rise, a peak around 15 minutes, and a return to baseline within 1–2 hours. In contrast, the IR glucose curve shows a higher peak at 15 minutes without fully returning to reference interval concentrations by the end of the test. (b) The insulin concentration parallels the glucose response curve with a peak at 30 minutes post infusion. The insulin response in the pony with IR is blunted and the insulin concentration remains slightly increased at the end of the testing period.

hypoglycemia should be detected and responded to promptly. Because glucose concentrations are being measured, it is important to separate the plasma or serum from the blood cells within an hour after collection or to use a NaF collection tube. If a glucometer is used for measurement of blood glucose, it should be a veterinary glucometer validated for horses (see section above on glucose measurement).

9.2.3.4.5 Insulin Response Test Insulin response tests are direct assessments of insulin sensitivity and insulin-dependent glucose uptake in response to exogenous insulin. The combined glucose–insulin test is difficult to perform in the field as it requires multiple blood samples over several hours. An alternative that is currently recommended is a two-step insulin response test that requires only two glucose measurements: one before and one 30 minutes after IV insulin administration [51]. The animal should be fed (pasture or hay) prior to testing. The two-step insulin response protocol is to give 0.1 IU/kg BM neutral insulin IV, followed by dextrose administration or a small feed, after 30 minutes to prevent hypoglycemia. In normal horses, blood glucose will decrease to less than half of the baseline concentration within 20–30 minutes after 0.02–0.125 IU/kg BM regular insulin IV and then return back to baseline levels within two hours [44]. If the blood glucose concentration does *not* decrease to <50% of baseline in an insulin response test, the result is considered indicative of insulin resistance.

9.2.4 Diseases Associated with Glucose Metabolic Defects

9.2.4.1 Pasture Laminitis

Risk factors for the development of pasture laminitis include IR states such as PPID and obesity (including regional adiposity) [17]. Nonstructural carbohydrates (e.g., simple sugars, starches, and fructose polymers) in pasture grass are implicated in the pathogenesis of pasture-associated laminitis, although insulin resistance is thought to be the predisposing factor. Carbohydrate overload is associated with the development and/or exacerbation of insulin resistance that might precipitate laminitis by interfering with glucose uptake by hoof keratinocytes or by altering blood flow to the hoof. However, several studies have thus far failed to implicate local tissue insulin resistance in the development of laminitis [22]. Carbohydrate overload may alter bacterial flora, causing the release of vasoactive endotoxins, exotoxins, or amines that potentially can alter hoof blood flow. Endotoxin activation of a systemic inflammatory response will also induce insulin resistance, although endotoxemia alone is not sufficient to induce laminitis [52].

Other pathogenetic mechanisms for pasture laminitis are proposed by recent studies of adiponectin. Feeding horses a diet high in carbohydrates has been shown to decrease plasma adiponectin compared with feeding horses an isocaloric diet high in fat [53]. Previously laminitic ponies had significantly lower adiponectin concentrations compared with nonlaminitic ponies irrespective of season, and an adiponectin concentration of <2.5 μg/mL was found to have a 78% sensitivity and 79% specificity to predict the occurrence of pasture-associated laminitis within three years [19].

Adiponectin is known to enhance insulin sensitivity and has antiinflammatory properties; decreased concentrations may contribute to ID and/or a decreased antiinflammatory state. Because low plasma adiponectin with high basal insulin or insulin post dexamethasone was shown to be a risk factor for laminitis [19], the authors hypothesized that hypoadiponectinemia and hyperinsulinemia could potentially combine to alter lamellar epithelial and endothelial insulin and insulin-like growth factor (IGF-1) receptor expression, resulting in epithelial proliferation and endothelial dysfunction and subsequent laminitis. Alternatively, adiponectin promotes vasorelaxation through increased vascular expression of endothelial nitric oxide (NO) synthase and prostacylin (PGI_2) synthase and it is possible that low adiponectin concentrations could increase the risk for future laminitis through decreased vasorelaxation of the equine digital vasculature [19].

Pasture-associated laminitis follows a seasonal pattern, with increased incidence of laminitis in the fall. Pasture grazing increases blood concentrations of glucose and insulin concomitant with seasonal upregulation of ACTH, which may be an important part of the development of laminitis, especially in PPID horses. There is a positive correlation between insulin concentration and simple sugar content of pasture grass [54].

9.2.4.2 Equine Metabolic Syndrome

In a recent consensus statement regarding the characterization of EMS, it was agreed that the three major components of the syndrome were obesity (generalized or regional), hyperinsulinemia, and insulin resistance with a predisposition to laminitis [40]. It is now recognized that although EMS is most often associated with obesity, it may manifest in nonobese animals. The fundamental characteristic of EMS is ID [39]. ID is defined by hyperinsulinemia or abnormal responses to glucose and/or insulin tolerance tests. It is currently uncertain whether these components alone are responsible for the susceptibility to laminitis or whether there is another as yet unidentified factor that precipitates laminitis in horses with EMS. Additional characteristics of EMS include hypertriglyceridemia (discussed above), arterial hypertension that is detected in the summer in laminitis-prone ponies, altered reproductive cycling in mares, increased systemic markers of inflammation in association with obesity, hyperleptinemia, and hypoadiponectinemia [39, 40]. The highest incidence of EMS is seen in pony breeds, Morgan horses, Paso Finos, Arabians, Saddlebreds, quarter horses, and Tennessee walking horses [15]. There is evidence of breed-associated differences in insulin dynamics independent of BCS [55].

Glucose concentrations may be within reference limits in EMS because hyperinsulinemia often maintains euglycemia. Hyperglycemia in the context of hyperinsulinemia suggests uncompensated insulin resistance (or type 2 DM). Obese horses with high serum leptin concentrations showed abnormal glucose tolerance test results compared with obese horses with lower leptin concentrations, suggesting that high leptin concentrations reflect insulin resistance and are a component of EMS [45]. However, leptin is more directly associated with fat mass than ID [42]. Concurrent hyperinsulinemia, hyperglycemia, hypoadiponectinemia, and hyperleptinemia are supportive of EMS. Since EMS is fundamentally the consequence of ID, horses and ponies should be screened for evidence of ID. Current recommendations for EMS screening [39] are summarized in Figure 9.6.

9.2.4.3 Pituitary Pars Intermedia Dysfunction (PPID)

Pituitary pars intermedia dysfunction is covered fully in Chapter 11 and will only be discussed here in the context of a glucose metabolic disorder. Insulin resistance associated with PPID is a consequence of hypercortisolemia. Cortisol is an insulin antagonist. The net effects of hypercortisolemia include enhanced gluconeogenesis in hepatocytes, increased hormone-sensitive lipase activity resulting in increased NEFA substrate for gluconeogenesis, and inhibition of insulin activity at the receptor and postreceptor level. It is thought that inhibition of GLUT-4-mediated glucose uptake in the laminar tissue may be integral to the development of laminitis in PPID and other IR conditions.

Localized obesity, insulin resistance, and laminitis are recognized components of PPID as well as EMS [56]. These two syndromes may occur alone or in conjunction. Given the clinical similarities, it is important to distinguish between these disorders. Clinical signs supportive of a diagnosis of PPID but not EMS include delayed shedding/retention of winter haircoat, hirsutism, excessive sweating, skeletal muscle atrophy, and polyuria/polydipsia. The patient's age is another distinguishing factor. EMS is generally first identified in younger horses whereas PPID is commonly diagnosed in older horses. And finally, laboratory results showing inappropriately increased plasma ACTH concentration is a feature of PPID and not EMS.

9.2.4.4 Systemic Inflammatory Response Syndrome

Systemic inflammatory disease is a well-documented cause of ID in multiple species, manifesting as peripheral insulin resistance, hyperinsulinemia, hyperglycemia, and impaired insulin-mediated glucose uptake. The pathogenetic mechanisms are posited to involve decreased availability of the insulin receptor as a result of cellular hypoxia, and oxidative stress causing activation of inflammatory pathways and inhibition of postreceptor insulin signaling pathways. Hyperglycemia is a known cause of oxidative stress.

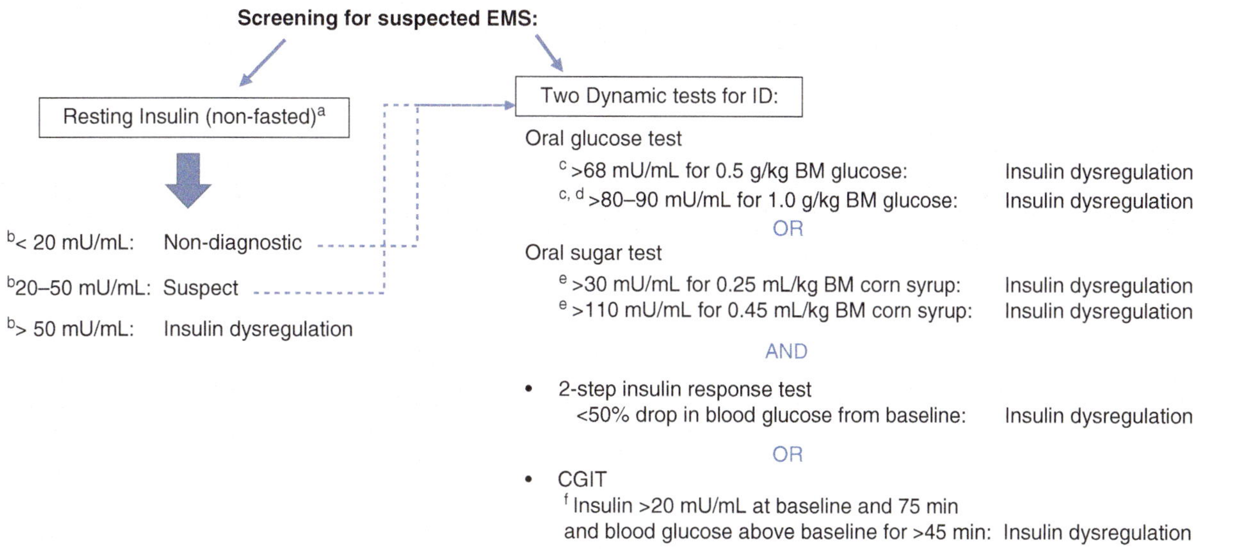

[a] Hay or pasture; not grain.
[b] Values are for insulin assayed on the Immulite1000 and Coat-a-Count and DSL-1600 insulin radioimmunoassays (RIA).
[c] Values are for insulin assayed on the Immulite1000.
[d] >65.5 mU/mL for 1.0 g/kg BM glucose using ADVIA Centaur luminescent assay.
[e] Using the RIA; a cut-off of >40 mU/mL for 0.45 mL/kg BM corn syrup is used for the Immulite1000.
[f] Insulin measured via RIA.

Figure 9.6 Current recommendations for EMS screening.

In horses, experimental lipopolysaccharide (LPS) infusion to induce an acute inflammatory response has been shown to result in peripheral tissue insulin resistance [25]. Acute gastrointestinal disease is associated with hyperglycemia much more frequently than hypoglycemia, also suggesting peripheral tissue insulin resistance. In a recent study, the majority of horses with signs of SIRS were hyperglycemic and over a third were hyperinsulinemic [29]. Horses with higher glucose:insulin ratios, an indicator of peripheral insulin resistance, were less likely to survive. Conversely, hyperinsulinemia in this context was positively correlated with survival, suggesting an appropriate response to SIRS-associated hyperglycemia. Similar to critically ill humans, hyperglycemia in horses with acute abdominal disease and in horses with SIRs is a negative prognostic indicator [29, 37, 57].

9.2.4.5 Diabetes Mellitus

Diabetes mellitus is characterized by persistent hyperglycemia due to reduced insulin secretion and/or insulin resistance. Hyperglycemia in type 1 DM is attributed to absolute hypoinsulinemia as a result of pancreatic beta-cell destruction, and is very rare in horses. Equine type 2 DM, which is initially a relative insulin deficiency, is gaining increasing recognition [26].

Type 2 DM is characterized in the early stage by normoglycemia with concurrent hyperinsulinemia (prediabetes), but in later stages manifests as hyperglycemia with normo- or hypoinsulinemia as pancreatic beta-cell function declines. Type 2 DM develops in humans as a result of prolonged insulin resistance and subsequent pancreatic beta-cell exhaustion. Diagnosis of type 2 DM requires confirmation of insulin resistance with an evaluation of beta-cell function for staging. Low serum insulin concentrations with poor pancreatic beta-cell response could indicate either type 1 or type 2 DM; quantitative measures of insulin sensitivity are therefore needed to distinguish between the types. Currently, these types of measurements are not feasible in the field and are used mainly in select clinical and research situations. Persistent hyperglycemia with low or normal insulin concentrations and clinical signs of polyuria, polydipsia, and weight loss are strongly suggestive of DM.

9.2.4.6 Other Diseases: Enhanced Glucose Metabolism

While most diseases of equine glucose metabolism are associated with IR states, often with hyperglycemia, there are three diseases associated with hypoglycemia: quarter horse polysaccharide storage myopathy (PSSM; discussed in Chapter 10), lipid storage myopathy (discussed in Chapter 10), and equine motor neuron disease. Oral and intravenous glucose tolerance testing in PSSM horses reveals increased sensitivity to insulin, which results in increased glucose uptake and storage and hypoglycemia relative to controls [58, 59]. Equine motor neuron disease is also associated with increased glucose clearance and decreased blood glucose concentrations relative to healthy control horses during glucose challenge. The mechanism is currently unclear [60, 61].

A single case report of lipid storage myopathy in a foal most similar to multiple acyl-CoA dehydrogenase deficiency was characterized by persistent hypoglycemia with increases in muscle and liver enzymes [62]. Multiple acyl-CoA dehydrogenase deficiency hypoglycemia is attributable to impaired activities of dehydrogenases involved in the oxidation of fatty acids and amino acids due to impaired beta-oxidation and ketogenesis [63].

References

1 Stockham, S.L. and Scott, M.A. (2002). Lipids. In: *Fundamentals of Veterinary Clinical Pathology* (eds. S.L. Stockham and M.A. Scott), 521–537. Ames: Wiley.

2 Rifai, N., Albers, J.J., and Bachorik, P.S. (2001). Lipids, lipoproteins, and apolipoproteins. In: *Tietz Fundamentals of Clinical Chemistry*, 5e (eds. C.A. Burtis and E.R. Ashwood), 462–493. Philadelphia: Saunders.

3 Watson, T.D., Burns, L., Love, S. et al. (1991). The isolation, characterisation and quantification of the equine plasma lipoproteins. *Equine Vet. J.* 23: 353–359.

4 Frank, N., Elliott, S.B., Brandt, L.E., and Keisler, D.H. (2006). Physical characteristics, blood hormone concentrations, and plasma lipid concentrations in obese horses with insulin resistance. *J. Am. Vet. Med. Assoc.* 228: 1383–1390.

5 Argenzio, R.A. and Hintz, H.F. (1972). Effect of diet on glucose entry and oxidation rates in ponies. *J. Nutr.* 102: 879–892.

6 McKenzie, H.C. (2011). Equine hyperlipidemias. *Vet. Clin. North Am. Equine Pract.* 27: 59–72.

7 Dunkel, B. and McKenzie, H.C. (2003). Severe hypertriglyceridaemia in clinically ill horses: diagnosis, treatment and outcome. *Equine Vet. J.* 35: 590–595.

8 Hughes, K.J., Hodgson, D.R., and Dart, A.J. (2004). Equine hyperlipaemia: a review. *Aust. Vet. J.* 82: 136–142.

9 Burden, F.A., Toit Du, N., Hazell-Smith, E., and Trawford, A.F. (2011). Hyperlipemia in a population of aged donkeys: description, prevalence, and potential risk factors. *J. Vet. Intern. Med.* 25: 1420–1425.

10 Shulman, G.I. (2000). Cellular mechanisms of insulin resistance. *J. Clin. Invest.* 106: 171–176.

11 Sato, T., Liang, K., and Vaziri, N.D. (2002). Down-regulation of lipoprotein lipase and VLDL receptor in rats with focal glomerulosclerosis. *Kidney Int.* 61: 157–162.

12 Mogg, T.D. and Palmer, J.E. (1995). Hyperlipidemia, hyperlipemia, and hepatic lipidosis in American miniature horses: 23 cases (1990–1994). *J. Am. Vet. Med. Assoc.* 207: 604–607.

13 Murray, M. (1985). Hepatic-lipidosis in a post parturient mare. *Equine Vet. J.* 17: 68–69.

14 Naylor, J.M., Kronfeld, D.S., and Acland, H. (1980). Hyperlipemia in horses: effects of undernutrition and disease. *Am. J. Vet. Res.* 41: 899–905.

15 Frank, N. (2011). Equine metabolic syndrome. *Vet. Clin. North Am. Equine Pract.* 27: 73–92.

16 Watson, T.D., Burns, L., Freeman, D.J. et al. (1993). High density lipoprotein metabolism in the horse (Equus caballus). *Comp. Biochem. Physiol., B* 104: 45–53.

17 Carter, R.A., Treiber, K.H., Geor, R.J. et al. (2009). Prediction of incipient pasture-associated laminitis from hyperinsulinaemia, hyperleptinaemia and generalised and localised obesity in a cohort of ponies. *Equine Vet. J.* 41: 171–178.

18 Treiber, K.H., Kronfeld, D.S., Hess, T.M. et al. (2006). Evaluation of genetic and metabolic predispositions and nutritional risk factors for pasture-associated laminitis in ponies. *J. Am. Vet. Med. Assoc.* 228: 1538–1545.

19 Menzies-Gow, N.J., Harris, P.A., and Elliott, J. (2017). Prospective cohort study evaluating risk factors for the development of pasture-associated laminitis in the United Kingdom. *Equine Vet. J.* 49: 300–306.

20 Ford, E.J. and Simmons, H.A. (1985). Gluconeogenesis from caecal propionate in the horse. *Br. J. Nutr.* 53: 55–60.

21 Kronfeld, D.S., Treiber, K.H., Hess, T.M., and Boston, R.C. (2005). Insulin resistance in the horse: definition, detection, and dietetics. *J. Anim. Sci.* 83 (Suppl 13): E22–E31.

22 Bertin, F.R. and de Laat, M.A. (2017). The diagnosis of equine insulin dysregulation. *Equine Vet. J.* 49: 570–576.

23 de Laat, M.A., McGree, J.M., and Sillence, M.N. (2016). Equine hyperinsulinemia: investigation of the enteroinsular axis during insulin dysregulation. *Am. J. Physiol. Endocrinol. Metab.* 310: 61–72.

24 Vick, M.M., Adams, A.A., Murphy, B.A. et al. (2007). Relationships among inflammatory cytokines, obesity, and insulin sensitivity in the horse. *J. Anim. Sci.* 85: 1144–1155.

25 Vick, M.M., Murphy, B.A., Sessions, D.R. et al. (2008). Effects of systemic inflammation on insulin sensitivity in horses and inflammatory cytokine expression in adipose tissue. *Am. J. Vet. Res.* 69: 130–139.

26 Durham, A.E., Hughes, K.J., Cottle, H.J. et al. (2009). Type 2 diabetes mellitus with pancreatic beta cell dysfunction in 3 horses confirmed with minimal model analysis. *Equine Vet. J.* 41: 924–929.

27 Garcia, M.C. and Beech, J. (1986). Equine intravenous glucose tolerance test: glucose and insulin responses of healthy horses fed grain or hay and of horses with pituitary adenoma. *Am. J. Vet. Res.* 47: 570–572.

28 Treiber, K.H., Kronfeld, D.S., and Geor, R.J. (2006). Insulin resistance in equids: possible role in laminitis. *J. Nutr.* 136 (7 Suppl): 2094S–2098S.

29 Bertin, F., Ruffin-Taylor, D., and Stewart, A.J. (2018). Insulin dysregulation in horses with systemic inflammatory response syndrome. *J. Vet. Intern. Med.* 32: 1420–1427.

30 Tóth, F., Frank, N., Elliott, S.B. et al. (2009). Optimisation of the frequently sampled intravenous glucose tolerance test to reduce urinary glucose spilling in horses. *Equine Vet. J.* 41: 844–851.

31 Coldman, M.F. and Good, W. (1967). The distribution of sodium, potassium and glucose in the blood of some mammals. *Comp. Biochem. Physiol.* 21: 201–206.

32 Goodwin, R.F. (1956). The distribution of sugar between red cells and plasma: variations associated with age and species. *J. Physiol.* 134: 88–101.

33 Hollis, A.R., Dallap Schaer, B.L., Boston, R.C., and Wilkins, P.A. (2008). Comparison of the Accu-Chek Aviva point-of-care glucometer with blood gas and laboratory methods of analysis of glucose measurement in equine emergency patients. *J. Vet. Intern. Med.* 22: 1189–1195.

34 Russell, C., Palmer, J.E., Boston, R.C., and Wilkins, P.A. (2007). Agreement between point-of-care glucometry, blood gas and laboratory-based measurement of glucose in an equine neonatal intensive care unit. *J. Vet. Emerg. Crit. Care* 17: 236–242.

35 Hackett, E.S. and McCue, P.M. (2010). Evaluation of a veterinary glucometer for use in horses. *J. Vet. Intern. Med.* 24: 617–621.

36 Stockham, S.L. and Scott, M.A. (2002). Glucose and related regulatory hormones. In: *Fundamentals of Veterinary Clinical Pathology* (eds. S.L. Stockham and M.A. Scott), 487–506. Ames: Blackwell.

37 Hassel, D.M., Hill, A.E., and Rorabeck, R.A. (2009). Association between hyperglycemia and survival in 228 horses with acute gastrointestinal disease. *J. Vet. Intern. Med.* 23: 1261–1265.

38 Oberg, J., Brojer, J., Wattle, O., and Lilliehook, I. (2012). Evaluation of an equine-optimized enzyme-linked immunosorbent assay for serum insulin measurement and stability study of equine serum insulin. *Comp. Clin. Pathol.* 21: 1291–1300.

39 Durham, A.E., Frank, N., McGowan, C.M. et al. (2019). ECEIM consensus statement on equine metabolic syndrome. *J. Vet. Intern. Med.* 33: 335–349.

40 Frank, N., Geor, R.J., Bailey, S.R. et al. (2010). Equine metabolic syndrome. *J. Vet. Intern. Med.* 24: 467–475.

41 Warnken, T., Huber, K., and Feige, K. (2016). Comparison of three different methods for the quantification of equine insulin. *BMC Vet. Res.* 12: 196.

42 Radin, M.J., Sharkey, L.C., and Holycross, B.J. (2009). Adipokines: a review of biological and analytical principles and an update in dogs, cats, and horses. *Vet. Clin. Pathol.* 38: 136–156.

43 Buff, P.R., Dodds, A.C., Morrison, C.D. et al. (2002). Leptin in horses: tissue localization and relationship between peripheral concentrations of leptin and body condition. *J. Anim. Sci.* 80: 2942–2948.

44 Caltabilota, T.J., Earl, L.R., Thompson, D.L. et al. (2010). Hyperleptinemia in mares and geldings: assessment of insulin sensitivity from glucose responses to insulin injection. *J. Anim. Sci.* 88: 2940–2949.

45 Cartmill, J.A., Thompson, D.L., Storer, W.A. et al. (2003). Endocrine responses in mares and geldings with high body condition scores grouped by high vs. low resting leptin concentrations. *J. Anim. Sci.* 81: 2311–2321.

46 de Laat, M.A. and Sillence, M.N. (2017). The repeatability of an oral glucose test in ponies. *Equine Vet. J.* 49: 238–243.

47 Meier, A.D., de Laat, M.A., Reiche, D.B. et al. (2018). The oral glucose test predicts laminitis risk in ponies fed a diet high in nonstructural carbohydrates. *Domest. Anim. Endocrinol.* 63: 1–9.

48 Jocelyn, N.A., Harris, P.A., and Menzies-Gow, N.J. (2018). Effect of varying the dose of corn syrup on the insulin and glucose response to the oral sugar test. *Equine Vet. J.* 50: 836–841.

49 Eiler, H., Frank, N., Andrews, F.M. et al. (2005). Physiologic assessment of blood glucose homeostasis via combined intravenous glucose and insulin testing in horses. *Am. J. Vet. Res.* 66: 1598–1604.

50 Dunbar, L.K., Mielnicki, K.A., Dembek, K.A. et al. (2016). Evaluation of four diagnostic tests for insulin dysregulation in adult light-breed horses. *J. Vet. Intern. Med.* 30: 885–891.

51 Bertin, F.R. and Sojka-Kritchevsky, J.E. (2013). Comparison of a 2-step insulin-response test to conventional insulin-sensitivity testing in horses. *Domest. Anim. Endocrinol.* 44: 19–25.

52 Tóth, F., Frank, N., Chameroy, K.A., and Bostont, R.C. (2009). Effects of endotoxaemia and carbohydrate overload on glucose and insulin dynamics and the development of laminitis in horses. *Equine Vet. J.* 41: 852–858.

53 Bamford, N.J., Potter, S.J., Harris, P.A., and Bailey, S.R. (2016). Effect of increased adiposity on insulin sensitivity and adipokine concentrations in horses and ponies fed a high fat diet, with or without a once daily high glycaemic meal. *Equine Vet. J.* 48: 368–373.

54 Frank, N., Elliott, S.B., Chameroy, K.A. et al. (2010). Association of season and pasture grazing with blood hormone and metabolite concentrations in horses with presumed pituitary pars intermedia dysfunction. *J. Vet. Intern. Med.* 24: 1167–1175.

55 Bamford, N.J., Potter, S.J., Harris, P.A., and Bailey, S.R. (2014). Breed differences in insulin sensitivity and insulinemic responses to oral glucose in horses and ponies of moderate body condition score. *Domest. Anim. Endocrinol.* 47: 101–107.

56 Schott, H. 2nd (2002). Pituitary pars intermedia dysfunction: equine Cushing's disease. *Vet. Clin. North Am. Equine Pract.* 18: 237.

57 Hollis, A.R., Boston, R.C., and Corley, K.T.T. (2007). Blood glucose in horses with acute abdominal disease. *J. Vet. Intern. Med.* 21: 1099–1103.

58 Annandale, E.J., Valberg, S.J., Mickelson, J.R., and Seaquist, E.R. (2004). Insulin sensitivity and skeletal muscle glucose transport in horses with equine polysaccharide storage myopathy. *Neuromuscul. Disord.* 14: 666–674.

59 de la Corte, F.D., Valberg, S.J., MacLeay, J.M. et al. (1999). Glucose uptake in horses with polysaccharide storage myopathy. *Am. J. Vet. Res.* 60: 458–462.

60 Benders, N.A., Dyer, J., Wijnberg, I.D. et al. (2005). Evaluation of glucose tolerance and intestinal luminal membrane glucose transporter function in horses with equine motor neuron disease. *Am. J. Vet. Res.* 66: 93–99.

61 van der Kolk, J.H., Rijnen, K.E.P.M., Rey, F. et al. (2005). Evaluation of glucose metabolism in three horses with lower motor neuron degeneration. *Am. J. Vet. Res.* 66: 271–276.

62 Pinn, T.L., Divers, T.J., Southard, T. et al. (2018). Persistent hypoglycemia associated with lipid storage myopathy in a paint foal. *J. Vet. Intern. Med.* 32: 1442–1446.

63 Peake, R.W.A. and Kozakewich, H.P.W. (2017). A term newborn with respiratory distress, acidosis, and hypoglycemia. *Clin. Chem.* 63: 613–615.

10

Laboratory Markers of Muscle Injury

Allison Billings[1], Jennifer K. Quinn[2], and Melanie S. Spoor[2]

[1] Veterinary Clinical Pathology, IDEXX Laboratories, Inc., Portland, OR, USA
[2] Veterinary Clinical Pathology, IDEXX Laboratories, Inc., Wetherby, UK

10.1 Laboratory Evaluation of Equine Muscle Disorders

Most laboratory tests directed to the evaluation of muscle measure the serum activity of enzymes released from muscle tissue after injury. Extramuscular factors contributing to increases in serum enzyme activity should be considered when interpreting changes in these enzymes. Other constituents released from muscle such as myoglobin and troponin I are also useful biomarkers of muscle injury. The cardiac isoform of troponin I is currently a valuable clinical tool in the assessment of myocardial injury.

10.1.1 General Causes of Increased Serum Enzymes

The basis of clinical enzymology of muscle is the measurement of enzyme activities that occur when muscle tissue has been damaged. A range of enzymes and biomarkers are available for use in clinical investigations to monitor the onset or progress of muscle disease. The concentrations of enzymes in serum or plasma can be determined by using the chemical reactions they catalyze or by an immunoassay.

The concentration of muscle enzymes in serum or plasma is usually low in healthy horses because the enzymes are located within the myofiber, with most present in the sarcoplasm. However, certain enzymes also have a mitochondrial form. In general, an increase in serum enzyme activity may be secondary to increased production of the enzyme (e.g., hyperplasia), increased release from damaged cells, or due to decreased removal of the enzyme from the blood. The major mechanism by which serum enzyme activity increases is through release from damaged myofibers at a rate that exceeds the rate of enzyme inactivation or removal from blood [1]. Cell necrosis and irreversible cell damage lead to release of enzymes and increased serum enzyme concentrations. Minor cell injury that causes reversible damage may also create increases in serum enzyme activities through formation of membrane blebs containing cytoplasmic enzymes. These blebs may rupture or be released into blood and lyze, producing an increase in serum enzyme activity [2].

The rate of enzyme loss (or its rate of rise in plasma) is affected by the severity of tissue damage, the enzyme concentration within the cell, the location of the enzyme within the cell, and how the enzyme enters the blood. Thus, the magnitude of increase does not depend *only* on the extent of muscle injury. The common muscle enzymes are cytoplasmic enzymes and their rate of increase is likely to be greater with more severe muscle damage. Because enzymes from myofibers are released into the interstitial space and enter the plasma via the lymphatics, there is a slower rate of enzyme increase than direct release into blood [3].

10.1.2 Serum Enzymes Detecting Muscle Injury

10.1.2.1 Aspartate Aminotransferase (AST)

Aspartate aminotransferase (AST), formerly known as glutamic oxaloacetic transaminase (GOT), catalyzes the reversible transamination of L-aspartate and 2-oxoglutarate (alpha-ketoglutarate) to oxaloacetate and glutamate and requires pyridoxal-5′-phosphate (PP) as a cofactor. The requirement of a cofactor is of note because assays including the cofactor may generate different results from those lacking the cofactor. Poor saturation of serum alanine aminotransferase (ALT) with endogenous PP caused underestimation

Equine Hematology, Cytology, and Clinical Chemistry, Second Edition.
Edited by Raquel M. Walton, Rick L. Cowell, and Amy C. Valenciano.

of the total enzyme activity in a study of horses post exercise; however, the same study showed the majority of AST (94%) was saturated with endogenous PP and thus not subject to the same underestimation [4]. AST is reported to be stable for days in serum at room temperature, refrigerated, or frozen [5]. A study of equine clotted blood and serum stored at room temperature revealed significant increases in enzyme activity after 48 hours [6]. Results are reported in international units per liter (U/L).

The half-life for equine AST is generally reported to be 7–8 days [7]. However, other studies suggest a shorter half-life of 3–4 days [7–9]. In either case, serum AST has a longer half-life than creatine kinase (CK). Peak values in the horse are reached within 24–48 hours [9–11].

Aspartate aminotransferase is present within the cytoplasm and in the mitochondria. In horses, the ratio of cytoplasmic AST (cAST) to mitochondrial AST (mAST) is greater than in other mammals [4, 12]. It is postulated that with severe or irreversible cell injury, there may be a greater magnitude of serum AST increase due to the release of mAST as well as cAST. Studies to confirm this suspicion are lacking.

In addition to skeletal muscle, AST is found within cardiac muscle cells, hepatocytes, and erythrocytes, therefore increases in serum AST activity can occur with myocyte injury, hepatocellular injury, and hemolysis [13]. Although an increase in AST activity may reflect some degree of myocyte injury, it does not specify a particular disease or disorder. Given the nonspecific nature of AST, assessment of additional organ-specific enzymes is often required to distinguish between myocyte and hepatocellular injury.

Serial measurement of AST in conjunction with CK can often be useful to indicate the time course of muscle injury. CK has a very short half-life, increases very quickly (peaks at 6–12 hours), and remains increased for only a couple of days following an episode of muscle injury. Continued increases suggest ongoing or active muscle injury. In contrast, AST has a more gradual rise to peak activity and decreases more slowly due to its longer half-life. It can be present for one to several weeks following an episode of muscle injury and thus may be increased with either persistent or resolved muscle injury. Therefore, serial measurements that initially show an increase in both AST and CK, and later show only an increased AST, indicate that the episode of myonecrosis has resolved (see Figure 10.1).

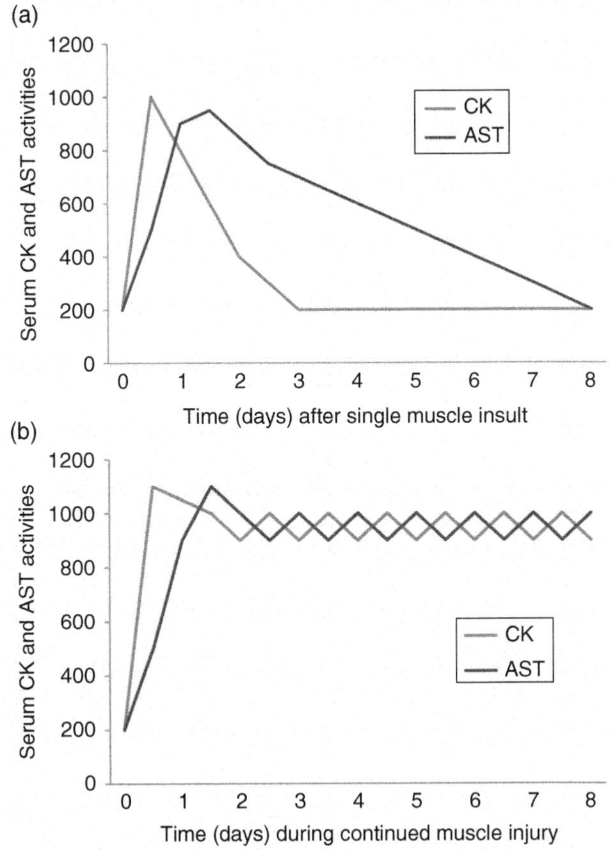

Figure 10.1 Increases in serum CK and AST activities after muscle injury. CK has an earlier rise to peak and shorter half-life than AST. Differences in CK and AST serum activities over time may be helpful in determining the time course of muscle injury. (a) After a single insult both CK and AST are initially increased. If measurements are repeated at day 3 following the insult, CK activity will likely be within or close to normal range while AST will still be increased. (b) Continued high levels of both CK and AST suggest repeated or ongoing muscle injury.

10.1.2.2 Creatine Kinase

Creatine kinase catalyzes the phosphorylation of creatine, utilizing ATP, to form phosphocreatine and adenosine diphosphate (ADP). In skeletal and cardiac myocytes, phosphocreatine serves as a reservoir for regeneration of ATP required for muscle contraction. CK is present in negligible amounts in many tissues throughout the body and in high concentrations within skeletal and cardiac muscle [14]. It is predominantly a cytoplasmic enzyme though a small amount is associated with the outer side of the inner mitochondrial membrane [15]. The enzyme is stable for seven days at 4 °C and one month at −20 °C in canine serum; published studies for refrigerated stored equine samples are lacking. Plasma collected from healthy foals and stored at −20 °C had a clinically insignificant decrease in CK activity after 12 weeks [16]. Equine samples (clotted blood and serum) stored at room temperature resulted in increases in CK after 72 hours [6]. Serum CK activity is higher than plasma CK activity in the dog due to release of CK with clot formation, but it is unknown if this is true in the horse [17]. Results are reported in international units per liter (U/L).

The half-life of CK is relatively short though specific times vary amongst studies. Intravenous and intramuscular injections of CK produce half-lives of approximately two hours and 12 hours, respectively [18]. The intramuscular administration is expected to be more reflective of actual physiological conditions as CK must be absorbed from the lymphatics into the blood after muscle injury and release from the myocyte. In more recent studies in horses, CK was shown to peak from six to 12 hours [10]. Return of CK to baseline values were reported at 24 hours, 2–3 days, and 3–4 days in each of the studies.

Creatine kinase has several isoenzymes. In most tissues, both cytoplasmic CK and mitochondrial CK isoenzymes are coexpressed. Cytoplasmic CK has a dimeric structure made of M (muscle) and B (brain) subunits. There are three cytosolic CK isoenzymes: CK-1 (or CK-BB) is found primarily in the brain and CK-2 (CK-MB) and CK-3 (CK-MM) are found in cardiac and skeletal muscle; CK-2 is present in overall low concentrations in the horse [19, 20]. Although it is possible to separate these isoenzymes, CK isoenzyme analysis has not been shown to be diagnostically useful in equine studies [21].

The majority of serum CK is of muscle origin. Therefore, CK is considered a muscle-specific marker and increases in serum CK activity are considered indicative of muscle injury. However, it is worthy of note that hemolysis can cause increases in measured CK, due to the release of adenylate kinase, glucose-6-phosphate, and ADP from erythrocytes which can interfere with the coupled reactions of CK assays [13, 22]. Adenosine monophosphate and diadenosine pentaphosphate may be used as inhibitors of adenylate kinase in CK assays [22]. As discussed above, serial measurements of AST and CK can be utilized to assess the time course of the muscle injury.

Extremely high serum CK activity (>10 000 IU/L) often requires dilution by a technician running the assay. Dilution of the serum results in dilution of endogenous CK inhibitors, so serial dilution of a sample with high CK activity may result in progressively higher activity levels. Thus, while the true activity level is high, it may be spuriously increased as a result of multiple dilutions to the sample [23].

10.1.2.3 Lactate Dehydrogenase

Lactate dehydrogenase (LDH) is a cytoplasmic enzyme that catalyzes the conversion of pyruvate to lactate at the end of anaerobic glycolysis. It is present in many tissues in the body and is therefore not specific to muscle. However, it is present in higher concentrations in skeletal and cardiac muscle, kidney, and liver [14]. In heparinized equine plasma samples, the enzyme is stable when stored at room temperature and −18 °C for seven days. However, storage of heparinized equine whole blood in the same conditions results in a marked increase in LDH activity [24]. In another study, storage of equine clotted blood and serum samples at room temperature produced increases in LDH activity after 24 hours [6]. Results are reported in international units per liter (U/L).

The half-life of LDH is reported to be seven days and peak concentrations are expected 24 hours after tissue injury [9]. More recent studies have produced different results for half-life, with return to normal values in three days in one study and 10–21 days in another [9, 11]. Perhaps these variations are due in part to the different half-lives of the LDH isoenzymes, which vary in concentration in any one tissue, as well as the variable half-lives of the same isoenzyme in different tissues [25, 26].

Lactate dehydrogenase is not organ specific and is present in a variety of tissues. Increases in serum LDH activity in the horse can suggest skeletal muscle injury, cardiac muscle injury, or hepatocellular insult; however, in the absence of isoenzyme analysis, utilization of other enzymes more specific for muscle and liver is recommended for interpretation. Erythrocytes contain a greater concentration of LDH than plasma, so hemolysis can cause increases in LDH as well [13].

10.1.2.4 Alanine Aminotransferase

Alanine aminotransferase catalyzes the reversible transamination of L-alanine and 2-oxoglutarate (alpha-ketoglutarate) to pyruvate and glutamate. This reaction requires PP as a cofactor. In horses, a considerable amount of serum ALT is reported to be in the apoenzyme form (inactive form that is not bound to the cofactor), which can generate an underestimation of the total serum ALT activity if PP is not added to the sample. In one study, the increase in serum ALT activity after the addition of PP ranged from an average of 27% in retired, non-Thoroughbred, unexercised horses to 61% in resting Thoroughbred racehorses and 72% in postexercise Thoroughbred racehorses [4].

Alanine aminotransferase is a cytoplasmic and mitochondrial enzyme, though the mitochondrial form is present in much smaller amounts. ALT activity is found in several organs in the horse, including muscle and liver. Based on studies of bovine blood, ALT is stable at room temperature in plasma for four days and serum for two days, though reports for human blood suggest a shorter stability of 24 hours at room temperature (and up to seven days at 4 °C) [27, 28]. Plasma ALT half-life in dogs is 2–3 days. Reports for values in the horse are lacking. Results are reported in international units per liter (U/L).

Many consider ALT to be a muscle-specific enzyme in the horse, as the liver has minimal ALT activity and is expected to contribute little to serum ALT activity [29].

Despite this specificity, it is often absent from large animal biochemical profiles, perhaps due to greater reliance on CK and AST for muscle injury assessment. Hemolysis in equine serum is reported to cause increases in ALT due to both spectral interference and the addition of ALT from erythrocytes [30].

10.1.3 Additional Factors Affecting CK and AST Enzyme Activity

10.1.3.1 Exercise and Training

The effect of exercise and training on serum muscle enzyme activity is difficult to determine. Results vary in the literature due to differences in protocols used by different studies (such as variations in exercise and training duration and intensity), fitness level of the study subjects, and the study interval.

Overall, the majority of studies find minimal to no increases in muscle enzymes during exercise. These studies include protocols of primarily submaximal intensity or short duration exercise [4, 7, 31]. In some studies that did report increases in muscle enzyme activity, these increases were attributed to muscle injury. For example, in one study, three horses had gluteal muscle injury and four had subclinical muscle damage. These horses were also exercised on a treadmill at an incline, which may have predisposed to injury [32].

In contrast to these results, studies in horses performing maximal or longer duration (endurance) exercise found significant increases in serum muscle enzymes (CK) activities, though these studies reported either no increase in AST or inconclusive AST results [33, 34]. Although CK and AST increases may occur with exercise, values are often not clinically significant and still within normal limits. Generally, with exercise there is a 50% increase in enzyme activity. CK increases can be attributed to plasma volume changes and muscle leakage and AST increases can be attributed to plasma volume change [35].

10.1.3.2 Sex, Age, and Pregnancy

Differences in CK and AST due to age and sex are inconsistent in the literature. One study of Thoroughbred mares between 2 and 4 years of age found no effects of age on resting CK or AST [36]. However, a separate study of 2- and 3-year-old Thoroughbreds in training revealed that fillies were more likely to have increased CK and AST than colts, and 2-year-olds tended to have higher AST than 3-year-olds. Thus, age was a factor for CK and both age and sex were factors for AST [37]. In addition, in another study, 2-year-old Thoroughbred fillies showed more marked fluctuations in AST and CK than 3-year-old Thoroughbred fillies and colts. No relationship was found between elevations in muscle enzymes and stage of the estrous cycle [38]. Some studies did find evidence that sex differences may be due to the effect of hormones such as progesterone and estradiol on CK and AST release [38, 39]. These findings suggest that age- and/or sex-specific reference intervals may be necessary.

In a study evaluating biochemical differences between pregnant and nonpregnant Lipizzaner mares, no significant differences were found in activities of AST, CK, or LDH between the two groups. However, AST activity was lower in late-term pregnant mares compared to those in early or mid-term pregnancy [40].

10.1.3.3 Venipuncture

Incorrect venipuncture can result in injury to connective tissue surrounding the vein and/or adjacent musculature and subsequent release of CK which mixes with the sample, thus increasing the CK activity measured. CK can increase over 125% above those values obtained via normal/correct venipuncture, yielding false-positive results [41].

10.1.4 Nonenzymatic Markers of Muscle Injury

10.1.4.1 Myoglobin

Myoglobin is a heme-containing, oxygen-carrying monomer protein expressed in muscle fibers that may be a useful biomarker of muscle fiber injury. Myoglobin is released into circulation immediately after muscle damage and its concentration peaks shortly (5–30 minutes) after muscle injury [42]. Myoglobin is cleared from the circulation faster than CK. Studies of horses with recurrent rhabdomyolysis show return to normal levels by 24–72 hours after exercise, though a study in humans suggests longer increases (of up to 19 days) may be possible with endurance exercise [42, 43].

Because myoglobin is cleared so quickly from the circulation, measurement of myoglobin in the urine may be of diagnostic value and helpful in situations where blood sampling soon after muscle injury is not possible. Myoglobin causes discoloration of the urine to a reddish-brown (port-wine-like) color (Figure 10.2). Pigmenturia can elicit suspicion for myoglobinuria; however, hematuria and hemoglobinuria must also be considered as possible differentials. Hematuria may be ruled out by sedimentation of erythrocytes after centrifugation of the urine sample for 30 seconds or by microscopic evaluation of the urine sample and detection of erythrocytes. In cases of hemoglobinuria, the plasma will be discolored as well (though it is more of a pink color), whereas myoglobin does not cause a change in plasma color because of its rapid clearance [44].

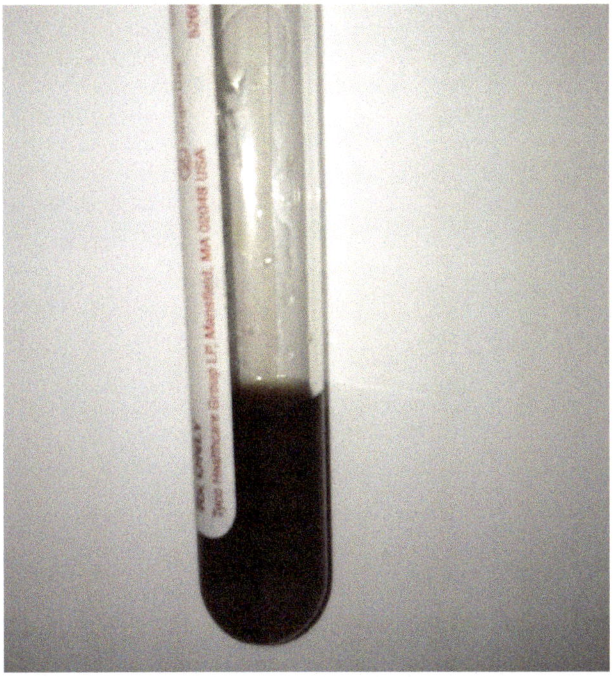

Figure 10.2 Urine sample with myoglobinuria. Unlike hemoglobinuria, a concurrent serum sample will be clear due to the rapid clearance of myoglobin from plasma.

Laboratory methods to detect myoglobin include urine dipstick tests, ammonium sulfate, spectrophotometric assays, and immunoassays. Cautious use of urine dipstick tests is recommended as many urine dipstick tests do not distinguish between myoglobin, hemoglobin, and hematuria. Ammonium sulfate, when added to urine, should precipitate the hemoglobin but not the myoglobin. Hemoglobin precipitates at 80% saturation with ammonium sulfate, whereas myoglobin precipitates at 100% saturation. However, because precipitation depends on the pH, temperature, time, and other factors, ammonium sulfate precipitation can give false results and is generally considered unreliable [45]. Spectrophotometric analysis can differentiate hemoglobinuria from myoglobinuria but some investigators consider it less reliable due to the rapid degradation of myoglobin to the met-myoglobin form (which changes the spectra). Immunoassays are the most sensitive and specific method for detection of myoglobin in both the blood and urine. Radial immunodiffusion, nephelometry/immunoturbidimetry, and radioimmunoassay have all been described. Radial immunodiffusion and nephelometric methods can detect very low concentrations of myoglobin in urine.

Of particular concern in horses with myoglobinuria is the development of acute tubular necrosis with acute or delayed renal failure due to tubular damage from the excretion of myoglobin. This sequela to muscle injury occurs only in rare cases, and appears to occur in horses with concurrent systemic acidosis and dehydration [46].

10.1.4.2 Troponin I

The troponins are proteins that regulate skeletal and cardiac muscle contraction by making actin–myosin interactions sensitive to cytosolic calcium levels. The troponin complex is composed of three different proteins: troponin C (TnC), which binds calcium, troponin I (TnI), which has an inhibitory function, and troponin T (TnT), which attaches troponin to tropomyosin [47]. The cardiac myocyte contains specific isoforms (cTnI and cTnT), which are used as biomarkers for cardiac myocyte injury due to their specificity and are discussed further in the cardiac muscle section.

Skeletal troponin I (sTnI) is a skeletal muscle-specific protein that has been proposed as a marker for skeletal myocyte injury. Significant sequence dissimilarity (40%) exists between sTnI and cTnI isoforms in humans [48]. If this difference is similar in horses, development of a commercial assay to detect skeletal muscle troponin could be useful in assessing muscle-specific injury. Studies in humans have shown the utility of sTnI to detect muscle injury and have even been successful in differentiating between slow- and fast-twitch muscle isoforms [49]. The enzyme rises in parallel to CK and stays increased for 1–2 days. Limited data in rats also show promise for skeletal muscle troponin as a biomarker for skeletal muscle injury [50]. However, studies in horses are lacking thus far.

10.2 Equine Muscle Diseases

Equine myopathies have many different etiopathogeneses (see Table 10.1). While many result in abnormal increases in laboratory biomarkers of muscle injury, some do not. Most show clinical signs attributable to myopathy that include abnormal function (e.g., tremors and fasciculations), muscle atrophy, and/or pain from muscle necrosis.

10.2.1 Immune-Mediated Myopathies

10.2.1.1 Immune-Mediated Myopathy with Muscle Atrophy

Immune-mediated myopathy in horses has been reported secondary to infection with or exposure to *Streptococcus equi* subsp. *equi*. Both development of a severe infarctive purpura hemorrhagica (IPH) and an acute, severe, rhabdomyolysis have been described secondary to infection with this bacterial agent [51, 52]. There are also reports of immune-mediated myositis in horses with a different clinical course (i.e., muscle atrophy).

Table 10.1 Equine myopathies.

Immune-mediated	Infectious	Traumatic	Inherited/congenital
Myopathy with muscle atrophy	Bacterial/rickettsial	Compartment syndrome	Glycogen branching enzyme deficiency
Infarctive purpura hemorrhagica	*Anaplasma phagocytophilum*	Postanesthetic myopathy	Hyperkalemic periodic paralysis
	Clostridial myositis	Extreme exercise	Malignant hyperthermia
	Clostridium botulinum		Myotonia
	Corynebacterium pseudotuberculosis		Polysaccharide storage myopathy
	Streptococcus equi		Myofibrillar myopathy
	Parasitic		Recurrent exertional rhabdomyolysis
	Otobius megnini		Lipid storage myopathy
	Sarcocystis spp.		Centronuclear myopathy
	Theileria equi		
	Babesia caballi		
	Viral		
	Equine herpesvirus I		
	Equine influenza virus 2		

Toxic	Nutritional	Unknown	Other
Hypoglycin A			
Blister beetle	Vit E/selenium deficiency	Acquired motor neuron disease	Pituitary pars intermedia dysfunction
Thiaminase-containing plants			Aortic iliac thrombosis
Senna occidentalis, obtusifolia		Systemic calcinosis	
Ionophores			
Ageratina altissima			
Malva parviflora			

One study in horses with this type of immune-mediated myositis revealed 39% had a history of exposure to *S. equi* or *S. zooepidemicus* within the three months prior to the onset of clinical signs; however, the remaining horses had no underlying trigger identified. The same study showed an overrepresentation of the quarter horse breed. A subsequent study identified an autosomal dominant missense mutation in the MYH1 gene encoding type 2X myosin heavy chain (substitution of glutamic acid for glycine at position 321), which is strongly associated with susceptibility to immune-mediated myositis in quarter horses [53, 54]. There appears to be a bimodal age distribution, with horses younger than 8 and older than 17 years more likely to be affected. Clinical signs include rapid onset of muscle atrophy (with the epaxial and gluteal muscles most severely affected), lethargy, stiffness, weakness, and fever. CK and AST levels are often persistently increased (between 1000 and 10 000 U/L), though in some cases are normal. Histological findings are consistent with immune-mediated myositis with cellular infiltrates of predominantly macrophages and lymphocytes [55].

10.2.1.2 Infarctive Purpura Hemorrhagica

Infarctive purpura hemorrhagica (IPH) has been reported as an uncommon sequela to infection or exposure to *S. equi equi*, *Corynebacterium pseudotuberculosis*, and vaccination against *S. equi equi*. Rare cases have occurred post infection with equine influenza virus, equine viral arteritis, equine herpesvirus type I, *S. equi zooepidemicus*, and *Rhodococcus equi*. However, around one-third of cases have no identified underlying etiology. Young to middle-aged horses are most commonly affected. Clinical signs often occur within

2–4 weeks after a respiratory infection. Most common signs include muscle swelling and edema of all the limbs, stiffness, lethargy, anorexia, hemorrhages on mucous membranes, and fever. Increases in CK ranging from 50000 to 280000 U/L and AST ranging from 1000 to 7000 U/L are common. Hematological changes include an inflammatory leukogram (leukocytosis characterized by a neutrophilia with left shift and toxic change), hyperfibrinogenemia, hyperglobulinemia, hypoalbuminemia, and abnormal clotting parameters. Histological findings show acute coagulative necrosis of affected tissue with leukocytoclastic (small vessel) vasculitis.

Immune complexes in horses with IPH are composed of IgM or IgA and streptococcal M protein (SeM). These complexes result in deposition of complement in vessel walls, cell destruction, and vascular occlusion. Enzyme-linked immunosorbent assay (ELISA) for detection of antibodies against SeM may be markedly increased (>1:1600) [51, 56, 57].

10.2.2 Infectious Myopathies

10.2.2.1 Bacterial

10.2.2.1.1 Anaplasma phagocytophilum Rhabdomyolysis associated with *Anaplasma phagocytophilum*, an obligate intracellular gram-negative bacterium, has been rarely reported in the literature. Clinical signs include fever, tachycardia, and stiffness. Increases in CK (>100000 U/L) and AST (>20000 U/L) are marked [58]. Microscopic blood smear evaluation may reveal morulae (or microcolonies) within neutrophils. Other methods of diagnosis include detection of antibodies via immunofluorescence assay (IFA), Western immunoblot (WIB), or ELISA, which require serial measurement and demonstration of an increasing titer, or detection of antigens in the blood via polymerase chain reaction (PCR) [59].

10.2.2.1.2 Clostridial Myositis *Clostridium perfringens* and *C. septicum* are the most common species reported in association with myonecrosis in the horse; other less commonly implicated species include *C. chauvoei*, *C. sordelli*, *C. novyi*, and *C. fallax*. The organisms are large, gram-positive, anaerobic bacteria that most commonly cause infection in horses by contamination of injection sites or puncture wounds. CK and AST may be mildly to moderately increased if sufficient muscle necrosis is present. Diagnosis may be by microscopic identification of organisms in affected tissue, anaerobic culture, or detection via a fluorescent antibody test [60, 61].

10.2.2.1.3 Clostridium botulinum (Botulism) *Clostridium botulinum* can also cause myopathy in horses due to type C toxin produced by the gram-positive anaerobic bacillus. The toxin may be ingested from contaminated feed, produced by ingested bacteria in the intestinal tract, or produced by the bacteria in wounds. Production of toxin within the intestines is the most common cause in foals, and usually occurs between 1 week and 6 months of age, while production in wounds is an uncommon cause in horses. The toxin cleaves SNARE proteins required for presynaptic vesicle exocytosis, prohibiting the release of acetylcholine and causing muscle weakness, tremors, and dysphagia. Signs often progress to generalized flaccid paralysis and recumbency. CK and AST are often normal but may eventually increase due to ischemic myopathy secondary to recumbency. Horses are extremely sensitive to the toxin and tests to detect and measure toxin levels may not be able to register such low amounts. Diagnosis can be based on analysis of stomach contents or feed but usually depends on clinical signs and elimination of other possible causes [62].

Equine grass sickness is a dysautonomia of unknown etiology, but may be a form of botulism in horses [63]. However, unlike botulism, equine grass sickness is associated with autonomic and enteric neurodegeneration and increased expression of SNARE proteins in neurons [64].

10.2.2.1.4* Corynebacterium pseudotuberculosis *(Pigeon Fever) *Corynebacterium pseudotuberculosis* is a gram-positive facultative intracellular pleomorphic bacterium. The bacteria may cause a diffuse infection of the limbs and internal or external abscesses. External abscesses are the most common presentation in the western United States. Intramuscular abscesses fall into this external abscess category and are commonly located in the pectoral region and along the ventral midline or abdomen. It is postulated that the bacteria enter the horse through skin abrasions and penetrating wounds. One study demonstrated that house flies may act as mechanical vectors of *C. pseudotuberculosis* in horses [65]. Infections usually occur in the fall and early winter. Both ELISA for detection of antibodies and PCR to identify bacteria isolated from abscesses have been reportedly used for the diagnosis of infection [61, 66].

10.2.2.1.5 Streptococcus equi Severe acute rhabdomyolysis is a rarely reported but often fatal complication of upper respiratory infections due to *S. equi* in the horse. Common signs of infection with this gram-positive bacterium include myalgia, stiffness, stilted gait (especially in the pelvic limbs), severe swelling and pitting edema of epaxial and gluteal muscles, recumbency, and myoglobinuria. Clinicopathological findings include a leukocytosis characterized by a neutrophilia, hyperfibrinogenemia, and markedly increased CK (over 100 000 U/L) and AST. Diagnostic methods include detection of cocci in affected skeletal muscle, bacterial culture of affected tissues, measurement of serum antibody titers to *S. equi* myosin binding protein via ELISA, immunofluorescent staining of skeletal muscle for *S. equi* myosin-binding protein, and *S. equi* PCR [52].

The exact mechanism of pathogenicity is unknown but may be due to cross-reacting streptococcal antibodies that target skeletal muscle myosin, direct muscle invasion by the bacteria, bacteremia with exotoxin and protease production within skeletal muscle, or nonspecific T-cell stimulation by streptococcal superantigens. Four *S. equi* superantigens have been identified that elicit immune responses similar to those in humans infected with *Streptococcus pyogenes* causing necrotizing myositis and toxic shock [52].

10.2.2.2 Parasitic

10.2.2.2.1 Otobius megnini (Equine Ear Tick) Infestation with the equine ear tick (Otobius megnini) is a rare cause of muscle tremors and muscle fasciculations in the horse. CK and AST may be mildly to moderately increased [67].

10.2.2.2.2* Sarcocystis *spp. *Sarcocystis* spp. are a common incidental finding in equine skeletal and cardiac muscle and are assumed to be rarely associated with clinical disease. However, this assumption is challenged by sporadic case reports linking *S. fayeri* infection with muscle degeneration and necrosis and eosinophilic myositis in the horse. Presenting clinical signs in these cases included weight loss, weakness, ataxia, and dysphagia (if tongue or esophagus was involved) [68–70]. One study identified a higher prevalence and burden of sarcocysts in the muscle of horses with neuromuscular disease compared to clinically healthy horses [71]. *Sarcocystis bertrami* is the species affecting horses and donkeys in Europe [72].

10.2.2.2.3 Piroplasmosis *Theileria equi* and *Babesia caballi* affect horses in tropical, subtropical, and temperate regions and are transmitted by ixodid ticks. An inflammatory myopathy has been described in horses with chronic piroplasmosis [73]. Clinical features include anorexia, weight loss, muscle atrophy, and poor performance. Endomysial lymphocytic infiltrates and autoantibodies directed against muscle antigens detected in horses with chronic piroplasmosis support an immune-mediated pathogenesis [73].

10.2.2.3 Viral

10.2.2.3.1 Equine Herpesvirus 1 (EHV-1) An outbreak of muscle stiffness in Thoroughbreds at a racing yard revealed a significant proportion of horses with antibody levels supportive of EHV-1 infection as well as increases in CK and AST [74].

10.2.2.3.2 Equine Influenza Virus A2 Equine influenza virus is reported as a rare cause of muscle degeneration in the horse. Clinical signs include upper respiratory infection and myalgia. Clinicopathological findings can include marked increases in muscle enzymes and myoglobinuria. The disease was rapidly progressive and fatal in all three of the reported cases in one study [68].

10.2.3 Traumatic Myopathies

Accidents or falls can cause significant muscle damage, including diaphragmatic rupture in the horse. Neurological disease can also cause myopathy in the horse, particularly during seizure activity or prolonged recumbency. Illness or trauma that results in prolonged recumbency has the potential to cause ischemic myopathy and rhabdomyolysis. In the horse, the gluteal muscles are often affected in dorsal recumbency and in lateral recumbency muscles such as the triceps group tend to be affected [75]. Trauma to muscle can also occur from medical treatments including surgical incisions and manipulation, injection of medications or irritating substances, and placement of tight casts or bandages. In horses, trauma to specific muscles such as the gastrocnemius muscle can occur during exercise or while struggling to rise.

10.2.3.1 Compartment Syndrome and Postanesthetic Myopathy

Compartment syndrome and postanesthetic myopathy develop when accumulation of fluid (edema or hemorrhage) creates high pressure within the enclosed fascial space surrounding the muscle. This high pressure results in reduced capillary blood flow to the muscle and ischemic damage. Placement of tight external bandages or casts can also result in a reduction of the compartment size and similar ischemic injury.

Compartment syndrome in horses undergoing anesthesia for surgical or nonsurgical procedures has also been reported and is referred to as postanesthetic myopathy. The most important contributing factors to development of inadequate muscle perfusion and myopathy are thought to include positioning (with the dependent muscles of recumbent horses often affected), increased intracompartmental muscle pressures, low arterial blood pressure, venous stasis, and a longer length of procedure [75–78]. Affected muscles may have increased intracompartmental pressures and increases in serum CK and AST are also reported [79].

10.2.3.2 Extreme Exercise/Overexertion

Extreme exercise and overexertion may cause myopathy and rhabdomyolysis in the horse. These cases are considered sporadic, versus the recurrent or chronic exertional rhabdomyolysis discussed later in this chapter. Sporadic exertional rhabdomyolysis occurs most often in cases of extreme exercise, heavy training/exercise after a period of decreased intensity training, or exercise/training in adverse environmental conditions (such as extreme heat). Dietary imbalances such as high nonstructural carbohydrate and low forage content or inadequate selenium and vitamin E can also be contributing factors [54]. Common clinicopathological findings include hemoconcentration, lactic acidosis, electrolyte changes, and increases in muscle enzymes (AST, CK, and LDH). Hypochloremia, hypokalemia, and hypocalcemia may all be seen with heavy sweating. Hyponatremia and hypernatremia have both been reported. Sporadic episodes may be subclinical to severe. In more severe cases, moderate to marked increases in muscle enzymes (up to 100 000 times the upper reference limit) and myoglobinuria may be seen. Calcium, magnesium, and potassium depletion can all contribute to stasis of the gastrointestinal tract and related clinical signs. Damage to the kidneys from myoglobin and/or inadequate tissue perfusion can result in renal failure, although this sequela is rare [80].

10.2.4 Inherited or Congenital Myopathies

10.2.4.1 Glycogen Branching Enzyme Deficiency

Glycogen branching enzyme deficiency is a fatal, autosomal-recessive disease of quarter horses and American Paint horses caused by a nonsense mutation of the glycogen branching enzyme I (GBE1) gene [81]. Approximately 8% of quarter horses and American Paint horses are carriers [82]. The enzyme is essential for the formation of alpha-1,6 glycosidic linkages to form branched glycogen, thus the enzyme deficiency limits the number of nonreducing ends at which glycogen can be formed and degraded. Polysaccharide with largely alpha-1,4 glycosidic linkages accumulates in skeletal and cardiac muscle, liver, and brain [81]. The inability to store and mobilize glycogen to maintain normal glucose homeostasis has catastrophic consequences. Affected foals may be aborted, stillborn, or weak at birth with contracted tendons. In surviving foals, rhabdomyolysis, hypoglycemic seizures, or cardiac failure occur and usually lead to euthanasia or death before 18 weeks of age [81]. Common laboratory findings include leukopenia, intermittent hypoglycemia, and moderate increases in CK, AST, and gamma-glutamyl transferase (GGT).

Analysis of peripheral blood or skeletal muscle for reduced activity of the enzyme or histopathological analysis of myocytes for detection of PAS-positive and amylase-resistant inclusions are supportive of the diagnosis. However, the most accurate method of diagnosis for carriers and affected foals is a DNA test performed on samples from pulled mane or tail hairs [83].

10.2.4.2 Hyperkalemic Periodic Paralysis

Hyperkalemic periodic paralysis (HYPP) is an autosomal-dominant trait found in quarter horses, Appaloosas, American Paint horses, and quarter horse cross-breeds. Approximately 4% of the quarter horse population carries the mutation [84]. It is caused by a missense point mutation in the skeletal muscle sodium channel gene (SCN4A). Affected horses are either homozygous or heterozygous for the disease.

The HYPP mutation results in a lower threshold for membrane depolarization in skeletal muscle and the failure of a subpopulation of sodium channels to inactivate after depolarization. The result is an excessive influx of sodium ions and outflux of potassium ions that generates a persistent depolarization of the myocyte [85].

Affected horses exhibit intermittent muscle fasciculations in the face, neck, shoulders, and flanks beginning around 2–3 years of age [81]. Fasciculations may cease after 15–20 minutes but can progress to weakness and recumbency. Horses heterozygous for HYPP are often less severely affected, with less frequent episodes than their homozygous counterparts, indicating a codominant mode of inheritance [81, 86]. Respiratory stridor, respiratory distress, and dysphagia may be evident with possible obstruction of the upper airway due to pharyngeal collapse or laryngeal paralysis. Upper airway obstruction tends to be seen more frequently in horses homozygous for the trait [87].

During an episode, clinicopathological abnormalities often include hyperkalemia (6–9 mEq/L), hemoconcentration, and mild hyponatremia. However, serum potassium concentrations are normal in between episodes and may be normal during mild episodes as well. CK values are usually normal, though mild increases in CK are occasionally seen a few hours after the episode [85, 86].

Episodes may be triggered by a variety of precipitating factors. One of the most important factors is consumption of high-potassium foods such as alfalfa, soybean, and molasses, as well as electrolyte supplements, and kelp-based supplements [88]. Other precipitating factors include sudden diet change, fasting, anesthesia, sedation, stress, transport, rest after exercise, exposure to cold, pregnancy, and concurrent disease [87]. Diagnosis is based on a DNA test for the mutation in the SCN4A gene using submitted mane or tail hairs. The test can distinguish between homozygous affected, heterozygous affected, and normal horses [85].

10.2.4.3 Malignant Hyperthermia

Malignant hyperthermia in horses is a pharmacogenetic disease of skeletal muscle. It has been reported in quarter horses, American Paint horses, Thoroughbreds, Appaloosas, ponies, and Arabians [54, 89, 90].

In quarter horses, a genetic basis for the disease has been linked to a mutation in the ryanodine receptor 1 gene (RyR1*)*. The prevalence of the mutation in quarter horses was reported to be 1.3% in one study [91]. Because the disease is inherited as an autosomal dominant trait, quarter horse-related breeds may also exhibit clinical signs [92]. The mutation causes dysfunction of the sarcoplasmic reticulum calcium release channel, resulting in massive release of calcium into the sarcoplasm and a hypermetabolic state characterized by hyperthermia and muscle rigidity.

Clinical signs are triggered by exposure to halogenated anesthetics (halothane, isoflurane), depolarizing muscle relaxants like succinylcholine, and stress or excitement [92]. Clinicopathological abnormalities include respiratory and metabolic acidosis, hyperkalemia, hyponatremia, hypocalcemia, hyperphosphatemia, hyperproteinemia, and azotemia. Marked elevations in CK and AST as well as myoglobinuria may also be noted [92, 93].

10.2.4.4 Myotonia Congenita and Dystrophica

Myotonia congenita is a nondystrophic form of myotonia, which occurs in foals and has also been described in humans and goats. Affected foals exhibit characteristic bulging of the thigh and rump muscles soon after birth and pelvic limb stiffness, which may improve with exercise. Percussion of affected muscles exacerbates muscle dimpling below the area of muscle contraction. Muscle relaxation can be delayed by a minute or more. Clinical signs usually do not progress beyond 6–12 months of age [81, 94]. A missense mutation in the same chloride channel gene (CLCN1) affected in myotonia congenita in humans and goats has recently been identified in one New Forest pony, but further studies are needed to confirm this as a causal mutation of myotonia congenita [95].

Myotonia dystrophica is a severe, progressive, neuromuscular disorder which has been reported in quarter horses, Thoroughbred foals, and Anglo-Arab-Sardinian foals [96–98]. Clinical signs of the disease may be apparent as early as 1 month of age and include generalized myotonia, proximal muscle hypertrophy and hypertonicity followed by stiffness, weakness, and atrophy. Horses may have marked exercise intolerance. Testicular hypoplasia, cataract formation, and glucose intolerance have also been reported.

Diagnosis of myotonia is based on age, clinical signs, prolonged muscle contraction after stimulation, and electromyographic (EMG) examination. Affected muscles produce pathognomonic crescendo–decrescendo, high-frequency, repetitive electrical bursts in EMG examination. Classic histopathological findings (sarcoplasmic masses, ringed fibers, internal positioning of sarcolemmal nuclei, and variation in fiber diameter size) are present in myotonia dystrophica which are not found in myotonia congenita [94].

10.2.4.5 Polysaccharide Storage Myopathy

Polysaccharide storage myopathy (PSSM) is characterized by accumulation of glycogen and abnormal complex polysaccharide inclusions in skeletal muscle. PSSM has been identified in many breeds. Quarter horses, American Paint horses, Appaloosas, Belgian and Percheron draught horses, and Warmbloods are the most commonly affected breeds. It is estimated that 5–12% of quarter horses and 36% of Belgian Draught horses are affected [99–101].

There are at least two types of PSSM. Type 1 (PSSM1) is caused by a gain of function mutation in the glycogen synthase 1 (GSY1) gene, which encodes the skeletal muscle isoform of glycogen synthase. The mutation causes constitutive activation of glycogen synthase 1, and consequently increased concentrations of glycogen in skeletal muscle [102]. Though the mutation was first identified in quarter horses, it has since been associated with PSSM in several other breeds. Prevalence of the mutation in one study ranged widely amongst breeds with approximately 80% of Belgian and Percheron draught horses, 50% of quarter horses and related breeds, and 8% of Warmbloods with histopathological diagnoses of PSSM demonstrating the mutation. In this same study, the mutation was not identified in any of the Standardbred, Thoroughbred, or Arabian Horses with PSSM [103].

Clinical signs range from sporadic or episodic rhabdomyolysis (exertional or nonexertional) to progressive weakness and muscle fasciculations, or less often muscle atrophy [99, 104]. Some horses may be asymptomatic [99]. CK and AST values may range from markedly elevated after an episode of rhabdomyolysis to mildly to moderately increased with exercise, recumbency, and possibly at rest. Values are often normal in draught breeds and Warmblood horses [99]. Myoglobinuria may also be seen after episodes of rhabdomyolysis. In rare cases, myoglobin may cause tubular damage and acute or delayed renal failure. Horses that develop renal failure usually have concurrent dehydration and metabolic acidosis [105].

Members of a family of quarter horses with a more severe and occasionally fatal expression of PSSM were demonstrated to have a mutation in the GYS1 gene as well as a mutation in the RYR1 gene (previously associated with malignant hyperthermia in quarter horses) [106]. Additionally, about 14% of halter quarter horses are affected by mutations of both the GYS1 and SCN4A (associated with HYPP) genes, predisposing them to severe, life-threatening rhabdomyolysis during an episode of HYPP [107]. Diagnosis may be based on histological evaluation of skeletal muscle biopsy and/or genetic testing for the mutation in GYS1.

Type 2 PSSM (PSSM2) characterizes horses with clinical signs of exercise intolerance and accumulations of abnormal polysaccharide in skeletal muscle which lack the GYS1 mutation. The abnormal polysaccharide is usually sensitive rather than resistant to amylase digestion, in contrast to PSSM1. Approximately 80% of Warmblood horses, 28% of quarter horses, and 20% of draught horses diagnosed with PSSM are classified with PSSM2 [54, 81, 108]. In one study, quarter horses with PSSM2 usually presented with chronic exertional rhabdomyolysis and elevations of CK and AST, while Warmblood horses with PSSM2 more frequently presented with stiffness and mild hindlimb lameness. Increases in CK and AST were less common in Warmblood horses with PSSM2 [54, 108]. This clinical variability suggests that PSSM2 is not one specific myopathy but represents multiple different disorders that share common histological changes.

10.2.4.6 Myofibrillar Myopathy

Myofibrillar myopathy (MFM) is a recently described condition affecting mature Arabian and Warmblood horses that has some similarities to MFM in humans and may be familial. Clinical features in Arabian horses include muscle stiffness, pain, or cramps, and muscle atrophy in some cases [109]. Most Warmblood horses identified with MFM presented with an insidious onset of exercise intolerance. Diagnosis is currently based on distinguishing histopathological and ultrastructural features, particularly cytoplasmic aggregates of desmin, as well as internalized myonuclei, anguloid atrophy, Z-disc degeneration, and myofibrillar disarray [109, 110].

10.2.4.7 Recurrent Exertional Rhabdomyolysis

Some sources refer to exertional rhabdomyolysis as an umbrella term that encompasses a variety of myopathies in different breeds, including PSSM in quarter horses and RER in Thoroughbreds. Though these myopathies manifest similarly, they differ in their etiopathogeneses.

Recurrent exertional rhabdomyolysis (RER) is a particular form of exertional rhabdomyolysis distinct from the sporadic exertional rhabdomyolysis discussed earlier. RER is prevalent in Thoroughbred and Standardbred horses and is estimated to affect 5% of the Thoroughbred population [111]. It has also been reported in quarter horses, Arabian, and Warmblood horses [54, 100]. In Thoroughbreds, RER is likely inherited as an autosomal dominant trait with variable expressivity [112, 113]. It is believed to be caused by a defect in intracellular calcium regulation or excitation-contraction coupling leading to excessive muscular contraction and necrosis with exercise, but the precise defect is yet to be identified [114, 115]. Several risk factors for the disease have been identified including young age, female sex, nervous disposition, rest one day prior to exercise, gallop during exercise, diets high in grain (>4.5 kg/day), and concurrent lameness [111, 116].

Clinical signs include muscle cramping, stiffness, lameness, and sweating during or shortly after exercise [81]. Most affected horses show clinical signs, but in some cases the disease can be hard to detect without analysis of muscle enzyme activity. Classic laboratory abnormalities include increases in serum muscle enzymes after exercise. Horses may also have myoglobinuria with moderate to severe episodes of muscle necrosis. In rare cases, myoglobin may damage renal tubules and lead to acute or delayed renal failure if there is concurrent dehydration and systemic acidosis [105].

A tentative diagnosis of RER may be based on clinical signs, risk factors, and increased muscle enzymes post exercise. In some cases, a muscle biopsy may be necessary for diagnosis but histological features of RER (e.g., increased numbers of central nuclei) are also nonspecific [81]. Muscle biopsy specimens have been shown to exhibit abnormal *in vitro* contracture response to potassium, caffeine, or halothane compared to control horses [114, 115].

10.2.4.8 Lipid Storage Myopathy

Lipid storage myopathy was suspected in a single case report of a <1-day-old foal, which presented with forelimb muscle fasciculations, weakness, and persistent hypoglycemia. Elevated serum muscle enzymes, serum free carnitine, serum acylcarnitines, and urine organic acids were detected, and muscle biopsy revealed numerous large lipid droplets within myofibers. Biochemical abnormalities were similar to multiple acyl-CoA dehydrogenase deficiency which may be congenital (described in humans) or acquired secondary to exposure to hypoglycin A (discussed later in this chapter) [117].

10.2.4.9 Centronuclear Myopathy

Weakness and severe progressive generalized muscle atrophy in an Arabian cross foal were suspected to be caused by centronuclear myopathy. This group of congenital myopathies is characterized by high numbers of myofibers with centrally located nuclei and abnormalities of the T-tubular system and triads [118].

10.2.5 Toxic Myopathies

10.2.5.1 Hypoglycin A (Seasonal Pasture Myopathy/Atypical Myopathy)

Hypoglycin A is a toxic compound found in seeds of trees belonging to the Sapindaceae family and is the cause of seasonal pasture myopathy, known as atypical myopathy in Europe. The box elder tree (*Acer negundo*) and sycamore tree (*Acer pseudoplatanus*) are the principal species implicated in hypoglycin A intoxication of horses in North America and Europe, respectively.

Hypoglycin A is metabolized to methylenecyclopropyl acetic acid (MCPA), which forms an ester with coenzyme A (MCPA-CoA) and subsequently inhibits multiple acyl-CoA dehydrogenases required for beta-oxidation of short and medium chain fatty acids in mitochondria. Consequently, acyl-CoAs accumulate in mitochondria and acyl moieties are scavenged by carnitine, resulting in the accumulation of acylcarnitines in plasma. MCPA also binds carnitine, disrupting the transport of long chain fatty acids into mitochondria, or may be conjugated with glycine. The toxin has the greatest impact on type I myofibers present in postural, cardiac, and respiratory muscles which are heavily dependent on beta-oxidation of fatty acids for energy. The inhibition of beta-oxidation leads to intracellular accumulation of fatty acids, increased anaerobic glycolysis, muscle glycogen depletion, and lactic acidosis [119–123].

Seasonal pasture myopathy/atypical myopathy most commonly occurs in horses grazing in autumn and spring. Typical clinical features are depression, profound muscular weakness progressing to recumbency, sweating, pigmenturia, bladder distension, tachypnea, and dyspnea [124]. The condition is rapidly fatal in approximately 75% of cases, the majority of which survive no more than three days after onset of clinical signs [125]. Markedly elevated CK values, hyperglycemia, and hypocalcemia are common. Hypocalcemia may contribute to development of dysrhythmias and is also a suggested prognostic marker. Horses with total calcium <2.69 mmol/L (RI 2.50-3.40) were reported to have a 70% chance of dying in one study [120]. Horses less than 5 years of age are less likely to survive than middle-aged horses [120, 124]. A single case report of atypical myopathy in a newborn foal suggests toxic metabolites of hypoglycin A may cross the placenta or be secreted in colostrum [126].

Diagnosis is often presumptive based on history, clinical signs, and biochemical changes. High-performance liquid chromatography (HPLC) and tandem mass spectrometry can be used to measure acylcarnitines, MCPA-carnitine, and/or MCPA-glycine conjugates in serum or urine to help confirm the diagnosis [127]. Profiling of acylcarnitines in serum shows promise for predicting survival in affected horses [120, 127]. Hypoglycin A can also be measured in serum to confirm exposure but has no prognostic value. Liquid chromatography and mass spectrometry can also be used to detect hypoglycin A in plant material [120, 127, 128]. Methylenecyclopropylglycine (MCPG), a structural analogue of hypoglycin A also found in *Acer* spp., is metabolized to methylenecyclopropylformyl-CoA (MCPF-CoA) which inhibits beta-oxidation at a different step from MCPA-CoA. MCPG, MCPF-CoA, as well as MCPF-carnitine and glycine conjugates, have also been identified in the serum and urine of horses with atypical myopathy [129].

10.2.5.2 Blister Beetle Toxicosis (Cantharidiasis)

Blister beetle toxicosis (cantharidiasis) in horses is most often due to ingestion of alfalfa hay or pellets contaminated with blister beetles (*Epicauta* spp.). Blister beetles secrete cantharidin, which can exert effects even in the absence of actual blister beetle bodies and can withstand degradation by heating and drying.

Gastrointestinal signs are the most common presenting signs (colic, irritability, restlessness, and diarrhea) though the toxin may also cause urinary tract signs (hematuria, stranguria, and pollakiuria). Cardiovascular signs and neuromuscular signs (aggressive behavior, seizure-like muscle fasciculations) are less commonly noted. Oral lesions (oral ulcers, profuse salivation) and synchronous diaphragmatic flutter (associated with hypocalcemia and hypomagnesemia) have been reported [130]. Laboratory abnormalities may include hypocalcemia (often marked), hypomagnesemia, increases in CK (within 24 hours of ingestion), and hyperglycemia. Urinalysis may reveal hyposthenuria, hematuria, and possibly myoglobinuria. Azotemia may be noted due to dehydration or secondary to toxin-mediated renal tubular necrosis.

The diagnosis can be confirmed via HPLC or gas chromatography and mass spectrometry to detect/quantify cantharidin in urine as well as liver, kidneys, and gastric contents [131].

10.2.5.3 Thiaminase: Bracken Fern (*Pteridium aquilinum*), Horsetail (*Equisetum arvense*), Rock Fern (*Cheilanthes sieberi*)

Thiamine (vitamin B1) is an essential component of energy metabolism and important in maintaining the myelin of peripheral nerves. Thiaminase cleaves the thiamine molecule and renders it inactive. Ingestion of thiaminase produces a thiamine deficiency, which results in metabolic abnormalities as well as myelin degeneration of peripheral nerves. The most common cause of intoxication in horses is ingestion of contaminated hay.

Clinical signs of thiamine deficiency include anorexia resulting in poor body condition and weight loss, as well as gait disturbances and uncoordinated movements that may progress to loss of muscle control (twitches and tremors) [132].

10.2.5.4 *Senna occidentalis* (Coffee Senna; Coffee Weed) and *Senna obtusifolia* (Sickle Pod; Coffee Bean; Coffee Weed)

The toxic effects of *Senna occidentalis* and *S. obtusifolia* are attributed to anthraquinones and their derivatives and alkaloids. Ingestion of the plants may cause liver degeneration, gastrointestinal signs (diarrhea), and muscle necrosis that manifests as muscular weakness progressing to recumbency and death. Increased serum CK and AST, hyperkalemia, and myoglobinuria are frequent findings [133].

10.2.5.5 Ionophore

Horses may suffer ionophore-induced myocardial and skeletal muscle degeneration with ingestion of monensin, lasalocid, maduramicin, narasin, or salinomycin. Ionophores are commonly used as coccidiostats in feed for food animals, and horses may be exposed by access to ruminant feed or by accidental contamination of horse feed. Intoxication may occur with very small doses because horses are highly sensitive to ionophores. The substances increase membrane permeability and cause abnormal movement of ions across cell membranes, thus disrupting normal ionic equilibrium [134–136].

Clinical signs initially include colic and anorexia that rapidly progresses to signs of myopathy/cardiomyopathy, recumbency, and death. Some cases may only present with neurological signs (ataxia and seizures) [135]. Horses that recover from the acute phase may suffer from cardiac damage and present with delayed signs of cardiomyopathy [137, 138]. Abnormal laboratory findings may include moderate to marked increases in CK and AST and myoglobinuria. Hypocalcemia and hypokalemia may be seen initially in the first 24 hours after exposure. Some cases also report mild hyponatremia, mild hypochloremia, mild hypomagnesemia, and severe hyperglycemia.

Diagnosis is usually based on clinical signs, history of exposure, and histopathological changes. Detection of ionophores may be difficult given the small dose that can cause intoxication; however, feed, stomach contents, and/or affected tissue can be analyzed.

10.2.5.6 *Ageratina altissima* (White Snakeroot)

The toxic component in this plant is tremetol, which can cause depression, muscle weakness and trembling, sweating, myoglobinuria, respiratory difficulty, and dysphagia. Progression of skeletal and heart muscle damage may result in recumbency and signs of cardiac failure. Elevations in CK and AST may be noted [139].

10.2.5.7 *Malva parviflora* (Marshmallow; Small-Flowered Mallow)

Four horses from one farm developed severe muscle fasciculations, tachycardia, sweating, and recumbency following ingestion of *Malva parviflora*. All cases died or were euthanized shortly after the onset of clinical signs. Cyclopropene fatty acids (malvalic and sterculic acid) are thought to be responsible for the toxic effects of this plant by interfering with fatty acid oxidation [140].

10.2.6 Nutritional Myopathies

10.2.6.1 Vitamin E/Selenium Deficiency

Vitamin E/selenium deficiency results in a myodegenerative condition affecting cardiac and skeletal muscle known as white muscle disease. This disease is most common in foals up to weanling age (especially from birth up to 2 weeks of age) though cases are occasionally reported in adults. The disease is most prevalent in areas where the soil selenium content is low. Because selenium uptake in foals mainly occurs via the placenta during gestation, most cases of white muscle disease in foals are due to a selenium-deficient dam. Predisposing factors such as diets high in unsaturated fat or unaccustomed exercise are reported [141, 142].

Selenium and vitamin E serve as antioxidants and prevent cellular damage from reactive oxygen species. Foals may present with a peracute form of the disease characterized by recumbency and struggling to rise with rapid progression to pulmonary edema, cardiovascular collapse, and death. Alternatively, they may present with a more insidious, subacute form of disease which manifests as severe weakness, muscle pain, muscle fasciculations, stiffness, and dysphagia [141]. Laboratory abnormalities include marked increases in CK and AST, hyperproteinemia, hyponatremia, hyperkalemia, hypocalcemia, hyperphosphatemia, and myoglobinuria [143]. Diagnosis is supported by low whole blood selenium and glutathione peroxidase activities. In some cases, plasma vitamin E levels are also decreased. Histological evaluation of muscle biopsies reveals muscle necrosis and regeneration with histiocytic inflammation and calcification [141, 142].

10.2.7 Myopathies of Unknown Cause

10.2.7.1 Acquired Equine Motor Neuron Disease (EMND)

Equine motor neuron disease (EMND) is characterized by degeneration of motor neurons in the spinal cord and brainstem that leads to neurogenic muscle atrophy, weight loss, and weakness. Clinical signs may include muscle fasciculations, trembling of the limbs, and frequent episodes of recumbency. Chronic vitamin E deficiency is a major contributing factor but the etiology is incompletely understood and other factors may contribute to development of the disease [144]. Vitamin E is a known antioxidant that helps in the neutralization of free radicals, and vitamin E deficiency is believed to lead to chronic oxidative stress and death of motor neurons.

Vitamin E deficiency may be attributed to limited access to pasture or access to poor-quality pasture (forage with low vitamin E content) or failure of horses to absorb or retain dietary vitamin E. Other factors that contribute to overall likelihood of EMND include age (older horses are more susceptible to the disease), turnout type and size, predominant type of concentrate fed, and rabies vaccination status [145, 146].

Clinicopathological abnormalities may include mildly to moderately increased serum muscle enzymes (CK and AST) as well as low plasma vitamin E levels [147]. A tentative diagnosis is based on suggestive clinical, epidemiological, and laboratory findings. A definitive diagnosis of EMND may be made on examination of muscle biopsy or spinal accessory nerve biopsy.

10.2.7.2 Systemic Calcinosis

Systemic calcinosis is a well-recognized syndrome of dystrophic calcification in humans and has more recently been suspected in horses. Affected horses present with lethargy, stiffness, and muscle atrophy particularly of the gluteal and epaxial muscles [148]. Respiratory signs and severe rhabdomyolysis are occasionally seen. Laboratory abnormalities include increased serum CK and AST, hyperphosphatemia with a serum calcium phosphorus product greater than 65, and hyperfibrinogenemia. Diagnosis is made on postmortem identification of dystrophic calcification of skeletal and cardiac myofibers, renal tubules, lungs, kidneys, and intestinal vessels [57, 61, 148]. The cause of systemic calcinosis in horses remains unknown, but it may be related to an underlying inflammatory condition. None of the horses reportedly affected had preexisting renal disease, hypercalcemia, or a history of exposure to excess vitamin D [57].

10.2.8 Other Myopathies

10.2.8.1 Cushing's Disease/PPID

Equine pituitary pars intermedia dysfunction (PPID) is a common neurodegenerative disease of aged horses and ponies that has an associated myopathy characterized by muscle atrophy and weakness. In horses with PPID, there is a loss of dopaminergic inhibitory input to the pituitary pars intermedia that results in increased melanotroph function and oversynthesis of proopiomelanocortin (POMC) derived peptides and chronic increases in endogenous glucocorticoids. Muscle enzymes are typically within normal range. Evaluation of muscle biopsies demonstrates type 2 myofiber atrophy [149].

10.2.8.2 Aortic-Iliac Thrombosis

Aortic-iliac thrombosis is occasionally reported in horses and causes decreased blood flow and ischemic damage to muscles. It is most commonly reported in racehorses but can occur in any breed, and males have a higher incidence than females [150]. Horses may have signs of hindlimb lameness (usually unilateral and often exercise-induced) and abdominal distress. The affected limb(s) may be cold and decreased distal pulses (femoral or plantar digital) may be palpated. Decreased blood flow to the hindlimbs, internal and external iliacs, and circumflex iliacs is responsible for the clinical signs. The severity of clinical signs varies depending on the degree of vascular occlusion, the presence of collateral circulation, and the length of time over which the occlusion forms. Diagnosis is based on history, clinical presentation, transrectal palpation, ultrasonography, thermography, and scintigraphy [151].

10.3 Laboratory Evaluation of Equine Cardiac Muscle Disorders

Markers used to monitor for underlying pathology or physiological process are typically leakage enzymes released from damaged cells or functional markers, which can increase or decrease in response to disease. Previously, lactate dehydrogenase (LDH-1 and LDH-2) and CK-myocardial band (CK-MB) were used to detect myocardial injury, but both can also be affected by skeletal muscle injury and chronic renal disease and are less sensitive than other cardiac biomarkers [152]. Troponins and natriuretic peptides, atrial natriuretic peptide (ANP) and brain natriuretic peptide (BNP), are the most used and studied markers. Endothelin-1 (ET-1) is a newer marker that may be shown to be valuable as well [153].

Troponins are leakage enzymes often released with myocardial necrosis/infarction while ANP and BNP are functional markers released in response to myocardial stretch, volume or pressure overload [154]. Diagnostic utility in horses depends on comparing the same assays, having appropriate sensitivity (such as high-sensitivity assays), and using standardized protocols, assay-specific validation, and reference intervals [155, 156]. They may be especially useful in horses for investigation of poor performance, monitoring therapeutic interventions, and distinguishing cardiac from respiratory disease when used in conjunction with echocardiogram, electrocardiogram, and radiology since cardiac diseases in horses often do not result in cardiomyocyte necrosis [154].

10.3.1 Cardiac Troponins

Troponins are composed of three globular proteins (troponin I, T, and C) in striated muscle. They bind together to form the troponin complex, which regulates the calcium-dependent myosin–actin interaction needed for muscle contraction [155–157]. Cardiac isoforms of troponin I and T are designated cTnI and cTnT, respectively. cTnI is not found in smooth muscle, fetal tissue or in significant amounts in normal or diseased striated skeletal muscle, making it useful to distinguish skeletal from cardiac muscle injury [152]. cTnT, however, is also expressed in slow-twitch skeletal muscle and may be increased in chronic skeletal muscular diseases such as polymyositis, muscular dystrophy, and rhabdomyolysis [152]. The proteins are highly conserved, thus human assays can often detect troponins in other species, especially mammals [152].

In the myocyte, the majority of the troponins are located within the myofibrils while a small proportion is within the cytosol. For example, only 2–4% of troponin I is in the cytosol. Approximately 1–2 hours post injury, the cytosolic troponins are released, resulting in a mild to moderate increase in troponin levels. Later on, with more severe injury, more troponins are released, resulting in a more substantial increase [156]. The magnitude of increase in troponin levels also correlates with the degree of severity of the myocardial injury. In humans, the increase in troponins after myocardial injury persists for 4–14 days (depending on the severity), allowing for delayed diagnosis [156–159].

10.3.2 Natriuretic Peptides

Atrial natriuretic peptide (ANP) and BNP are functional markers produced by the cardiac atria (ANP) and ventricles (BNP) in response to myocardial stretch, volume, or pressure overload, which occurs in many heart diseases such as atrial dilation, valvular disease, and heart failure. Elevations of ANP and BNP appear proportional to the severity of disease and atrial size [154, 160–163], but also may be increased during prolonged strenuous exercise [164]. They play a role in blood pressure regulation, diuresis, and natriuresis in order to help regulate volume overload. In dogs, they have also been shown to distinguish dyspnea due to heart failure from dyspnea due to extracardiac causes [165].

Natriuretic peptides are hormones, which are stored as prohormones (proANP and proBNP) and cleaved into the inactive N-terminal peptides (NT-proANP and NT-proBNP) and active ANP and BNP forms [160, 164]. NT-proANP, NT-proBNP, proANP, and proBNP are more stable than the active counterparts [164, 166]. ANP is highly conserved between species and assays are directed at conserved parts, which are similar between horses and humans [167], while BNP is species specific [160, 164]. Although ANP is highly conserved, in horses results between assays are not comparable and some underestimate plasma ANP [161]. Additionally, the coefficient of variation is higher than recommended at lower ANP levels [161]. Therefore, results are not directly comparable between different assays. Some of the variation between ANP assays may be related to ANP stability. Measuring proANP, which is more stable, may be more valuable and has been shown to be increased in horses with atrial dilation [166]. Currently, a species-specific BNP or NT-proBNP test is not available in horses.

10.3.3 Endothelin-1

Currently, there is only one paper evaluating ET-1 in horses [153]. ET-1 is produced primarily by vascular endothelial cells and is a potent vasoconstrictor. It was found to be significantly increased in horses with cardiac disease and normal heart dimensions as well as horses with enlarged left atria. ET-1 also increased significantly in horses with heart disease after exercise [153].

10.4 Specific Cardiac Biomarkers in Horses

10.4.1 Cardiac Troponin I

Cardiac troponin I (cTnl) is considered a highly specific and sensitive biomarker for detecting myocardial injury due to many different causes. It is cleared through the kidneys, therefore impaired renal function can also lead to increased cTnI levels [156]. The *in vivo* half-life of cTn1 in horse is estimated to be 6.4 hours [168].

There are many different immunoassays for cTn1, which vary in the amount they detect, cross-reactivity and sensitivity, so it is important that reference intervals and diagnostic cut-offs are assay specific [155, 169]. The difference between the assays makes direct comparison of results difficult; when comparing samples for a patient, use of the same type of sample on the same immunoassay is recommended [158]. Additionally, these tests need to be appropriately validated to ensure they are reliable and accurate [155]. There may also be a difference in results of the same assay depending on the type of sample used, as heparinized plasma may result in lower values compared to serum samples [158].

For many of the assays, studies showed that many horses are below the limit of detection (LOD). This may have affected the ability to detect differences between groups in earlier studies and may limit interpretation of the results. There are now high-sensitivity assays available, which means the test must have a coefficient of variability of less than 10% at the 99th percentile and a measurable concentration of cTnI should be obtained in ≥50% of healthy individuals [168].

Earlier studies have not shown significant differences in cTnI concentrations in healthy pastured compared to race-training Thoroughbred horses, or due to age [157], sex, gait, or race classification [169]. However, there was a weak positive correlation with cTnI concentration and age in one study looking at racing Standardbreds [169]. Winning racing Standardbreds had undetectable levels 1–2 hours after racing [169] and clinically normal racing Thoroughbreds also had undetectable levels [158]. However, four hours post race, there was a significant increase in cTnI in Thoroughbred race horses that received furosemide. cTnI was at baseline at 24 hours [170]. cTnI was found to be significantly increased shortly after and during recovery following a long-distance endurance ride [171, 172].

Using a validated high-sensitivity assay, Standardbred racehorses had detectable cTnI levels at rest, with all horses having an increase in cTnI post exercise [168]. The peak increase was between two and six hours and remained increased for almost 24 hours. The magnitude of the increase varied widely, from 1.72 to 23.76 ng/L. This variability may have been physiological and related to working at the edge of aerobic capacity or due to myocardial tissue injury. Therefore, exercise should be taken into account when evaluating a horse for cardiac injury. Serial samples beyond the first 24 hours following exercise are recommended [168].

10.4.2 Troponin T

Cardiac troponin T (cTnT) is cardiac specific, but cTnT may be upregulated with chronic muscle injury [152]. Far fewer assays are available for this analyte, which means different laboratories are more likely to use the same assay, resulting in more directly comparable results than cTnI assays discussed earlier. A high-sensitivity cTnT assay (hscTnT) has been validated and upper reference limits were established for use in horses [173]. It was also shown to be significantly increased in two horses with presumed cardiac pathology [173].

In one equine study [174], both cTnI and cTnT (using the hscTnT) were useful at detecting myocardial disease although the sample size was too small to directly compare the sensitivity and specificity of the assays. The hscTnT was also increased in short-distance, high-intensity chuckwagon races [159]. Peak level increases were similar to cTnI and were increased 2–6 hours post race. They also returned to baseline by 12–24 hours. Throughout the period, all were less than 23.2 ng/L [159].

10.4.3 Natriuretic Peptides

Atrial natriuretic peptide and NT-proANP have been evaluated in a few studies with variable results. They have been shown to be specific and increase with left atrial enlargement, valve regurgitation and congestive heart failure, although the sensitivity and reproducibility were sometimes poor such that some horses with heart disease were not identified [153, 160–163, 175, 176]. As previously stated, ProANP may be more useful because it is more stable [166]. At this time, using the same validated assay is essential for measuring ANP in order for results to be comparable.

10.5 Myocardial Diseases

Cardiac disease in horses is rare and often subclinical. Arrhythmias and murmurs are common. When arrhythmias are found, they are often physiological or due to systemic disease such as colitis, colic, sepsis, and intoxications. They may be due to hemostatic disturbance rather than myocardial injury though myocardial injury may be present as well [156, 177].

Cardiac TnI has been shown to be increased with many systemic diseases in horses such as sepsis [178], pyometra [179], colic [180], piroplasmosis (babesiosis) [181], rattlesnake envenomation [182], and transiently with equine influenza virus [183]. Other conditions that can directly affect the myocardium include toxic injury such as caused by ionophore antibiotics (sodium monensin toxicity [184, 185], lasalocid toxicity [186]), rayless golden rod (*Isocoma pluriflora*) toxicity [187], hypoglycin A (*Acer* spp.) [188], oleander, and blister beetle. Additional etiologies include infectious pericarditis/endocarditis, equine herpesvirus, African horse sickness, and equine arteritis, as well as trauma, nutritional imbalances (selenium deficiency), and neoplasia [156, 157].

References

1 Boyd, J.W. (1983). The mechanisms relating to increases in plasma enzymes and isoenzymes in diseases of animals. *Vet. Clin. Pathol.* 12 (2): 9–24.

2 Mair, J. (1999 Jan 18). Tissue release of cardiac markers: from physiology to clinical applications. *Clin. Chem. Lab. Med.* 37 (11–12): 1077–1084.

3 Lindena, J., Küpper, W., Friedel, R., and Trautschold, I. (1979). Lymphatic transport of cellular enzymes from muscle into the intravascular compartment. *Enzyme* 24 (2): 120–131.

4 Rej, R., Rudofsky, U., Magro, A., and Prendergast, J. (1990 May). Effects of exercise on serum aminotransferase activity and pyridoxal phosphate saturation in thoroughbred racehorses. *Equine Vet. J.* 22 (3): 205–208.

5 Hoffmann, W.E. and Solter, P.F. (2008). Diagnostic enzymology of domestic animals. In: *Clinical Biochemistry of Domestic Animals*, 6e (eds. J. Kaneko, J. Harvey and M. Bruss), 351–378. Burlington: Academic Press.

6 Rendle, D.I., Heller, J., Hughes, K.J. et al. (2009 May). Stability of common biochemistry analytes in equine blood stored at room temperature. *Equine Vet. J.* 41 (5): 428–432.

7 Cardinet, G.H., Littrell, J.F., and Freedland, R.A. (1967). Comparative investigations of serum creatine phosphokinase and glutamic-oxaloacetic transaminase activities in equine paralytic myoglobinuria. *Res. Vet. Sci.* 8 (2): 219–226.

8 Noonan, N. (1981). Variations of plasma enzymes in the pony and the dog after carbon tetrachloride administration. *Am. J. Vet. Res.* 42 (4): 674–678.

9 Teixeira-Neto, A.R., Ferraz, G.C., Moscardini, A.R.C. et al. (2008). Alterations in muscular enzymes of horses competing long-distance endurance rides under tropical climate. *Arq. Bras. Med. Veterinária e Zootec.* 60 (3): 543–549.

10 Dabareiner, R.M., Schmitz, D.G., Honnas, C.M., and Carter, G.K. (2004). Gracilis muscle injury as a cause of lameness in two horses. *J. Am. Vet. Med. Assoc.* 224 (10): 1630–1633, 1605–1606.

11 Ricketts, S. (2004). Hematologic and biochemical abnormalities in athletic horses. In: *Equine Sports Medicine and Surgery: Basic and Clinical Sciences of the Equine Athlete* (eds. K. Hinchcliff, A. Kaneps and R. Geor), 949–966. Philadelphia: Saunders.

12 Krueger, C.R., Ruple-Czerniak, A., and Hackett, E.S. (2014). Evaluation of plasma muscle enzyme activity as an indicator of lesion characteristics and prognosis in horses undergoing celiotomy for acute gastrointestinal pain. *BMC Vet. Res.* 10 (Suppl 1): 1–7.

13 Almeida, B.F.M., Zucatto, A.S., Vieira, R.F.C. et al. (2011). *Medicina Veterinária. Vol. 5, Medicina Veterinária (Brasil)*, 12–17. Departamento de Medicina Veterinária: Universidade Federal Rural de Pernambuco.

14 Thornton, J.R. and Lohni, M.D. (1979). Tissue and plasma activity of lactic dehydrogenase and creatine kinase in the horse. *Equine Vet. J.* 11 (4): 235–238.

15 Jacobus, W.E. and Lehninger, A.L. (1973). Creatine kinase of rat heart mitochondria. Coupling of creatine phosphorylation to electron transport. *J. Biol. Chem.* 248 (13): 4803–4810.

16 Forsyth, S., Lopez-Villalobos, N., and Rogers, C. (2006). The effect on creatinine kinase activity of freezing plasma from healthy foals. *N. Z. Vet. J.* 54 (5): 235–236.

17 Hall, R. and Bender, H. (2011). Muscle. In: *Duncan and Prasse's Veterinary Laboratory Medicine: Clinical Pathology*, 5e (ed. K.S. Latimer), 283–289. Ames: Wiley.

18 Toutain, P.L., Lassourd, V., Costes, G. et al. (1995). A non-invasive and quantitative method for the study of tissue injury caused by intramuscular injection of drugs in horses. *J. Vet. Pharmacol. Ther.* 18 (3): 226–235.

19 Anderson, M.G. (1976). The effect of exercise on the lactic dehydrogenase and creatine kinase isoenzyme composition of horse serum. *Res. Vet. Sci.* 20 (2): 191–196.

20 Argiroudis, S.A., Kent, J.E., and Blackmore, D.J. (1982). Observations on the isoenzymes of creatine kinase in equine serum and tissues. *Equine Vet. J.* 14 (4): 317–321.

21 Slack, J.A., McGuirk, S.M., Erb, H.N. et al. (2005). Biochemical markers of cardiac injury in normal, surviving septic, or nonsurviving septic neonatal foals. *J. Vet. Intern. Med.* 19 (4): 577–580.

22 Szasz, G., Gerhardt, W., Gruber, W., and Bernt, E. (1976). Creatine kinase in serum: 2. Interference of adenylate kinase with the assay. *Clin. Chem.* 22: 1806–1811.

23 Lassen, E. (2006). Laboratory evaluation of muscle injury. In: *Veterinary Hematology and Clinical Chemistry* (eds. M. Thrall, D. Baker and T. Campbell), 417. Ames: Blackwell Publishing.

24 Lindner, A. and Hatzipanagiotou, A. (1993). Effect of the storage temperature and time and the test sample materials on the LDH isoenzyme activity and protein fractions in horse blood. *Zentralbl. Veterinarmed. A* 40 (2): 128–133.

25 Boyd, J.W. (1967). The rates of disappearance of l-lactate dehydrogenase isoenzymes from plasma. *Biochim. Biophys. Acta, Enzymol.* 132 (2): 221–231.

26 Don, M. and Masters, C.J. (1976). On the comparative turnover rates of the lactate dehydrogenase isozymes in rat tissues. *Int. J. Biochem.* 7 (5): 215–220.

27 Jones, D.G. (1985). Stability and storage characteristics of enzymes in cattle blood. *Res. Vet. Sci.* 38 (3): 301–306.

28 Williams, A.E., Kline, L.M., and Dodd, R.Y. (1987). Stability of serum alanine aminotransferase activity. *Transfusion* 27 (5): 431–433.

29 Cornelius, C.E., Bishop, J., Switzer, J., and Rhode, E.A. (1959). Serum and tissue transaminase activities in domestic animals. *Cornell Vet.* 49 (1): 116–126.

30 Stockham, S. and Scott, M. (2008). Enzymes. In: *Fundamentals of Veterinary Clinical Pathology*, 2e, 640–663. Ames: Blackwell Publishing.

31 Hamlin, M.J., Shearman, J.P., and Hopkins, W.G. (2010). Changes in physiological parameters in overtrained Standardbred racehorses. *Equine Vet. J.* 34 (4): 383–388.

32 Robertson, I.D., Bolton, J.R., Mercy, A.R. et al. (1996). Haematological and biochemical values in 12 Standardbred horses during training. *Aust. Equine Vet.* 14 (2): 72–76.

33 Anderson, M.G. (1975). The influence of exercise on serum enzyme levels in the horse. *Equine Vet. J.* 7 (3): 160–165.

34 Lucke, J.N. and Hall, G.M. (1980 Dec 6). A biochemical study of the Arab horse society's marathon race. *Vet. Rec.* 107 (23): 523–525.

35 Freestone, J.F., Kamerling, S.G., Church, G. et al. (1989). Exercise induced changes in creatine kinase and aspartate aminotransferase activities in the horse: effects of conditioning, exercise tests and acepromazine. *J. Equine Vet. Sci.* 9 (5): 275–280.

36 Gigli, I., Aguero, A., Maizon, D.O., and Carou, N.E. (1996). Serum muscular enzymes (CPK/AST) and plasma progesterone in Thoroughbred mares in training. *Pferdeheilkunde* 12: 496–498.

37 Harris, P.A., Snow, D.H., Greet, T.R., and Rossdale, P.D. (1990). Some factors influencing plasma AST/CK activities in thoroughbred racehorses. *Equine Vet. J. Suppl.* 9: 66–71.

38 Frauenfelder, H.C., Rossdale, P.D., Ricketts, S.W. et al. (1986). Changes in serum muscle enzyme levels associated with training schedules and stage of the oestrous cycle in thoroughbred racehorses. *Equine Vet. J.* 18 (5): 371–374.

39 Amelink, G.J., Koot, R.W., Erich, W.B.M. et al. (1990). Sex-linked variation in creatine kinase release, and its dependence on oestradiol, can be demonstrated in an in-vitro rat skeletal muscle preparation. *Acta Physiol. Scand.* 138 (2): 115–124.

40 Vincze, B., Kutasi, O., Baska, F., and Szenci, O. (2015). Pregnancy-associated changes of serum biochemical values in Lipizzaner broodmares. *Acta Vet. Hung.* 63 (3): 303–316.

41 Rayolle, P., Lefebvre, H., and Braun, J. (1992). Effects of incorrect venepuncture on plasma creatine kinase activity in the dog and horse. *Br. Vet. J.* 148: 161–162.

42 Valberg, S., Jönsson, L., Lindholm, A., and Holmgren, N. (1993). Muscle histopathology and plasma aspartate aminotransferase, creatine kinase and myoglobin changes with exercise in horses with recurrent exertional rhabdomyolysis. *Equine Vet. J.* 25 (1): 11–16.

43 Neubauer, O., König, D., and Wagner, K.-H. (2008). Recovery after an ironman triathlon: sustained inflammatory responses and muscular stress. *Eur. J. Appl. Physiol.* 104 (3): 417–426.

44 Boulton, F.E. and Huntsman, R.G. (1971). The detection of myoglobin in urine and its distinction from normal and variant haemoglobins. *J. Clin. Pathol.* 24 (9): 816–821.

45 Hamilton, R.W., Hopkins, M.B., and Shihabi, Z.K. (1989). Myoglobinuria, hemoglobinuria, and acute renal failure. *Clin. Chem.* 35 (8): 1713–1720.

46 Arighi, M., Baird, J., and Hulland, T. (1984). Equine exertional rhabdomyolysis. *Compend. Cont. Educ. Pract. Vet.* 6: S726–S733.

47 Gordon, A.M., Homsher, E., and Regnier, M. (2000). Regulation of contraction in striated muscle. *Physiol. Rev.* 80 (2): 853–924.

48 Onuoha, G.N., Alpar, E.K., Dean, B. et al. (2001). Skeletal troponin-I release in orthopedic and soft tissue injuries. *J. Orthop. Sci.* 6 (1): 11–15.

49 Simpson, J.A., Labugger, R., Collier, C. et al. (2005). Fast and slow skeletal troponin I in serum from patients with various skeletal muscle disorders: a pilot study. *Clin. Chem.* 51 (6): 966–972.

50 Vassallo, J.D., Janovitz, E.B., Wescott, D.M. et al. (2009). Biomarkers of drug-induced skeletal muscle injury in the rat: troponin I and myoglobin. *Toxicol. Sci.* 111 (2): 402–412.

51 Kaese, H.J., Valberg, S.J., Hayden, D.W. et al. (2005). Infarctive purpura hemorrhagica in five horses. *J. Am. Vet. Med. Assoc.* 226 (11): 1893–1898, 1845.

52 Sponseller, B.T., Valberg, S.J., Tennent-Brown, B.S. et al. (2005). Severe acute rhabdomyolysis associated with Streptococcus equi infection in four horses. *J. Am. Vet. Med. Assoc.* 227 (11): 1800–1807. 1753–1754.

53 Finno, C.J., Gianino, G., Perumbakkam, S. et al. (2018). A missense mutation in MYH1 is associated with susceptibility to immune-mediated myositis in quarter horses. *Skelet. Muscle* 8 (1): 1–13.

54 Valberg, S.J. (2018). Muscle conditions affecting sport horses. *Vet. Clin. North Am. Equine Pract.* 34 (2): 253–276.

55 Lewis, S.S., Valberg, S.J., and Nielsen, I.L. (2007). Suspected immune-mediated myositis in horses. *J. Vet. Intern. Med.* 21 (3): 495–503.

56 Pusterla, N., Watson, J.L., Affolter, V.K. et al. (2003). Purpura haemorrhagica in 53 horses. *Vet. Rec.* 153 (4): 118–121.

57 Durward-Akhurst, S.A. and Valberg, S.J. (2018). Immune-mediated muscle diseases of the horse. *Vet. Pathol.* 55 (1): 68–75.

58 Hilton, H., Madigan, J.E., and Aleman, M. (2008). Rhabdomyolysis associated with Anaplasma phagocytophilum infection in a horse. *J. Vet. Intern. Med* 22 (1064): 1061–1064.

59 Lillini, E., Macri, G., Proietti, G., and Scarpulla, M. (2006). New findings on anaplasmosis caused by infection with anaplasma phagocytophilum. *Ann. N. Y. Acad. Sci.* 1081 (1): 360–370.

60 Peek, S.F., Semrad, S.D., and Perkins, G.A. (2003). Clostridial myonecrosis in horses (37 cases 1985–2000). *Equine Vet. J.* 35 (1): 86–92.

61 Quist, E.M., Dougherty, J.J., Chaffin, M.K., and Porter, B.F. (2011). Diagnostic exercise: equine rhabdomyolysis. *Vet. Pathol.* 48 (6): E52–E59.

62 Gerber, V., Straub, R., and Frey, J. (2006). Equine botulism and acute pasture myodystrophy: new soil-borne emerging diseases in Switzerland? *Schweiz. Arch. Tierheilkd.* 148 (10): 553–559.

63 McCarthy, H.E., French, N.P., Edwards, G.B. et al. (2004). Equine grass sickness is associated with low antibody levels to clostridium botulinum: a matched case-control study. *Equine Vet. J.* 36 (2): 123–129.

64 McGorum, B.C., Scholes, S., Milne, E.M. et al. (2016). Equine grass sickness, but not botulism, causes autonomic and enteric neurodegeneration and increases soluble N-ethylmaleimide-sensitive factor attachment receptor protein expression within neuronal perikarya. *Equine Vet. J.* 48 (6): 786–791.

65 Barba, M., Stewart, A.J., Passler, T. et al. (2015). Experimental transmission of Corynebacterium pseudotuberculosis biovar equi in horses by house flies. *J. Vet. Intern. Med.* 29 (2): 636–643.

66 Aleman, M., Spier, S.J., Wilson, W.D., and Doherr, M. (1996). Corynebacterium pseudotuberculosis infection in horses: 538 cases (1982–1993). *J. Am. Vet. Med. Assoc.* 209 (4): 804–809.

67 Madigan, J.E., Valberg, S.J., Ragle, C., and Moody, J.L. (1995). Muscle spasms associated with ear tick (Otobius megnini) infestations in five horses. *J. Am. Vet. Med. Assoc.* 207 (1): 74–76.

68 Freestone, J.F. and Carlson, G.P. (1991). Muscle disorders in the horse: a retrospective study. *Equine Vet. J.* 23 (2): 86–90.

69 Herd, H.R., Sula, M.M., Starkey, L.A. et al. (2015). Sarcocystis fayeri-induced granulomatous and eosinophilic myositis in 2 related horses. *Vet. Pathol.* 52 (6): 1191–1194.

70 Traub-Dargatz, J.L., Schlipf, J.W., Granstrom, D.E. et al. (1994). Multifocal myositis associated with Sarcocystis sp in a horse. *J. Am. Vet. Med. Assoc.* 205 (11): 1574–1576.

71 Aleman, M., Shapiro, K., Sisó, S. et al. (2016). Sarcocystis fayeri in skeletal muscle of horses with neuromuscular disease. *Neuromuscul. Disord.* 26 (1): 85–93.

72 Tenter, A.M. (1995). Current research on Sarcocystis species of domestic animals. *Int. J. Parasitol.* 25 (11): 1311–1330.

73 Pasolini, M.P., Pagano, T.B., Costagliola, A. et al. (2018). Inflammatory myopathy in horses with chronic piroplasmosis. *Vet. Pathol.* 55 (1): 133–143.

74 Harris, P.A. (1990). An outbreak of the equine rhabdomyolysis syndrome in a racing yard. *Vet. Rec.* 127 (19): 468–470.

75 Johnston, G.M., Eastment, J.K., Taylor, P.M., and Wood, J.L.N. (2004). Is isoflurane safer than halothane in equine anaesthesia? Results from a prospective multicentre randomised controlled trial. *Equine Vet. J.* 36 (1): 64–71.

76 Franci, P., Leece, E.A., and Brearley, J.C. (2006). Post anaesthetic myopathy/neuropathy in horses undergoing magnetic resonance imaging compared to horses undergoing surgery. *Equine Vet. J.* 38 (6): 497–501.

77 Grandy, J.L., Steffey, E.P., Hodgson, D.S., and Woliner, M.J. (1987). Arterial hypotension and the development of postanesthetic myopathy in halothane-anesthetized horses. *Am. J. Vet. Res.* 48 (2): 192–197.

78 Lindsay, W.A., Robinson, G.M., Brunson, D.B., and Majors, L.J. (1989). Induction of equine postanesthetic myositis after halothane-induced hypotension. *Am. J. Vet. Res.* 50 (3): 404–410.

79 Lindsay, W.A., McDonell, W., and Bignell, W. (1980). Equine postanesthetic forelimb lameness: intracompartmental muscle pressure changes and biochemical patterns. *Am. J. Vet. Res.* 41 (12): 1919–1924.

80 Carlson, G. (1987). Hematology and body fluids in the equine athlete: a review. In: *Equine Exercise Physiology*, 2e (eds. J. Gillespie and N. Robinson), 393–425. Davis: ICEEP Publications.

81 Mickelson, J.R. and Valberg, S.J. (2014). The genetics of skeletal muscle disorders in horses. *Annu. Rev. Anim. Biosci.* 3 (1): 197–217.

82 Wagner, M.L., Valberg, S.J., Ames, E.G. et al. (2006). Allele frequency and likely impact of the glycogen branching enzyme deficiency gene in quarter horse and paint horse populations. *J. Vet. Intern. Med.* 20 (5): 1207–1211.

83 Valberg, S.J., Ward, T.L., Rush, B. et al. (2001). Glycogen branching enzyme deficiency in quarter horse foals. *J. Vet. Intern. Med.* 15 (6): 572–580.

84 Bowling, A.T., Byrns, G., and Spier, S. (2009). Evidence for a single pedigree source of the hyperkalemic periodic paralysis susceptibility gene in quarter horses. *Anim. Genet.* 27 (4): 279–281.

85 Finno, C.J., Spier, S.J., and Valberg, S.J. (2009). Equine diseases caused by known genetic mutations. *Vet. J.* 179 (3): 336–347.

86 Meyer, T.S., Fedde, M.R., Cox, J.H., and Erickson, H.H. (1999). Hyperkalaemic periodic paralysis in horses: a review. *Equine Vet. J.* 31 (5): 362–367.

87 Carr, E.A., Spier, S.J., Kortz, G.D., and Hoffman, E.P. (1996). Laryngeal and pharyngeal dysfunction in horses homozygous for hyperkalemic periodic paralysis. *J. Am. Vet. Med. Assoc.* 209 (4): 798–803.

88 Reynolds, J.A., Potter, G.D., Greene, L.W. et al. (1998). Genetic-diet interactions in the hyperkalemic periodic paralysis syndrome in quarter horses fed varying amounts of potassium: part II–symptoms of HYPP. *J. Equine Vet. Sci.* 18 (10): 655–661.

89 Hildebrand, S.V. and Howitt, G.A. (1983). Succinylcholine infusion associated with hyperthermia in ponies anesthetized with halothane. *Am. J. Vet. Res.* 44 (12): 2280–2284.

90 Manley, S.V., Kelly, A.B., and Hodgson, D. (1983). Malignant hyperthermia-like reactions in three anesthetized horses. *J. Am. Vet. Med. Assoc.* 183 (1): 85–89.

91 Nieto, J.E. and Aleman, M. (2009). A rapid detection method for the ryanodine receptor 1 (C7360G) mutation in quarter horses. *J. Vet. Intern. Med.* 23 (3): 619–622.

92 Aleman, M., Nieto, J.E., and Magdesian, K.G. (2009). Malignant hyperthermia associated with ryanodine receptor 1 (C7360G) mutation in quarter horses. *J. Vet. Intern. Med.* 23 (2): 329–334.

93 Aleman, M., Brosnan, R.J., Williams, D.C. et al. (2005). Malignant hyperthermia in a horse anesthetized with halothane. *J. Vet. Intern. Med.* 19 (3): 363–366.

94 Valberg, S.J. (2019). *Myotonic Disorders in Horses. Merck Veterinary Manual.* Whitehouse Station: Merck & Co.

95 Wijnberg, I.D., Owczarek-Lipska, M., Sacchetto, R. et al. (2012). A missense mutation in the skeletal muscle chloride channel 1 (CLCN1) as candidate causal mutation for congenital myotonia in a new forest pony. *Neuromuscul. Disord.* 22 (4): 361–367.

96 Hegreberg, G.A. and Reed, S.M. (1990). Skeletal muscle changes associated with equine myotonic dystrophy. *Acta Neuropathol.* 80 (4): 426–431.

97 Montagna, P., Liguori, R., Monari, L. et al. (2001). Equine muscular dystrophy with myotonia. *Clin. Neurophysiol.* 112 (2): 294–249.

98 Reed, S.M., Hegreberg, G.A., Bayly, W.M. et al. (1988). Progressive myotonia in foals resembling human dystrophia myotonica. *Muscle Nerve* 11 (4): 291–296.

99 Firshman, A.M., Baird, J.D., and Valberg, S.J. (2005). Prevalences and clinical signs of polysaccharide storage myopathy and shivers in Belgian draft horses. *J. Am. Vet. Med. Assoc.* 227 (12): 1958–1964.

100 Hunt, L.M., Valberg, S.J., Steffenhagen, K., and McCue, M.E. (2008). An epidemiological study of myopathies in warmblood horses. *Equine Vet. J.* 40 (2): 171–177.

101 McCue, M.E. and Valberg, S.J. (2007). Estimated prevalence of polysaccharide storage myopathy among overtly healthy quarter horses in the United States. *J. Am. Vet. Med. Assoc.* 231 (5): 746–750.

102 Maile, C.A., Hingst, J.R., Mahalingan, K.K. et al. (2017). A highly prevalent equine glycogen storage disease is explained by constitutive activation of a mutant glycogen synthase *Biochim. Biophys. Acta, Gen. Subj.* 1861 (1): 3388–3398.

103 McCue, M.E., Valberg, S.J., Lucio, M., and Mickelson, J.R. (2008). Glycogen synthase 1 (GYS1) mutation in diverse breeds with polysaccharide storage myopathy. *J. Vet. Intern. Med.* 22 (5): 1228–1233.

104 McCue, M.E., Valberg, S.J., Miller, M.B. et al. (2008). Glycogen synthase (GYS1) mutation causes a novel skeletal muscle glycogenosis. *Genomics* 91 (5): 458–466.

105 Andrews, F. (1994). Acute rhabdomyolysis. *Vet. Clin. North Am. Equine Pract.* 10: 567–573.

106 McCue, M.E., Valberg, S.J., Jackson, M. et al. (2009). Polysaccharide storage myopathy phenotype in quarter horse-related breeds is modified by the presence of an RYR1 mutation. *Neuromuscul. Disord.* 19 (1): 37–43.

107 Tryon, R.C., Penedo, M.C.T., McCue, M.E. et al. (2009). Evaluation of allele frequencies of inherited disease genes in subgroups of American quarter horses. *J. Am. Vet. Med. Assoc.* 234 (1): 120–125.

108 Lewis, S.S., Nicholson, A.M., Williams, Z.J., and Valberg, S.J. (2017). Clinical characteristics and muscle glycogen concentrations in warmblood horses with polysaccharide storage myopathy. *Am. J. Vet. Res.* 78 (11): 1305–1312.

109 Valberg, S.J., McKenzie, E.C., Eyrich, L.V. et al. (2016). Suspected myofibrillar myopathy in Arabian horses with a history of exertional rhabdomyolysis. *Equine Vet. J.* 48 (5): 548–556.

110 Valberg, S.J., Nicholson, A.M., Lewis, S.S. et al. (2017). Clinical and histopathological features of myofibrillar myopathy in warmblood horses. *Equine Vet. J.* 49 (6): 739–745.

111 MacLeay, J.M., Sorum, S.A., Valberg, S.J. et al. (1999). Epidemiologic analysis of factors influencing exertional rhabdomyolysis in thoroughbreds. *Am. J. Vet. Res.* 60 (12): 1562–1566.

112 MacLeay, J.M., Valberg, S.J., Sorum, S.A. et al. (1999). Heritability of recurrent exertional rhabdomyolysis in thoroughbred racehorses. *Am. J. Vet. Res.* 60 (2): 250–256.

113 Dranchak, P.K., Valberg, S.J., Onan, G.W. et al. (2005). Inheritance of recurrent exertional rhabdomyolysis in thoroughbreds. *J. Am. Vet. Med. Assoc.* 227 (5): 762–767.

114 Lentz, L.R., Valberg, S.J., Herold, L.V. et al. (2002). Myoplasmic calcium regulation in myotubes from horses with recurrent exertional rhabdomyolysis. *Am. J. Vet. Res.* 63 (12): 1724–1731.

115 Lentz, L.R., Valberg, S.J., Balog, E.M. et al. (1999). Abnormal regulation of muscle contraction in horses with recurrent exertional rhabdomyolysis. *Am. J. Vet. Res.* 60 (8): 992–999.

116 MacLeay, J.M., Valberg, S.J., Pagan, J.D. et al. (2000). Effect of ration and exercise on plasma creatine kinase activity and lactate concentration in thoroughbred horses with recurrent exertional rhabdomyolysis. *Am. J. Vet. Res.* 61 (11): 1390–1395.

117 Pinn, T.L., Divers, T.J., Southard, T. et al. (2018). Persistent hypoglycemia associated with lipid storage myopathy in a paint foal. *J. Vet. Intern. Med.* 32 (4): 1442–1446.

118 Polle, F., Andrews, F.M., Gillon, T. et al. (2014). Suspected congenital centronuclear myopathy in an Arabian-cross foal. *J. Vet. Intern. Med.* 28 (6): 1886–1891.

119 Medina, S.G. (2015). Update on the cause of equine atypical myopathy. *Vet. Rec.* 176 (6): 143–145.

120 Boemer, F., Amory, H., van Galen, G. et al. (2017). Acylcarnitines profile best predicts survival in horses with atypical myopathy. *PLoS One* 12 (8): e0182761.

121 Valberg, S.J., Sponseller, B.T., Hegeman, A.D. et al. (2013). Seasonal pasture myopathy/atypical myopathy in North America associated with ingestion of hypoglycin a within seeds of the box elder tree. *Equine Vet. J.* 45 (4): 419–426.

122 Lemieux, H., Boemer, F., van Galen, G. et al. (2016). Mitochondrial function is altered in horse atypical myopathy. *Mitochondrion* 30: 35–41.

123 Westermann, C.M., van Leeuwen, R., van Raamsdonk, L.W.D., and Mol, H.G.J. (2016). Hypoglycin a concentrations in maple tree species in the Netherlands and the occurrence of atypical myopathy in horses. *J. Vet. Intern. Med.* 30 (3): 880–884.

124 González-Medina, S., Ireland, J.L., Piercy, R.J. et al. (2017). Equine atypical myopathy in the UK: epidemiological characteristics of cases reported from 2011 to 2015 and factors associated with survival. *Equine Vet. J.* 49 (6): 746–752.

125 Van Galen, G., Marcillaud Pitel, C. et al. (2012). European outbreaks of atypical myopathy in grazing equids (2006–2009): spatiotemporal distribution, history and clinical features. *Equine Vet. J.* 44 (5): 614–620.

126 Karlíková, R., Široká, J., Mech, M. et al. (2018). Newborn foal with atypical myopathy. *J. Vet. Intern. Med.* 32 (5): 1768–1772.

127 Sander, J., Cavalleri, J.M.V., and Terhardt, M. (2016). Rapid diagnosis of hypoglycin a intoxication in atypical myopathy of horses. *J. Vet. Diagn. Invest.* 28 (2): 98–104.

128 Medina, S.G., Hyde, C., Lovera, I., and Piercy, R.J. (2018). Detection of equine atypical myopathy-associated hypoglycin a in plant material: optimisation and validation of a novel lc-ms based method without derivatisation. *PLoS One* 13 (7): 13–15.

129 Terhardt, M., Ziegler, J., and Janzen, N. (2019). Detection of MCPG metabolites in horses with atypical myopathy. *PLoS One* 14 (2): e0211698.

130 Helman, R.G. and Edwards, W.C. (1997). Clinical features of blister beetle poisoning in equids: 70 cases (1983–1996). *J. Am. Vet. Med. Assoc.* 211 (8): 1018–1021.

131 Ray, A.C., Kyle, A.L., Murphy, M.J., and Reagor, J.C. (1989). Etiologic agents, incidence, and improved diagnostic methods of cantharidin toxicosis in horses. *Am. J. Vet. Res.* 50 (2): 187–191.

132 Knight, A. and Walter, R. (2001). *A Guide to Plant Poisoning of Animals in North America*, 194–197. Jackson, WY: Teton New Media, 222–224.

133 Martin, B.W., Terry, M.K., Bridges, C.H., and Bailey, E.M. (1981). Toxicity of Cassia occidentalis in the horse. *Vet. Hum. Toxicol.* 23 (6): 416–417.

134 Aleman, M., Magdesian, K.G., Peterson, T.S., and Galey, F.D. (2007). Salinomycin toxicosis in horses. *J. Am. Vet. Med. Assoc.* 230 (12): 1822–1826.

135 Dawson, D.R. (2011). Toxins and adverse drug reactions affecting the equine nervous system. *Vet. Clin. North Am. Equine Pract.* 27 (3): 507–526.

136 Hall, J.O. (2001). Toxic feed constituents in the horse. *Vet. Clin. North Am. Equine Pract.* 17 (3): 479–489, vii.

137 Aleman, M., Magdesian, K.G., Peterson, T.S., and Galey, F.D. (2007). Salinomycin toxicosis in horses. *J. Am. Vet. Med. Assoc.* 230 (12): 1822–1826.

138 Peek, S.F., Marques, F.D., Morgan, J. et al. Atypical acute monensin toxicosis and delayed cardiomyopathy in belgian draft horses. *J. Vet. Intern. Med.* 18 (5): 761–764.

139 Olson, C.T., Keller, W.C., Gerken, D.F., and Reed, S.M. (1984). Suspected tremetol poisoning in horses. *J. Am. Vet. Med. Assoc.* 185 (9): 1001–1003.

140 Bauquier, J., Stent, A., Gibney, J. et al. (2017). Evidence for marsh mallow (Malva parviflora) toxicosis causing myocardial disease and myopathy in four horses. *Equine Vet. J.* 49 (3): 307–313.

141 Löfstedt, J. (1997). White muscle disease of foals. *Vet. Clin. North Am. Equine Pract.* 13 (1): 169–185.

142 Delesalle, C., Bruijn, M., Wilmink, S. et al. (2017). White muscle disease in foals: focus on selenium soil content. A case series. *BMC Vet. Res.* 13 (1): 1–10.

143 Perkins, G., Valberg, S.J., Madigan, J.M. et al. (1998). Electrolyte disturbances in foals with severe rhabdomyolysis. *J. Vet. Intern. Med.* 12 (3): 173–177.

144 Mohammed, H.O., Divers, T.J., Summers, B.A., and de Lahunta, A. (2007). Vitamin E deficiency and risk of equine motor neuron disease. *Acta Vet. Scand.* 49 (1): 17.

145 De la Rúa-Domènech, R., Mohammed, H.O., Cummings, J.F. et al. (1997). Association between plasma vitamin E concentration and the risk of equine motor neuron disease. *Vet. J.* 154 (3): 203–213.

146 De La Rúa-Domènech, R., Mohammed, H.O., Cummings, J.F. et al. (1997). Intrinsic, management, and nutritional factors associated with equine motor neuron disease. *J. Am. Vet. Med. Assoc.* 211 (10): 1261–1267.

147 Divers, T.J., Mohammed, H.O., Cummings, J.F. et al. (1994). Equine motor neuron disease: findings in 28 horses and proposal of a pathophysiological mechanism for the disease. *Equine Vet. J.* 26 (5): 409–415.

148 Tan, J.-Y., Valberg, S.J., Sebastian, M.M. et al. (2010). Suspected systemic calcinosis and calciphylaxis in 5 horses. *Can. Vet. J.* 51 (9): 993–999.

149 Aleman, M., Watson, J.L., Williams, D.C. et al. (2006). Myopathy in horses with pituitary pars intermedia dysfunction (Cushing's disease). *Neuromuscul. Disord.* 16 (11): 737–744.

150 Maxie, M.G. and Physick-Sheard, P.W. (1985). Aortic-iliac thrombosis in horses. *Vet. Pathol.* 22 (3): 238–249.

151 Brama, P.A., Rijkenhuizen, A.B., van Swieten, H.A., and Warmerdam, E.P. (1996). Thrombosis of the aorta and the caudal arteries in the horse; additional diagnostics and a new surgical treatment. *Vet. Q.* 18 (Suppl 2): S85–S89.

152 O'Brien, P.J., Landt, Y., and Ladenson, J.H. (1998). Differential reactivity of cardiac and skeletal muscle from various species in a cardiac troponin I immunoassay. *Res. Vet. Sci.* 65: 135–137.

153 Gehlen, H., Shety, T., El-Zahar, H., and Hofheinz, I. (2018). Measurement of plasma endothelin-1 concentration in healthy horses and horses with cardiac disease during rest and after exercise. *J. Vet. Med. Sci.* 81 (2): 263–268.

154 Jesty, S.A. (2012). Cardiac biomarkers in equine medicine. *Vet. J.* 192 (2): 131–132.

155 Rossi, T.M., Kavsak, P.A., Maxie, M.G. et al. (2018). Analytical validation of cardiac troponin I assays in horses. *J. Vet. Diagn. Invest.* 30 (2): 226–232.

156 Rossi, T.M., Pyle, W.G., Maxie, M.G. et al. (2014). Troponin assays in the assessment of the equine myocardium. *Equine Vet. J.* 46: 270–275.

157 Phillips, W., Giguè, S., Franklin, R.P. et al. (2003). Cardiac troponin I in pastured and race-training thoroughbred horses. *J. Vet. Intern. Med.* 17: 591–599.

158 Begg, L.M., Hoffmann, K.L., and Begg, A.P. (2006). Serum and plasma cardiac troponin I concentrations in clinically normal thoroughbreds in training in Australia. *Aust. Vet. J.* 84: 336–337.

159 Shields, E., Seiden-Long, I., Massie, S., and Leguillette, R. (2018). 24-hour kinetics of cardiac troponin-T using a "high-sensitivity" assay in thoroughbred Chuckwagon racing geldings after race and associated clinical sampling guidelines. *J. Vet. Intern. Med.* 32 (1): 433–440.

160 Van der Vekens, N., Decloedt, A., de Clercq, D. et al. (2016). Atrial natriuretic peptide vs. N-terminal-pro-atrial natriuretic peptide for the detection of left atrial dilatation in horses. *Equine Vet. J.* 48 (1): 15–20.

161 Trachsel, D.S., Schwarzwald, C.C., Grenacher, B., and Weishaupt, M.A. (2014). Analytic validation and comparison of three commercial immunoassays for measurement of plasma atrial/A-type natriuretic peptide concentration in horses. *Res. Vet. Sci.* 96 (1): 180–186.

162 Leroux, A.A., Al Haidar, A., Remy, B. et al. (2014). Atrial natriuretic peptide as an indicator of the severity ofvalvular regurgitation and heart failure in horses. *J. Equine Vet. Sci.* 34 (10): 1226–1233.

163 Trachsel, D.S., Grenacher, B., Weishaupt, M.A., and Schwarzwald, C.C. (2012). Plasma atrial natriuretic peptide concentrations in horses with heart disease: a pilot study. *Vet. J.* 192 (2): 166–170.

164 Leroux, A.A. (2015). Using natriuretic peptides to detect cardiac diseases in horses. *Vet. Rec.* 177 (24): 622–623.

165 Ettinger, S.J., Farace, G., and Forney, S.D. (2012). Circulating concentrations of BNP. *J. Am. Vet. Med. Assoc.* 240 (2): 171–180.

166 Van Der Vekens, N., Hunter, I., Timm, A. et al. (2015). Total plasma proANP increases with atrial dilatation in horses. *Vet. Rec.* 117 (24): 624.

167 Richter, R., Mägert, H.-J., Mifune, H. et al. (1998). Equine cardiodilatin/atrial natriuretic peptide. *Cells Tissues Organs* 162 (4): 185–193.

168 Rossi, T.M., Kavsak, P.A., Maxie, M.G. et al. (2019). Post-exercise cardiac troponin I release and clearance in normal standardbred racehorses. *Equine Vet. J.* 51 (1): 97–101.

169 Slack, J., Boston, R.C., Soma, L., and Reef, V.B. (2012). Cardiac troponin I in racing standardbreds. *J. Vet. Intern. Med.* 26 (5): 1202–1208.

170 Gunther-Harrington, C.T., Arthur, R., Estell, K. et al. (2018). Prospective pre- and post-race evaluation of biochemical, electrophysiologic, and echocardiographic indices in 30 racing thoroughbred horses that received furosemide. *BMC Vet. Res.* 14 (1): 1–10.

171 Flethøj, M., Schwarzwald, C.C., Haugaard, M.M. et al. (2016). Left ventricular function after prolonged exercise in equine endurance athletes. *J. Vet. Intern. Med.* 30 (4): 1260–1269.

172 Holbrook, T.C., Birks, E.K., Sleeper, M.M., and Durando, M. (2006). Endurance exercise is associated with increased plasma cardiac troponin I in horses. *Equine Vet. J.* 38 (Suppl.36): 27–31.

173 Shields, E., Seiden-Long, I., Massie, S. et al. (2016). Analytical validation and establishment of reference intervals for a "high-sensitivity" cardiac troponin-T assay in horses. *BMC Vet. Res.* 12 (1): 504–509.

174 Van der Vekens, N., Decloedt, A., Ven, S. et al. (2015). Cardiac troponin I as compared to troponin T for the detection of myocardial damage in horses. *J. Vet. Intern. Med.* 29 (1): 348–354.

175 Trachsel, D.S., Grenacher, B., and Schwarzwald, C.C. (2015). Plasma atrial/A-type natriuretic peptide (ANP) concentration in horses with various heart diseases. *J. Vet. Cardiol.* 17 (3): 216–228.

176 Gehlen, H., Sundermann, T., Rohn, K., and Stadler, P. (2007). Plasma atrial natriuretic peptide concentration in warmblood horses with heart valve regurgitations. *J. Vet. Cardiol.* 9 (2): 99–101.

177 Keen, J.A. (2019). Examination of horses with cardiac disease. *Vet. Clin. North Am. Equine Pract.* 35 (1): 23–42.

178 Slack, J.A., Mcguirk, S.M., Erb, H.N. et al. (2005). Biochemical markers of cardiac injury in Normal, surviving septic, or nonsurviving septic neonatal foals. *J. Vet. Intern. Med.* 19: 577–580.

179 El-Bahr, S.M. and El-Deeb, W.M. (2016). Acute-phase proteins, oxidative stress biomarkers, proinflammatory cytokines, and cardiac troponin in Arabian mares affected with pyometra. *Theriogenology* 86 (4): 1132–1136.

180 Díaz, O.M.S., Durando, M.M., Birks, E.K., and Reef, V.B. (2014). Cardiac troponin I concentrations in horses with colic. *J. Am. Vet. Med. Assoc.* 245 (1): 118–125.

181 Diana, A., Guglielmini, C., Candini, D. et al. (2007). Cardiac arrhythmias associated with piroplasmosis in the horse: a case report. *Vet. J.* 174 (1): 193–195.

182 Gilliam, L.L., Holbrook, T.C., Ownby, C.L. et al. (2012). Cardiotoxicity, inflammation, and immune response after rattlesnake envenomation in the horse. *J. Vet. Intern. Med.* 26 (6): 1457–1463.

183 Durando, M.M., Birks, E.K., Hussey, S.B., and Lunn, D.P. (2011). Cardiac troponin I concentrations in ponies challenged with equine influenza virus. *J. Vet. Intern. Med.* 25 (2): 339–344.

184 Divers, T.J., Kraus, M.S., Jesty, S.A. et al. (2009). Clinical findings and serum cardiac troponin I concentrations in horses after intragastric administration of sodium monensin. *J. Vet. Diagn. Invest.* 21: 338–343.

185 Kraus, M.S., Jesty, S.A., Gelzer, A.R. et al. (2010). Concentration by use of a point-of-care analyzer with experimentally induced cardiac disease. *Am. J. Vet. Res.* 71 (1): 55–59.

186 Decloedt, A., Verheyen, T., de Clercq, D. et al. (2012). Acute and long-term cardiomyopathy and delayed neurotoxicity after accidental lasalocid poisoning in horses. *J. Vet. Intern. Med.* 26 (4): 1005–1011.

187 Davis, T.Z., Stegelmeier, B.L., Lee, S.T. et al. (2013). Experimental rayless goldenrod (*Isocoma pluriflora*) toxicosis in horses. *Toxicon* 73: 88–95.

188 Votion, D.-M. (2012). The story of equine atypical myopathy: a review from the beginning to a possible end. *ISRN Vet. Sci.* 2012: 1–14.

11

Endocrine Evaluation

Jill Beech[1], Raquel M. Walton[2], and Melissa Blauvelt[3]

[1] School of Veterinary Medicine, University of Pennsylvania, Kennett Square, PA, USA
[2] IDEXX Laboratories, Inc., Langhorne, PA, USA
[3] IDEXX Laboratories, Inc., Worthington, OH, USA

Abbreviations

ACTH, adrenocorticotropic hormone; alpha-MSH, alpha-melanocyte stimulating hormone; DST, dexamethasone suppression test; fT4D, free thyroxine dialysis method; fT4, free thyroxine; fT3, free triiodothyronine; L-T4, levothyroxine sodium; ODST, overnight dexamethasone suppression test; PPID, pituitary pars intermedia dysfunction; PI, pars intermedia; PTU, propylthiouracil; rT3, reverse T3; T3, triiodothyronine; T4, thyroxine; TT3, total triiodothyronine; TT4, total thyroxine; TRH, thyrotropin-releasing hormone; TSH, thyroid-stimulating hormone (thyrotropin).

Equine endocrinology research over the past few decades has contributed greatly to our current understanding of mechanisms, triggers and disease manifestations, and it will likely remain a very active area of ongoing investigation. The intentions of this chapter are to characterize selected equine endocrinopathies and to provide a brief overview of these diseases and the diagnostics that are currently available.

11.1 Pituitary Pars Intermedia Dysfunction (PPID)

The hypothalamus functions as the interface between the nervous and endocrine systems. The pituitary gland interacts closely with the hypothalamus and orchestrates the signaling needed for initiating and terminating many endocrine functions. Pituitary pars intermedia disease was previously known as equine Cushing's disease. The disease is now referred to as PPID to more accurately reflect the pathophysiology of the disease which, unlike Cushing's disease, is not typically characterized by hypercortisolemia.

11.1.1 General Overview

An abnormal haircoat is considered the most common and specific clinical presentation of PPID (Figure 11.1) [1]. Hypertrichosis or other changes in the haircoat (e.g., retention of guard hairs; failure to shed; lightening of color), laminitis, and muscle wasting are characteristic clinical manifestations of PPID. A recent study of 301 laminitic horses identified PPID in 38% [2]. Other clinical findings can include obesity, polyuria/polydipsia (PU/PD), abnormal hidrosis, and lethargy [3].

Pituitary pars intermedia dysfunction occurs in horses, ponies, and donkeys. In horses, it is usually a disease seen in patients over 15 years of age, but has been documented in horses as young as 8 years. It is believed to occur in approximately 3% of the entire equine population and in approximately 20–30% in horses over the age of 20 years [3, 4]. No predisposing factors are known except for age.

The general pathogenetic mechanism of PPID is rooted in the loss of periventricular dopaminergic neurons located mostly in the hypothalamus, which serve as inhibitory regulators for the pars intermedia [5]. With the loss of tonic inhibition, there is hyperplasia and hypertrophy of the pars intermedia with either a single macroadenoma or multiple microadenomas with concomitant increases in the production of pars intermedia hormones such as ACTH, alpha-melanocyte stimulating hormone (α-MSH), corticotropin-like intermediate lobe peptide (CLIP), and proopiomelanocortin (POMC) peptides, amongst others

Equine Hematology, Cytology, and Clinical Chemistry, Second Edition.
Edited by Raquel M. Walton, Rick L. Cowell, and Amy C. Valenciano.

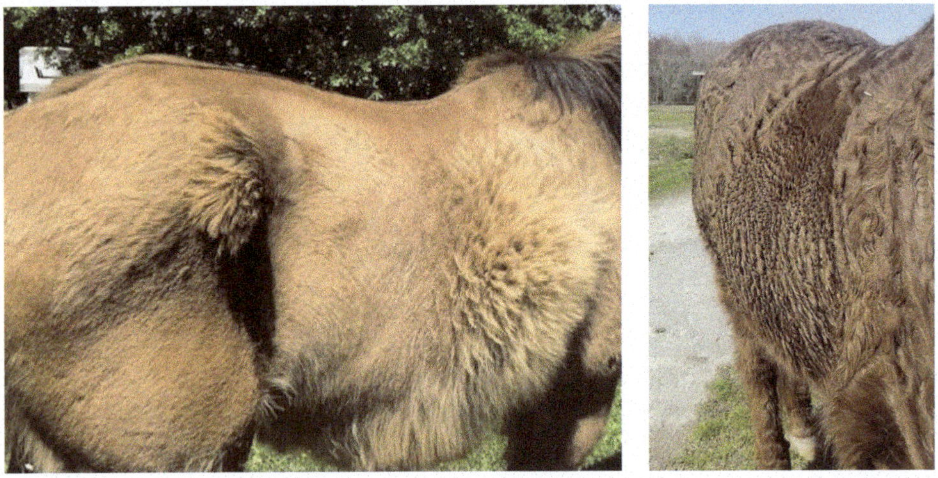

Figure 11.1 (*Left panel*) PPID horse showing poor coat shedding. *Source:* Photo courtesy of Dina Duplantis DVM. (*Right panel*) Abnormal coat in a horse with PPID. *Source:* Photo courtesy of Cathy Lombardi DVM.

[1]. Unlike ACTH release by corticotropes of the pars distalis, ACTH release by melanotropes in the pars intermedia does not stimulate adrenal hyperplasia or cortisol production and this seems to be the reason that hypercortisolemia is not a common finding in these patients [6].

11.2 Testing for PPID

Over the years, a number of endocrine tests have been introduced as diagnostic tests for PPID. Although horses with PPID may have hyperglycemia, hypertriglyceridemia, and other changes in serum biochemical analysis, and measuring nonhormonal blood components may help in managing individual patients with PPID, the data are not specific or sensitive for diagnosis. A leading group of equine endocrinology experts (the Equine Endocrinology Group; https://sites.tufts.edu/equineendogroup) has generated recommendations regarding the diagnosis and treatment of PPID. This chapter presents the individual hormone tests that most commonly have been used to diagnose PPID, with emphasis on those currently accepted as the most accurate by the Equine Endocrinology Group. It is important to remember that most of the tests have been evaluated in small populations, and it is possible that they may not represent large diverse equine populations in different geographic regions.

11.2.1 Cortisol Concentrations

11.2.1.1 Baseline Cortisol Concentration

Plasma cortisol concentration is usually measured by radioimmunoassay (RIA) (Diagnostic Products Corp., Los Angeles, CA) or chemiluminescent immunoassay (Immulite, Siemens, Los Angeles, CA). Concentrations are affected by stress, including transport, exercise, stage of pregnancy, drugs, and disease states such as colic [7–10]. Cortisol concentrations in donkeys are reported to be similar to those of horses [11]. Normal horses may have diurnal variation with higher concentrations in the morning than afternoon but this variation can be eliminated if a horse is moved to a novel environment [12]. In a study of 50 healthy horses, 64% had less than a 30% difference between the a.m. and p.m. cortisol concentrations [6]. A lack of rhythmicity has also been reported in horses with various health problems.

Basal cortisol concentrations and diurnal variation do not reliably distinguish between normal horses and those with PPID; horses with PPID may have basal cortisol concentrations that are lower than those in normal horses [13–15]. These tests are not appropriate for diagnosis of PPID.

11.2.1.2 Salivary Cortisol Concentrations

Salivary cortisol concentrations measure free, not total, cortisol concentrations. Free cortisol is believed to be metabolically active while protein-bound cortisol is not. Saliva contains only free cortisol and has been examined to determine if free levels in equine patients correlated with serum levels in response to ACTH. Although the study population was very small (five horses), and did not include patients with endocrine disease, free salivary and total serum cortisol ratios appeared to correlate [16]. A recent study showed measurement of free cortisol increased in horses with PPID, equine metabolic syndrome (EMS), obesity, and hyperinsulinemia [17], but there are insufficient studies to determine whether a high free cortisol is useful in identifying specific endocrine disorders. At present, their measurement is not recommended as a diagnostic test for PPID.

11.2.1.3 Urinary Corticoids: Creatinine Ratio and Cortisol

The urinary cortisol concentration and the cortisol: creatinine ratio have been reported to be higher in horses with PPID compared to normal horses [18, 19]. Reports comparing seven healthy normal horses and seven with PPID indicated a 100% sensitivity for the urinary corticoid:creatinine ratio in horses, with ratios greater than 16×10^{-6} seen only in horses with PPID; however, there were also some false-negative test results [19]. Another report comparing clinically normal horses with horses with PPID and with dysautonomia found no difference in the ratios between the groups, but reported that a diagnostic cut-off in the cortisol:creatinine ratio of $\geq 6.9 \times 10^{-6}$ gave positive results in 3/12 healthy horses, 12/13 horses with PPID, and 7/8 horses with dysautonomia. An increase in the cut-off value to $>12.5 \times 10^{-6}$ (the highest ratio in the normal animals) resulted in positive classification in 8/13 horses with PPID and 6/8 horses with dysautonomia [18]. The low specificity and sensitivity limit the value of the test in diagnosing PPID. The test has not become widely used, especially with the availability of plasma ACTH assays, which are more sensitive and specific.

11.2.1.4 ACTH Stimulation of Endogenous Cortisol Concentration

Administering ACTH elicits cortisol release from the adrenal cortex, the magnitude of which depends on the number of adrenal cortical cells and their activity [20, 21]. Responses in horses with PPID have been variable. Although PPID horses as a group have been reported to have a greater response than a group of normal horses, the test does not determine whether an individual horse is affected and the test is not appropriate for diagnosing PPID.

11.2.1.5 Dexamethasone Suppression of Cortisol Concentrations

For many years, the overnight dexamethasone suppression test (ODST) was considered the gold standard for diagnosing PPID. Administration of dexamethasone in healthy horses suppresses ACTH secretion, resulting in decreased cortisol concentrations. However, both false-negative and false-positive tests have been reported and repeated testing can yield varying responses in the same horse. Positive ODST results have been reported in clinically normal horses between May and October, and abnormal cortisol responses have been reported in normal and in previously laminitic ponies in all seasons except spring [13, 22–24]. Individual horses with PPID can have inconsistent test responses. For these reasons and because of the current availability of an ACTH assay, this test is not advocated as a primary test for diagnosis of PPID.

The potential link between the dexamethasone suppression test (DST) and laminitis is of concern to some. Although the test has been widely used without apparent problems, the risk has not been adequately studied.

11.2.1.6 Thyrotropin-Releasing Hormone (TRH) Stimulation with Measurement of Cortisol

The TRH stimulation test was originally used based on the premise that TRH stimulates the release of ACTH; cortisol was initially measured because of a lack of any commercially available ACTH assay [14]. The TRH stimulation test is based on the observation that horses with PPID have a 30–50% increase in serum cortisol concentration following administration of TRH, whereas normal horses do not respond [14]. The initial report of a significant increase in cortisol from baseline following TRH administration was attributed by other investigators to the lower baseline level of cortisol in the PPID horses, and a diminution in response was later reported in PPID horses with high baseline cortisol concentrations [25, 26]. The validity of this test was questioned and it is not considered appropriate for PPID diagnosis.

11.2.1.7 Combined Dexamethasone Suppression and TRH Stimulation Test

The DST/TRH administration test was reported to have a high specificity and sensitivity in differentiating between normal horses and those with PPID [15, 25]. In this test, blood is obtained before dexamethasone administration (40 μg/kg IV), a blood sample is obtained three hours later, and 1 mg of TRH is administered intravenously; blood samples are then obtained at 15, 30, 45, 60, 90 minutes, and 21 hours after TRH administration. The test is considered positive if (i) plasma cortisol concentration is ≥1 μg/dL (10 ng/mL) at 24 hours, or (ii) plasma cortisol concentration is increased ≥66% above the three-hour baseline 30 minutes after TRH. A comparison of 17 PPID and 25 clinically normal horses with no pituitary pathology reported a sensitivity of 88%, specificity of 76%, positive predictive value of 71%, and negative predictive value of 90%. Two out of 17 PPID horses had a negative test and 6/25 normal horses had a positive test [15]. Currently, this test is not recommended for PPID testing.

11.2.2 Adrenocorticotropic Hormone (ACTH) Concentrations

11.2.2.1 Basal Plasma ACTH Concentration

With the availability of commercial laboratories measuring ACTH, measuring basal plasma ACTH concentrations has become widely used to test for PPID. Normal reference interval depends on the laboratory and methodology. Both RIAs and chemiluminescent immunoassays (CIAs) are used for measurement of ACTH concentration in horses, but one study showed poor agreement and only moderate correlation between a commercial RIA and CIA [27]. Thus, ACTH measurements using different methodologies should not be considered interchangeable. The chemiluminescent immunoassay (Immulite, Siemens, Los Angeles, CA) is commonly used by commercial laboratories in the United States and current cut-offs recommended for diagnosis of PPID are based on ACTH values obtained using this assay (Figure 11.2).

Veterinarians should determine the basis for the reference interval of the laboratory they expect to use. In the US, generally the same reference interval (9–35 pg/mL) is used for both horses and ponies. One study reported ACTH concentrations were more likely to exceed the reference interval in ponies than in horses in late summer/autumn, which is in contrast to a study in England on ponies where ACTH concentrations were generally within the reference interval in summer but above reference range in winter [28, 29]. Normal mammoth donkeys (n = 45) tested in May/June were reported to have ACTH concentrations that ranged from 36 to 115 pg/mL, which was higher than the laboratory's normal horse range (11.9–25.5 pg/mL) [11]. Larger numbers of donkeys in other geographic locations should be tested to further clarify normal ranges.

Variable seasonal increases in basal ACTH concentrations in both ponies and horses have been reported from various geographic locations [23, 24, 30–34]. Concentrations can exceed the reference interval from mid-August to mid-October in normal horses and ponies, particularly in the latter. In one study on clinically normal equids, ACTH concentrations sometimes exceeded 200 pg/mL, and in another study several ponies had ACTH concentrations greater than 65 pg/mL between August and mid-October [23, 29]. A study in the UK on circannual variation in ACTH concentrations in normal equids (n = 156) and those clinically suspected to have PPID (n = 941) suggested a normal upper reference value of 47 pg/mL between August and October and 29 pg/mL from November to July [30]. Another UK study with a smaller group of animals suggested an appropriate cut-off value in March and June of 40–50 pg/mL with a value almost doubled in September and December [32]. As the same CIA was used in these studies, albeit in different laboratories, different populations probably explain the differing results amongst studies.

As ACTH levels vary with season, season-dependent reference intervals are determined. Better sensitivity and specificity are reported during nonfall months (80% sensitive and 83% specific) and are recommended for testing, but reference intervals for autumn months are established [35]. Current cut-offs recommended by the Equine Endocrinology Group are different for fall and nonfall months (see Figure 11.2).

Although basal concentrations of ACTH can be useful for diagnosing PPID, false-negative tests can also occur [13, 29]. In one study in the UK, 556 of 1497 plasma samples submitted from untreated horses suspected to have PPID were within

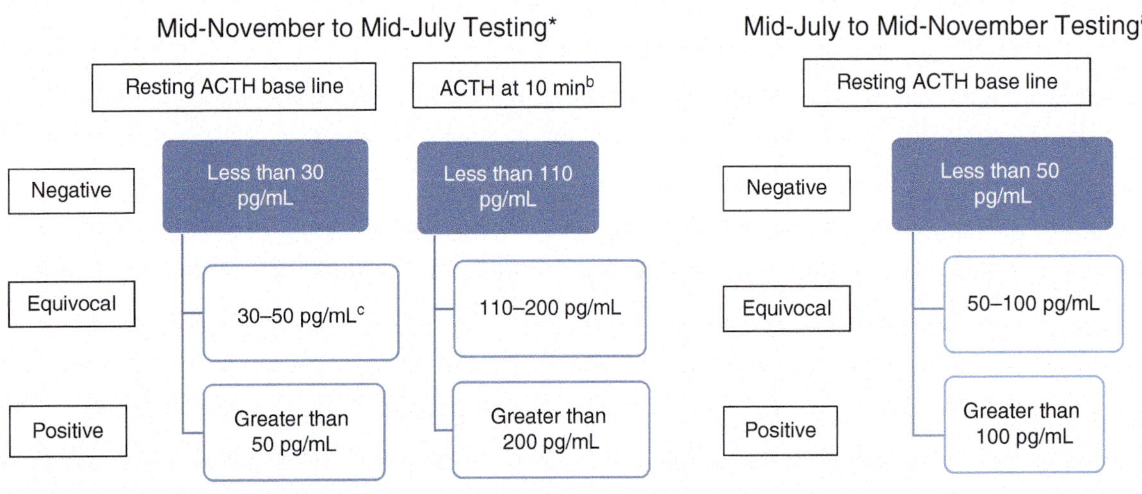

*ACTH cutoff recommendations are appropriate only for values obtained using the Immulite-TM immunoassay or assays that are strongly correlated with this assay.

[a]There is currently insufficient data available to determine accurate cut-offs for TRH stimulation testing in fall months.

[b]ACTH measurement from blood taken 10 minutes after intravenous administration of TRH (TRH stimulation test).

[c]DoTRH stimulation testing.

Based on the Equine Endocrine Group recommendations: https://sites.tufts.edu/equineendogroup/files/2019/12/2019-PPID_EEGbooklet.pdf

Figure 11.2 Schema for PPID diagnosis using the TRH stimulation test measuring plasma ACTH.

the reference interval [30]. Also, some horses with PPID may have basal ACTH concentrations that vary quite widely within a very short time period and there appears to be greater variability when concentrations are high [13, 29]. When measuring basal ACTH concentrations, collection of paired sampling did not improve sensitivity or specificity of the test [36]. If a horse suspected to have PPID has normal basal plasma ACTH concentrations, measuring the ACTH concentration change in response to TRH administration is advised (see Figure 11.2).

11.2.2.2 TRH Stimulation with Measurement of ACTH

The TRH stimulation test measuring plasma ACTH following intravenous administration of TRH is currently recommended for diagnosis of PPID in horses with early clinical signs or equivocal resting ACTH results (see Figure 11.2). Horses can eat hay prior to testing, but no grain within 12 hours of the test. It is recommended that horses less than 250 kg receive 0.5 mg and horses greater than 250 kg should receive 1.0 mg intravenously (https://sites.tufts.edu/equineendogroup/files/2019/12/2019-PPID_EEGbooklet.pdf). Blood should be collected into plastic or silicon-coated glass EDTA tubes and refrigerated prior to plasma separation. It is currently recommended to spin blood and collect plasma within eight hours of collection, although a recent study demonstrated ACTH concentrations remained stable when collected in EDTA and refrigerated prior to plasma separation for up to 36 hours [37]; plasma may also be frozen. A preinjection blood ACTH sample should be collected and then a second sample for ACTH measurement collected 10 minutes after TRH administration.

The magnitude of the increase in plasma ACTH at 10 minutes after stimulation is an indication of the hormone content stored in both the pars intermedia melanotropes and pars distalis corticotropes [38]. Measuring TRH-stimulated ACTH concentrations has been shown to be useful in the identification of PPID and pituitary hyperplasia, including in some subclinically affected horses [13, 39]. However, because of the large variability in TRH response among horses in the fall, seasonal reference intervals may not be useful in the diagnosis of PPID. To date, there are insufficient data to permit establishment of accurate cut-offs for the diagnosis of PPID in the fall and TRH stimulation testing is recommended in nonfall months.

11.2.2.3 Domperidone Stimulation of ACTH

Domperidone is a dopamine (D2) receptor antagonist and its administration should release ACTH and α-MSH secreting cells (melanotrophs) from dopaminergic inhibition, resulting in increased concentrations of these hormones in the blood. An advantage of using domperidone is that its administration PO is approved for treating mares with agalactia and it is more readily available than TRH. Disadvantages are variable blood levels, potentially due to altered gastrointestinal absorption, delayed gastric emptying, and variable food within the stomach.

Both age and pituitary pathology have been reported to correlate with domperidone response [40]. Horses with PPID were reported to have greater increases in ACTH concentration compared to normal horses four and eight hours following administration of doses ranging from 1.25 to 5 mg/kg domperidone PO [40, 41]. An increase ≥2-fold basal concentrations was considered a positive response and it was suggested that the basal and the four hours postdomperidone administration samples were best for differentiating between PPID and clinically normal horses [41]. In another study, a ≥2-fold increase in ACTH concentration was seen in 3/15 clinically normal and 4/12 PPID horses at two hours and in 4/16 clinically normal and 3/12 PPID horses at four hours, leading the authors to conclude that the test did not appear as accurate as measuring ACTH or α-MSH response to TRH administration [39]. If one looked at ACTH concentrations >36 pg/mL as a cut-off for diagnosing PPID, administering domperidone did not increase sensitivity or specificity for making the diagnosis above using baseline ACTH concentrations [39]. Further evaluation of the test using larger numbers of horses is needed to determine its clinical value, but currently the test is not recommended (https://sites.tufts.edu/equineendogroup/files/2019/12/2019-PPID_EEGbooklet.pdf).

11.2.3 α-MSH Concentrations

α-MSH is considered a more specific marker of pars intermedia secretion than is ACTH as it is secreted by the melanotropes of the pars intermedia, whereas ACTH is secreted by both pars intermedia melanotropes and pars distalis corticotropes [38]. The assay is not commercially available to date; however, as this may change, information on its use as a marker for PPID follows.

Studies cited in this chapter reporting its use have quantified the hormone using a RIA (American Laboratory Products Co., Windham, NH). A positive correlation has been found between α-MSH and obesity/body mass index in healthy horses greater than 10 years of age, although there was huge individual variation [42]. Concentrations also rise significantly in autumn [33, 43]. As the pars intermedia (PI) area, PI:total pituitary ratio, and total pituitary area increase in the fall, the observed increase in α-MSH is not unexpected [44]. A greater seasonal effect was reported for α-MSH than for ACTH [6, 24, 29, 31]. Although greater increases were reported in ponies than in horses in one study, reports are inconsistent and geographic location and body condition scores could have affected results [29, 44].

It is apparent that the range of α-MSH concentration that is considered normal may vary geographically and potentially with the populations being studied. Stabling does not appear to influence seasonal changes [29, 33]. α-MSH concentration does not appear to be affected by circadian rhythm [43]. Reports comparing seasonal increases in α-MSH with ACTH have varied, and both geographic location and breed appear influential [29, 33]. Whether α-MSH appears superior to ACTH for diagnosing PPID appears unresolved at this time as reports have varied regarding comparative sensitivity and specificity [29, 33, 35, 39].

11.2.4 ACTH and α-MSH Concentration Responses Following TRH Administration

Increases in both ACTH and α-MSH concentration after TRH administration have been documented to be higher in horses with PPID compared to normal horses and can identify horses with PPID that have normal basal hormone concentrations [13, 29, 38, 39]. The protocol is to obtain two baseline plasma samples (5–10 minutes apart), administer 1 mg TRH intravenously, and then obtain a sample 30 minutes later. Although additional samples can be obtained (e.g., at 15 and 45 minutes), sampling at 30 minutes appears to be sensitive and specific for differentiating between clinically normal horses and those with PPID using a cut-off of <36 pg/mL for normal ACTH concentration and ≤50 pmol/L for α-MSH concentration [29, 39]. Although concentrations of both hormones increase after administration of TRH, in normal horses they have usually returned to baseline by 30 minutes after TRH administration.

In one study on 53 clinically normal horses and 25 horses with PPID, at baseline 10/60 tests from normal horses and 26/37 tests from PPID horses had ACTH concentrations >36 pg/mL; at 30 minutes post TRH administration, these respective numbers were 16/60 and 36/38. Numbers of clinically normal horses with ACTH >36 pg/mL were decreased when the group was limited to horses without pituitary histological changes; ACTH >36 pg/mL was seen in only 1/23 baseline and 2/23 30-minute samples. For α-MSH, a concentration >50 pmol/L was seen in 1/30 baseline samples and 9/30 30-minute samples in clinically normal horses and in 12/18 baseline samples and 18/18 30-minute samples in PPID horses. In the clinically normal horses without pituitary changes, no baseline samples and only 1/15 30-minute samples had α-MSH >50 pmol/L [39]. It is unknown whether the TRH stimulation test will identify horses with subclinical PPID that potentially might benefit from early dopaminergic treatment prior to onset of overt signs of PPID.

The advantages of measuring α-MSH or ACTH response to TRH compared to measuring the cortisol response to the combined DST/TRH test are that the hormones of interest are being measured, fewer samples over a shorter period of time during one patient visit are needed, and dexamethasone administration is avoided. Results from one study evaluating cortisol response to the combined DST/TRH test and another evaluating ACTH response to the TRH test showed 15/17 PPID horses and 6/25 normal horses (with no PI hyperplasia or adenomas) had a positive response to the former test and 36/38 tests in PPID horses and 1/23 tests in clinically and pathologically normal horses had a positive response to the latter test [15, 39]. However, as different populations were included in each of these studies, further studies would be needed to adequately compare the two tests.

Chemical-grade TRH has been used in published reports of the test, although it is not approved for this use. Acquisition, storage, and preparation of TRH may limit its use among veterinarians. Most studies have not reported side-effects, but minor transient to generalized moderate muscle trembling for several minutes after administration of TRH has been seen in a few horses. This response was inconsistent when the test was repeated in the same horses, and the cause of the trembling remains speculative. Transient licking, yawning, and sometimes flehmen have been seen in a few horses [29, 39].

In summary, currently the best screening test for PPID is measurement of basal ACTH concentration in horses with moderate to severe clinical signs of PPID, and TRH stimulation testing in horses with equivocal signs or an equivocal ACTH concentration but appropriate clinical signs (see Figure 11.2).

11.2.5 Insulin Concentrations

Adiposity associated with insulin resistance has been reported in 15–30% of horses with PPID and hyperinsulinemia has been reported in some horses with PPID [6, 33]. One study reported that although insulin concentrations differed between normal horses and those with PPID, hyperinsulinemia was rare [45]. Normal ponies were reported to have more variable concentrations than horses and more individual clinically normal ponies had insulin concentrations above the reference interval (24/48 tests in six normal ponies versus 0/48 tests in 14 normal horses); however, this could be associated with the greater body condition score in the ponies [29].

When evaluating donkeys, it is important to know that they are reported to have lower insulin concentrations than horses. In one study on 45 healthy donkeys, all but five had insulin concentrations below the normal horse reference limit [11]. Nonobese donkeys were reported to have lower insulin concentrations than nonobese horses. Concentrations were significantly higher in obese donkeys and those with a history of laminitis or current laminitis compared to nonobese donkeys. Veterinarians evaluating donkeys should ascertain whether the laboratory they use has reference intervals for donkeys.

There has been growing interest in better defining hyperinsulinemia and equine metabolic syndrome (see Chapter 9) and investigating the relationship with PPID. It may be useful to monitor insulin concentrations in horses as high concentrations have been predictive for the development of laminitis and low insulin concentrations have been associated with improved survival [46, 47]. Factors such as diet can explain hyperinsulinemia and insulin resistance (see Chapter 9), and this combined with highly variable concentrations throughout the day complicates interpretation of values from single samples.

11.3 Testing Thyroid Function in Horses

Despite very few documented cases of thyroid dysfunction in horses and the unreliability of single measurements of thyroid hormones, basal serum concentrations of total triiodothyronine (TT3) and total thyroxine (TT4) are frequently evaluated by veterinarians. This section provides information on tests that have been used to evaluate thyroid function and factors that can influence results.

11.3.1 Thyroid Dysfunction

There appear to be few studies documenting the prevalence of primary thyroid dysfunction in horses. Naturally occurring hypothyroidism is reported in foals and there are several case reports of mature/aged horses with hyperthyroidism [48–51]. Low thyroid hormone concentrations have been measured in horses with various conditions in the absence of evidence of hypothyroidism. Although hypothyroidism has been implicated as a contributing cause of laminitis, it should be noted that no evidence has been found to support measurement of thyroid hormones as a predictor of pasture-associated laminitis in horses, and horses with experimentally induced hypothyroidism have not developed laminitis [52–56]. Horses that have been thyroidectomized have shown various clinical signs, most frequently haircoat abnormalities and decreased tolerance to cold. In younger animals, stature is affected. Mares can continue to show normal estrous cycles, conceive and deliver normal foals, and although stallions have decreased libido, they are fertile [55, 57, 58]. Propylthiouracil (PTU)-induced hypothyroidism has changed serum hormone concentrations in the absence of clinical signs [52, 54]. Severe signs have been reported in neonatal foals with naturally occurring hypothyroidism and in foals that have been partially thyroidectomized *in utero* [49, 59, 60].

11.3.2 Thyroid Hormones

Secretion of thyroid hormones is stimulated by thyrotropin (thyroid-stimulating hormone – TSH) released from the anterior pituitary gland. TSH is regulated by TRH secretion from the hypothalamus. The cuboidal to low columnar thyroid epithelial cells secrete thyroglobulin, a glycoprotein containing multiple tyrosine residues. Iodine is oxidized within the gland and bound to tyrosine on thyroglobulin to produce monoiodotyrosine and diiodotyrosine. Thyroxine (T4) and triiodothyronine (T3) result from mono- and diidodotyrosine couplings. Thyroglobulin undergoes proteolysis to release T3 and T4 into the blood. The majority of thyroid hormone released into the blood is in the form of T4 because much more T4 is formed in the thyroid gland than T3.

Once in the blood, 99% of T4 and T3 is bound to transport proteins (thyroid hormone-binding globulin, transthyretin, and albumin). Only the unbound free fractions are metabolically active; free T3 is more metabolically active than T4 because it binds much more avidly to thyroid hormone receptors. The majority of T3 is produced outside the thyroid gland, via deiodination of T4 in the peripheral tissues by deiodinases. Production of reverse T3 (rT3), a metabolically inactive form of T3, also occurs in peripheral tissues through the action of iodinases, and is important in thyroid hormone regulation.

11.3.3 Hypothyroidism in Foals

A syndrome in foals known as congenital hypothyroidism and dysmaturity (CHD) is described primarily in the Pacific North West of the United States and western Canada [49, 60]. These foals generally have a prolonged gestation, and have physical characteristics such as a short silky haircoat, tendon laxity, angular limb deformities, prognathism, and poor carpal mineralization. They have thyroid hyperplasia with often normal T3 and T4 levels at birth, but with a diminished response to TSH [61].

11.3.3.1 Congenital Goiter

A goiter is a nonspecific enlargement of the thyroid gland that can be due to thyroid hyperplasia, colloid accumulation, or neoplasia. Goiters are most commonly seen in foals (congenital goiter) and are most often due to thyroid hyperplasia associated with low serum thyroid hormone concentrations.

Foals may present with only a goiter, but musculoskeletal abnormalities such as tendon contracture and delayed bone development and ossification (especially of the carpus and tarsus) are sometimes seen in conjunction with weakness, hypothermia, and poor suckling ability [61].

Congenital goiters are usually linked to the mare's diet while pregnant; both excessive and inadequate iodine concentrations are reported to induce goiter [62, 63]. Iodine plays a vital role in thyroid hormone production. Without iodine, T3 and T4 levels decrease and the pituitary secretes increased TSH, resulting in thyroid hyperplasia. The mechanism of goiter development in association with excessive iodine is not fully understood, but it is suspected that excess iodine inhibits effective production and release of thyroid hormone, resulting in a functional hypothyroid state [64].

Plants and iodine-based wound treatments are causes of abnormal iodine concentrations in horses. Kelp contains high levels of iodine and iodine in kelp supplements crosses the placenta in pregnant mares, resulting in fetal hypothyroidism and goiter [61]. Ingestion of endophyte (*Acremonium coenophialum*)-infected fescue plants by pregnant mares from gestation day 300 (or throughout gestation) was shown to cause congenital goiter in foals. Foals with goiter had significantly decreased mean T3 concentration relative to foals born from mares that had not ingested infected fescue [65].

11.3.4 Extrathyroidal Effects on Thyroid Hormones

One should always inquire about whether a horse is receiving medications or supplements and avoid testing if drugs have recently been administered. Drugs that are highly protein bound and could displace thyroid hormones from protein-binding sites are of the greatest concern. Free T3 and T4 (fT3 and fT4) are readily excreted via the kidneys, thus increased concentrations of unbound fT3 and fT4 may result in increases or decreases in thyroid hormone concentrations depending upon whether total hormone (TT3 and TT4) or free hormone concentrations are measured. Systemic administration of dexamethasone (0.04 mg/kg SID for five days) resulted in significant increases in rT3 and sometimes also fT3, and also blunted response to TSH administration [66]. Topical dexamethasone and neomycin applied on the shaved side of horses' necks (8.5 mg of dexamethasone every 12 hours per 470–660 kg body weight for 10 days) resulted in a significant decline in TT3 by day 2 and this remained less than baseline for at least 20 days after treatment; TT4 concentrations showed a mild but nonsignificant decrease [67].

Phenylbutazone administration decreases thyroid hormone concentration [68–70]. The duration of effect of phenylbutazone treatment (4.4 mg/kg IV BID for five days) was reported to last for 10 days for TT4 and two days for fT4 [70]. However, these dosages of phenylbutazone are rarely used in clinical practice and the effect of lower or oral dosage regimens has not been reported.

Administration of synthetic thyroid hormone (levothyroxine sodium or L-T4) affects both basal concentrations of thyroid hormones and the response to TRH injections [71]. Dose and duration of treatment with L-T4 affect the magnitude of change in hormones and probably affect the length of drug-free interval required prior to testing a horse that has been receiving L-T4 [71].

Diet can affect thyroid hormone concentration [72–74]. Exercising horses fed high sugar and starch diets were reported to have higher TT3 and fT3 concentrations than horses fed fat and fiber diets. Blood samples should not be obtained close to feeding a high-energy and protein meal and an interval of at least 4–6 hours is advised [73]. Food deprivation in healthy horses was reported to result in a 42% decrease in TT3 and a 30% decrease in fT3 after two days, a 38% decrease in TT4 and 24% increase in fT4 after four days, and an increase of 31% in rT3 after one day [74]. However, no differences in TT3 and TT4 were reported in weanling horses fed restricted diets [72].

Age also influences thyroid hormone concentrations [75–79]. Premature foals have lower serum concentrations of total and free thyroid hormones compared to normal foals. A number of studies have reported that young foals have much higher TT3 and TT4 concentrations than mature horses. Table 11.1 shows concentrations in neonatal foals published in two different reports [61, 80]. Concentrations of both TT4 and TT3 are reported to be greatest in foals within one hour of birth (prior to colostrum ingestion) and may be 14- and 12-fold greater, respectively, than in blood from mature horses [79]. A study on Thoroughbred foals (eight males and five females) from 30 to 390 days of age showed an insignificant decrease in TT4 between 1 and 6 months of age, but a marked decrease between 7 and 13 months of age. The fT4 decreased significantly by the third month. The TT3 values were more variable, while the fT3 usually decreased over time [76]. Another study on six foals reported that TT3 and TT4 dropped after one month but TT4 remained higher for 12 months [77]. In Standardbred females, plasma TT3 was reported to decline from a mean of 7.9 ng/mL on day 1 to 2.4 ng/mL on day 14 and TT4 declined from 233 to 49 ng/mL in the same time period, with insignificant differences reported between samples obtained between 1 month and 22 years [78]. It appears that consensus amongst the studies exists for changes in young foals, but reports on animals older than 1 month appear variable. If one is evaluating foals for thyroid dysfunction, comparison with age- and preferably sex-matched controls is prudent.

Table 11.1 Concentrations of thyroid hormones in neonatal foals.

	<12 h[a] (n = 18)		12 to 36 h[b] (n = 25)	
	Median	Range	Median	Range
TT4 nmol/L	277	238–337	712	295–1012
fT4 pmol/L	78	46–118	NA	NA
fT4D pmol/L	106	78–184	50.2	27–70
TT3 nmol/L	8.2	3.4–10.8	7.9	3.2–9.5
fT3 pmol/L	7.8	2.4–20.3	21.2	6.9–34.3
rT3 pmol/L	NA	NA	6.6	5.2–8.1
TSH ng/mL	0.22	0.12–0.72	NA	NA

[a] [61].
[b] [80].

The effect of gender on thyroid hormone levels is unclear as reports have been inconsistent. There is usually no gender effect on thyroid hormone concentrations except that males sometimes have significantly higher TT4 concentrations. Estrus and pregnancy do not appear to affect TT3 or TT4 [81, 82].

Thyroid hormone concentrations are affected by ambient temperature and/or season and these factors should be considered when taking blood samples from horses. A negative relationship for serum TT3 (but not TT4) and temperature has been reported, with significantly higher concentrations in December through May and significantly lower concentrations from July to October [82]. TT4 was reported to have a slight but significant negative association with photoperiod, but this appears unlikely to affect diagnostic testing. Reports on diurnal variation in TT3 and TT4 vary [77, 83, 84]. In clinical practice, diurnal rhythm does not appear to be a major influence on deciding when one obtains samples for measuring thyroid hormones.

Exercise can affect thyroid hormone levels, but studies on horses performing endurance exercise have shown no changes or only transient decreases after rides between 40 and 56 km and decreased concentrations following 160 km rides that return to normal by 24 hours [85]. Basal concentrations of TT3 and TT4 were reported to be within reference range for competitive showjumping horses [86]. To avoid any possible influence of exercise, one should avoid measuring thyroid hormone concentrations within several days of strenuous exercise.

11.3.5 Nonthyroidal Illness Syndrome

Nonthyroidal illness syndrome (NTIS) or euthyroid sick syndrome may result in central hypothyroidism via decreased secretion of TRH by lowering set points for feedback inhibition and inhibition of TSH by glucocorticoids and inflammatory cytokines. Nonthyroidal illness may also decrease thyroid hormone-binding protein as well as binding affinity and capacity. The syndrome is characterized by low TT3, increased rT3, and/or low TT4 with normal fT4 [80]. With thyroid-dependent hypothyroidism, rT3 is typically decreased whereas T4 metabolism is altered in NTIS so that the inactivating pathway producing rT3 is upregulated. TSH concentrations are normal, distinguishing NTIS from hypothyroidism in which TSH is increased.

Nonthyroidal illness syndrome is documented in critically ill foals [75, 80], as well as in adult horses [87]. Critically ill foals were reported to have decreased concentrations of all thyroid hormones except rT3 and concentrations correlated with the sepsis score in septic foals [80]. Another study reported sick term foals had lower TT3 than normal foals but their TT4 concentration was intermediate between premature and normal foals [75]. TT3 and fT3 decreased first, even in mild disease.

In adult horses, TT4 and fT4D decreased significantly in horses with moderate disease, and decreases were more pronounced in horses with severe disease. Median TT4 was below the normal reference interval in horses with moderate or severe disease, but fT4 by dialysis (fT4D) remained within the reference interval. These findings suggest that fT4D may be a good indicator of true thyroid status in ill horses. In contrast to the decreases seen in T3 and T4 with increasing disease severity, TSH remained within reference limits, which suggests hypothalamic–pituitary axis dysregulation [87].

11.3.6 Thyroid Hormone Evaluation

Many commercial laboratories assay TT3 and TT4. Because single measurements of TT3 and TT4 are difficult to interpret as a result of extrathyroidal effects on protein binding, it is important to consider concentrations of fT3 and fT4. It has been suggested that measuring fT3 and fT4 and fT4D is superior to measuring TT3 and TT4, although in normal horses measurement of fT4 (by single RIA) was reported to offer no additional information compared to measuring TT4 [52, 61, 84]. Similar to dogs and humans, measuring fT4 concentrations directly instead of by dialysis appears to underestimate fT4 concentrations in horses. Free T4 by dialysis can be useful to differentiate hypothyroidism from NTIS. With NTIS, fT4D is usually within reference limits whereas TT4 and TT3 may be low [87, 88].

In a study of PTU-induced hypothyroidism, TT3 and fT3 fell abruptly whereas TT4 and fT4 did not decrease dramatically until weeks 5 and 4 of PTU administration, respectively [52]. This suggests that measuring TT3 and fT3 is superior to measuring TT4 and fT4 in a horse suspected to be acutely hypothyroid.

The use of blood collection tubes with additives (i.e., gel separator and clot activator) should be avoided due to potential interference with test results. Free T4 can be falsely increased if the sample is warmed, so whole-blood specimens and processed samples (serum/plasma) should be kept refrigerated, while frozen sample storage is recommended if the time between obtaining the sample and shipping is ≥12 hours. However, veterinarians should consult the laboratory they use to determine the requirements regarding handling of samples and also the source of the laboratory's reference intervals. As shown in Table 11.2, reference intervals vary and results from different laboratories are not interchangeable.

11.3.7 TSH Concentration

An assay for TSH has been validated for use in horses, but has not become widely available or used [52, 89]. TSH has been shown to steadily increase in horses given PTU to induce hypothyroidism, with a dramatic increase by weeks 5 and 6 [54]. Concentration decreases in horses receiving L-T4 [71]. Concentrations of TSH were reported to be greater in anestrus mares during winter than in estrus mares during summer [83]. To the authors' knowledge, further studies on the effect of season and estrus cycle on TSH have not been published. As natural cases of true hypothyroidism or hyperthyroidism appear to be rare, the ranges of serum levels of TSH in these conditions have not been described.

11.3.8 TRH Stimulation

Exogenous TRH stimulates release of thyroxine in euthyroid horses [82, 84, 90, 91]. Studies on the TT3 and TT4 responses following administration of intravenous TRH have shown a maximum response at four hours for TT4 and two hours for TT3. Ponies have responded to 0.5 mg and the usual dose used in horses is 1 mg. In one study, both TT3 and TT4 remained significantly increased at six hours but in another study TT3 was similar to baseline concentration [14, 92, 93].

Since both TT3 and TT4 increase significantly from baseline by two hours and remain increased for four hours, in clinical practice, collecting a second sample within this 2–4-hour period should suffice to show whether the horse has a normal response. A 2–3-fold increase from baseline is normal although individuals may vary especially with regard to T3 [61]. In a study of 36 normal mature horses, at four hours post TRH administration, TT4 increased 1.3–3.8 times and fT4 and fT4D increased 1.1–2.1 and 1.1–2.8 times baseline, respectively. At two hours, TT3 had increased 1.1–10.3 (mean = 3) times and fT3 increased 1–53 (mean = 4.2) times baseline [61]. These wide variations

Table 11.2 Range of concentrations of thyroid hormones in mature horses from different diagnostic laboratories.

	A (n = 71)		B	C
	Value ranges	95% confidence interval	Value ranges	Value ranges
TT4 nmol/L	6–46	18–22	7–27	13–39
fT4 pmol/L	6–21	10–12	6–24	NA
fT4D pmol/L	7–47	21–25	8–39	15–23
TT3 nmol/L	0.3–2.9	0.9–1.1	0.7–2.5	0.5–1.2
fT3 pmol/L	0.1–5.9	1.8–2.4	1.7–5.2	NA
TSH ng/mL	0.02–0.97	0.21–0.37	NA	NA

A, Breuhaus [61]; B, Diagnostic Center for Population and Animal Health, Michigan State University, Lansing MI; C, Animal Health Diagnostic Center, Endocrinology Laboratory, Cornell University College of Veterinary Medicine, Ithaca, NY.

NA, not available.

can complicate interpretation of an individual horse's response. It appears that resting baseline levels can affect responses; high resting TT3 or TT4 appeared to have blunted responses or altered the time of peak concentration, and low baseline concentrations were associated with greater responses [61]. An inadequate response can be seen in primary or secondary hypothyroidism.

Other factors may influence response to TRH. Variable effects of exercise on the TRH response test have been reported. Obese hyperinsulinemic horses with laminitis were reported to have greater TT3 and fT3 responses compared to horses with chronic lameness due to other musculoskeletal disorders [94]. Medication may also affect response. Administration of oral L-T4 was associated with decreased concentrations of TT4, TT3, fT3, and TSH in response to intravenous TRH, but the fT4 response was unaffected [71]. The chemical form of TRH used in the test is not approved for use in horses although it has been used in hundreds of horses without significant adverse effects.

11.3.9 TSH Stimulation Test

There is no equine TSH available and no approved form for use in horses. This test has been evaluated in research but appears less utilized in clinical medicine than the TRH stimulation test [68, 91, 95, 96]. Following 5 IU TSH intravenously, baseline TT3 values were reported to double by 30 minutes, and peak at five times baseline value at two hours; TT4 doubled between two and three hours and peaked at four hours (2.4 × baseline concentration) [68]. As the TT3 response is of greater magnitude and occurs earlier than the rise in TT4, measurement of TT3 before and one hour after 5 IU TSH has been suggested [95, 96].

A greater increase in TT3 than TT4 was documented after IM administration of TSH [68]. Due to variable response to IM administration of TSH, intravenous administration has been advised [91, 95, 96]. Phenylbutazone decreased baseline TT3 and TT4, but did not decrease response to TSH [68]. In contrast, after five days of dexamethasone (0.04 mg/kg IM every 24 hours), the response of thyroid hormones to TSH was blunted [66].

The clinical value of this test is unclear, and some individual clinically normal horses have failed to respond with a doubling of TT4. In a study in 12 mature horses, only six horses' TT4 increased more than twice baseline at six hours after TSH, although mean serum concentrations of TT3, TT4, rT3, and fT4 were significantly increased from baseline in all horses. In the group of horses that failed to have a twofold increase in TT4, although the fT3 more than doubled, the increase for the groups was not significant [66]. Currently this test is not recommended for clinical use.

11.3.10 T3 Suppression Test

This test is performed to confirm hyperthyroidism in a horse with high baseline thyroid hormone concentrations. To the authors' knowledge, there are only two published case reports using this test [48, 51]. The protocols used are not clinically practical as they require intramuscular administration of T3 over multiple days with blood collection up to nearly a week later. Hyperthyroid horses fail to show a suppression of thyroid hormones whereas normal horses showed a prompt suppression which persisted for at least five days after the last dose of T3 [48, 51].

Baseline concentrations of thyroid hormones can be influenced by the many factors described, and low baseline TT4 or TT3 levels by themselves may be inadequate for diagnosis of hypothyroidism. While evaluation of thyroid hormone changes in response to TRH administration is helpful in evaluating thyroid function, the chemical grade of TRH that has most frequently been used is not approved for this use in horses.

11.4 Parathyroid Disease

The parathyroid gland functions to regulate serum calcium within a narrow range. Most horses have four parathyroid glands: two in the cranial thyroid and two in variable locations in the ventral neck. These glands can often be located by scintigraphy but sometimes cannot be found, even when an adenoma is present [97, 98].

The parathyroid chief cells (C-cells) secrete parathyroid hormone (PTH) in response to low blood calcium levels. Parathyroid hormone increases blood calcium by (i) liberating it from bone; (ii) decreasing renal excretion; and (iii) decreasing GI absorption. Release of calcium from bone is achieved by increased osteoclastic activity resulting in bone resorption and loss with replacement by fibrous connective tissue (osteodystrophia fibrosa). The secretion of PTH is also magnesium dependent. Low blood magnesium levels have an inhibitory effect on PTH release and are associated with PTH resistance [99], resulting in hypocalcemia. PTH acts to lower phosphorus concentration by decreasing renal phosphorus reabsorption.

11.4.1 Hyperparathyroidism

Hyperparathyroidism can be primary (due to hyperplasia or neoplasia of the gland) or secondary. Reported cases of primary hyperparathyroidism in horses are rare and have been due to parathyroid adenoma [100–102]. Presenting signs most often reported include lethargy, weakness, lameness, anorexia, and facial swelling (osteodystrophia fibrosa). The clinical signs of primary hyperparathyroidism are attributable to hypercalcemia and hypophosphatemia from the autonomous secretion of PTH by neoplastic chief cells. A diagnosis can be made when there is persistent hypercalcemia (total and ionized), increased PTH, and normal or low phosphorus concentration (Table 11.3). Urinary fractional excretion is characterized by hypocalciuria and hyperphosphaturia as a result of increased PTH. Serum alkaline phosphatase (ALP) may be increased as a result of bone resorption and loss if osteodystrophia fibrosa is present.

Ionized calcium concentration should be measured in serum. EDTA will chelate calcium, and an ionized calcium concentration is often undetectable in an EDTA plasma sample. PTH is also measured in serum and has been validated for use in horses [103]. Equine PTH testing is offered through commercial veterinary diagnostic laboratories and at Michigan State University Veterinary Diagnostic Laboratory.

Hypercalcemia of malignancy is a paraneoplastic phenomenon typically mediated by a PTH-related peptide (PTHrp; see Chapter 7). PTHrp can be measured in horses and is often part of a diagnostic hypercalcemia panel with PTH. PTHrp acts via PTH receptors and will thus result in hypercalcemia and hypophosphatemia with hypocalciuria and hyperphosphaturia. However, PTH concentration will be normal or low.

11.4.1.1 Secondary Hyperparathyroidism

Secondary hyperparathyroidism results from any disorder that causes chronic hypocalcemia. Renal secondary hyperparathyroidism is one of the most common types of secondary hyperparathyroidism in other species but is not recognized in horses [104]. Many species in chronic renal failure are hyperphosphatemic (and usually hypocalcemic), resulting in increased PTH production. In contrast, horses with chronic renal failure typically are hypercalcemic and often hypophosphatemic (see Chapters 6 and 7). As a consequence of the hypercalcemia, PTH in horses with chronic renal failure is usually normal or low [105].

Nutritional secondary hyperparathyroidism (NSH) is well characterized in equids and occurs when horses are maintained on a diet with an inappropriately increased phosphorus to calcium ratio or graze on plants with high oxalate content. Excessive dietary phosphorus (typified by a phosphorus to calcium ratio of 3:1 or greater) inhibits intestinal calcium absorption and results in hyperphosphatemia. Grazing on plants with high oxalate content may result in NSH because the oxalates complex with calcium and interfere with intestinal calcium absorption [104]. Thus, in contrast to primary hyperparathyroidism, secondary hyperparathyroidism is characterized by increased PTH with hyperphosphatemia and normal (or rarely low) calcium concentrations (see Table 11.3). High phosphorus, low calcium diets stimulate PTH secretion in horses, and decreases in calcitriol concentrations due to hyperphosphatemia further enhance PTH secretion since calcitriol is an inhibitor of parathyroid cell function [104]. PTH-mediated release of calcium from bone usually maintains calcium concentrations within reference limits in the face of inhibited intestinal calcium absorption, but leads to osteodystrophia fibrosa ("big head"). Serum ALP may be increased as a result of bone resorption and loss if osteodystrophia fibrosa is present.

11.4.2 Hypoparathyroidism

Hypoparathyroidism may be the result of decreased production of PTH by chief cells due to primary cell dysfunction or a secondary decrease in production associated with sepsis and endotoxemia [106, 107]. Secondary hypoparathyroidism may occur with hypomagnesemia as magnesium is required for the release of PTH from chief cells [99]; in these cases, parenteral administration of magnesium rapidly restores PTH secretion.

Primary hypoparathyroidism is rare in horses, but has been described [108–110]. The clinical signs are indicative of hypocalcemia: weakness, muscle twitching, labored breathing, synchronous diaphragmatic flutter, ileus, and seizures. The characteristic laboratory findings include hypocalcemia (ionized and total), hyperphosphatemia, decreased or normal PTH, and hypomagnesemia with hypophosphaturia and hypercalciuria (see Table 11.3). Hypomagnesemia can both cause and be a consequence of hypoparathyroidism. However, if the hypoparathyroidism is secondary to hypomagnesemia, the PTH levels should normalize rapidly in response to parenteral magnesium administration.

The pathogenetic mechanism of hypocalcemia associated with endotoxemia and sepsis in horses is multifactorial but includes parathyroid gland dysfunction, as well as intracellular calcium sequestration and intestinal losses [106, 107]. PTH concentrations in critically ill horses with hypocalcemia may be increased or decreased; decreased PTH with concurrent hypocalcemia is inappropriate and indicates dysfunction. Parathyroid chief cell dysfunction is attributed to the effects of increased inflammatory mediators associated with gastrointestinal disease, sepsis, and endotoxemia [107]. Because hypocalcemia is frequently accompanied by hypomagnesemia in critically ill horses [107, 111], the hypomagnesemia may also be a cause of decreased PTH concentrations.

Table 11.3 Laboratory findings in parathyroid disorders.

	Primary hyperparathyroidism	Secondary nutritional hyperparathyroidism	Hypercalcemia of malignancy	Primary hypoparathyroidism
Ionized calcium	Increased	Normal (can be decreased)	Increased	Decreased
Phosphorus	Normal or decreased	Increased	Normal or decreased	Increased (can be normal)
PTH	Increased	Increased	Normal or decreased	Decreased or normal
PTHrp	Not present	Not present	Present	NA
Magnesium	Usually normal	Usually normal	Usually normal	Decreased
Urinary calcium	Decreased	Decreased	Decreased	Increased
Urinary phosphorus	Increased	Increased	Increased	Decreased

NA, not applicable; PTH, parathyroid hormone; PTHrp, PTH-related peptide.

References

1 McFarlane, D. (2014). Pathophysiology and clinical features of pituitary pars intermedia dysfunction. *Equine Vet. Educ.* 26 (11): 592–598.

2 de Laat, M.A., Sillence, M.N., and Reiche, D.B. (2019). Phenotypic, hormonal, and clinical characteristics of equine endocrinopathic laminitis. *J. Vet. Intern. Med.* 33 (3): 1456–1463.

3 Ireland, J.L. and McGowan, C.M. (2018). Epidemiology of pituitary pars intermedia dysfunction: a systematic literature review of clinical presentation, disease prevalence and risk factors. *Vet. J.* 235: 22–33.

4 McGowan, T.W., Pinchbeck, G.P., and McGowan, C.M. (2013). Prevalence, risk factors and clinical signs predictive for equine pituitary pars intermedia dysfunction in aged horses. *Equine Vet. J. Suppl.* 45 (1): 74–79.

5 McFarlane, D. (2019). Diagnostic testing for equine endocrine diseases: confirmation versus confusion. *Vet. Clin. North Am. Equine Pract.* 35 (2): 327–338.

6 McFarlane, D. (2011). Equine pituitary pars intermedia dysfunction. *Vet. Clin. North Am. Equine Pract.* 27 (1): 93–113.

7 Ayala, I., Martos, N.F., Silván, G. et al. (2012). Cortisol, adrenocorticotropic hormone, serotonin, adrenaline and noradrenaline serum concentrations in relation to disease and stress in the horse. *Res. Vet. Sci.* 93 (1): 103–107.

8 Fazio, E., Medica, P., Aronica, V. et al. (2008). Circulating beta-endorphin, adrenocorticotrophic hormone and cortisol levels of stallions before and after short road transport: stress effect of different distances. *Acta Vet. Scand.* 50 (1): 6–7.

9 Hinchcliff, K.W., Rush, B.R., and Farris, J.W. (2005). Evaluation of plasma catecholamine and serum cortisol concentrations in horses with colic. *J. Am. Vet. Med. Assoc.* 227 (2): 276–280.

10 Niinistö, K.E., Korolainen, R.V., Raekallio, M.R. et al. (2010). Plasma levels of heat shock protein 72 (HSP72) and beta-endorphin as indicators of stress, pain and prognosis in horses with colic. *Vet. J.* 184 (1): 100–104.

11 Dugat, S.L., Taylor, T.S., Matthews, N.S., and Gold, J.R. (2010). Values for triglycerides, insulin, cortisol, and ACTH in a herd of normal donkeys. *J. Equine Vet. Sci.* 30 (3): 141–144.

12 Irvine, C.H. and Alexander, S.L. (1994). Factors affecting the circadian rhythm in plasma cortisol concentrations in the horse. *Domest. Anim. Endocrinol.* 11 (2): 227–238.

13 Beech, J., Boston, R., Lindborg, S., and Russell, G.E. (2007). Adrenocorticotropin concentration following administration of thyrotropin-releasing hormone in healthy horses and those with pituitary pars intermedia dysfunction and pituitary gland hyperplasia. *J. Am. Vet. Med. Assoc.* 231 (3): 417–426.

14 Beech, J. and Garcia, M. (1985). Hormonal response to thyrotropin-releasing hormone in healthy horses and in horses with pituitary adenoma. *Am. J. Vet. Res.* 46 (9): 1941–1943.

15 Frank, N., Andrews, F.M., Sommardahl, C.S. et al. (2006). Evaluation of the combined dexamethasone suppression/thyrotropin-releasing hormone stimulation test for detection of pars intermedia pituitary adenomas in horses. *J. Vet. Intern. Med.* 20 (4): 987–993.

16 Schwinn, A.-C., Sauer, F.J., Gerber, V. et al. (2018). Free and bound cortisol in plasma and saliva during ACTH challenge in dairy cows and horses. *J. Anim. Sci.* 96 (1): 76–84.

17 Hart, K.A., Wochele, D.M., Norton, N.A. et al. (2016). Effect of age, season, body condition, and endocrine status on serum free cortisol fraction and insulin concentration in horses. *J. Vet. Intern. Med.* 30 (2): 653–663.

18 Chandler, K.J. and Dixon, R.M. (2002). Urinary cortisol:creatinine ratios in healthy horses and horses with hyperadrenocorticism and non-adrenal disease. *Vet. Rec.* 150 (25): 773–776.

19 van der Kolk, J.H., Kalsbeek, H.C., Wensing, T., and Breukink, H.J. (1994). Urinary concentration of corticoids in normal horses and horses with hyperadrenocorticism. *Res. Vet. Sci.* 56 (1): 126–128.

20 Glover, C.M., Miller, L.M., Dybdal, N.O. et al. (2009). Extrapituitary and pituitary pathological findings in horses with pituitary pars intermedia dysfunction: a retrospective study. *J. Equine Vet. Sci.* 29 (3): 146–153.

21 Heinrichs, M., Baumgärtner, W., and Capen, C.C. (1990). Immunocytochemical demonstration of proopiomelanocortin-derived peptides in pituitary adenomas of the pars intermedia in horses. *Vet. Pathol.* 27 (6): 419–425.

22 Borer, K.E., Menzies-Gow, N.J., Berhane, Y. et al. (2010). Seasonal influence on insulin and cortisol results from overnight dexamethasone suppression tests (DST) in normal and previously laminitic ponies. *J. Equine Vet. Sci.* 2 (30): 103.

23 Donaldson, M.T., McDonnell, S.M., Schanbacher, B.J. et al. (2005). Variation in plasma adrenocorticotropic hormone concentration and dexamethasone suppression test results with season, age, and sex in healthy ponies and horses. *J. Vet. Intern. Med.* 19 (2): 217–222.

24 Schreiber, C.M., Stewart, A.J., Kwessi, E. et al. (2012). Seasonal variation in results of diagnostic tests for pituitary pars intermedia dysfunction in older, clinically normal geldings. *J. Am. Vet. Med. Assoc.* 241 (2): 241–248.

25 Eiler, H., Oliver, J.W., Andrews, F.M. et al. (1997). Results of a combined dexamethasone suppression/thyrotropin-releasing hormone stimulation test in healthy horses and horses suspected to have a pars intermedia pituitary adenoma. *J. Am. Vet. Med. Assoc.* 211 (1): 79–81.

26 Hillyer, M.H., Taylor, F.G.R., Mair, T.S. et al. (1992). Diagnosis of hyperadrenocorticism in the horse. *Equine Vet. Educ.* 4 (3): 131–134.

27 Banse, H.E., Schultz, N., McCue, M. et al. (2018). Comparison of two methods for measurement of equine adrenocorticotropin. *J. Vet. Diagn. Investig.* 30 (2): 233–237.

28 Bailey, S.R., Habershon-Butcher, J.L., Ransom, K.J. et al. (2008). Hypertension and insulin resistance in a mixed-breed population of ponies predisposed to laminitis. *Am. J. Vet. Res.* 69 (1): 122–129.

29 Beech, J., Boston, R.C., McFarlane, D., and Lindborg, S. (2009). Evaluation of plasma ACTH, alpha-melanocyte-stimulating hormone, and insulin concentrations during various photoperiods in clinically normal horses and ponies and those with pituitary pars intermedia dysfunction. *J. Am. Vet. Med. Assoc.* 235 (6): 715–722.

30 Copas, V.E.N. and Durham, A.E. (2012). Circannual variation in plasma adrenocorticotropic hormone concentrations in the UK in normal horses and ponies, and those with pituitary pars intermedia dysfunction. *Equine Vet. J. Suppl.* 44 (4): 440–443.

31 Funk, R.A., Stewart, A.J., Wooldridge, A.A. et al. (2011). Seasonal changes in plasma adrenocorticotropic hormone and α-melanocyte-stimulating hormone in response to thyrotropin-releasing hormone in normal, aged horses. *J. Vet. Intern. Med.* 25 (3): 579–585.

32 Lee, Z.-Y., Zylstra, R., and Haritou, S.J.A. (2010). The use of adrenocorticotrophic hormone as a potential biomarker of pituitary pars intermedia dysfunction in horses. *Vet. J.* 185 (1): 58–61.

33 McFarlane, D., Paradis, M.R., Zimmel, D. et al. (2011). The effect of geographic location, breed, and pituitary dysfunction on seasonal adrenocorticotropin and α-melanocyte-stimulating hormone plasma concentrations in horses. *J. Vet. Intern. Med.* 25 (4): 872–881.

34 Place, N.J., McGowan, C.M., Lamb, S.V. et al. (2010). Seasonal variation in serum concentrations of selected metabolic hormones in horses. *J. Vet. Intern. Med.* 24 (3): 650–654.

35 McGowan, T.W., Pinchbeck, G.P., and McGowan, C.M. (2013). Evaluation of basal plasma α-melanocyte-stimulating hormone and adrenocorticotrophic hormone concentrations for the diagnosis of pituitary pars intermedia dysfunction from a population of aged horses. *Equine Vet. J. Suppl.* 45 (1): 66–73.

36 Rendle, D.I., Duz, M., Beech, J. et al. (2015). Investigation of single and paired measurements of adrenocorticotropic hormone for the diagnosis of pituitary pars intermedia dysfunction in horses. *J. Vet. Intern. Med.* 29 (1): 355–361.

37 Shepard, K.N., Haffner, J.C., Neal, D.L. et al. (2019). Effect of delayed plasma centrifugation on equine adrenocorticotropic hormone concentration. *J. Vet. Diagn. Invest.* 31 (4): 585–587.

38 McFarlane, D., Beech, J., and Cribb, A. (2006). Alpha-melanocyte stimulating hormone release in response to thyrotropin releasing hormone in healthy horses, horses with pituitary pars intermedia dysfunction and equine pars intermedia explants. *Domest. Anim. Endocrinol.* 30 (4): 276–288.

39 Beech, J., McFarlane, D., Lindborg, S. et al. (2011). α-Melanocyte-stimulating hormone and adrenocorticotropin concentrations in response to thyrotropin-releasing hormone and comparison with adrenocorticotropin concentration after domperidone administration in healthy horses and horses with pituitary pars intermedia dysfunction. *J. Am. Vet. Med. Assoc.* 238 (10): 1305–1315.

40 Miller, M.A., Pardo, I.D., Jackson, L.P. et al. (2008). Correlation of pituitary histomorphometry with adrenocorticotrophic hormone response to domperidone administration in the diagnosis of equine pituitary pars intermedia dysfunction. *Vet. Pathol.* 45 (1): 26–38.

41 Sojka, J.E., Jackson, L.P., Moore, G. et al. (2006). Domperidone causes an increase in endogenous ACTH concentration in horses with pituitary pars intermedia dysfunction (equine Cushing's disease). *Proc. Am. Assoc. Equine Pract.* 52: 320–323.

42 Donaldson, M.T., McFarlane, D., Jorgensen, A.J.R., and Beech, J. (2004). Correlation between plasma alpha-melanocyte-stimulating hormone concentration and body mass index in healthy horses. *Am. J. Vet. Res.* 65 (11): 1469–1473.

43 McFarlane, D., Donaldson, M.T., McDonnell, S.M., and Cribb, A.E. (2004). Effects of season and sample handling on measurement of plasma alpha-melanocyte-stimulating hormone concentrations in horses and ponies. *Am. J. Vet. Res.* 65 (11): 1463–1468.

44 Cordero, M., McFarlane, D., Breshears, M.A. et al. (2012). The effect of season on the histologic and histomorphometric appearance of the equine pituitary gland. *J. Equine Vet. Sci.* 32 (2): 75–79.

45 Frank, N., Elliott, S.B., Chameroy, K.A. et al. (2010). Association of season and pasture grazing with blood hormone and metabolite concentrations in horses with presumed pituitary pars intermedia dysfunction. *J. Vet. Intern. Med.* 24 (5): 1167–1175.

46 Carter, R.A., Treiber, K.H., Geor, R.J. et al. (2009). Prediction of incipient pasture-associated laminitis from hyperinsulinaemia, hyperleptinaemia and generalised and localised obesity in a cohort of ponies. *Equine Vet. J. Suppl.* 41 (2): 171–178.

47 McGowan, C.M., Frost, R., Pfeiffer, D.U., and Neiger, R. (2004). Serum insulin concentrations in horses with equine Cushing's syndrome: response to a cortisol inhibitor and prognostic value. *Equine Vet. J. Suppl.* 36 (3): 295–298.

48 Alberts, M.K., McCann, J.P., and Woods, P.R. (2000). Hemithyroidectomy in a horse with confirmed hyperthyroidism. *J. Am. Vet. Med. Assoc.* 217 (7): 1051–1054.

49 Allen, A.L., Doige, C.E., Fretz, P.B., and Townsend, H.G. (1994). Hyperplasia of the thyroid gland and concurrent musculoskeletal deformities in western Canadian foals: reexamination of a previously described syndrome. *Can. Vet. J.* 35 (1): 31–38.

50 Ramirez, S., McClure, J.J., Moore, R.M. et al. (1998). Hyperthyroidism associated with a thyroid adenocarcinoma in a 21-year-old gelding. *J. Vet. Intern. Med.* 12 (6): 475–477.

51 Tan, R.H.H., Davies, S.E., Crisman, M.V. et al. (2008). Propylthiouracil for treatment of hyperthyroidism in a horse. *J. Vet. Intern. Med.* 22 (5): 1253–1258.

52 Breuhaus, B.A. (2002). Thyroid-stimulating hormone in adult euthyroid and hypothyroid horses. *J. Vet. Intern. Med.* 16 (1): 109–115.

53 Frank, N., Sojka, J.E., and Latour, M.A. (2004). Effect of hypothyroidism on the blood lipid response to higher dietary fat intake in mares. *J. Anim. Sci.* 82 (9): 2640–2646.

54 Johnson, P.J., Messer, N.T., Ganjam, V.K. et al. (2003). Effects of propylthiouracil and bromocryptine on serum concentrations of thyrotrophin and thyroid hormones in normal female horses. *Equine Vet. J. Suppl.* 35 (3): 296–301.

55 Lowe, J.E., Foote, R.H., Baldwin, B.H. et al. (1987). Reproductive patterns in cyclic and pregnant thyroidectomized mares. *J. Reprod. Fertil. Suppl.* 35: 281–288.

56 Vischer, C.M., Foreman, J.H., Constable, P.D. et al. (1999). Hemodynamic effects of thyroidectomy in sedentary horses. *Am. J. Vet. Res.* 60 (1): 14–21.

57 Lowe, J.E., Baldwin, B.H., Foote, R.H. et al. (1975). Semen characteristics in thyroidectomized stallions. *J. Reprod. Fertil. Suppl.* 23: 81–86.

58 Messer, N.T. and Johnson, P.J. (2007). Evidence-based literature pertaining to thyroid dysfunction and Cushing's syndrome in the horse. *Vet. Clin. North Am. Equine Pract.* 23 (2): 329–264.

59 Allen, A.L., Fretz, P.B., Card, C.E., and Doige, C.E. (1998). The effects of partial thyroidectomy on the development of the equine fetus. *Equine Vet. J. Suppl.* 30 (1): 53–59.

60 Allen, A.L., Townsend, H.G., Doige, C.E., and Fretz, P.B. (1996). A case-control study of the congenital hypothyroidism and dysmaturity syndrome of foals. *Can. Vet. J.* 37 (6): 349–358.

61 Breuhaus, B.A. (2011). Disorders of the equine thyroid gland. *Vet. Clin. North Am. Equine Pract.* 27 (1): 115–128.

62 Durham, A.E. (1995). Congenital goitre in two colt foals born to mares fed excess iodine during pregnancy. *Equine Vet. Educ.* 7 (5): 239–241.

63 Osame, S. and Ichijo, S. (1994). Clinicopathological observations on thoroughbred foals with enlarged thyroid gland. *J. Vet. Med. Sci.* 56 (4): 771–772.

64 Zimmermann, M.B., Aeberli, I., Andersson, M. et al. (2013). Thyroglobulin is a sensitive measure of both deficient and excess iodine intakes in children and indicates no adverse effects on thyroid function in the UIC range of 100-299 μg/L: a UNICEF/ICCIDD study group report. *J. Clin. Endocrinol. Metab.* 98 (3): 1271–1280.

65 Boosinger, T.R., Brendemuehl, J.P., Bransby, D.L. et al. (1995). Prolonged gestation, decreased triiodothyronine concentration, and thyroid gland histomorphologic features in newborn foals of mares grazing *Acremonion coenophialum*-infected fescue. *Am. J. Vet. Res.* 56 (1): 66–69.

66 Messer, N.T., Ganjam, V.K., Nachreiner, R.F., and Krause, G.F. (1995). Effect of dexamethasone administration on serum thyroid hormone concentrations in clinically normal horses. *J. Am. Vet. Med. Assoc.* 206 (1): 63–66.

67 Abraham, G., Allersmeier, M., Schusser, G.F., and Ungemach, F.R. (2011). Serum thyroid hormone, insulin, glucose, triglycerides and protein concentrations in normal horses: association with topical dexamethasone usage. *Vet. J.* 188 (3): 307–312.

68 Morris, D.D. and Garcia, M. (1983). Thyroid-stimulating hormone: response test in healthy horses, and effect of phenylbutazone on equine thyroid hormones. *Am. J. Vet. Res.* 44 (3): 503–507.

69 Morris, D.D. and Garcia, M.C. (1985). Effects of phenylbutazone and anabolic steroids on adrenal and thyroid gland function tests in healthy horses. *Am. J. Vet. Res.* 46 (2): 359–364.

70 Ramirez, S., Wolfsheimer, K.J., Moore, R.M. et al. (1997). Duration of effects of phenylbutazone on serum total thyroxine and free thyroxine concentrations in horses. *J. Vet. Intern. Med.* 11 (6): 371–374.

71 Sommardahl, C.S., Frank, N., Elliott, S.B. et al. (2005). Effects of oral administration of levothyroxine sodium on serum concentrations of thyroid gland hormones and responses to injections of thyrotropin-releasing hormone in healthy adult mares. *Am. J. Vet. Res.* 66 (6): 1025–1031.

72 Glade, M.J., Gupta, S., and Reimers, T.J. (1984). Hormonal responses to high and low planes of nutrition in weanling thoroughbreds. *J. Anim. Sci.* 59 (3): 658–665.

73 Glade, M.J. and Reimers, T.J. (1985). Effects of dietary energy supply on serum thyroxine, tri-iodothyronine and insulin concentrations in young horses. *J. Endocrinol.* 104 (1): 93–98.

74 Messer, N.T., Johnson, P.J., Refsal, K.R. et al. (1995). Effect of food deprivation on baseline iodothyronine and cortisol concentrations in healthy, adult horses. *Am. J. Vet. Res.* 56 (1): 116–121.

75 Breuhaus, B.A. (2014). Thyroid function and dysfunction in term and premature equine neonates. *J. Vet. Intern. Med.* 28 (4): 1301–1309.

76 Fazio, E., Medica, P., Cravana, C. et al. (2007). Total and free iodothyronine levels of growing thoroughbred foals: effects of weaning and gender. *Livest. Sci.* 110 (3): 207–213.

77 Komosa, M., Flisinska-Bojanowska, A., and Gill, J. (1990). Development of diurnal rhythm in some metabolic parameters in foals. *Comp. Biochem. Physiol. A Comp. Physiol.* 95 (4): 549–552.

78 Malinowski, K., Christensen, R.A., Hafs, H.D., and Scanes, C.G. (1996). Age and breed differences in thyroid hormones, insulin-like growth factor (IGF)-I and IGF binding proteins in female horses. *J. Anim. Sci.* 74 (8): 1936–1942.

79 Murray, M.J. and Luba, N.K. (1993). Plasma gastrin and somatostatin, and serum thyroxine (T4), triiodothyronine (T3), reverse triiodothyronine (rT3) and cortisol concentrations in foals from birth to 28 days of age. *Equine Vet. J. Suppl.* 25 (3): 237–239.

80 Himler, M., Hurcombe, S.D.A., Griffin, A. et al. (2012). Presumptive nonthyroidal illness syndrome in critically ill foals. *Equine Vet. J. Suppl.* 41: 43–47.

81 Berg, E.L., McNamara, D.L., and Keisler, D.H. (2007). Endocrine profiles of periparturient mares and their foals. *J. Anim. Sci.* 85 (7): 1660–1668.

82 Johnson, A.L. (1986). Serum concentrations of prolactin, thyroxine and triiodothyronine relative to season and the estrous cycle in the mare. *J. Anim. Sci.* 62 (4): 1012–1020.

83 Duckett, W.M., Manning, J.P., and Weston, P.G. (1989). Thyroid hormone periodicity in healthy adult geldings. *Equine Vet. J. Suppl.* 21 (2): 123–125.

84 Sojka, J.E., Johnson, M.A., and Bottoms, G.D. (1993). Serum triiodothyronine, total thyroxine, and free thyroxine concentrations in horses. *Am. J. Vet. Res.* 54 (1): 52–55.

85 Graves, E.A., Schott, H.C. II, Marteniuk, J.V. et al. (2006). Thyroid hormone responses to endurance exercise. *Equine Vet. J. Suppl.* 38 (36): 32–36.

86 Cravana, C., Medica, P., Prestopino, M. et al. (2010). Effects of competitive and noncompetitive showjumping on total and free iodothyronines, β-endorphin, ACTH and cortisol levels of horses. *Equine Vet. J. Suppl.* 42 (38): 179–184.

87 Hilderbran, A.C., Breuhaus, B.A., and Refsal, K.R. (2014). Nonthyroidal illness syndrome in adult horses. *J. Vet. Intern. Med.* 28 (2): 609–617.

88 Breuhaus, B.A., Refsal, K.R., and Beyerlein, S.L. (2006). Measurement of free thyroxine concentration in horses by equilibrium dialysis. *J. Vet. Intern. Med.* 20 (2): 371–376.

89 Sticker, L.S., Thompson, D.L., and Gentry, L.R. (2001). Pituitary hormone and insulin responses to infusion of amino acids and N-methyl-D,L-aspartate in horses. *J. Anim. Sci.* 79 (3): 735–744.

90 Gentry, L.R., Thompson, D.L., and Stelzer, A.M. (2002). Responses of seasonally anovulatory mares to daily administration of thyrotropin-releasing hormone and(or) gonadotropin-releasing hormone analog. *J. Anim. Sci.* 80 (1): 208–213.

91 Harris, P., Marlin, D., and Gray, J. (1992). Equine thyroid function tests: a preliminary investigation. *Br. Vet. J.* 148 (1): 71–80.

92 Chen, C.L. and Li, W.I. (1986). Effect of thyrotropin releasing hormone (TRH) on serum levels of thyroid hormones in thoroughbred mares. *J. Equine Vet. Sci.* 6 (2): 58–61.

93 Lothrop, C.D. and Nolan, H.L. (1986). Equine thyroid function assessment with the thyrotropin-releasing hormone response test. *Am. J. Vet. Res.* 47 (4): 942–944.

94 Graves, E.A., Schott, H.C. II, Johnson, P. et al. (2002). Thyroid function in horses with peripheral Cushing's syndrome. *Proc. Am. Assoc. Equine Pract.* 48: 178–180.

95 Held, J.P. and Oliver, J.W. (1984). A sampling protocol for the thyrotropin-stimulation test in the horse. *J. Am. Vet. Med. Assoc.* 184 (3): 326–327.

96 Oliver, J.W. and Held, J.P. (1985). Thyrotropin stimulation test – new perspective on value of monitoring triiodothyronine. *J. Am. Vet. Med. Assoc.* 187 (9): 931–934.

97 Frank, N., Hawkins, J.F., Couëtil, L.L., and Raymond, J.T. (1998). Primary hyperparathyroidism with osteodystrophia fibrosa of the facial bones in a pony. *J. Am. Vet. Med. Assoc.* 212 (1): 84–86.

98 Wong, D., Sponseller, B., Miles, K. et al. (2004). Failure of technetium Tc 99m sestamibi scanning to detect abnormal parathyroid tissue in a horse and a mule with primary hyperparathyroidism. *J. Vet. Intern. Med.* 18 (4): 589–593.

99 Agus, Z.S. (1999). Hypomagnesemia. *J. Am. Soc. Nephrol.* 10 (7): 1616–1622.

100 Cottle, H.J., Hughes, K.J., Thompson, H. et al. (2016). Primary hyperparathyroidism in a 17-year-old Arab × welsh cob pony mare with a functional parathyroid adenoma. *Equine Vet. Educ.* 28 (9): 477–485.

101 Peauroi, J.R., Fisher, D.J., Mohr, F.C., and Vivrette, S.L. (1998). Primary hyperparathyroidism caused by a functional parathyroid adenoma in a horse. *J. Am. Vet. Med. Assoc.* 212 (12): 1915–1918.

102 Tomlinson, J.E., Johnson, A.L., Ross, M.W. et al. (2014). Successful detection and removal of a functional parathyroid adenoma in a pony using technetium Tc 99m sestamibi scintigraphy. *J. Vet. Intern. Med.* 28 (2): 687–692.

103 Estepa, J.C., Aguilera-Tejero, E., Mayer-Valor, R. et al. (1998). Measurement of parathyroid hormone in horses. *Equine Vet. J. Suppl.* 30 (6): 476–481.

104 Toribio, R.E. (2011). Disorders of calcium and phosphate metabolism in horses. *Vet. Clin. North Am. Equine Pract.* 27 (1): 129–147.

105 Brobst, D.F., Bayly, W.M., Reed, S.M. et al. (1982). Parathyroid hormone evaluation in normal horses and horses with renal failure. *J. Equine Vet. Sci.* 2 (5): 150–157.

106 Toribio, R.E., Kohn, C.W., Chew, D.J. et al. (2001). Comparison of serum parathyroid hormone and ionized calcium and magnesium concentrations and fractional urinary clearance of calcium and phosphorus in healthy horses and horses with enterocolitis. *Am. J. Vet. Res.* 62 (6): 938–947.

107 Toribio, R.E., Kohn, C.W., Hardy, J., and Rosol, T.J. (2005). Alterations in serum parathyroid hormone and electrolyte concentrations and urinary excretion of electrolytes in horses with induced endotoxemia. *J. Vet. Intern. Med.* 19 (2): 223–231.

108 Couëtil, L.L., Sojka, J.E., and Nachreiner, R.F. (1998). Primary hypoparathyroidism in a horse. *J. Vet. Intern. Med.* 12 (1): 45–49.

109 Durie, I., van Loon, G., Hesta, M. et al. (2010). Hypocalcemia caused by primary hypoparathyroidism in a 3-month-old filly. *J. Vet. Intern. Med.* 24 (2): 439–442.

110 Hudson, N.P., Church, D.B., Trevena, J. et al. (1999). Primary hypoparathyroidism in two horses. *Aust. Vet. J.* 77 (8): 504–508.

111 Johansson, A.M., Gardner, S.Y., Jones, S.L. et al. (2003). Hypomagnesemia in hospitalized horses. *J. Vet. Intern. Med.* 17 (6): 860–867.

12

Cytology of Cutaneous and Subcutaneous Lesions

Amy C. Valenciano[1], Andrew Burton[2], Angela Borchers[3], and Rick L. Cowell[4]

[1] IDEXX Laboratories, Inc., Dallas, TX, USA
[2] IDEXX Laboratories, Inc., North Grafton, MA, USA
[3] School of Veterinary Medicine, University of California, Davis, CA, USA
[4] Stillwater, OK, USA

12.1 Introduction

Cytological examination can be very useful when a cutaneous or subcutaneous lesion is not easily diagnosed by clinical evaluation, and when there is lack of response to initial therapy. Cutaneous and subcutaneous lesions in the equine are easily accessible, and there are no significant contraindications for aspiration, scraping, or impression smear collection. Tranquilization and/or anesthesia is seldom needed. The cytological specimen can be collected, prepared, stained, and microscopically evaluated in minutes, often providing a diagnosis, prognosis, indication of appropriate therapy, and/or indication of the next diagnostic procedure.

12.2 Collection Techniques

Lesions may be swabbed, imprinted, scraped, and/or aspirated. Ulcerated or eroded masses should be imprinted initially to characterize the superficial pathology, then cleaned and dried followed by scraping or deep aspiration, to characterize the deeper pathology. Nonulcerated masses require only aspiration. If the mass is large or complex, aspiration from various angles or depths should be performed. If the lesion is cystic, aspiration from both the cystic contents and the solid portion should be performed. This is important, as often, cystic components are nonspecific.

Swabs are collected only when imprints, scrapings, and aspirates cannot be made, as this method often results in low cell yield. If the lesion is dry, a cotton swab can be moistened with sterile isotonic fluid, such as 0.9% NaCl, to minimize cell damage during collection and slide preparation, but is unnecessary if the lesion is moist or exudative. After sample collection, gently roll the swab along the flat surface of the slide. Do not rub the swab across the slide surface, as this will result in excessive cell damage. Imprints are made by removing any scab covering the lesion and then touching the surface of a clean glass slide to the surface of the lesion. If *Dermatophilus congolensis* infection is suspected, the underside of the scab is imprinted as well. The lesion can then be cleaned with a nonirritating antiseptic, wiped dry with a sterile gauze sponge, and reimprinted.

High-quality cytological smears can also be made by imprinting biopsy specimens. The biopsied tissue surface is gently blotted on a clean gauze until dry and the tissue gently sticks to the gauze, then, the tissue is gently but firmly pressed onto a glass slide multiple times. Scrapings of cutaneous lesions are made by rubbing the edge of a blunt instrument, such as a glass slide or the back of a scalpel blade, across the lesion. This results in accumulation of cells along the edge of the blunt instrument. The cells can then be gently spread onto a clean, dry glass slide.

Aspirates are obtained by using a 20–25 gauge needle attached to a 3–20 mL syringe. If microbiological evaluation is to be performed, the area of aspiration should be surgically prepared. Otherwise, an alcohol swab can be used to clean the area. Hold the mass to be aspirated firmly to aid penetration of the skin and mass and to control the direction of the needle. Introduce the needle, attached to a syringe, into the center of the mass and apply strong negative pressure by withdrawing the plunger about one-half to three-fourths the volume of the syringe. If the lesion is large enough, redirect the needle to sample different angles and depths of the mass without removing the needle, and relieve the negative pressure first (apply negative pressure

Equine Hematology, Cytology, and Clinical Chemistry, Second Edition.
Edited by Raquel M. Walton, Rick L. Cowell, and Amy C. Valenciano.

only when the needle is static). When aspiration is complete (often, high-quality collections do not have sample showing in the syringe and sometimes not even in the hub of the needle), release negative pressure from the syringe and remove the needle from the mass. This step is important to avoid aspirating blood and surrounding normal tissue and to avoid the sample from being aspirated from the barrel and needle hub into the syringe itself, making expulsion of material onto slides difficult. Once the negative pressure has been fully released, remove the needle from the mass and skin. Then, remove the needle from the syringe and aspirate air into the syringe. Next, replace the needle onto the syringe and expel the material onto a glass slide by rapidly depressing the plunger.

Alternatively, a nonaspiration or tattoo technique may be used. This method is useful in very hemorrhagic lesions when adequate numbers of cells are difficult to retrieve without contaminating the sample with peripheral blood or when aspiration yield is low, which can happen with very firm and solid lesions. The nonaspiration technique collects cells within the needle by capillary action after shearing cells from the tissue with small, repeated movements of the needle tip. Using just the needle itself or the needle attached to a syringe filled with air and no negative pressure applied, rapidly and repeatedly advance the needle through most of the thickness of the mass, using an action like a sewing machine. Next, withdraw the needle from the mass and expel the material onto a glass slide as described above.

12.3 Slide Preparation

Gently spray the aspirated material onto the center of a glass slide, and place a second glass slide on top. Let the material spread between the two slides with only the weight of the second glass slide. Next, gently pull the slides apart from each other horizontally using a smooth technique with no downward pressure. If excessive cellular lysis is noted from cursory review of a stained slide, use a coverslip to spread the material instead of another glass slide.

For fluid-filled and cystic lesions, make a few direct smears of the fluid component, using a blood smear technique with a small drop of fluid at one end of the slide and a second slide at a 45° angle to spread the fluid into a monolayer containing a feathered edge. A small drop of fluid can also be placed onto the middle of a slide, with a second slide on top and gently pulling the slides apart horizontally. If the fluid is clear and poorly cellular then, in addition to a direct smear, centrifugation and slide preparation from the sediment may also be performed. Fluid can also be sent to the laboratory for cytospin concentrated slides to be made. It is important to also aspirate the wall or solid portion of the mass, which can be sent in together with the fluid slides and fluid specimen.

12.4 General Evaluation of Cytological Smears

The first step in cytological evaluation of a smear is to determine whether sufficient numbers of intact cells are present and whether the sample is spread and stained adequately. If repeated collection attempts fail to yield sufficient numbers of cells, biopsy may be necessary.

Once a suitable cytological preparation has been produced, the smears are evaluated for evidence of inflammation and/or neoplasia. If all the cells from a solid mass are tissue cells (i.e., no inflammatory cells are present), the lesion is caused by neoplasia or hyperplasia. If all the cells are inflammatory cells, an inflammatory process is most likely the primary cause, but an inflamed, poorly exfoliative neoplasm cannot be ruled out. An admixture of inflammatory cells and tissue cells can be caused by inflammation with secondary tissue cell hyperplasia or dysplasia, or could be consistent with an inflamed neoplasm. Therefore, caution must be exercised in diagnosing neoplasia if evidence of inflammation is detected, as in the face of inflammation, tissue cells can become dysplastic and be mistaken for neoplasia.

12.5 Evaluation of Inflammatory Cell Populations

Figure 12.1 provides an algorithm to aid evaluation of the inflammatory cell component of cutaneous and subcutaneous lesions. Table 12.1 gives some general considerations for inflammatory responses.

If most of the inflammatory cells are neutrophils (Figures 12.2 and 12.3) but no bacteria are found, a covert infection may be present or the neutrophilic inflammatory response may be due to one of the conditions listed under *Marked predominance of neutrophils* in Table 12.1. The lesion should be cultured to identify a covert infection. If culture results reveal an infectious agent, appropriate therapy can be instituted. If culture results do not reveal an infectious agent or if therapy for the infectious agent identified by culture is not effective, cytological evaluation can be repeated or a biopsy can be submitted for histopathological evaluation.

When >15% of the inflammatory cells are macrophages (Figure 12.4) and/or giant inflammatory cells, fungal

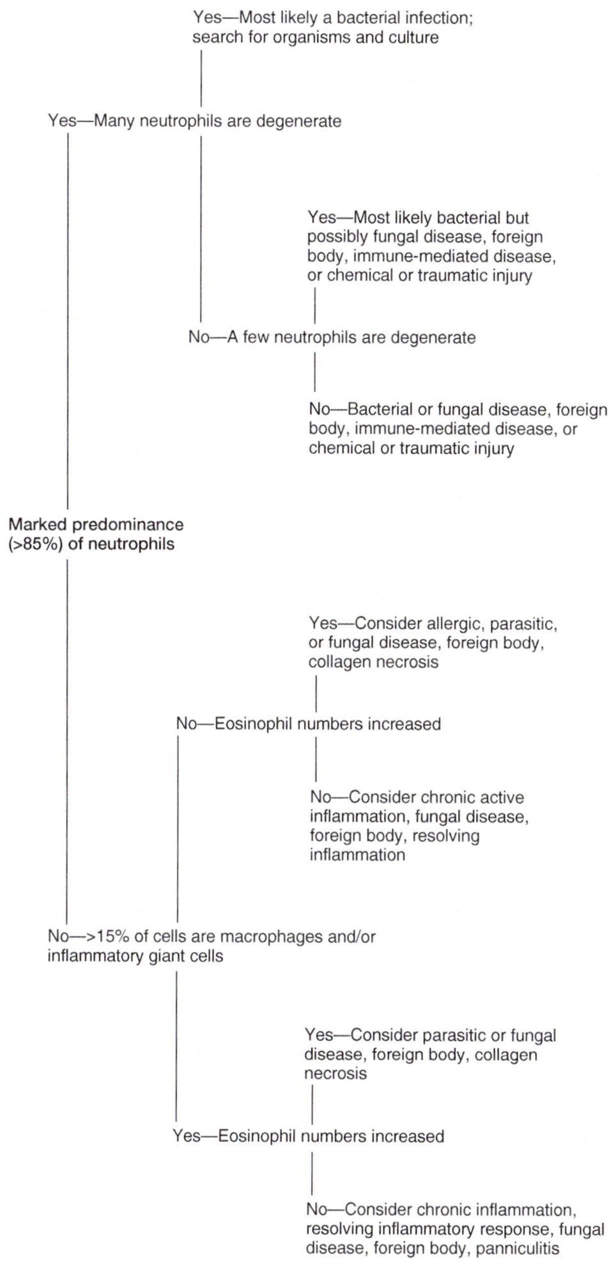

Figure 12.1 Algorithm to aid in evaluation of aspirates containing a preponderance of inflammatory cells.

infection or foreign body granuloma should be considered. The slide should be carefully perused for organisms or signs of foreign material, such as refractile debris or eosinophilic material typical of adjuvant. Also, historical information concerning possible introduction of foreign material should be sought. If no organisms or foreign materials are found and there is no historical information indicating introduction of a foreign substance into the area, the tissue can be cultured or a biopsy can be submitted for histopathological examination.

If the proportion of eosinophils exceeds 10% (Figures 12.5 and 12.6), an allergic, parasitic, foreign body reaction or fungal infection should be considered. Again, the slide should be carefully searched for organisms or signs of foreign material. If none are found, the lesion can be cultured for bacteria and/or fungal organisms and a biopsy can be submitted.

12.6 Cytological Characteristics of Select Infectious Agents

Lesions characterized by >85% neutrophils (Figures 12.7 and 12.8), which are often degenerate, with fewer macrophages, are often associated with bacterial infection. Fungal infections tend to produce lesions containing prominent numbers of macrophages but often with a predominance of neutrophils. With certain fungal infections, eosinophils can be numerous. Bacterial and fungal infections can also contain lesser numbers of mature lymphocytes and plasma cells. Fibroblasts (spindle-shaped tissue cells) can also be present and consistent with a reactive and reparative component. The cellular composition is also influenced by the type of infectious agent, location of the lesion, duration of the lesion and immune status of the patient.

12.6.1 Bacterial Cocci

Most pathogenic bacterial cocci are gram positive and of the genus *Staphylococcus* or *Streptococcus* (Figures 12.9 and 12.10). Staphylococci usually occur in clusters of 4–12 bacteria, whilst streptococci tend to occur in short or long chains. When cocci are identified in cytological preparations, aerobic and anaerobic culture and sensitivity should be performed to identify the organism and appropriate antibacterial therapy. As most pathogenic cocci are gram positive, antibacterial therapy effective against gram-positive organisms should be used when it is necessary to initiate therapy before culture and sensitivity results are received.

12.6.2 Dermatophilus congolensis

Dermatophilus congolensis is a facultative anaerobic actinomycete that infects the superficial epidermis, causing exudative, crusty lesions. Infection occurs in humid, tropical, and subtropical locations, after significantly prolonged rainfall and concurrent with other skin diseases. Removal of crusts reveals eroded to ulcerated skin underneath. Cytological preparations from the undersurface

Table 12.1 Some conditions suggested by certain proportions of inflammatory cells.

Inflammatory cell population	First considerations	Second considerations
Marked predominance (85%) of neutrophils		
Many degenerate neutrophils	Gram-negative bacteria Gram-positive bacteria	Abscess secondary to neoplasia, foreign bodies, etc.
Few degenerate neutrophils	Gram-positive bacteria Gram-negative bacteria Higher bacteria (*Nocardia*, *Actinomyces*, etc.)	Fungi Protozoa Foreign body Immune mediated Chemical or traumatic injury Abscess secondary to neoplasia
No degenerate neutrophils	Gram-positive bacteria Higher bacteria (*Nocardia*, *Actinomyces*, etc.) Chemical or traumatic injury Panniculitis	Abscess secondary to neoplasia Fungi Foreign body
Admixture of inflammatory cells		
15–40% macrophages	Higher bacteria (*Nocardia*, *Actinomyces*, etc.) Fungi Protozoa Neoplasia Foreign body Panniculitis Any resolving inflammatory lesions	Nonfilamentous gram-positive bacteria Parasites Chronic allergic inflammation
>40% macrophages	Fungi Foreign body Protozoa Neoplasia Panniculitis Any resolving inflammatory lesions	Parasites Chronic allergic inflammation
Giant inflammatory cells present	Fungi Foreign body Protozoa Collagen necrosis Panniculitis Parasites (if eosinophils are present)	
>10% eosinophils	Allergic inflammation Parasites Collagen necrosis Mast cell tumor	Neoplasia Foreign body Hyphating fungi

of scabs are most rewarding in demonstrating organisms. These preparations usually contain mature epithelial cells, keratin bars, debris, and organisms. A few neutrophils may also be found. If the undersurface of the scab is dry and does not yield adequate cytological preparations, crusts and scabs may be minced in saline and smears made for cytological evaluation. *D. congolensis* replicates by transverse and longitudinal division, producing chains of cocci arranged in 2–8 parallel rows resembling small, blue railroad tracks (Figure 12.11). Also, many individual coccoid cells may be seen cytologically. Dermatophilosis can be acute, subacute, and chronic. Organisms may not be seen on cytology in some chronic cases, or in cases in which cytology is negative and infection is clinically suspected. In these instances, other testing such as RT-qPCR may be necessary [1]. Diagnosis can also be obtained by biopsy and histopathology and culture. Dermatophilosis is a zoonotic agent and caution in handling infected animals and skin lesions/crusts is warranted.

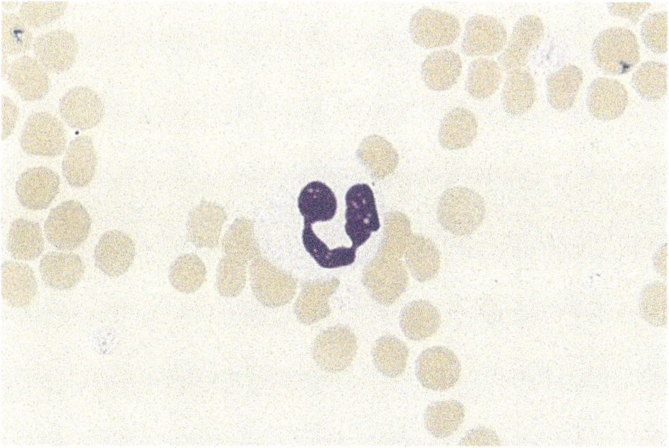

Figure 12.2 Nondegenerate neutrophil. Note the tightly clumped, dark-staining (basophilic) nuclear chromatin. Wright's stain, original magnification 250×.

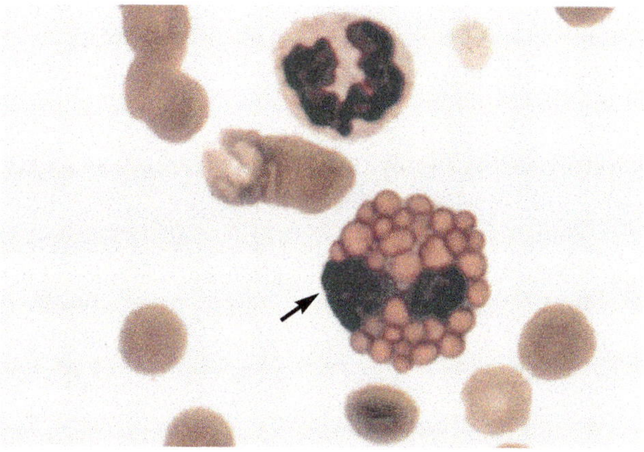

Figure 12.5 Equine eosinophils (*arrow*) are characterized by large, round, eosinophilic (red) intracytoplasmic granules. Wright's stain, original magnification 250×. *Source:* Courtesy of Oklahoma State University.

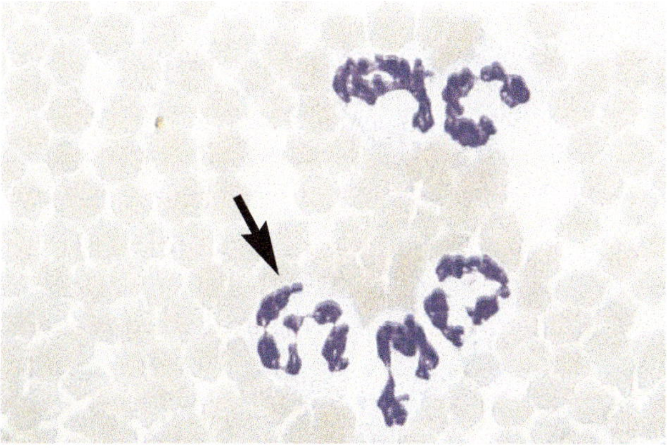

Figure 12.3 A hypersegmented neutrophil (*arrow*). Hypersegmentation is an age-related change. Wright's stain, original magnification 250×.

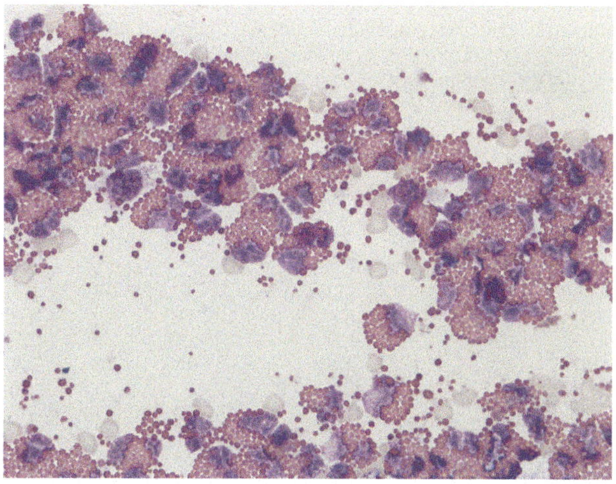

Figure 12.6 Large numbers of equine eosinophils with few red blood cells.

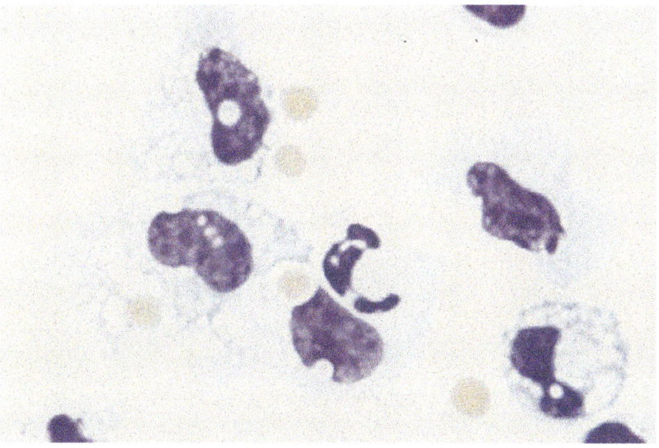

Figure 12.4 Foamy macrophages from peritoneal fluid. Wright's stain, original magnification 100×.

12.6.3 Small Bacterial Rods

Most small bacterial rods are gram negative but some, such as *Corynebacterium* spp., are gram positive. Some gram-negative rods can be recognized cytologically as bipolar (Figures 12.12 and 12.13). All pathogenic bipolar bacterial rods are gram negative. Rod bacterial infections are usually associated with a marked neutrophilic inflammatory response. When small bacterial rods are recognized in cytological preparations, the lesion should be cultured to identify the organism and sensitivity tests performed to determine appropriate antibacterial therapy. If it is necessary to institute antibacterial therapy before culture and sensitivity results are received, therapy employed should be effective against gram-negative organisms since most pathogenic small rods are gram negative.

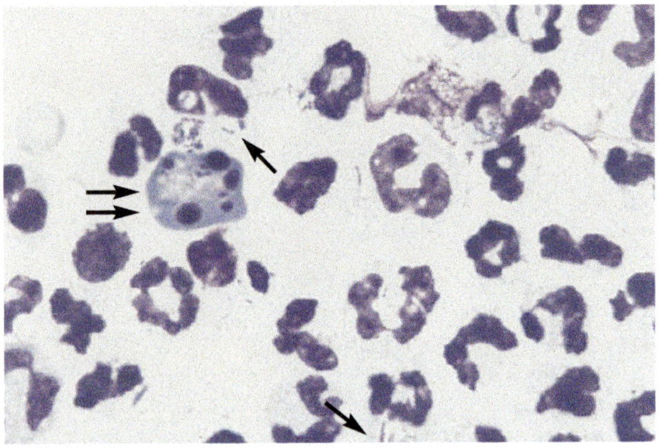

Figure 12.7 Neutrophils showing hydropic degeneration (degenerative neutrophils). Hydropic degeneration develops in neutrophils after they have migrated from the blood into an area of inflammation. Degeneration is caused by toxins such as endotoxin. Note the nuclear chromatin is spread out, fills up more of the cytoplasm, and stains more eosinophilic than that of the nondegenerate neutrophil. Bacterial rods (*arrows*) are present within the cytoplasm of some of the neutrophils. A pyknotic cell with round, somewhat eosinophilic spheres of nuclear chromatin is also present (*double arrow*). Wright's stain, original magnification 250×.

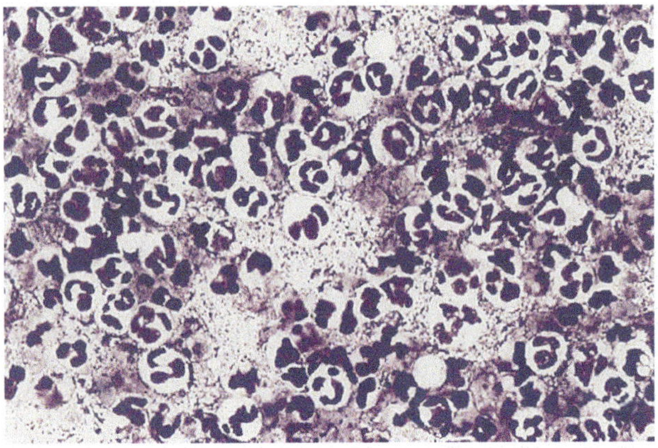

Figure 12.8 Purulent inflammation is characterized by a predominance of neutrophils. Many of the neutrophils in this preparation are degenerate. Diff-Quik stain, original magnification 125×.

12.6.4 Filamentous Rods

Filamentous rods that can cause cutaneous infections include *Nocardia* spp., *Actinomyces* spp., *Mycobacterium* spp., and certain anaerobes such as *Fusobacterium* spp. Because these organisms are often refractory to common antibacterial therapy and reliable culture of these organisms requires special conditions, cytological evaluation is very useful in indicating the need for special cultures. Rarely, the pathogenic filamentous rods of *Nocardia* spp. and *Actinomyces* spp. (Figure 12.14) may cause cutaneous or subcutaneous lesions (abscesses, ulcers, draining tracts, masses) in horses. Cutaneous infection

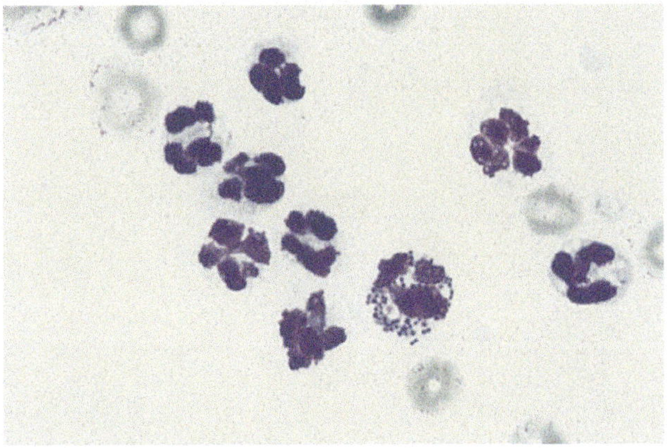

Figure 12.9 A neutrophil containing phagocytized cocci. Wright's stain, original magnification 250×.

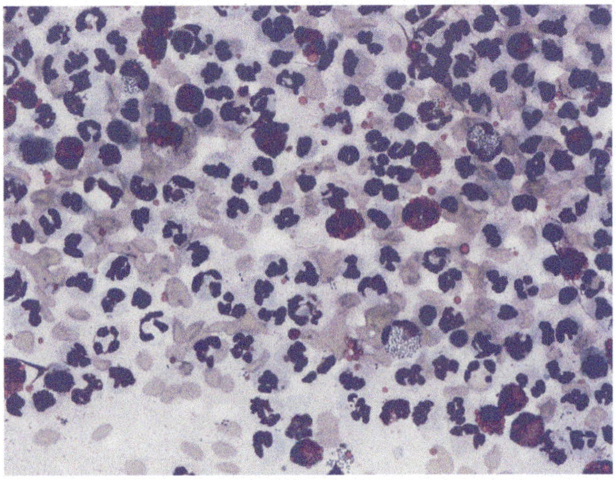

Figure 12.10 Large numbers of variably degenerate neutrophils. Some are filled with phagocytosed coccoid bacteria which are also found extracellularly in low numbers. There are fewer eosinophils present.

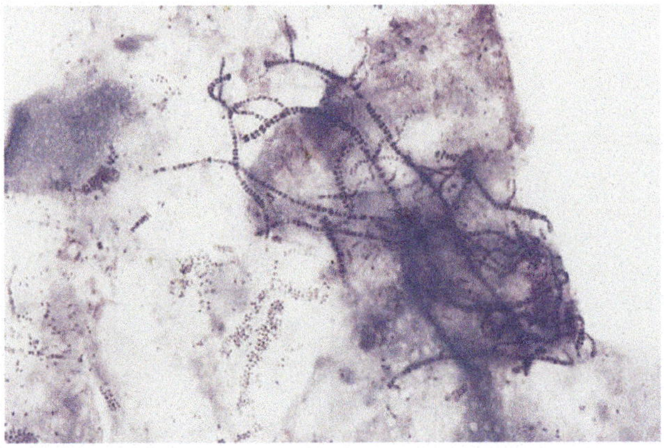

Figure 12.11 Imprint from underside of scab secondary to *Dermatophilus congolensis* infection. There is a background of squamous debris and numerous chains of bacterial doublets. Scattered individual bacteria are also present. Wright's stain, original magnification 250×.

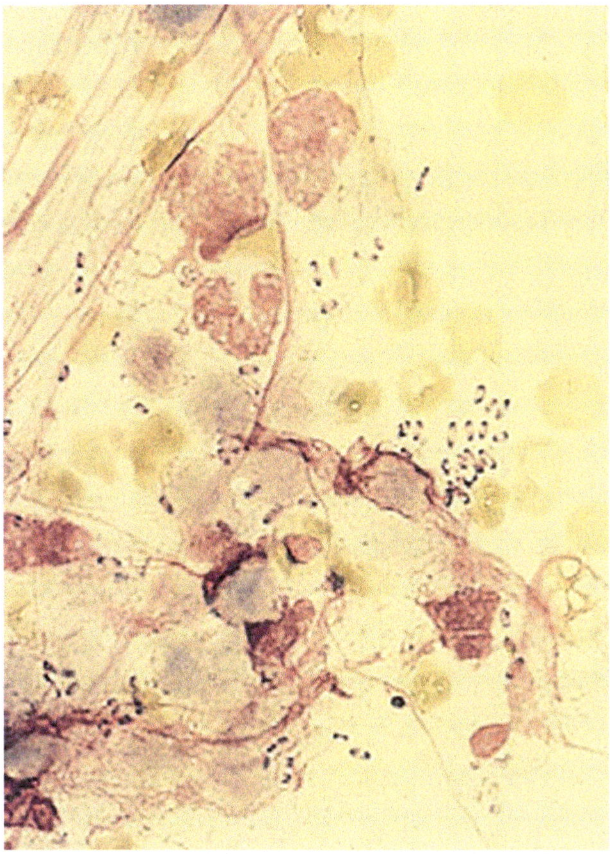

Figure 12.12 Numerous small, bipolar bacterial rods are present extracellularly. Wright's stain, original magnification 250×.

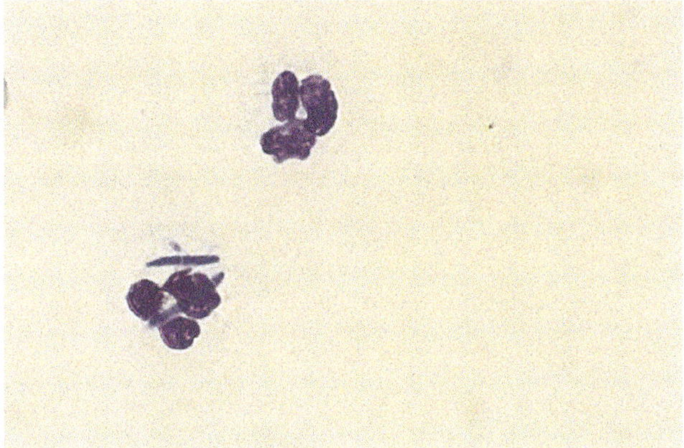

Figure 12.13 A neutrophil containing phagocytized bacilli. Wright's stain, original magnification 250×.

with these agents is uncommon and usually occurs secondary to contamination of an existing wound. *Mycobacterium* spp. and some anaerobes, such as *Fusobacterium*, rarely may be filamentous. *Nocardia* and *Actinomyces* generally have a distinctive morphology in cytological preparations stained with Romanowsky-type stains. They are characterized by long, slender (filamentous) strands that stain pale blue and have intermittent, small, pink to purple areas, giving the rods a beaded appearance. This morphology is characteristic of both *Nocardia* and *Actinomyces* spp. and the filamentous form of *Fusobacterium* spp. When these features are recognized cytologically, cultures should be performed specifically for *Nocardia*, *Actinomyces*, and anaerobes.

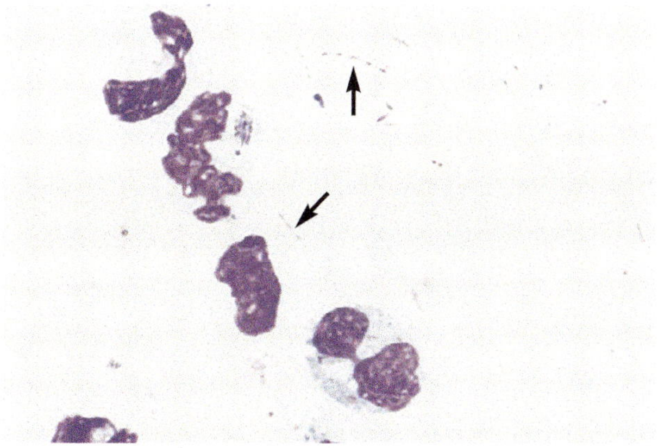

Figure 12.14 Degenerate neutrophils and bacteria. The long filamentous bacterial rods that stain blue with reddish dots are characteristic of the Actinomyces family (*arrow*). Wright's stain, original magnification 250×.

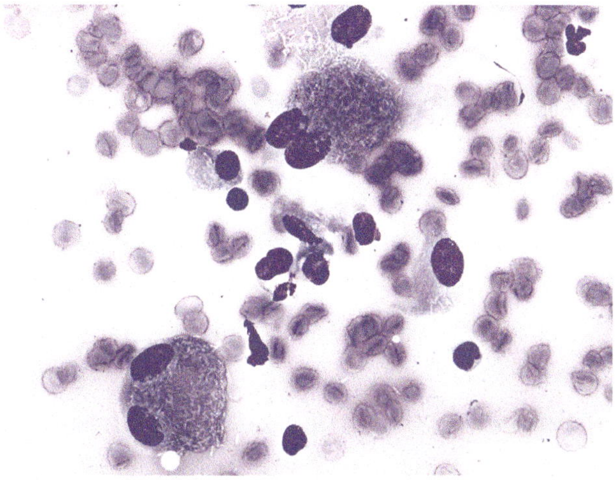

Figure 12.15 Note two large binucleate macrophages filled with phagocytosed negative-staining mycobacteria.

Mycobacterium spp. (atypical mycobacterial infections and cutaneous tuberculosis), on the other hand, often do not stain with Romanowsky-type stains. As a result, negative images (Figures 12.15 and 12.16) may be observed in the cytoplasm of macrophages and free in the extracellular space. *Mycobacterium* spp. stain bright pink with acid-fast stains (Figure 12.17). Therefore, when negative images are encountered or when the character of the lesion suggests mycobacteria infection, an acid-fast stain can be performed to demonstrate the organism and/or cultures for *Mycobacterium* spp. can be performed to identify the organism.

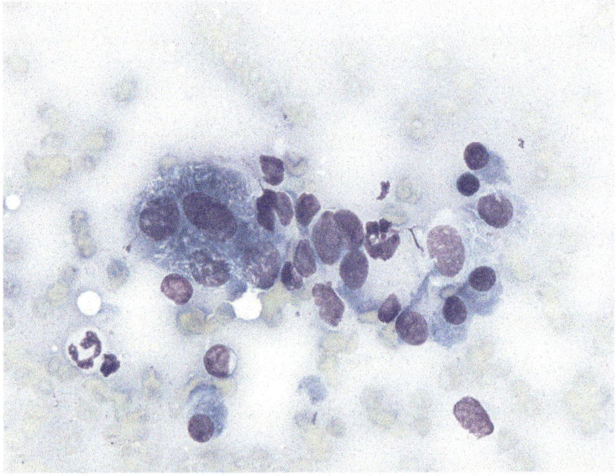

Figure 12.16 Few macrophages with intracytoplasmic negative-staining mycobacteria and few admixed neutrophils, mature lymphocytes, and plasma cells.

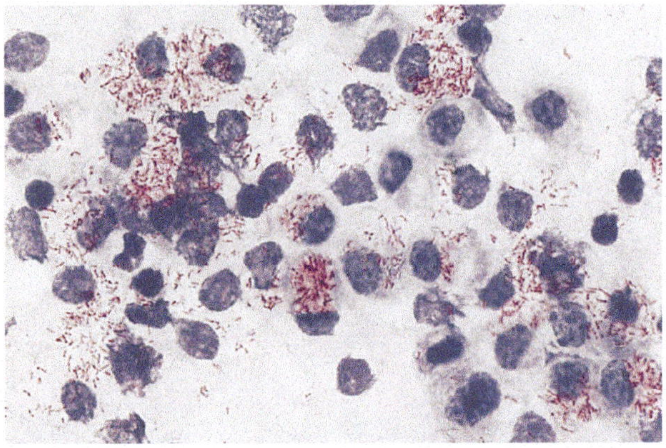

Figure 12.17 Acid-fast stain showing red filamentous mycobacteria.

12.6.5 Large Bacterial Rods

Large bacterial rods found in cytological preparations may be pathogenic or nonpathogenic. Those that are pathogenic and sometimes infect cutaneous and subcutaneous tissues include *Clostridium* spp. and, infrequently, *Bacillus* spp. When large bacterial rods are thought to be pathogenic, both aerobic and anaerobic cultures should be performed. Also, the smears should be inspected for large bacterial rods that contain spores.

12.6.6 *Sporothrix schenckii*

Sporothrix schenckii infection (sporotrichosis) most commonly occurs in a cutaneolymphatic form; however, a primary cutaneous form with no lymphatic involvement is seen occasionally. In the cutaneolymphatic form, hard subcutaneous nodules develop along lymphatics and the lymphatics may become *corded*. The nodules may ulcerate. In horses, the organisms are scarce and cytological preparations must be perused carefully. If organisms are not found, the lesion should be cultured and a biopsy of the lesion should be submitted for histopathological evaluation. In cytological preparations stained with Romanowsky stains, *S. schenckii* organisms are round to oval to fusiform (cigar shaped). They are 3–9 μ long and 1–3 μ wide and stain pale to medium blue with a slightly eccentric pink to purple nucleus (Figure 12.18). They may be confused with *Histoplasma capsulatum* if only a few organisms are found and the classic fusiform (cigar shape) is not seen.

12.6.7 Histoplasma capsulatum, Blastomyces dermatitidis, Cryptococcus neoformans, and Coccidioides immitis

Cutaneous lesions secondary to infection with *Histoplasma*, *Blastomyces*, *Cryptococcus*, and *Coccidioides* organisms are rare in the equine. Infection of the skin can be secondary to hematogenous and/or lymphatic spread from primary pulmonary infection. However, these organisms may rarely produce a primary cutaneous lesion from direct trauma and inoculation.

Characteristics of these organisms in cytological preparations stained with Romanowsky-type stains are as follows: *H. capsulatum* organisms (Figure 12.19) are round to slightly oval but are not fusiform or cigar shaped. They are 2–4 μ in diameter (about half the size of a RBC), stain pale to medium blue, and contain an eccentric pink to purple nucleus. A thin, clear capsule surrounds the yeast. Accompanying inflammation is pyogranulomatous. *B. dermatitidis* organisms

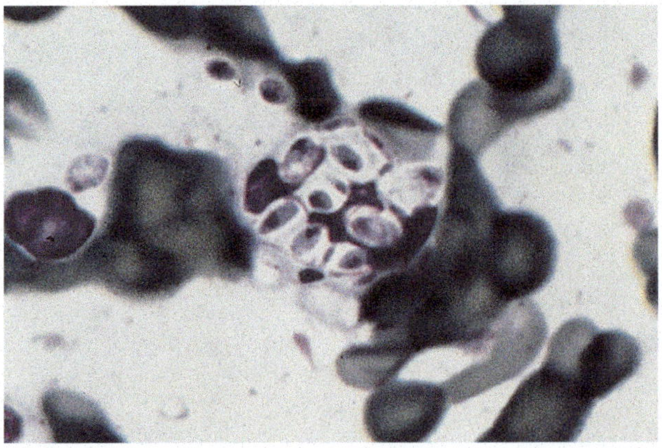

Figure 12.18 A neutrophil containing numerous *Sporothrix schenckii* organisms is in the center of the field. *Sporothrix schenckii* organisms are small (1–4 μ in diameter) and round to oblong, with a thin, clear halo. They are about the same size as *Histoplasma* organisms. They can be differentiated by identifying the fusiform or oblong (cigar) shape that some, but not all, of the organisms have. Wright's stain, original magnification 250×.

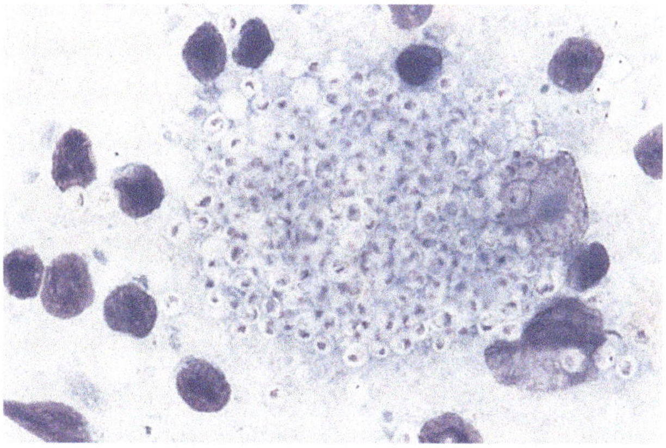

Figure 12.19 A large macrophage containing numerous *Histoplasma* organisms is shown. *Histoplasma* organisms are small (1–4 μ in diameter), round to oval, yeast-like organisms. They have a dark blue/purple-staining nucleus surrounded by a thin, clear halo. Wright's stain, original magnification 250×.

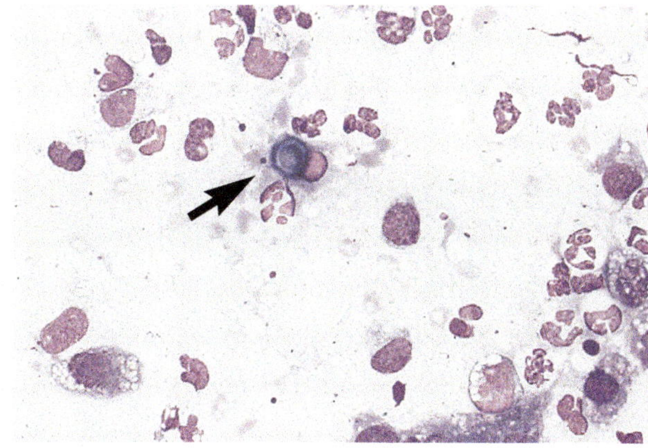

Figure 12.20 Pyogranulomatous inflammation. A *Blastomyces dermatitidis* organism (*arrow*) is in the center of the field. Neutrophils, macrophages, and an inflammatory giant cell are present. Wright's stain, original magnification 250×.

are blue, spherical, 8–20 μ in diameter, and thick walled. Budding is occasionally seen and is broad based (Figures 12.20–12.23). Inflammation is primarily pyogranulomatous with few to many organisms. *C. neoformans* organisms are spherical and usually have a thick mucoid capsule; occasionally, poorly encapsulated (rough) forms are found. Poorly encapsulated forms measure 4–8 μ in diameter and capsulated forms are 8–40 μ in diameter. The internal structures stain light pink to blue-purple and may be slightly granular (Figures 12.24–12.26). The capsule usually is clear and homogeneous, but it may stain light to medium pink. Cryptococcal infection usually evokes a minor granulomatous response of epithelioid macrophages and/or inflammatory giant cells. In some cytological preparations, *Cryptococcus* organisms may outnumber inflammatory and tissue cells. Poorly encapsulated forms tend to elicit a greater inflammatory response than heavily encapsulated forms. *C. immitis* organisms are large, 10–100 μ in diameter, contoured, blue to blue-green spheres (Figures 12.27–12.30). Budding is not seen. The spherules are filled with numerous endospores measuring 2–5 μ in diameter, which may be seen in larger organisms, and if the yeast is broken open, endospores may be seen spilling out. Inflammation is primarily neutrophilic with a lesser granulomatous component. *Coccidioides* organisms are often scarce in cytological preparations. The tremendous variation in size, presence of endospores, and pale blue/green tint to the organism differentiate *C. immitis* from nonbudding *B. dermatitidis*.

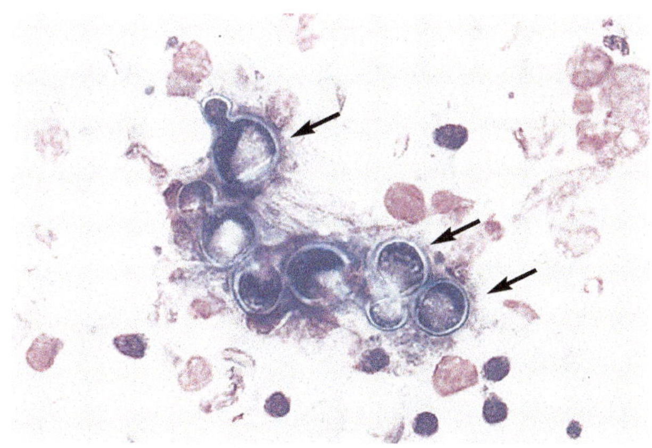

Figure 12.21 *Blastomyces dermatitidis* (*arrows*) is a bluish, spherical, thick-walled, yeast-like organism in Romanowsky-stained smears. The organisms are 8–20 μ in diameter. Occasionally a single broad-based bud may be present. Wright's stain, original magnification 250×.

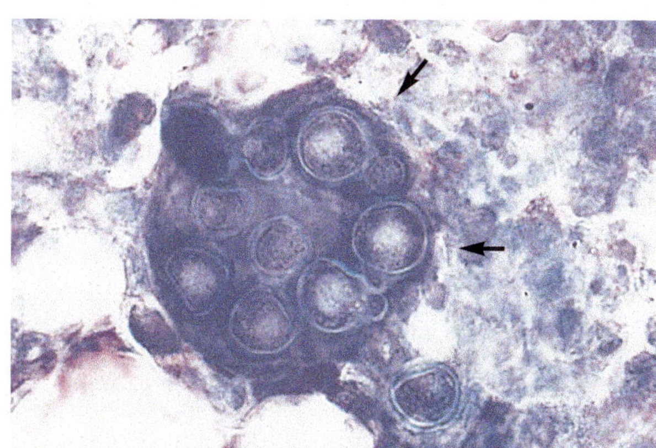

Figure 12.22 *Blastomyces dermatitidis* organisms in a macrophage (*arrows*). Wright's stain, original magnification 250×.

12.6.8 Dermatophytes

The dermatophytes *Trichophyton* spp. and *Microsporum* spp. cause cutaneous lesions that may have a typical ringworm-like appearance or appear as gray to yellow-brown crusty

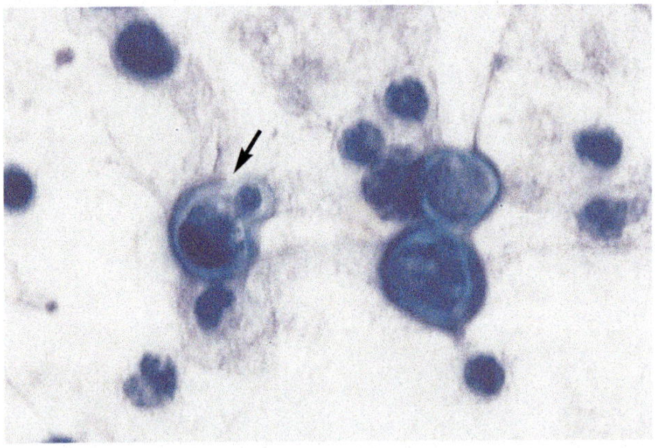

Figure 12.23 A budding *Blastomyces dermatitidis* organism (*arrow*). Wright's stain, original magnification 100×.

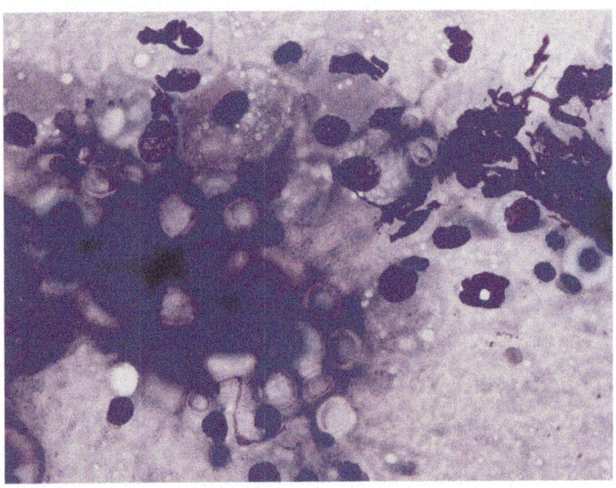

Figure 12.24 Large cluster of several extracellular, round, heavily encapsulated *Cryptococcus* yeast surrounded by few neutrophils and macrophages.

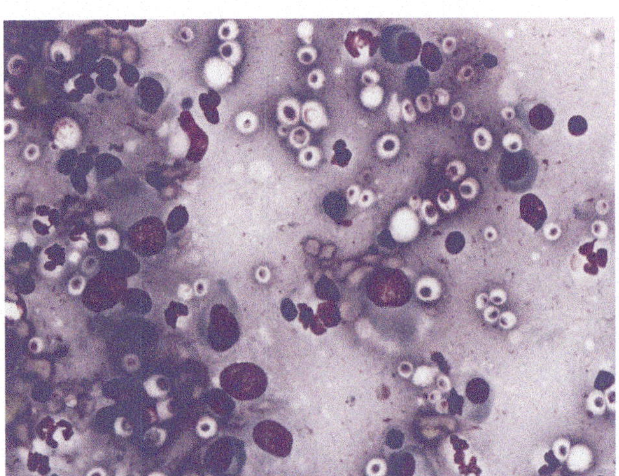

Figure 12.25 Many extracellular *Cryptococcus* yeasts. The large capsule appears clear, with a central round basophilic nucleus.

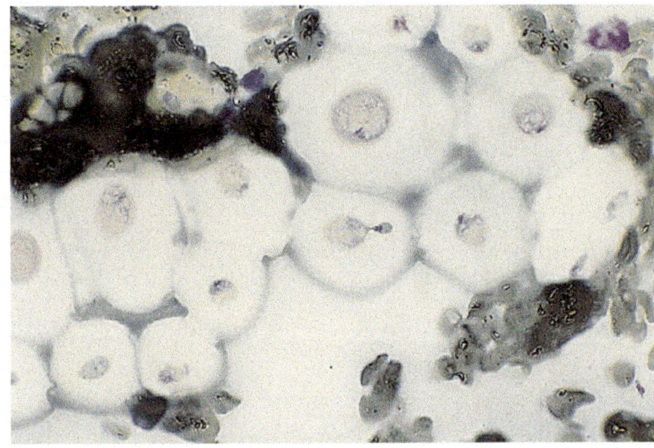

Figure 12.26 *Cryptococcus neoformans* is a spherical, yeast-like organism that frequently has a thick, clear-staining, mucoid capsule. The organism with its capsule ranges in size from 8 to 40 μ. Occasionally a single narrow-based bud may be present. Numerous budding and nonbudding *C. neoformans* organisms with prominent nonstaining capsules are shown. Wright's stain, original magnification 250×.

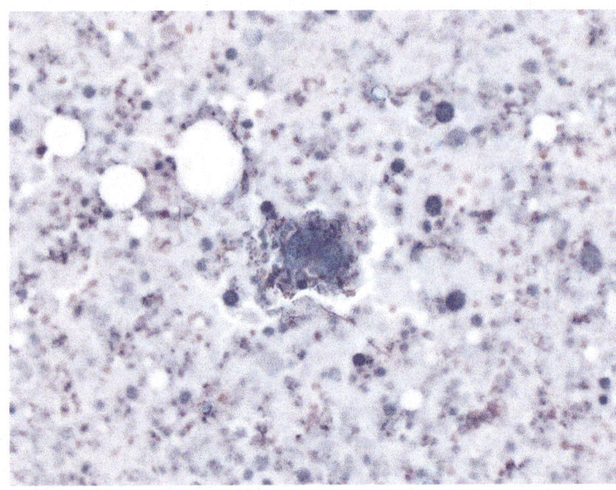

Figure 12.27 In the center of the field is a singular, large, round, basophilic *Coccidioides* yeast which is filled with several small, round, blue endospores. In the background (out of focus to highlight the yeast) are large numbers of neutrophils.

lesions or as follicular papules. Scrapings from the edge of the lesion are most rewarding when searching for dermatophytes. Dermatophytes can be identified in cytological preparations using the standard 20% potassium hydroxide in wet mount preparations stained with new methylene blue, or in air-dried preparations stained with Romanowsky-type stains. Cytologically, very small, spherical conidia are found free within the smears as well as within hair shafts (endothrix invasion) or on the hair shaft surface (ectothrix invasion). With Romanowsky-type stains, conidia stain medium to dark blue with a thin clear halo (Figure 12.31). An inflammatory reaction composed of an admixture of neutrophils, macrophages, lymphocytes, eosinophils, and plasma cells

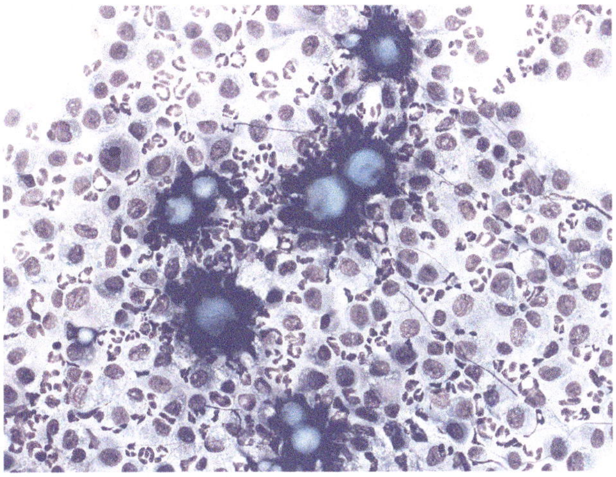

Figure 12.28 Many large, round, blue *Coccidioides* yeast are in the extracellular space and surrounded by neutrophils and macrophages.

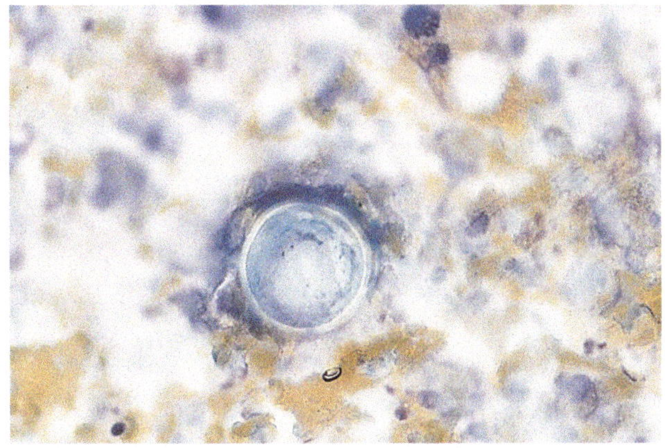

Figure 12.30 *Coccidioides immitis* organisms are large, double-contoured, blue-staining spherical yeasts (10–100 μ in diameter). Occasionally, endospores varying from 2 to 5 μ in diameter may be seen within some of the larger spherules. Wright's stain, original magnification 125×.

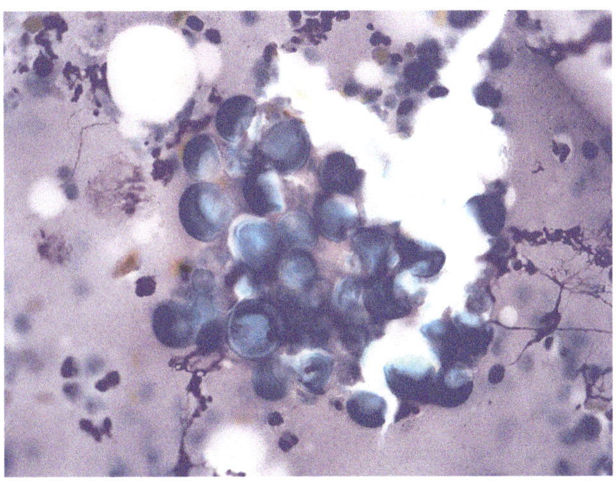

Figure 12.29 Large cluster of *Coccidioides* yeast. Note the thin but defined capsule. Some of the organisms are folded or crinkled.

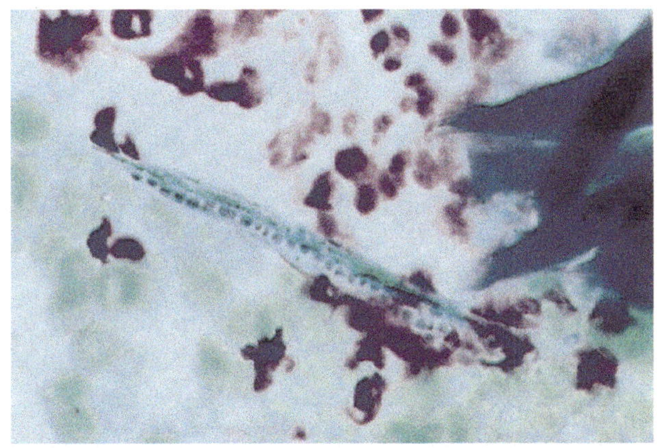

Figure 12.31 Scraping from animal with ringworm. Several degenerate neutrophils are present, along with red blood cells and a row of dermatophyte organisms attached to a hair shaft. Wright's stain, original magnification 330×.

may be seen in cytological preparations from skin scrapings. Fungal culture of hair and crusts can also be helpful to diagnose dermatophytosis.

12.6.9 Fungi That Form Hyphae in Cutaneous and Subcutaneous Tissues

Many fungi can infect and form hyphae in cutaneous and subcutaneous tissues. They may cause single or multiple, small to very large lesions that range from nodules to ulcers to draining tracts. These fungi induce a granulomatous inflammatory response characterized by epithelioid macrophages and inflammatory giant cells. Neutrophil, lymphocyte, plasma cell, and eosinophil numbers are variable. Pheohyphomycosis refers to infections by pigmented fungi. Whilst most fungi stain well with Romanowsky-type stains (Figure 12.32), some do not and are recognized as negative images (Figure 12.33). Fungal culture or histopathological examination with special immunohistochemical stains may be used to definitively classify the fungus.

12.6.10 Leishmania

Leishmania spp. are protozoans which can infect skin and subcutaneous tissues of horses, involving any part of the body but often the head, neck, and ears. Lesions range from small to very large, are thickened, nodular, crusty, and may be ulcerated or nonulcerated. Imprints, scrapings, and aspirates yield a variable inflammatory mixture of neutrophils, macrophages, lymphocytes, and plasma cells. Usually, numerous, small (2–4 μ), round to oval amastigotes with

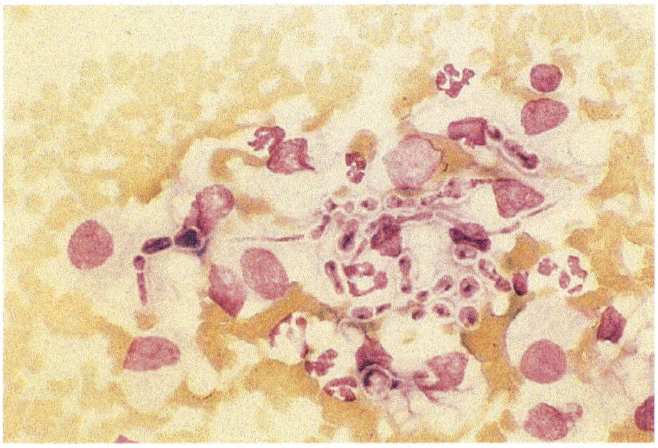

Figure 12.32 Numerous fungal hyphae are present. Many macrophages and neutrophils indicate a pyogranulomatous response. Wright's stain, original magnification 250×.

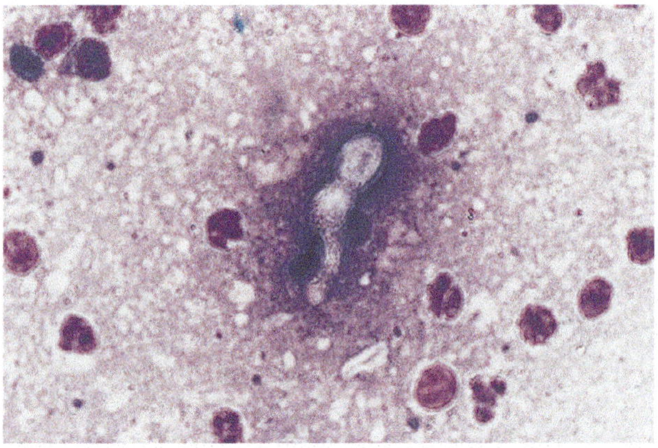

Figure 12.33 The negative image of a nonstaining fungal hyphae can be seen in the background. Some fungi do not stain with routine Romanowsky stains. Wright's stain, original magnification 250×.

light blue cytoplasm, a red oval eccentric nucleus, and a small dark (red-purple) kinetoplast at right angles to the nucleus are found within macrophages and free in the preparation [2] (Figures 12.34 and 12.35).

12.7 Noninfectious Inflammatory Lesions

Inflammatory lesions not caused by infectious agents include immune-mediated diseases, allergic and hypersensitivity reactions, and sterile foreign body reactions. Cytological evaluation along with clinical evaluation may be helpful in diagnosing noninfectious inflammatory lesions.

12.7.1 Allergic/Hypersensitivity Inflammatory Reactions

Allergic or hypersensitivity reactions in horses can have many different etiologies and presentations. Hypersensitivity reactions may be due to exposure to allergens from food,

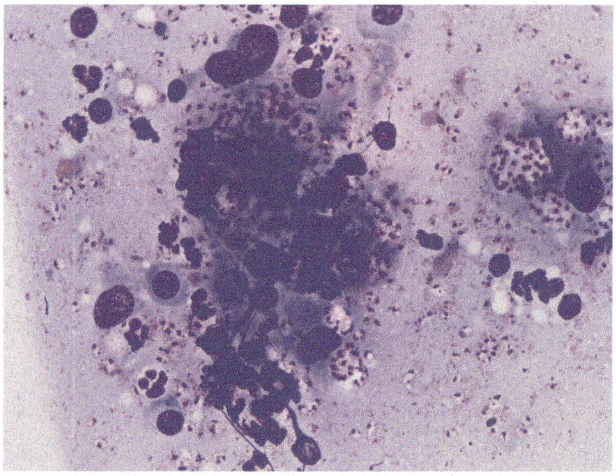

Figure 12.34 Many extracellular and phagocytosed (within macrophages) *Leishmania* organisms are present.

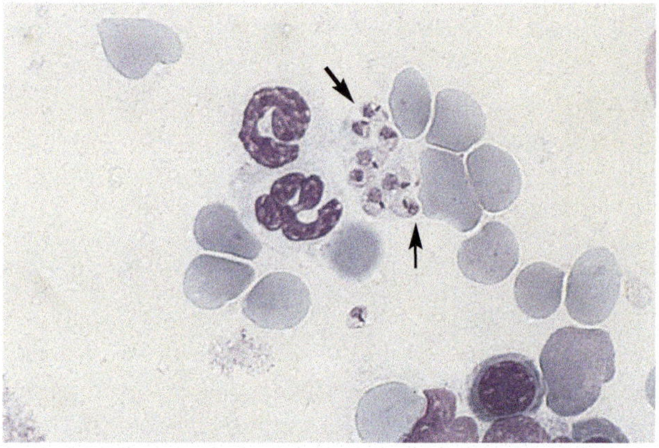

Figure 12.35 Numerous *Leishmania donovani* organisms (*arrows*). *Leishmania donovani* organisms are small and round to oval. They have clear to very light blue cytoplasm, an oval nucleus, and a small, dark, ventral kinetoplast. Wright's stain, original magnification 330×.

inhalation, insect hypersensitivity, contact allergens, drug reactions or atopy. The clinical manifestation of these reactions results in many different gross presentations including formation of hives, nodules, wheals, and papules, which can progress to alopecia, crusting, and hypopigmentation (e.g., secondary to chronic irritation associated with insect bite hypersensitivity). Urticaria and angioedema are also common manifestations of hypersensitivity in horses.

Lesions secondary to allergic or hypersensitivity disease typically contain a predominance of eosinophils, particularly in type I hypersensitivity reactions such as those associated with contact allergens or arthropod bites, largely mediated through release of cytokines such as interleukin (IL)-5 [3, 4]. Mast cells and basophils are variably present, and may predominate in type III hypersensitivity reactions that most commonly manifest with urticaria and angioedema. Neutrophils may be present, especially in ulcerated or crusted lesions. Additionally, macrophages, lymphocytes, and plasma cells may be present in lesser numbers in chronic lesions. A predominance of eosinophils may be seen in other lesions and correlation with other clinical findings and diagnostic tests is imperative.

12.7.2 Eosinophilic Granuloma with Collagen Degeneration

This condition, also termed nodular necrobiosis, nodular collagenolytic granuloma, collagenolytic granuloma, eosinophilic granuloma, or acute collagen necrosis, is the most common cause of nonneoplastic nodular disease in horses. Many cases of eosinophilic granuloma are considered to represent a form of hypersensitivity reaction, such as that secondary to arthropod bites or injection reactions [5]. Atopic dermatitis has also been proposed as a possible pathogenesis. Lesions are characterized by single or multiple nodules that are generally well circumscribed and firm. Predilection sites include the neck, withers, and girth. Lesions typically occur in warmer months, and males are more frequently affected [6]. Nodules are firm, ranging in size from 1 to 10 cm in diameter. They do not typically present with alopecia, ulceration, or pigmentation but some lesions may ulcerate or become cystic.

Collagen degeneration elicits an inflammatory response characterized by marked infiltration of eosinophils and monocytes, with development of epithelioid macrophages and inflammatory giant cells. As a result, cytological preparations from areas of collagen degeneration contain numerous eosinophils and variable numbers of macrophages, epithelioid macrophages, and inflammatory giant cells. Eosinophilic, amorphous debris representing necrosis may be found. Lymphocytes and plasma cells are scarce and no microorganisms are seen. Mineralized debris secondary to dystrophic mineralization may be present in chronic lesions.

History, clinical presentation, and cytological findings are highly suggestive for eosinophilic granulomas although histopathology is required for definitive diagnosis. These lesions are characterized histologically by a granulomatous reaction and flame figures comprising infiltrates of eosinophils and eosinophil granules around collagen bundles [7].

12.7.3 Multisystemic Eosinophilic Epitheliotropic Disease (MEED)

This is an uncommon, idiopathic disease in equids in which eosinophils infiltrate various tissues such as the skin, gastrointestinal tract, liver, and bile ducts, lymph nodes, pancreas and pancreatic duct, kidney, and respiratory tract. A peripheral eosinophilia may or may not be present. Most cases of MEED include skin lesions, which are pruritic and characterized by a generalized exfoliative dermatitis seen as raised papules and nodules which may be ulcerated. The inflammatory infiltrate consists of eosinophils, lymphocytes, and plasma cells [8, 9].

12.7.4 Parasite-Induced Inflammatory Reactions

Parasite-induced inflammatory reactions are characterized by numerous eosinophils and few to many neutrophils. Macrophages may be present in large numbers as well. Variable numbers of lymphocytes and plasma cells may be present; occasionally, the parasitic organism is found. Habronemiasis, also known as "summer sores," results from larvae of *Habronema majus*, *H. muscae*, or *Draschia megastoma*. Flies frequently deposit these larvae in wounds or areas with increased moisture and predisposed areas include the eyes, penile sheath, and distal extremities [10]. Lesions secondary to habronemiasis present as chronic, exuding, nonhealing nodules and wounds. Grossly, material aspirated ranges from brown to yellow with gritty, calcified material. Microscopically, many inflammatory cells are seen, ranging from a predominance of macrophages, with multinucleated cells, to a predominance of eosinophils. Occasionally, parasitic organisms may be seen. *Onchocerca* spp. (especially *O. cervicalis*) cause a seasonal dermatitis, seen in summer months. Microfilaria in the skin cause lesions such as alopecia, swellings, nodules, and papules that may be exudative and calcified. They are associated with chronic eosinophilic dermatitis.

12.7.5 Immune-Mediated Skin Lesions

Pemphigus foliaceus is the most common immune-mediated skin disease in horses [11, 12]. The disease results from autoantibody production against cell adhesion proteins, particularly desmoglein 1 (DSG1), of stratified squamous epithelium, inciting acantholysis. Grossly, pemphigus lesions typically appear as alopecic crusts, erosions, and pustules. Lesions often affect the face and limbs initially prior to spread. Cytological samples from immune-mediated lesions typically contain a large population of nondegenerative neutrophils. Whilst these lesions are sterile, ulceration with secondary infection may be present.

The presence of acantholytic squamous epithelial cells should raise suspicion for immune-mediated disease, especially pemphigus foliaceus. Acantholytic squamous epithelial cells are large, ovoid, and not keratinized. They have deep blue cytoplasm and round, centrally located nuclei with stippled chromatin. They are often scattered individually (due to loss of cohesion) amongst the inflammatory cells.

A few lymphocytes and plasma cells may be present. Acantholytic squamous epithelial cells are highly suggestive of pemphigus foliaceus but they are not pathognomonic for this disease, and can be seen in chronic inflammatory lesions and secondary to infectious disease such as *Trichophyton equinum* [13]. As such, histopathological examination and special stains (e.g., for fungi, and immunohistochemical stains) are recommended for diagnosis.

12.7.6 Traumatic Skin Lesions

Traumatic skin lesions may be caused by physical, thermal, or chemical injury. Cytological preparations from these lesions usually contain numerous neutrophils and may contain abundant necrotic material and/or bacteria from secondary infection. History and physical examination usually help establish the suspicion of either physical, thermal, or chemical injury.

12.7.7 Sterile Foreign Body-Induced Inflammation

Cytological preparations from inflammatory lesions induced by sterile foreign bodies usually contain an admixture of neutrophils and macrophages. Many of the macrophages in foreign body reactions may be epithelioid (seen in sheets/tight aggregates) and multinucleated giant macrophages (also known as foreign body macrophages) are frequently present. Occasionally, eosinophils are present, especially if there is a concurrent allergic response to the foreign body. Mature lymphocytes and plasma cells may occur in variable numbers as well (Figure 12.36). Sometimes, refractile material can be found phagocytized within macrophages and in the extracellular space. When a sterile foreign body is suspected, the smear can be viewed under polarized light. Some foreign material refracts polarized light, whereas endogenous breakdown products, such as hemosiderin, that might be mistaken as particulate foreign body material, do not refract polarized light.

12.7.8 Injection Site Reactions

Vaccinations or other injections can result in foreign body reactions, and often have a delayed onset due to a delayed immune response. Cytologically, there is a mixed population of inflammatory cells, with neutrophils often predominating in the early phase and a mixture of lymphocytes, plasma cells and macrophages in the later stages. A characteristic finding in some vaccine reactions is bright purple/eosinophilic globular material (vaccine adjuvant) phagocytosed by macrophages and/or seen in the background of the slides. The absence of this material does not preclude a vaccine reaction, but is helpful when present to increase suspicion for this etiology (Figure 12.37).

12.7.9 Fat Necrosis/Steatitis/Panniculitis

Necrosis and inflammation of adipose tissue (steatitis/panniculitis) rarely occur in horses. It may present as single or multiple nodules that may wax and wane and/or plaque-like lesions. Panniculitis may be due to sterile inflammatory disease such as sterile nodular panniculitis [14]. Less commonly, panniculitis may be seen secondary to nutri-

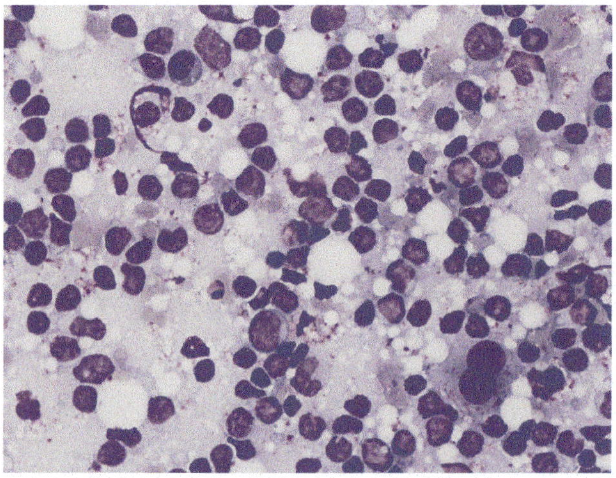

Figure 12.36 Vaccination reaction. Large numbers of mononuclear inflammatory cells are present, with extracellular and phagocytosed (within binucleate macrophage at bottom right corner) stippled pink to magenta staining material suggestive of adjuvant. Most of the inflammatory cells are mature lymphocytes, with a few plasma cells and macrophages. Droplets of clear lipid are also present with minimal hemodilution.

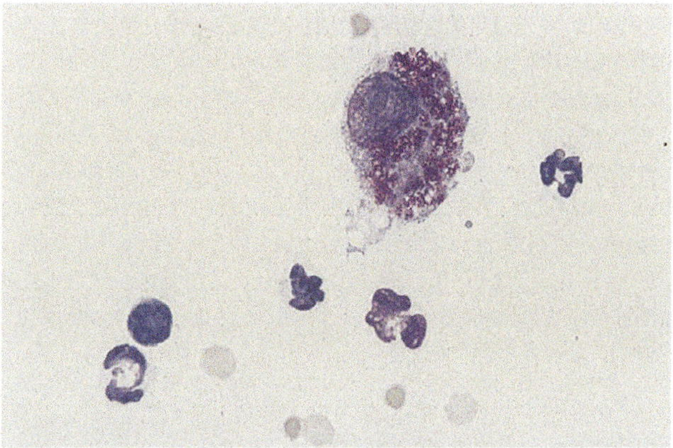

Figure 12.37 Aspirate from an injection site reaction in a gelding. Large macrophage contains bright eosinophilic noncellular material typical of adjuvant. Scattered neutrophils are also present. Wright's stain, original magnification 125×.

tional deficiencies (nutritional panniculitis or "yellow fat disease") or secondary to peripancreatitis [15, 16]. Cellulitis most commonly affects the limbs [17, 18]. Cytological preparations from areas of fat necrosis/steatitis/panniculitis usually contain variable numbers of inflammatory cells intermixed with numerous lipid droplets and often with aggregates of adipocytes (Figure 12.38). The inflammatory cells are predominantly macrophages and a few to many large, multinucleated, inflammatory giant cells may be observed (Figure 12.39). Reactive spindle cells may be present. Often, the spindle cells are dysplastic, with pleomorphic features, and caution is warranted to avoid misclassification as neoplasia. Lymphocytes and plasma cells are common in chronic lesions. There may also be aggregates of mineralized debris if there is dystrophic mineralization.

Note that cellulitis may be due to infectious disease, including *Staphylococcus* spp., *Streptococcus* spp., *Rhodococcus equi*, and *Corynebacterium pseudotuberculosis* [17–20]. Thus, careful microscopic evaluation is recommended to identify bacteria with culture.

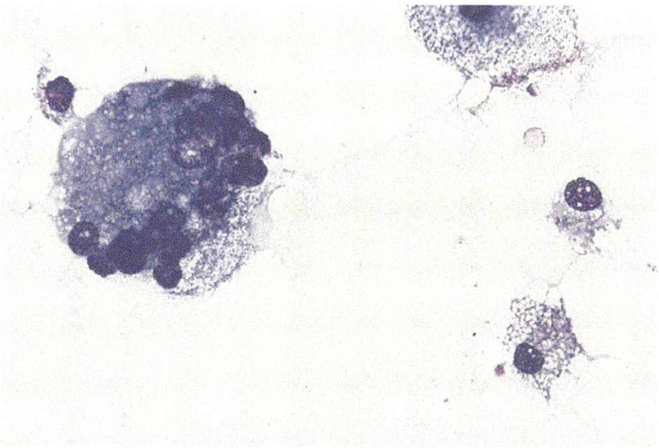

Figure 12.39 Cytological preparation from area of fat necrosis. Large multinucleated inflammatory giant cell and scattered macrophages. Wright's stain, original magnification 125×.

12.7.10 Granulation Tissue

Granulation tissue forms in healing wounds, and is composed of proliferating fibroblasts and vessel formation (neovascularization). Excessive formation of granulation tissue in wounds, especially those on the distal limbs, is referred to as "proud flesh." Because granulation tissue contains proliferating fibroblasts, these cells frequently appear dysplastic and may contain numerous criteria of malignancy, especially anisocytosis and anisokaryosis. It is therefore difficult to differentiate these cells from neoplastic processes such as a fibrosarcoma or other mesenchymal tumors, and histopathology may be required for appreciation of tissue architecture for characterization of the biological behavior of the cells.

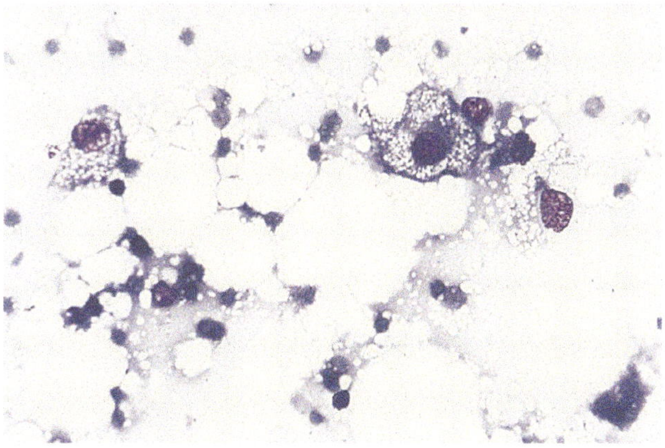

Figure 12.38 Cytological preparation from area of fat necrosis. Numerous macrophages interspersed amongst fat droplets. Macrophages contain many fine clear cytoplasmic vacuoles. Wright's stain, original magnification 50×.

12.7.11 Insect Bites

Cytological preparations from wheals caused by acute allergic reactions, such as bee stings, usually contain only a few local tissue cells and a few neutrophils and/or eosinophils. Older bumps caused by insect bites may contain a few neutrophils, eosinophils, macrophages, lymphocytes, and plasma cells, along with a few local tissue cells. Rarely, moderate to high numbers of basophils may be present due to cutaneous basophil hypersensitivity (Jones–Mote reaction).

12.7.12 Snake Bites

The muzzle, head, and legs are sites most commonly bitten by snakes. Cytological preparations from recent snake bites tend to be of low cellularity. The cells present are local tissue cells and a few neutrophils. However, neutrophil infiltration of the bitten area is very rapid. Within a few hours of a bite, neutrophil numbers begin to increase markedly. Within a couple of days, lesions contain necrotic debris, numerous neutrophils, and variable numbers of macrophages.

12.8 Round Cell Tumors

Round cell tumors are characterized by discrete cells, which are usually found individually and not in cohesive sheets; however, in highly cellular samples, the neoplastic cells may be pushed into aggregates that can mimic epithelial tumors. The most common equine round cell tumors of the skin are lymphoma and mast cell tumors.

12.8.1 Lymphoma

Lymphoma is the most common malignant neoplasm in the horse. Cutaneous manifestation of lymphoma has been reported in up to 19% cases of equine lymphoma [21]; however, in comparison to other equine skin tumors, cutaneous lymphoma only accounts for 1.7–3% of reported cases [22–24].

T-cell rich, large B-cell lymphoma (TBL) is the most common subtype of equine cutaneous lymphoma followed by epitheliotropic cutaneous T-cell lymphoma (CTL) [21, 24, 25]. Quarter horses most frequently develop TBL whilst CTL is common in Thoroughbreds. Horses with TBL typically develop multiple, widespread masses, with the head, neck, trunk, proximal extremities, and eyelids most commonly affected [24, 25]. TBL tumors also tend to be larger than CTL tumors. CTL tumors are more likely to arise as solitary masses but may also manifest as generalized, exfoliative dermatitis with or without pruritus [24, 25]. Waxing and waning of the skin masses have been described in mares, possibly due to fluctuation in progesterone [26]. Weight loss, anorexia, depression, ventral edema with/without hypoproteinemia, pyrexia, anemia, diarrhea, and colic are the most common signs of systemic manifestation of lymphoma in horses [21, 24]. Reported survival times of horses with cutaneous lymphoma vary between weeks and years but overall, the long-term prognosis appears to be poor [24]. Horses with TBL appear to have a higher survival rate and surgical excision without recurrence may be an effective treatment modality in over 50% of reported cases [25].

Cytology samples from cutaneous lymphoma frequently are highly cellular. The samples may have a variable background of blood, and may contain cytoplasmic fragments from lysis of fragile lymphocytes. The neoplastic lymphocytes are discrete and seen individually, but may be pushed into crowded sheets. The cells typically have large nuclei, approximately 2–3 red blood cells in diameter, and have finely stippled chromatin with prominent nucleoli (Figures 12.40 and 12.41). The cells mostly have a small volume of pale blue cytoplasm that may encircle the cell or wrap halfway around the cell. The cells are uniform (consistent with a monoclonal expansion of neoplastic cells) with minimal anisocytosis/anisokaryosis. Samples from TBL can be more difficult to diagnose on cytology due to the heavy infiltrate of small mature lymphocytes that can mimic inflammatory lesions.

Histopathology is required to distinguish between epitheliotropic and nonepitheliotropic cutaneous lymphoma.

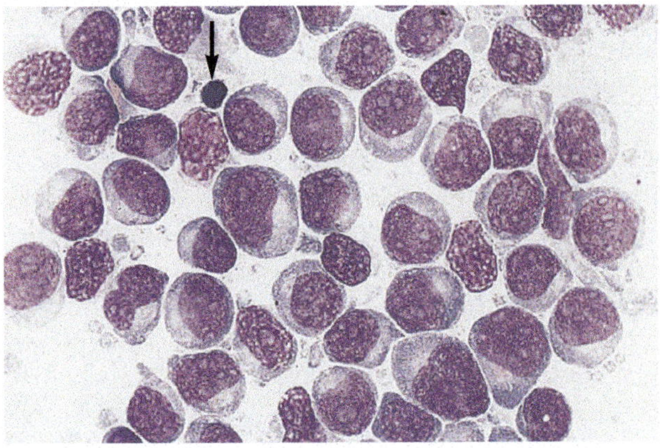

Figure 12.40 Cutaneous lymphosarcoma. Note large numbers of lymphoblasts. A single small lymphocyte (*arrow*) is also present. Wright's stain, original magnification 250×. *Source:* Courtesy of Oklahoma State University.

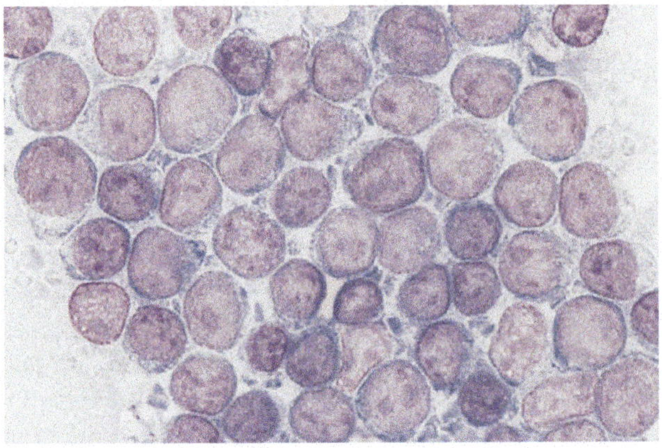

Figure 12.41 Lymphoblasts, characterized by a small amount of blue cytoplasm, eccentric round nucleus containing finely stippled chromatin and a visible nucleolus. Wright's stain, original magnification 250×.

TBL histopathology is consistent with sheets of large round cells with a small amount of basophilic cytoplasm as well as many small, mature lymphocytes with nuclei approximately the size of red blood cells. The nuclei of the large lymphocytes are round to oval and 2–3 times the diameter of a red blood cell. CTL exhibits epitheliotropism with nests of cells within the epidermis or the basal layers of the epidermis. Neoplastic round cells have scant cytoplasm, nuclei are approximately 1.5–2.5 times the diameter of a red blood cell, are highly and pleomorphic and contain up to 2–5 prominent basophilic nucleoli. Mitoses are abundant [21, 25].

12.8.2 Mast Cell Neoplasia

Mast cell tumors in horses are uncommon and often benign; however, more aggressive behavior has also been reported [27–29]. These tumors account for 2–6.9% of cutaneous neoplasms in the horse [22–24]. Cutaneous mast cell tumors are usually solitary and firm but can also be fluctuant, with or without caseous discharge. The overlying skin may be normal, alopecic, or ulcerated and is typically nonpruritic [24]. Tumors often involve the head, neck, trunk, and limbs with the head being most commonly affected [23, 24, 29, 30]. There appears to be a wide age spread with a breed predilection towards Arabian horses, and male horses seem to be overrepresented [29, 30]. Limb lesions are often found in proximity to joints, are firm and nonmovable and may cause lameness [24, 29]. More aggressive tumor behavior reported includes sentinel lymph node metastasis and eosinophilia [29], draining tracts on multiple limbs [28], and metastasis to the thoracic and abdominal cavity [31]. Regardless, the prognosis for mast cell tumors in horses is generally good, with surgical excision typically curative and many lesions may resolve spontaneously [24].

Mast cell tumors mostly are highly exfoliative. The background of samples often contains many extracellular mast cell granules due to rupture of mast cells during collection or smear preparation. The samples contain discrete cells seen individually, with a moderate to abundant amount of pale cytoplasm that frequently contains metachromatic granules. Nuclear details may be obscured by large numbers of granules. When visible, nuclei are round and centrally located and have reticulated chromatin with small basophilic nucleoli (Figures 12.42–12.44). Some mast cell tumors (especially poorly differentiated neoplasms) may contain cells with faint granulation or agranular cells; however, the majority of equine mast cells tumors are well differentiated [30] or moderately differentiated [27]. It is important to note that Diff-Quik® stain may sometimes fail to stain mast cell granules appropriately, making visualization difficult.

12.8.3 Histiocytic Sarcoma

Histiocytic sarcoma is a rare neoplasm of the skin, arising from histiocytes of dendritic origin. In one horse, the disease manifested with multiple subcutaneous tumors and wide metastatic disease involving skeletal muscle, mediastinal lymph nodes, bladder, and pericardium [32].

Histiocytic sarcoma exfoliates well for cytology, and comprises a population of large discrete round cells. These cells have a variable volume of cytoplasm that may contain clear punctate vacuoles. Nuclei are ovoid to ameboid and have finely stippled chromatin with multiple prominent, basophilic nucleoli. Multinucleation is a characteristic finding in histiocytic sarcoma, and many mitotic figures typically are seen. Anisocytosis/anisokaryosis are marked, and nuclear:cytoplasmic (N:C) ratios are variable.

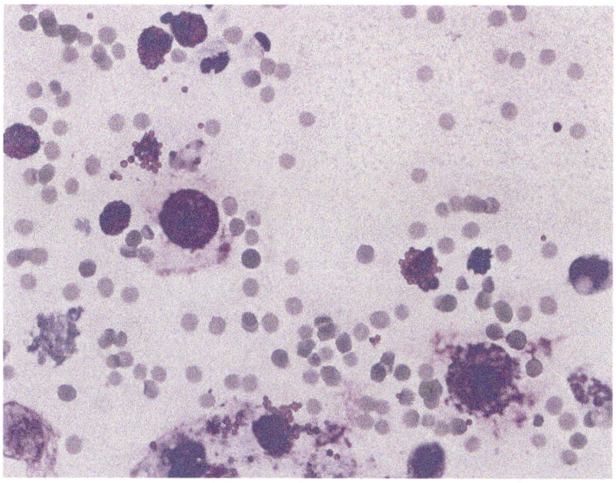

Figure 12.42 Left of center is a round mast cell filled with metachromatic (purple) granules. There are a few eosinophils also present.

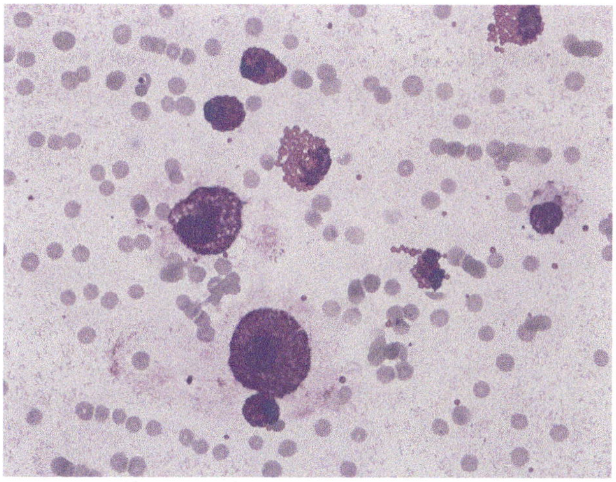

Figure 12.43 Two large mast cells and several eosinophils.

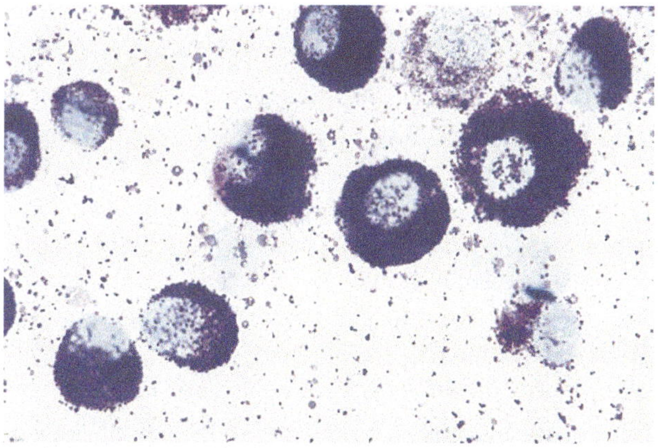

Figure 12.44 Mast cells are recognized by their round to oval nucleus and numerous red-purple intracytoplasmic granules. Wright's stain, original magnification 100×. *Source:* Courtesy of Oklahoma State University.

12.9 Epithelial Tumors

Epithelial cells tend to adhere to each other in cytological samples and often appear in cellular sheets with prominent intercellular boundaries. Normal epithelial cells vary in size from small to large depending on the type and maturation. Cell shapes may be round, polygonal, columnar or caudate. Acinar or ductal arrangements may be identified with adenomas or adenocarcinomas. In neoplastic lesions, epithelial cells have variable degrees of pleomorphism; however, it is important to note that epithelial cells can undergo hyperplasia or dysplasia secondary to inflammation that may mimic neoplasia and histopathology may be necessary for further characterization of biological behavior.

12.9.1 Papilloma

Papillomas are common, benign squamous epithelial tumors induced by equine papillomavirus, accounting for ~4.3–10.5% of equine cutaneous tumors [22–24]. Papillomavirus-induced clinical disease in horses may present as one of three clinical disorders: classic equine papillomatosis (warts), genital papillomatosis, or aural papillomatosis/plaques. There appears to be no breed or sex predilection. Lesions typically appear as single, multiple, or coalescing sessile, papillomatous to pedunculated, gray to white masses with a hyperkeratotic surface and frond-like projections [24, 33].

Classic equine papillomatosis is a contagious disease caused by *E. caballus* papillomavirus type 1 (EcPV-1). This form typically affects horses <3 years old. Transmission occurs via direct contact or contaminated fomites on injured skin. Sites most commonly affected include the muzzle and lips and less commonly external genitalia and distal legs. Lesions usually spontaneously resolve within 3–4 months unless the animal is immunosuppressed. No treatment is usually required [24, 33].

Aural papillomatosis/plaques can affect horses of any age and EcPV-3, EcPV-4, EcPV-5, and EcPV-6 have been isolated from lesions [33]. Lesions often affect the concave aspect of the pinna but may also cover the entire surface of the pinna. Affected animals usually are asymptomatic but head hypersensitivity has been reported. This type of papillomatous disease usually does not resolve spontaneously, though treatment may not be required as animals are usually asymptomatic.

Genital papillomatosis has been associated with infection with EcPV-2 and EcPV-7, and affected horses are often older. Lesions are most commonly seen on the tip of the penis or glans penis in male horses as well as the vulvar lips, the clitoris or vestibular walls in mares. These lesions typically do not resolve spontaneously and there is increasing evidence that some genital papillomas may evolve into squamous cell carcinoma [33, 34]. Recently, generalized papillomatosis associated with a novel EcPV-8 has been described [35].

Equine papillomatosis is visually distinct and further diagnostic work is rarely pursued for the classic equine papillomatous and aural forms. Due to the tendency of some genital papillomas to evolve into squamous cell carcinoma, caution should be exercised and more diagnostics undertaken. Cytological samples of papillomas are often composed of mature squamous epithelial cells. However, some cells may be large, ovoid to fusiform with abundant cytoplasm, which may be stippled, pink to purple or vacuolated in appearance. The nucleus is often eccentrically placed with coarse, reticulated chromatin and a small nucleolus (Figures 12.45 and 12.46).

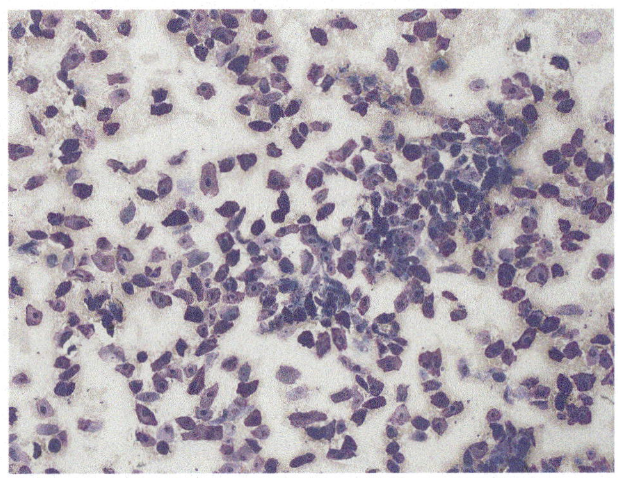

Figure 12.45 Aspirate of a papilloma. Low-power view of large numbers of individualized, angulated koilocytes. Note bright pink cytoplasm.

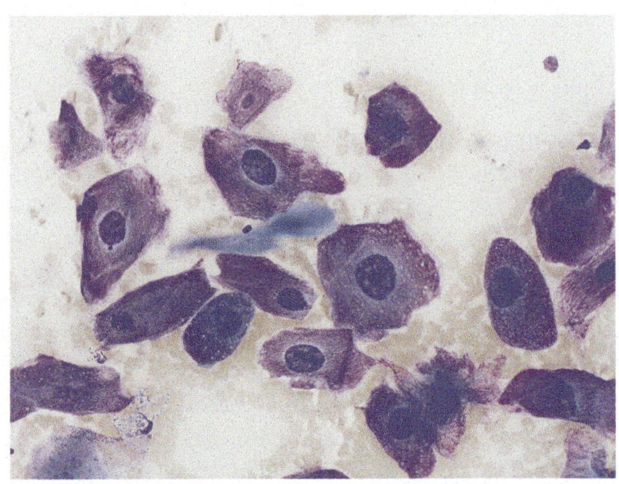

Figure 12.46 Aspirate of a papilloma. Higher power view of koilocytes. There is bright pink cytoplasm and a singular, central ovoid nucleus and mild anisocytosis and anisokaryosis.

12.9.2 Basal Cell Tumors

These are rare, benign cutaneous tumors in horses, accounting for approximately 0.4–5.7% of equine cutaneous neoplasia [22–24]. There appears to be a wide age range and no apparent sex predilection, but ponies and Morgan horses may be predisposed to development of basal cell tumors [22]. Basal cell tumors are usually evenly distributed affecting the head, limbs, trunk, ventrum, tail, and perianal areas [22]; however, a retrospective study found a possible predisposition for the extremities in horses [36]. The masses usually are well circumscribed, freely movable, round, and firm. The overlying skin may be normal, hyperpigmented, alopecic, or ulcerated [24, 36]. Complete surgical excision appears to be curative [36].

Basal cell tumors often exfoliate well for cytology, with numerous cells present in sheets, rows, or ribbons, as well as individually. The cells are cuboidal to round, with centrally located, round nuclei that have stippled to finely clumped chromatin and indistinct nucleoli. They have a small to moderate volume of cytoplasm that stains clear to pale blue (Figures 12.47 and 12.48). Based on findings of a retrospective study, which identified cell differentiation towards follicular structures, occasional sebaceous cells amongst basal cells and arrangement of cells towards outer root sheets, basal cell tumors are possibly of follicular origin in the horse and the cytological diagnosis of trichoblastoma might be more correct [36].

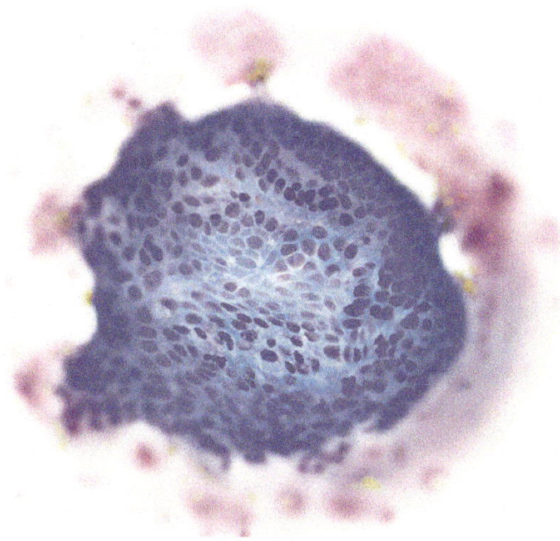

Figure 12.47 Aspirate of a neoplasm of basilar epithelial origin. Note large sheet of compact, uniform basaloid epithelial cells. The top right edge shows rowing of the cells. Observe the scant amount of basophilic cytoplasm and central round nucleus.

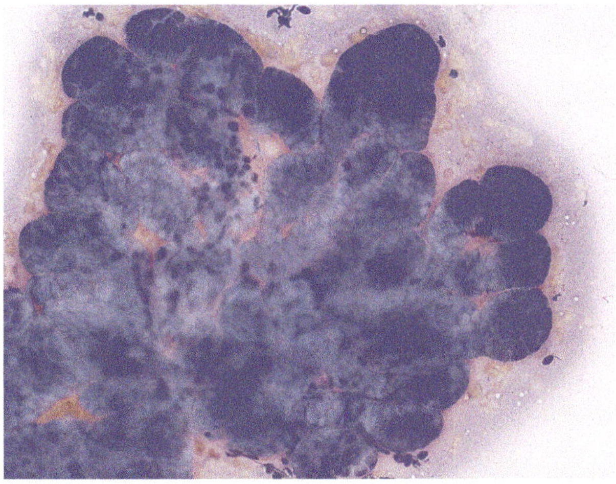

Figure 12.48 Aspirate of a neoplasm of basilar epithelial origin. Large, compact, lobulated sheet of basaloid cells forming ribbons and rows.

12.9.3 Squamous Cell Carcinoma

Squamous cell carcinoma is one of the most frequently diagnosed cutaneous malignancies in horses, reported in 18.9–37% of all reported malignant tumors. There appears to be a higher incidence in geographic regions with higher exposure to UV radiation [22–24].

This type of cancer is characterized by locally destructive lesions most commonly confined to the mucocutaneous junctions on the penis, perianal region, eyelids, or vulva. Lesions are usually solitary, poorly circumscribed masses and have a cauliflower-like or ulcerated appearance [24]. Appaloosas and American paint horses appear to be overrepresented, likely due to the high frequency of white hair and pink skin in these breeds. Affected horses are usually older, with an age range of 12–29 years [22–24]. Chronic exposure to UV radiation appears to be a strong trigger for the development of this tumor; however, squamous cell carcinoma may also arise from chronic, nonhealing wounds, burn scars or other areas of chronic inflammation [24]. Squamous cell carcinomas of the urogenital tract may also be associated with *E. caballus* papillomavirus type 2 (EcPV-2) infection [33, 34]. Squamous cell carcinoma is an aggressive neoplasm and local metastasis to regional lymph nodes has been reported in over 20% of affected horses [24, 36]. The long-term prognosis varies depending on the location and presence of metastasis [24].

Cytological interpretation may be impaired by exuberant local inflammation and superficial bacterial infection, hence deep aspirates may be very helpful for the diagnosis. Neoplastic cells can be found individually, in clusters or in sheets. Individual cells vary in shape from round to polygonal and angular. The cells often have marked criteria of malignancy with marked anisocytosis and anisokaryosis, multinucleation and prominent basophilic nucleoli. Additionally, the cells frequently have nuclear to cytoplasmic dissociation, with keratinization of cells with immature nuclei (Figures 12.49–12.51). It is important to note that squamous cell dysplasia is common in inflammatory lesions, and the marked paraneoplastic inflammatory response that often accompanies squamous cell carcinoma may pose a diagnostic dilemma.

12.9.4 Sebaceous Tumors

Sebaceous gland tumors are rare skin tumors in horses arising from sebocytes. These tumors are grouped into adenomas, epitheliomas, and carcinomas. Sebaceous tumors are single, raised, smooth to lobular or wart-like in appearance. A sebaceous carcinoma with abdominal metastasis and an eyelid sebaceous carcinoma have been reported in horses [37, 38].

Samples from sebaceous tumors usually are highly cellular, and may have keratinized debris in the background. Cells are ovoid, frequently with abundant, clear, foamy cytoplasm. The nucleus is small, with coarse chromatin, and indistinct or inapparent nucleoli that are central or slightly eccentrically located (Figure 12.52). Sebaceous epitheliomas are of similar cytological appearance but are admixed with basal epithelial cells, which are smaller, and have high N:C ratios. Cytological characteristics of sebaceous carcinoma include cohesive sheets of epithelial cells, which display criteria of malignancy with moderate anisocytosis and anisokaryosis. The cytoplasm is clear to medium blue with fine clear vacuoles with a central nuclei, stippled chromatin and prominent nucleoli (Figure 12.53).

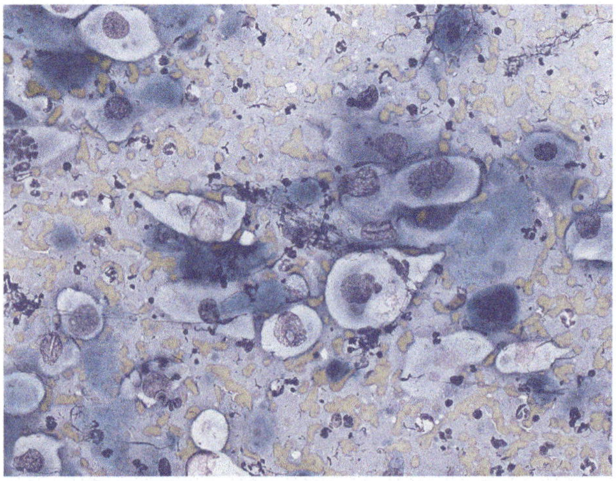

Figure 12.49 Aspirate of a squamous cell carcinoma. Note individualized, very large neoplastic cells, with abundant cytoplasm ranging from pale to medium blue. Note large, prominent nuclei, open chromatin, and occasional large nucleoli.

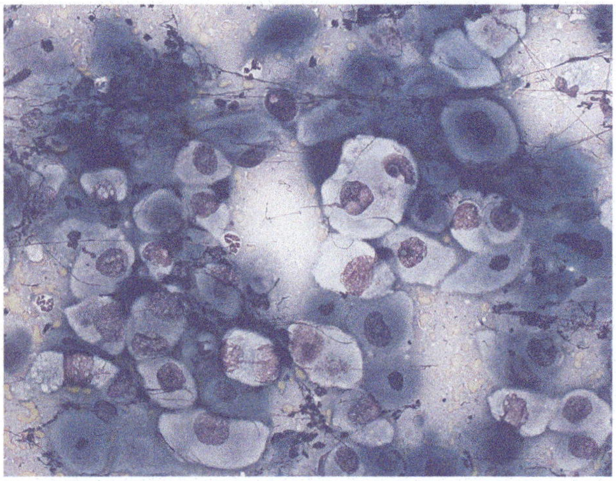

Figure 12.50 Aspirate of a squamous cell carcinoma. Neoplastic squamous cells range from round to ovoid to angular to irregular. Some cells have small pyknotic nuclei, and others have large nuclei. The cells exhibit moderate to marked anisocytosis and anisokaryosis.

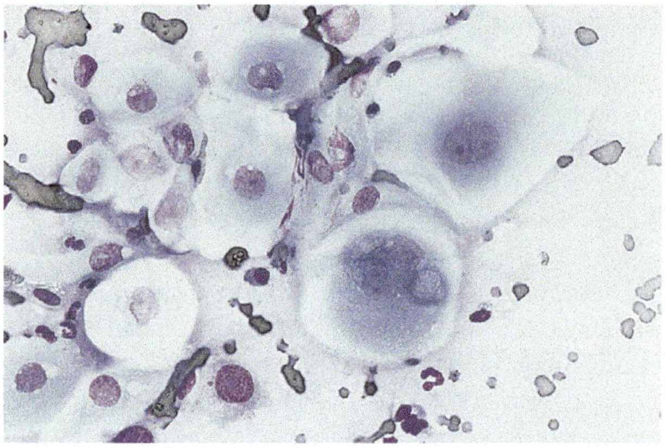

Figure 12.51 Aspirate from a squamous cell carcinoma. Several squamous epithelial cells with nuclear to cytoplasmic asynchrony and visible nucleoli. Wright's stain, original magnification 132×.

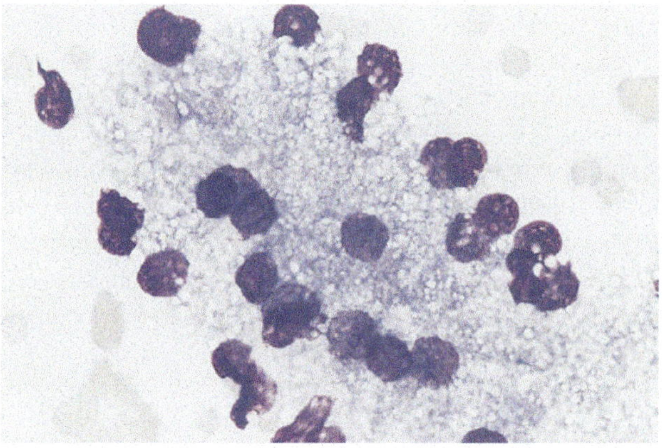

Figure 12.52 Aspirate from a sebaceous adenoma. A cluster or acinus of sebaceous cells is shown. Wright's stain, original magnification 250×.

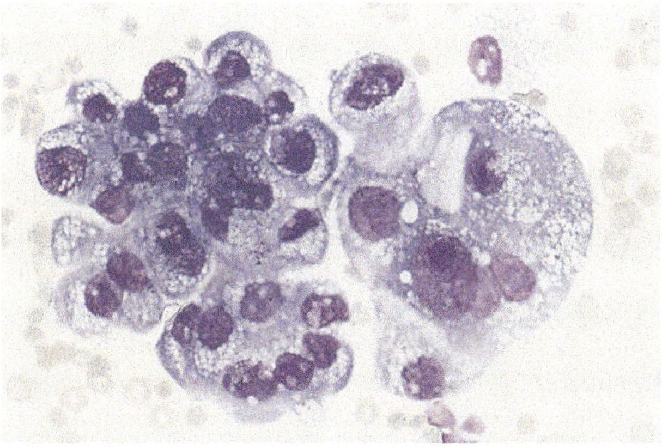

Figure 12.53 A cluster of malignant glandular epithelial cells is shown. Note the acinar arrangement and numerous vacuoles suggesting glandular origin. Also notice the coarse chromatin pattern, anisocytosis, anisokaryosis, and prominent large nucleoli. One of the cells has a nucleolus that is larger than the RBC present. Wright's stain, original magnification 125×.

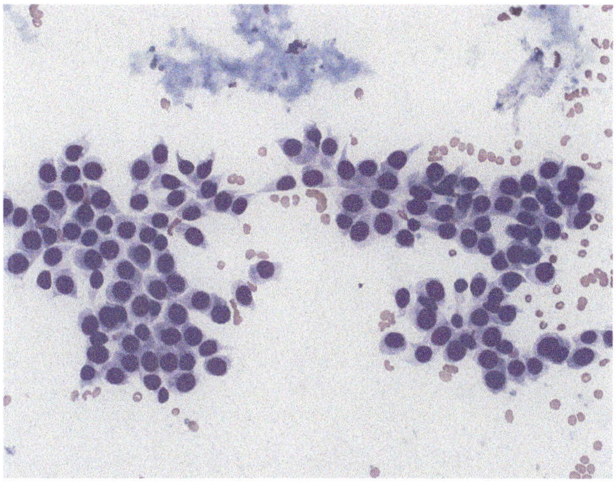

Figure 12.54 Aspirate from an apocrine adenoma. Large cluster of cohesive neoplastic epithelial cells, some with a columnar shape. A small amount of basophilic stippled secretory material is noted in the cytoplasm of some of the cells. Above the sheet of cells is a large clump of basophilic, amorphous, extracellular secretory material.

12.9.5 Sweat Gland Tumors

Epitrichial adenoma or carcinomas are rare cutaneous tumors of the secretory or ductal epithelium of glands. Sweat gland tumors are mostly benign and reported on the pinna and vulva [24]. In a case report, one horse developed recurrent, multiple epitrichial carcinomas on the distal extremities. Despite the tumors, the horse was systemically healthy and no regional metastasis was reported [39]. These tumors are usually described as solitary, firm to cystic, well-circumscribed nodules. The overlying skin may be normal, alopecic, or ulcerated [24].

Cytological preparations usually contain many sheets of cells that may also be noted individually. The cells are round to ovoid with a slightly eccentric nucleus. The cytoplasm is pale and may contain basophilic, globular secretory material (Figure 12.54). Sweat gland adenocarcinomas have moderate to marked criteria of malignancy, with higher N:C ratios, moderate to marked anisocytosis/anisokaryosis and prominent basophilic nucleoli.

12.9.6 Thyroid Tumors

Thyroid adenomas are common incidental necropsy findings in older horses with a prevalence of 75% in horses aged 20 years or older. Thyroid adenomas can arise from the follicular thyroid epithelium or medullary, parafollicular C-cells, and both origins have been described in the horse [40–44]. Thyroid tumors often present as a palpable swelling in the cranial cervical region. Occasionally, horses may be physically impaired by the size of the mass and may have breathing or gulping due to compression of the trachea and/or esophagus [41, 45]. Most equine thyroid tumors are nonfunctional, but a calcitonin-secreting medullary parafollicular C-cell tumor has been described with no apparent clinical signs of increased calcitonin levels such as hypocalcemia and lameness due to osteosclerosis [41]. Distant metastases to the lungs, eye, kidney, and heart were described in a horse with follicular thyroid carcinoma [45].

Thyroid tissue consists of follicles lined with cuboidal to columnar epithelial cells filled with colloid. Thyroid adenoma aspirates are variably cellular and may have excessive blood contamination and nucleated cells may be ruptured with many bare nuclei. Bright pink colloid may be seen in the background. Cells are uniform with a moderate amount of basophilic cytoplasm and a round to oval nuclei with clumped chromatin. Intracytoplasmic blue-black tyrosine granules may be present (Figure 12.55). Thyroid adenocarcinoma may be difficult to distinguish from thyroid adenoma if well differentiated. Smears tend to be highly cellular with excessive blood contamination. Criteria of malignancy with anisocytosis and anisokaryosis vary from subtle to completely lacking in thyroid carcinoma (Figure 12.56). Follicular thyroid carcinomas stain positive for thyroglobulin whilst parafollicular C-cell tumor cells stain positive for calcitonin [40–42, 44]. With increasing use of immunohistochemical stains, more parafollicular C-cell tumors have been identified in the horse [40, 41, 44].

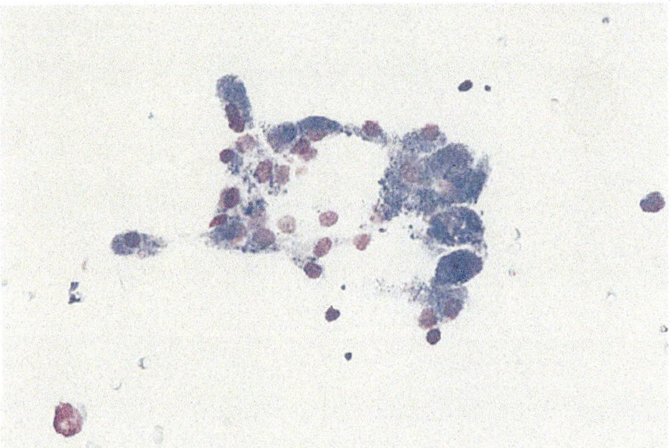

Figure 12.55 Aspirate from thyroid gland. Note small cluster of thyroid epithelial cells containing numerous blue-black tyrosine cytoplasmic granules. Wright's stain, original magnification 100×. *Source:* Courtesy of Oklahoma State University.

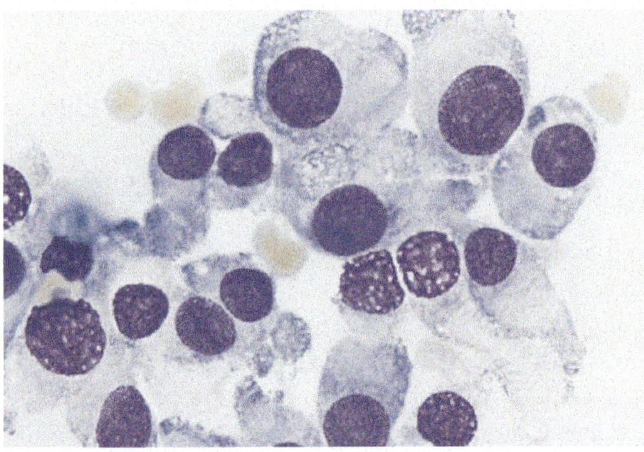

Figure 12.56 Aspirate of thyroid adenocarcinoma from an aged gelding. The neoplastic epithelial cells are less cohesive than those in Figure 12.55 and show moderate anisocytosis, anisokaryosis, and a variable N:C ratio. No tyrosine granules are present. Wright's stain, original magnification 250×.

12.9.7 Mammary Tumors

Mammary neoplasia is uncommon in horses. The majority of the published cases are malignant (solid carcinoma, tubular adenocarcinoma, papillary ductal adenocarcinoma, invasive ductal adenocarcinoma) [46–54]. However, a case of malignant, fibrous histiocytoma of the mammary gland [55] and a case of mammary melanoma [56] have also been described. Benign mammary adenomas are rare [57].

Mares commonly present with unilateral or bilateral swelling of the mammary gland with pain, redness, and often serous to purulent discharge, often resembling mastitis. The overlying skin may be ulcerated or necrotic [58]. Metastasis to regional and distant lymph nodes and tissues are common [48, 49, 53, 56]. The prognosis for mares with mammary tumors is poor as complete surgical excision is often impossible due to invasiveness of the tumor and metastasis is common [58].

Mammary tumors exfoliate variably well for cytological analysis. They may have a variably thick blue background if there is a concurrent cystic component, which is common in such tumors. The tumors may also be accompanied by an infiltrate of inflammatory cells. Nucleated cells are seen in cohesive sheets, and cells vary from cuboidal to ovoid, with a variable volume of pale to medium blue cytoplasm. Nuclei are round to ovoid with stippled chromatin and variably prominent nucleoli. Malignant tumors may have marked criteria of malignancy but well-differentiated carcinomas may be cytologically bland, and histopathology is recommended for appreciation of tissue architecture for evaluation of biological behavior.

Immunohistochemistry staining of mammary carcinomas typically is positive for cytokeratin 18, vimentin and alpha-smooth muscle actin. In contrast, an invasive ductal adenocarcinoma was negative for alpha-smooth muscle actin, indicating variation between carcinomas, whilst staining for vimentin and cytokeratin 18 appears to be more consistently positive [53, 59]. A subset of equine mammary carcinoma also exhibited strong nuclear staining for estrogen receptor alpha [59]. No upregulation of the oncogene cMyc was observed in one study, and tumor suppressor gene p53 was significantly downregulated [54].

12.10 Mesenchymal Tumors

Mesenchymal tumors exfoliate variably well for cytology. They are characterized by cells that are spindloid or fusiform but some mesenchymal tumors may have a round to ovoid shape. The cells often are seen individually or in aggregates which may be associated with pink extracellular matrix. Fibroblasts have a tendency to undergo reactive fibroplasia secondary to inflammation, trauma, or irritation, causing cytological changes that can mimic neoplasia. Samples should therefore be interpreted with consideration of history and clinical impressions, and histopathology may be required for appreciation of tissue architecture for further characterization of biological behavior.

12.10.1 Fibroma

Fibromas are uncommon skin tumors in horses, mostly affecting adult to aged animals. They mostly present as solitary, haired masses that vary from soft (fibroma molle) to firm (fibroma durum). Fibromas most commonly affect the

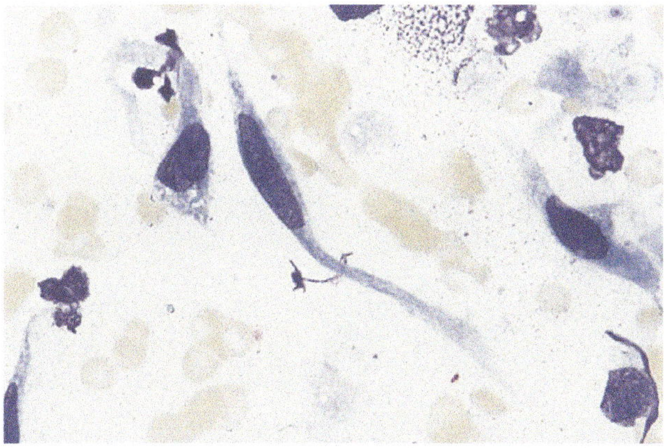

Figure 12.57 Fibrocytes have long slender nuclei, with long tails of cytoplasm streaming away from the nuclei. Wright's stain, original magnification 250×.

head, around the orbit, mandible, and maxilla [60–62], and frequently are ossifying. Fibromas rarely affect the limbs [63].

Fibromas are variably exfoliative, and many cytological samples will be acellular (often with hemodilution) or contain only low numbers of cells for review. When present, the cells are seen mostly individually, with loose aggregates of a few cells occasionally present, that may be associated with pink extracellular matrix. They are spindloid, with a small to moderate volume of pale blue cytoplasm that forms unipolar or bipolar tendrils. Nuclei are elongated, with stippled chromatin and small basophilic nucleoli. The population of spindle cells is uniform, with minimal anisocytosis/anisokaryosis (Figure 12.57). When low numbers of well-differentiated spindle cells are seen, multiple differentials are possible, including reactive processes (reactive fibroplasia, granulation tissue, etc.) or neoplastic lesions (such as fibroma, peripheral nerve sheath tumor, hemangioma, etc.).

Additionally, these lesions can be very difficult to distinguish from sarcoids, and histopathology is required for appreciation of tissue architecture for further characterization of origin and biological behavior.

12.10.2 Fibrosarcoma

Fibrosarcomas arise from fibroblasts and may be seen in cutaneous or subcutaneous tissues. In one study including 54 fibrosarcomas, 12.5% were found in the skin. They can be seen in horses of any age, including juveniles. Some tumors may be congenital, and some have been reported at sites of previous trauma, burns, or vaccination [64, 65]. Fibrosarcomas typically present as solitary masses that may ulcerate and become secondarily infected. They are locally invasive and may recur after surgical excision, especially with marginal excision. They typically have low metastatic potential, but can metastasize widely [66].

For cytology, these tumors are variably exfoliative and may be highly cellular. Neoplastic cells are seen individually and in aggregates, that may be associated with pink extracellular matrix. The cells vary from ovoid to spindloid/stellate, with short tapering ends or long tendrils of cytoplasm. Nuclei are ovoid to elongated and have finely stippled chromatin, with multiple basophilic nucleoli that may vary in size and shape. Mitotic figures and multinucleation may be seen. Anisocytosis/anisokaryosis often are marked, and N:C ratios are variable.

12.10.3 Sarcoid

Sarcoids are the most common tumors and dermatological neoplasms in horses [67, 68]. Most are benign but malignant variants are seen that are locally aggressive, and transformation of benign lesions to malignant neoplasms is possible. It is believed that delta papillomaviruses (bovine papillomavirus [BPV] types 1 and 2 [subgroup A] and 3) are responsible for the development of sarcoid disease, mainly through the activity of E5 oncogene, and through alteration in DNA methylation and oxidative stress [69, 70].

Sarcoids are seen more commonly in donkeys and mules than horses, though Appaloosas, Arabians and quarter horses may be predisposed [71, 72]. Standardbreds are less likely to develop sarcoids, possibly due to decreased expression of MHC class II antigen W13 ELA [73]. Young geldings (1–7 years of age) are most frequently affected.

The lesions may be solitary or multiple. They tend to occur in regions subject to trauma or chronic irritation such as that seen secondary to tack or insect bites, with predisposed sites including the chest, legs, and around the face (periocular and muzzle).

Sarcoids can be classified into many different types [74].

- *Occult (superficial)*: lesions are flat, annular, and alopecic with scaling. Typically affect the neck, face/periocular region, medial thigh, and shoulder.
- *Verrucous*: lesions have a wart-like appearance and affect the head/neck, groin, and axillary regions.
- *Nodular*: subcutaneous masses with normal overlying hair. Affected regions include periocular areas, groin, and penile sheath.
- *Fibroblastic*: these lesions typically are fast growing and have a fleshy/ulcerated appearance that may clinically mimic proud flesh or granulation tissue. Type 1 lesions are pedunculated, whilst type 2 have a broad base. They are found most commonly around the legs, groin, and periocular. Occult, verrucous, and nodular lesions subjected to trauma may stimulate formation of the fibroblastic type.
- *Malignant type*: lesions extend into surrounding skin and subcutaneous tissues. They are most commonly found over elbows and the jaw.

It is important to note that mixed forms may be seen that contain components of different sarcoid types.

Sarcoids exfoliate variably well for cytology. When present, mesenchymal cells are well differentiated, with a small volume of cytoplasm forming tapering ends and tendrils. Nuclei are ovoid to elongated and have stippled chromatin with small or inapparent nucleoli. Anisocytosis/anisokaryosis are mild to moderate, and N:C ratios are moderate to high. Sarcoids may ulcerate, and inflammation may be a prominent finding, or possibly the only finding on cytology. An increased number of eosinophils may be seen. Additionally, epithelial hyperplasia may be present, with sheets of well-differentiated epithelial cells variably present.

The well-differentiated nature of the spindle cells raises multiple differential diagnoses for sarcoid lesions including granulation tissue, fibroma, or peripheral nerve sheath tumor, and histopathology is recommended for appreciation of deep tissue architecture for characterization.

12.10.4 Lipoma

Lipomas are benign tumors of adipocytes. Whilst intraabdominal lipomas are most common, tumors in subcutaneous or other soft tissue accounted for 44% of lipomas in one study [75]. Predilection sites for subcutaneous tumors include the neck, hindlimbs, and thorax [76, 77]. In the subcutis, lipomas are variably well demarcated and can be large, firm tumors. Infiltrative lipomas are rare variants, mostly reported in younger patients (~2 years of age) [78]. Whilst local infiltration can be extensive, metastatic disease is not reported for these tumors.

Aspiration of lipomas often yields greasy material, that does not dry and can dissolve from the slide during staining, especially using alcohol-based stains, and samples from lipomas may be devoid of cells and/or contain clear vacuoles where lipid has dissolved. When present, mature, fat-laden adipocytes are seen in aggregates and have ballooning, clear cytoplasm, with small, round nuclei that often are pushed to the periphery of the cells (Figure 12.58).

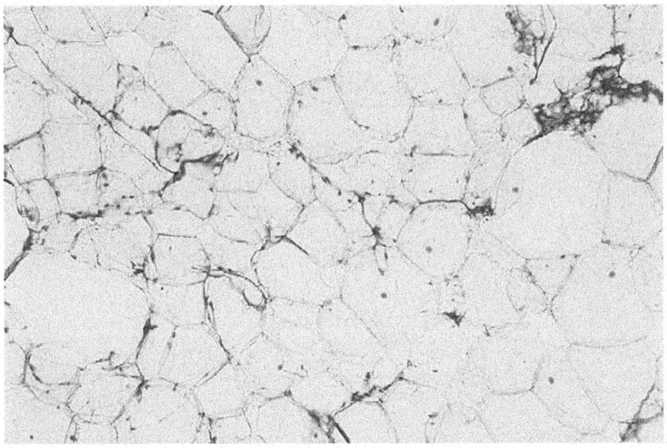

Figure 12.58 Aspirate from a lipoma containing numerous adipocytes which are large and round, with pyknotic nuclei and clear cytoplasm. Wright's stain, original magnification 25×.

12.10.5 Liposarcoma

Liposarcomas are rarely reported in the skin of horses [75]. They are malignant tumors arising from adipocytes and are regionally invasive but rarely metastasize. Cytologically, the samples may contain abundant clear lipid vacuoles in the background. Neoplastic cells typically have pale cytoplasm with indistinct cell borders. The cytoplasm often contains coarse, clear vacuoles. Nuclei are ovoid, with finely granular chromatin and multiple prominent basophilic nucleoli. Anisocytosis/anisokaryosis are moderate to marked, and N:C ratios are variable.

12.10.6 Hemangioma

Hemangiomas are benign tumors arising from endothelial cells. Cutaneous hemangiomas typically are solitary, raised, hairless, and have a red/purple/blue appearance. Verrucous hemangiomas are a rare variant that have a warty, verrucous surface that may ulcerate [79]. They are most commonly seen on the distal limbs, and most frequently affect young horses [80].

Cytological preparations frequently will have a dense background of blood, that may include many aggregates of platelets or clotted material. Hemangiomas often exfoliate poorly, with only rare spindloid cells available for review. The cells have a scant volume of cytoplasm that forms small tendrils and wisps. Nuclei are ovoid to elongated, with stippled chromatin and small basophilic nucleoli. Anisocytosis/anisokaryosis are mild, and N:C ratios are high (Figure 12.59).

Given the inherent vascular nature of these tumors, there may also be evidence of chronic hemorrhage within cytological samples such as macrophages that are erythrophagocytic or contain heme breakdown pigments such as hemosiderin or hematoidin (Figures 12.60 and 12.61). This poses a diagnostic dilemma, as the low numbers of well-differentiated spindle cells may represent a neoplastic process (i.e., hemangioma, fibroma, etc.), or reactive fibroblasts secondary to trauma within a hematoma, or granulation tissue, which is also highly vascular. Whilst the gross appearance of the mass may be helpful to further increase suspicion for a hemangioma, histopathology may be required for appreciation of tissue architecture for further characterization of biological behavior.

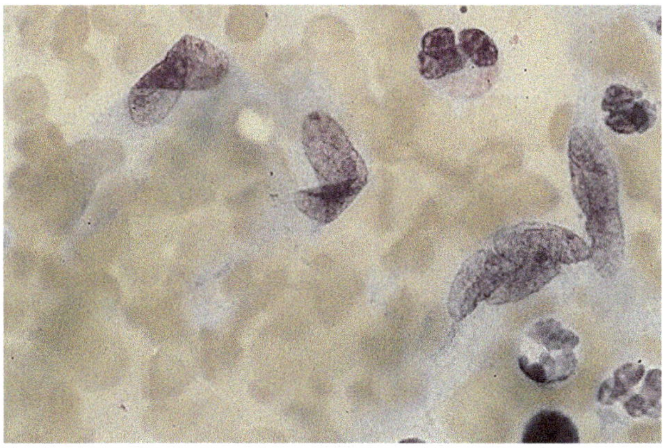

Figure 12.59 Aspirate from a hemangioma shows several spindle-shaped cells. Note how the nuclei appear very thin and capable of folding over upon themselves. Wright's stain, original magnification 250×. *Source:* Courtesy of Oklahoma State University.

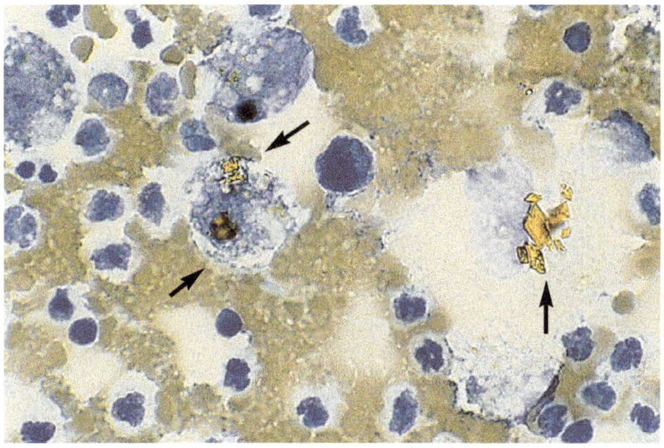

Figure 12.60 Large foamy macrophage with intracytoplasmic golden, hematoidin crystals (*arrows*). Hematoidin is a product of erythrocyte breakdown and is often referred to as tissue bilirubin. It indicates intratissue or intracavity hemorrhage. Wright's stain, original magnification 250×.

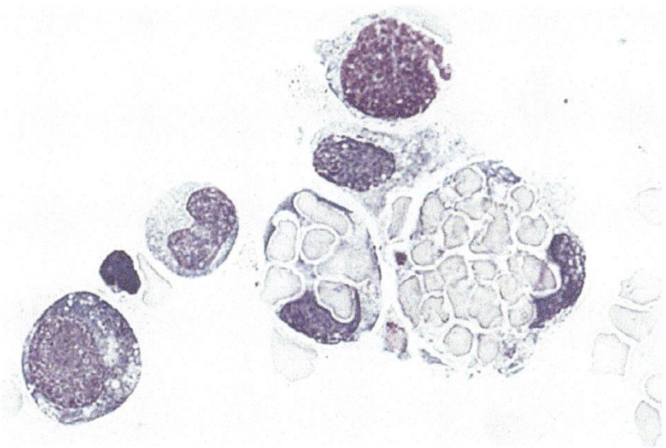

Figure 12.61 Macrophages showing erythrophagocytosis. Wright's stain, original magnification 250×. *Source:* Courtesy Oklahoma State University.

12.10.7 Hemangiosarcoma

Hemangiosarcomas are rare tumors of the skin in horses, with a prevalence of 0.02% in one study [81]. They are malignant tumors, arising from vascular endothelium. They often are rapidly growing lesions in adult to aged patients, but congenital tumors have been reported in young animals. In foals, congenital cutaneous and subcutaneous hemangiosarcomas are reported that may be multiple or regionally extensive [82]. They may also be seen in periocular locations [83]. Hemangiosarcomas are highly aggressive tumors that frequently metastasize widely, including to regional lymph nodes, liver, and lungs.

Hemangiosarcomas often are highly vascular, and cytological samples frequently have a dense background of blood, that may contain aggregates of platelets and clotted material. Cellularity is variable, with some samples containing only blood while others may contain small or large numbers of cells distributed individually or in tight aggregates/sheets. The cells vary from ovoid to polygonal/spindloid and have a moderate volume of pale to medium blue cytoplasm. Nuclei are ovoid, with finely stippled, immature chromatin, and often multiple basophilic nucleoli of varying size and shape (Figure 12.62).

12.10.8 Myxoma

Myxomas and myxosarcomas are neoplasms of fibroblastic origin that produce matrix rich in glycosaminoglycans.

In cytological samples from myxomas, samples often have a thick streaming background of pink mucinous material. The cells may be found individually or in small

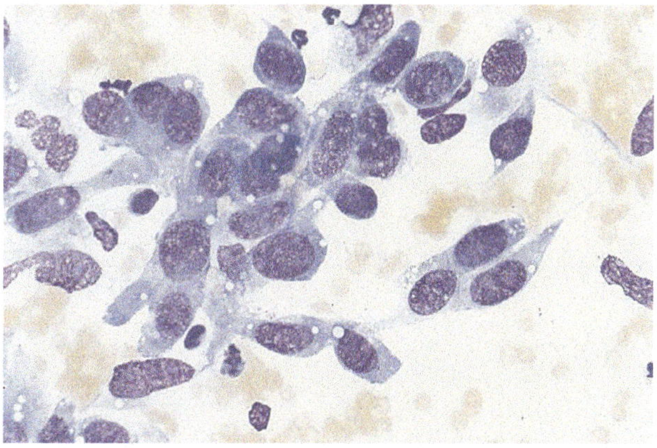

Figure 12.62 Aspirate from a malignant spindle cell tumor. Spindle cells show criteria of malignancy including anisocytosis; coarse chromatin; prominent, variably sized, and occasionally angular nucleoli; and increased N:C ratio. Wright's stain, original magnification 250×.

loose aggregates, often in a prominent streaming arrangement. The samples contain a variable number of uniform spindloid cells. These cells have a small volume of pale blue cytoplasm, that may contain pink granules. Nuclei are ovoid to elongated, with stippled chromatin, and small to inapparent nucleoli. Anisocytosis/anisokaryosis are mild, and N:C ratios are moderate to high.

12.10.9 Myxosarcoma

Myxosarcomas exfoliate variably well for cytological analysis. They often have a thick background of streaming pink mucinous material. The cells may be present individually or in loose aggregates, and individualized cells often are pulled into rows (Figure 12.63). The cells are spindloid, with a moderate volume of pale blue cytoplasm, that may contain fine pink granules. Nuclei are ovoid to elongated, with finely stippled chromatin, and multiple prominent nucleoli. Mitotic figures may be seen. Anisocytosis/anisokaryosis are moderate to marked, and N:C ratios are moderate to high (Figure 12.64). Well-differentiated myxosarcomas also are possible, which may have only mild criteria of malignancy that can mimic myxomas, and histopathology for appreciation of tissue architecture may be warranted for assessment of biological behavior.

12.10.10 Peripheral Nerve Sheath Tumor

Peripheral nerve sheath tumors encompass a group of neoplasms, typically referring to schwannomas and neurofibromas. Cutaneous peripheral nerve sheath tumors mostly are solitary neoplasms, found around the head and neck, as well as the limbs [84]. In horses, there is a predilection for peripheral nerve sheath tumors (neurofibromas) to affect the eyelids [76]. The vast majority of these tumors are benign but malignant variants have been reported, especially affecting the periocular region [85, 86].

Grossly, peripheral nerve sheath tumors typically are well-demarcated, potentially lobulated, firm masses, ranging from 1 to 4 cm in diameter [84]. These tumors exfoliate variably well for cytology, and some samples may be highly cellular. The cells are spindloid, with a small to moderate volume of cytoplasm that forms bipolar tendrils and wisps. Nuclei are ovoid to elongated, with stippled chromatin and often multiple, small nucleoli. Anisocytosis/anisokaryosis typically are mild to moderate, and N:C ratios are moderate. Multinucleate forms may be seen with peripheralized nuclei (Figure 12.65). Differentiating these cells from

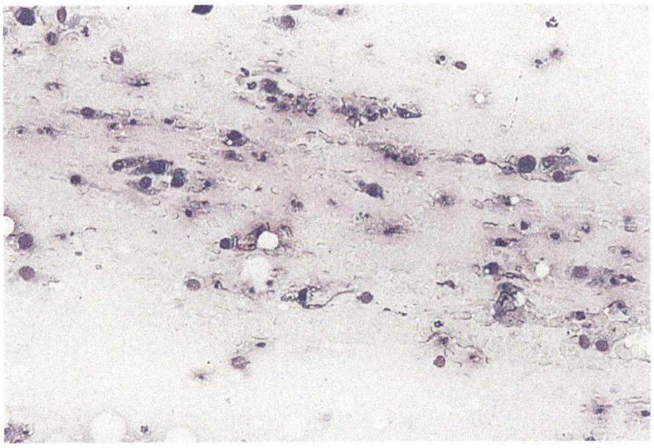

Figure 12.63 Aspirate from myxosarcoma. Low magnification shows mesenchymal cells and erythrocytes present in rows, suggesting a viscous nature to the material being spread. Note lightly eosinophilic nature to background. Wright's stain, original magnification 50×.

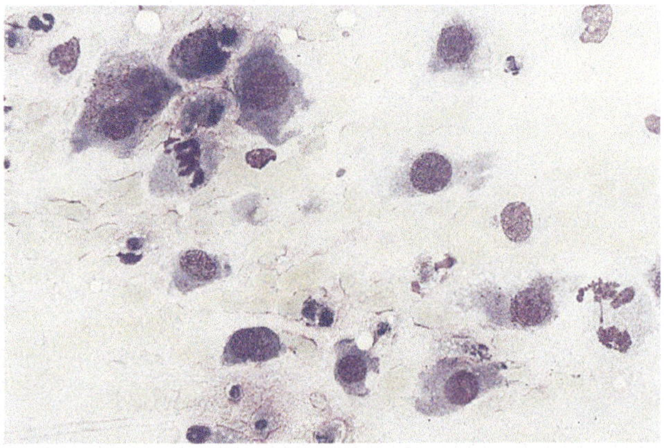

Figure 12.64 Aspirate from myxosarcoma. Higher magnification shows pleomorphic population of spindle-shaped mesenchymal cells. Cytoplasmic granules of eosinophilic secretory material are visible in the cell in the lower right. Wright's stain, original magnification 125×.

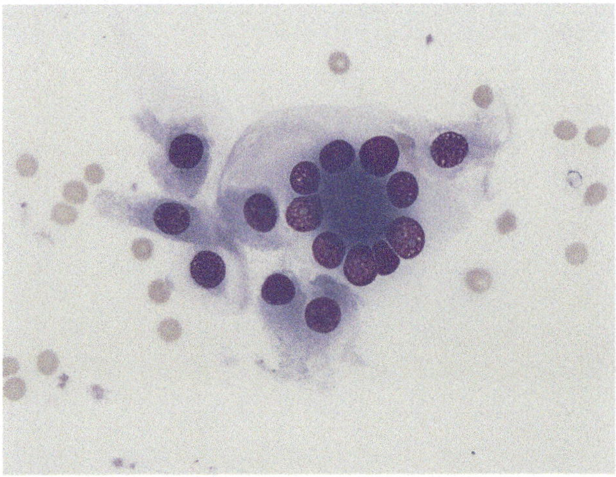

Figure 12.65 Aspirate from a peripheral nerve sheath tumor. Note large multinucleate neoplastic cell with peripheralized nuclei (crown cell) surrounded by several spindle cells with singular nuclei.

reactive fibroblasts or from other mesenchymal tumors such as fibroma/fibrosarcoma requires histopathology for appreciation of tissue architecture.

12.10.11 Giant Cell Tumor of Soft Parts

Giant cell tumors of soft parts are rare tumors of the skin in horses, representing approximately 1% of cutaneous neoplasms [67]. These tumors mostly affect older horses (>10 years of age), and present as solitary, raised, firm masses that may ulcerate. They have a predilection for the hindlimbs, but have also been reported on the thorax, shoulder, abdomen, muzzle, and jugular groove [87, 88]. The tumors have low metastatic potential and whilst surgical excision may be curative, local recurrence has been reported in tumors with incomplete or minimal excision [87].

Cytological samples from such tumors are variably cellular, and contain a population of spindloid cells with pale to medium blue cytoplasm forming tapering ends and wisps. The tumors are characterized by the presence of multinucleated giant cells. These cells have abundant medium blue cytoplasm that frequently forms tails and wisps. Multiple nuclei are present (up to 50) that have little variation in size (Figure 12.66) [88]. Anisocytosis/anisokaryosis typically are moderate to occasionally marked. There may also be an infiltrate of mixed inflammatory cells, including neutrophils, lymphocytes, and plasma cells, as well as evidence of chronic hemorrhage within the samples (e.g., macrophages that are erythrophagocytic or contain heme breakdown pigment).

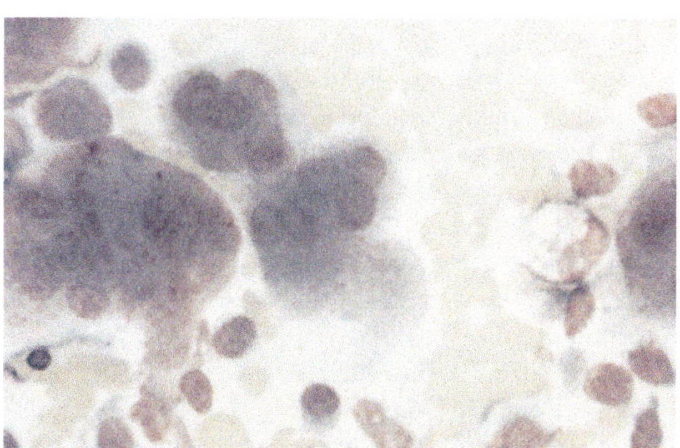

Figure 12.66 Aspirate from malignant fibrous histiocytoma (giant cell tumor). Several multinucleated cells and a few histiocytic cells are present. One cell has a tail of cytoplasm trailing away from it. Wright's stain, original magnification 200×.

12.11 Melanocytic Tumors

The skin is the most common site for melanomas in horses. Melanocytic tumors comprise a diverse category with differing biological behavior and clinical syndromes. These categories include melanocytic nevus (melanocytoma), dermal melanoma, dermal melanocytosis, and anaplastic malignant melanoma [89].

12.11.1 Melanocytic Nevus/Melanocytoma

These tumors occur in the superficial dermis or epidermal–dermal junction. They typically are solitary, heavily pigmented tumors, mostly seen around the head, legs, and trunk. They are seen in horses of any color and >70% occur in horses ≤6 years of age [89].

12.11.2 Dermal Melanoma and Dermal Melanocytosis

Dermal melanomas arise in the deep dermis. Dermal melanocytosis refers to multiple or coalescing tumors. They are most common in older, gray horses. They have malignant potential, with 8–14 horses available for follow-up in one study showing evidence of metastatic disease [89]. In a study of gray horses, they were most commonly found on the ventral tail (93.9%), the perianal region (43%), lips (33%), and eyelids (24%) [90].

12.11.3 Anaplastic Malignant Melanoma

These tumors typically occur in horses of any color and are seen in older animals.

The cytological appearance of melanocytic tumors is variable, based on type and differentiation. The background of the samples often contains abundant green to black granules, that are often elongated. Melanomas mostly exfoliate well, with moderate to marked numbers of cells available for review. The cells may be seen individually, or in tight aggregates, and the shape is highly variable, ranging from ovoid to polygonal or spindloid. The cells typically have an abundant volume of cytoplasm. In melanocytic nevus/melanocytomas, the cytoplasm contains many melanin pigment granules that may obscure the nucleus (Figures 12.67 and 12.68). Dermal melanomas are variably granular, and anaplastic malignant melanomas frequently are poorly granular, with cells that contain a fine dusting of pigment, or agranular variants. Nuclei are ovoid with finely stippled chromatin and often prominent nucleoli. Many mitotic figures are seen in anaplastic malignant melanomas. Anisocytosis/anisokaryosis vary from mild (melanocytomas) to marked (anaplastic malignant melanoma).

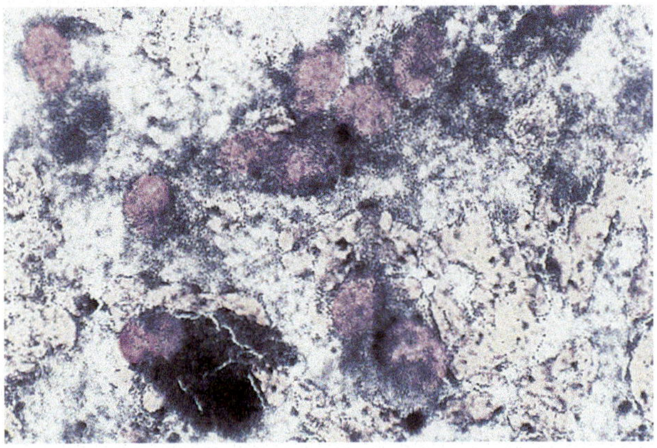

Figure 12.67 Aspirate from melanoma. Neoplastic cells contain abundant amount of intracytoplasmic green-black pigment. Background contains abundant pigment released from cells ruptured during aspiration and slide preparation. Wright's stain, original magnification 250×. *Source:* Courtesy of Oklahoma State University.

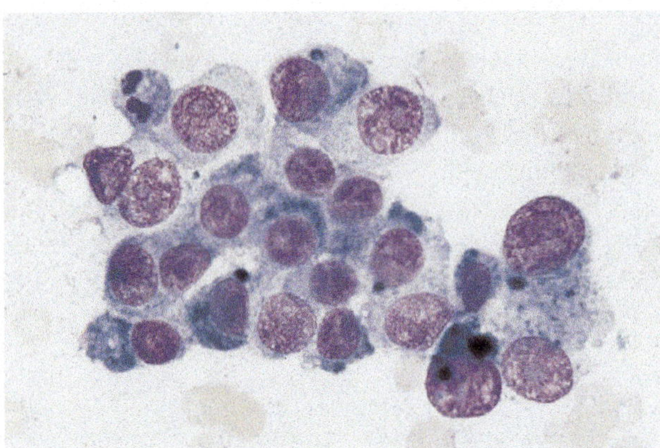

Figure 12.68 Aspirate from a malignant melanoma shows several neoplastic cells containing melanin pigment. Numerous criteria of malignancy are seen. These include anisocytosis; coarse chromatin; increased nucleus to cytoplasm ratio; and prominent, variably sized, and angular nucleoli. Wright's stain, original magnification 250×.

It may be difficult to distinguish well-differentiated melanocytes from melanophages (macrophages containing phagocytosed melanin pigment) and hemosiderophages (macrophages containing hemosiderin) in cytological preparations. The pigment within melanophages often is more aggregated than that seen in melanocytes, and may be seen within vacuoles. Hemosiderin in hemosiderophages is also often aggregated, and may vary from black to golden brown. Distinguishing these cells can be particularly problematic when assessing lymph nodes for metastatic disease, as melanophages may be present (phagocytosing draining melanin pigment from a tumor) that can mimic metastatic disease. Special stains on histopathology may be helpful to characterize the cells. Melanocytes will stain positively with PNL2 which is a sensitive marker for melanocytic tumors in horses, whilst macrophages will not stain. It is interesting to note that monoclonal antibody to Melan A does not react with equine melanoma [91]. Fontana–Mason stain can also be used to highlight iron within hemosiderophages.

12.12 Evaluation of Fluid-Filled Lesions

Fluid-filled skin lesions may represent a primary or secondary process. Primary fluid-filled lesions may include seroma, hematoma, or abscess formation, whereas fluid may also accumulate secondary to other underlying pathology such as a neoplastic process. Indeed, some tumors may be predisposed to having a fluid component, such as hemangiomas, myxomas, or cyst formation in adenocarcinomas.

Evaluation of the fluid component of fluid-filled lesions may be highly supportive of a diagnosis (such as keratinized material in epidermoid cysts), but it is important to remember that underlying pathology may not exfoliate into the fluid component of the lesion. For example, the finding of hemorrhage may indicate a hematoma but hemorrhage around a nonexfoliating vascular tumor such as a hemangioma may also be possible. It is therefore ideal to also try and aspirate material from a more solid component of a lesion if possible, to try and assess deeper tissues. Histopathology may be required for appreciation of deep tissue architecture for further characterization of fluid-filled lesions of the skin.

12.12.1 Epidermal Cyst

The material aspirated from epidermal cysts often has a creamy white to gray or brown appearance, and may be chunky or gritty if the lesion is mineralized. They mostly present as single lesions, but multiple tumors and generalized disease have been reported [92].

Cytologically, epidermal cysts may have a clear background, or a medium to thick blue proteinaceous background (Figure 12.69). Many cholesterol crystals or cholesterol clefts (negatively staining areas left by dissolved cholesterol crystals during staining with alcohol-based Romanowsky-type stains) are characteristic of cystic lesions due to degeneration of cells within the cystic fluid (Figure 12.70). Cholesterol crystals are clear, rectangular, and have notched borders, and may be seen in any cystic lesion. Epidermal cysts are characterized by abundant, variably sized aggregates of keratinized debris which appears as amorphous, blue/gray material. This debris may be studded with mineralized aggregates due to dystrophic

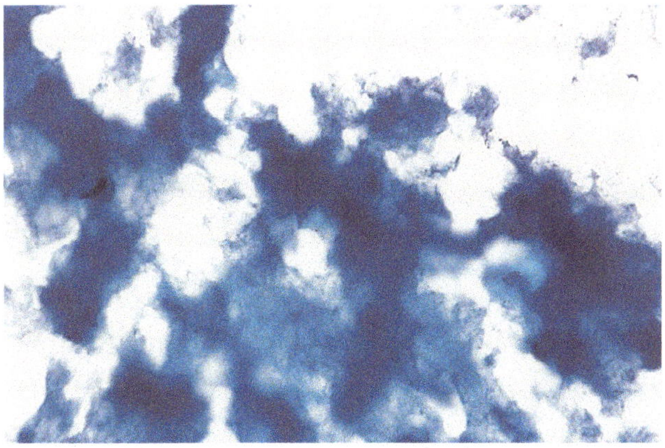

Figure 12.69 Aspirate from an epidermal cyst. Note abundant blue amorphous debris. Wright's stain, original magnification 50×.

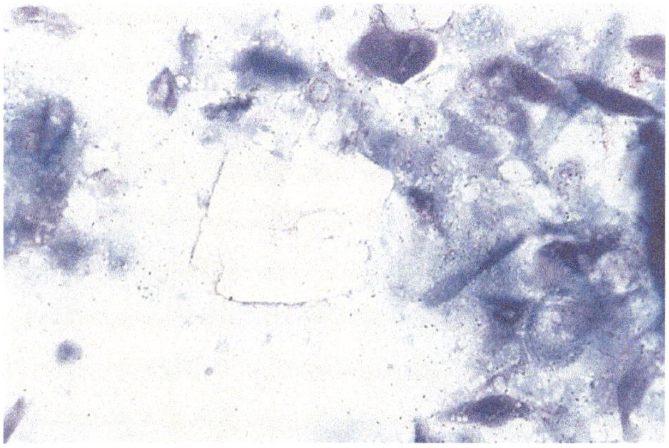

Figure 12.70 Aspirate from an epidermal cyst. A cholesterol crystal is present in a background of degenerating squamous cells and basophilic cell debris. Wright's stain, original magnification 50×.

mineralization in chronic lesions. Polygonal squamous epithelial cells may be present, that typically are anucleated or have pyknotic nuclei. Inflammatory cells may also be present in these lesions, which may be due to rupture of the mass or leakage of keratin into the dermis, which incites a foreign body-type reaction. Macrophages often predominate and frequently are multinucleated. Neutrophils may also be present in large numbers, and will be nondegenerative if the response is sterile, or degenerative if the lesion is secondarily infected.

12.12.2 Hematoma

Hematomas commonly form in the skin secondary to traumatic events, which may include at the site of injections or trauma secondary to dystocia-associated birth [93, 94]. The fluid aspirated from hematomas is deep red to red-brown, and often will not clot after aspiration. The samples have a dense background of blood that usually is devoid of platelets, unless there has been acute hemorrhage into the area, or peripheral blood is also collected at the time of aspiration. Nucleated cells comprise mostly a mixture of blood-associated leukocytes, with a variable number of nondegenerative neutrophils and reactive macrophages. In cases of chronic hemorrhage, the macrophages will contain phagocytosed red blood cells or heme breakdown products including hemosiderin or hematoidin. Cytology alone cannot differentiate a hematoma from hemorrhage around a deeper, nonexfoliating process, and these findings should be correlated with history, clinical impressions, and further diagnostic tests as appropriate.

12.12.3 Seroma/Hygroma

Seromas may form secondary to blunt trauma, or around surgical wounds, especially if there is abundant dead space for fluid to accumulate [95]. Hygromas are most common around pressure points, areas subject to chronic irritation/trauma or over joints [96]. Fluid aspirated from seromas or hygromas typically is clear to amber colored, and may be thin or viscous. The fluid usually has an increased total protein concentration (>2.5 g/dL). The fluid is variably cellular, and may be of very low cellularity, requiring sediment examination to evaluate cells present. Cellularity may be high in acutely inflamed lesions. The cells typically comprise a mixture of nondegenerative neutrophils and macrophages. Neutrophils dominate in acute lesions, whereas macrophages predominate when the process is chronic.

12.12.4 Abscess

Grossly, the fluid aspirated from abscesses often has a thick, creamy, and chunky texture. The protein concentration of abscess fluid often cannot be determined due to its thick nature, but if quantifiable is usually >4.0 g/dL. The colour can be variable, often depending on the cells present, with yellow/brown fluid when neutrophils predominate or green if eosinophils are present in large numbers. The fluid will often have a putrid smell.

The samples are highly cellular. Neutrophils most commonly predominate and may account for >90% of the cells in the sample. If the neutrophils are degenerative, with poorly segmented nuclei that appear puffy, an infectious etiology is more likely, and close examination of the samples for intracellular bacteria of other infectious agents is recommended, and microbial culture and susceptibility testing may also be warranted. Whilst nondegenerative neutrophils are present in sterile lesions, they do not rule out an infectious etiology. Macrophages may be seen in large numbers within some abscesses or with granuloma formation. They may also predominate in abscesses that form secondary to foreign material or some infectious organisms such as fungal agents [97].

It is important to consider that aspiration of fluid with septic inflammation may represent a primary process (i.e., abscess) or secondary infection/abscessation of a deeper, nonexfoliating pathological lesion. Reevaluation of the area after treatment of the septic inflammation is prudent, with aspiration for cytological evaluation or histopathology for appreciation of deep tissue architecture warranted if the lesion does not completely resolve.

References

1 Frank, L., Kania, S., and Weyant, E. (2016). RT-qPCR for the diagnosis of dermatophilosis in horses. *Vet. Dermatol.* 27 (5): 431.

2 Ramos-Vara, J.A., Ortiz-Santiago, B., Segales, J., and Dunstan, R.W. (1996). Cutaneous leishmaniasis in two horses. *Vet. Pathol.* 33: 731–734.

3 Fettelschoss-Gabriel, A., Fettelschoss, V., Olomski, F. et al. (2019). Active vaccination against interleukin-5 as long-term treatment for insect-bite hypersensitivity in horses. *Allergy* 74 (3): 572–585.

4 van der Haegen, A., Griot-Wenk, M., Welle, M. et al. (2001). Immunoglobulin-E-bearing cells in skin biopsies of horses with insect bite hypersensitivity. *Equine Vet. J.* 33 (7): 669–706.

5 Slovis, N.M., Watson, J.L., Affolter, V.K. et al. (1999). Injection site eosinophilic granulomas in 3 horses. *J. Vet. Intern. Med.* 13 (6): 606–612.

6 Valentine, B.A. (2005). Equine cutaneous non-neoplastic nodular and proliferative lesions in the Pacific Northwest. *Vet. Dermatol.* 16 (6): 425–428.

7 Fernandez, C.J., Scott, D.W., and Erb, H.N. (2000). Staining abnormalities of dermal collagen in eosinophil or neutrophil-rich inflammatory dermatoses of horses and cats as demonstrated with Masson's trichrome stain. *Vet. Dermatol.* 11 (1): 43–48.

8 Pucheu-Haston, C.M. and del Piero, F. (2013). Equine multi-systemic eosinophilic epitheliotropic disease. *Equine Vet. Educ.* 25 (12): 614–617.

9 Bosseler, L., Verryken, K., Bauwens, C. et al. (2013). Equine multisystemic eosinophilic epitheliotropic disease: a case report and review of the literature. *N. Z. Vet. J.* 61 (3): 177–182.

10 Pusterla, N., Watson, J.L., Wiolson, W.D. et al. (2003). Cutaneous and ocular habronemiasis: 63 cases (1988–2002). *J. Am. Vet. Med. Assoc.* 222 (7): 978–982.

11 Vandenabeele, S.I.J., White, S.D., Affolter, V.K. et al. (2004). Pemphigus foliaceus in the horse: retrospective study of 20 cases. *Vet. Dermatol.* 15 (6): 381–388.

12 Zabel, S., Mueller, R.S., Fieseler, K.V. et al. (2005). Review of 15 cases of pemphigus foliaceus in horses and a survey of the literature. *Vet. Rec.* 157 (17): 505–509.

13 Scott, D.W. (1994). Marked acantholysis associated with dermatophytosis due to *Trichophyton equinum* in two horses. *Vet. Dermatol.* 5 (3): 105–110.

14 Karcher, L.F., Scott, D.W., Paradis, M. et al. (1990). Sterile nodular panniculitis in five horses. *J. Am. Vet. Med. Assoc.* 196 (11): 1823–1826.

15 Suárez-Bonnet A, de los Monteros, E., A., Herráez, P. et al. (2008). Fat embolism secondary to yellow fat disease in an Appaloosa horse. *J. Vet. Diagn. Invest.* 20 (5): 684–687.

16 Waitt, L.H., Cebra, C.K., Tornquist, S.J. et al. (2006). Panniculitis in a horse with peripancreatitis and pancreatic fibrosis. *J. Vet. Diagn. Invest.* 18 (4): 405–408.

17 Adam, E.N. and Southwood, L.L. (2007). Primary and secondary limb cellulitis in horses: 44 cases (2000–2006). *J. Am. Vet. Med. Assoc.* 231 (11): 1696–1703.

18 Fjordbakk, C.T., Arroyo, L.G., and Hewson, J. (2008). Retrospective study of the clinical features of limb cellulitis in 63 horses. *Vet. Rec.* 162 (8): 233–236.

19 Perdrizet, J.A. and Scott, D.W. (1987). Cellulitis and subcutaneous abscesses caused by *Rhodococcus equi* infection in a foal. *J. Am. Vet. Med. Assoc.* 190 (12): 1559–1561.

20 Farstvedt, E.G., Hendrickson, D.A., Dickenson, C.E. et al. (2004). Treatment of suppurative facial cellulitis and panniculitis caused by Corynebacterium pseudotuberculosis in two horses. *J. Am. Vet. Med. Assoc.* 224 (7): 1139–1142.

21 Durham, A.C., Pillitteri, C.A., San Myint, M. et al. (2013). Two hundred three cases of equine lymphoma classified according to the World Health Organization (WHO) classification criteria. *Vet. Pathol.* 50 (1): 86–93.

22 Schaffer, P.A., Wobesser, B., Martin, L.E. et al. (2013). Cutaneous neoplastic lesions of equids in the Central United States and Canada: 3351 biopsy specimens from 3272 equids (2000–2010). *J. Am. Vet. Med. Assoc.* 242 (1): 99–104.

23 Valentine, B.A. (2006). Survey of equine cutaneous neoplasia in the Pacific Northwest. *J. Vet. Diagn. Invest.* 18 (1): 123–126.

24 Scott, D.W. (2011). Lymphohistiocytic neoplasms. In: *Equine Dermatology*, 2e, 499–504. St Louis: Elsevier.

25 Miller, C.A., Durham, A.C., Schaffer, P.A. et al. (2015). Classification and clinical features in 88 cases of equine cutaneous lymphoma. *J. Vet. Diagn. Invest.* 27 (1): 86–91.

26 Henson, K.L., Alleman, A.R., Kelley, L.C. et al. (2000). Immunohistochemical characterization of estrogen and progesterone receptors in lymphoma of horses. *Vet. Clin. Pathol.* 29 (2): 40–46.

27 Ressel, L., Ward, S., and Kipar, A. (2015). Equine cutaneous mast cell tumors exhibit variable differentiation, proliferation activity and KIT expression. *J. Comp. Pathol.* 153 (4): 236–243.

28 Millward, L.M., Hamberg, A., Mathews, J. et al. (2010). Multicentric mast cell tumors in a horse. *Vet. Clin. Pathol.* 39 (3): 365–370.

29 Reppas, G.P. and Canfield, P.J. (1996). Malignant mast cell neoplasia with local metastasis in a horse. *N. Z. Vet. J.* 44 (1): 22–25.

30 Clarke, L., Simon, A., Ehrhart, E.J. et al. (2014). Histologic characteristics and KIT staining patterns of equine cutaneous mast cell tumors. *Vet. Pathol.* 51 (3): 560–562.

31 Tan, R.H., Crisman, R.V., Clark, S.P. et al. (2007). Multicentric mastocytoma in a horse. *J. Vet. Intern. Med.* 21 (2): 340–343.

32 Beusker, N., Muller, J.M.V., Seehusen, F. et al. (2010). Histiocytic sarcoma in a 16-year-old pony gelding. *Pferdeheilkunde* 26 (5): 680–684.

33 Torres, S.M. and Koch, S.N. (2013). Papillomavirus-associated diseases. *Vet. Clin. North Am. Equine Pract.* 29 (3): 643–655.

34 Lange, C.E., Tobler, K., Lehner, A. et al. (2013). EcPV2 DNA in equine papillomas and in situ and invasive squamous cell carcinomas supports papillomavirus etiology. *Vet. Pathol.* 50 (4): 686–692.

35 Lindner, K.E., Bizikova, P., Luff, J. et al. (2018). Generalized papillomatosis in three horses associated with a novel equine papillomavirus (EcPV8). *Vet. Dermatol.* 29 (1): 72–e30.

36 Slovis, N.M., McEntee, M.C., Fairley, R.A. et al. (2001). Equine basal cell tumors: 6 cases (1985–1999). *J. Vet. Intern. Med.* 15 (1): 43–46.

37 McMartin, D.N. and Gruhn, R.F. (1977). Sebaceous carcinoma in a horse. *Vet. Pathol.* 14 (5): 532–534.

38 Guerel, A., Haktanir, D., Kurban, I. et al. (2018). A case of sebaceous carcinoma detected on the eyelid of a horse. *Acta Vet. Eurasia* 44 (2): 101–104.

39 Cihocki, L.M., Divers, T.J., Johnson, A.L. et al. (2007). A case of multiple epitrichial sweat gland ductal carcinomas in a horse. *Vet. Dermatol.* 18 (2): 134–137.

40 Ueki, H., Kowatari, Y., Oyamada, T. et al. (2004). Non-functional C-cell adenoma in aged horses. *J. Comp. Pathol.* 131 (2–3): 157–165.

41 Dittus, N., Hahn, K., Stokar-Regenscheit, N. et al. (2018). Calcitonin as a potential tumor marker for medullary thyroid carcinoma in an 11-year old Spanish pure-bred gelding with two independent carcinomas. *Equine Vet. Educ.* 30 (12): 658–663.

42 Bradley, A.E., Pirie, R.S., and MacIntyre, N. (2010). Thyroid carcinoma with multiple metastases in a horse. *Equine Vet. Educ.* 12 (4): 170–174.

43 Chiba, S., Okada, K., Namakunai, S. et al. (1987). A case of equine thyroid follicular carcinoma accompanied with adenohypophysial adenoma. *Nihon Juigaku Zasshi.* 49 (3): 551–554.

44 Saulez, M.N., Viljoen, A., Kafka, U. et al. (2013). The use of nuclear imaging for a mixed C cell microfollicular carcinoma of the thyroid gland in a mature horse. *Equine Vet. Educ.* 25 (3): 118–125.

45 Perez-Ecija, A., Toribio, R.E., and Mendoza, F.J. (2018). Endocrine tumors in equids. *Equine Vet. Educ.* 30 (12): 664–670.

46 Schalk, W. (1972). Solid mammary carcinoma in a horse. *Berl Munch Tierartzl Wochenschr* 85 (8): 141–142.

47 Acland, H.M. and Gillette, D.M. (1982). Mammary carcinoma in a mare. *Vet. Pathol.* 19 (1): 93–95.

48 Munson, L. (1987). Carcinoma of the mammary gland in a mare. *J. Am. Vet. Med. Assoc.* 191 (1): 71–72.

49 Foreman, J.H., Weidner, J.P., and Parry, B.W. (1990). Pleural effusion secondary to thoracic metastatic mammary adenocarcinoma in a mare. *J. Am. Vet. Med. Assoc.* 197 (9): 1193–1195.

50 Reppas, G.P., McClintock, S.A., Canfield, P.J. et al. (1996). Papillary ductal adenocarcinoma in the mammary glands of two horses. *Vet. Rec.* 138 (21): 518–519.

51 Kato, M., Higuchi, T., Hata, H. et al. (1998). Lactalbumin-positive mammary carcinoma in a mare. *Equine Vet. J.* 30 (4): 358–360.

52 Prendergast, M., Bassett, H., and Larkin, H.A. (1999). Mammary carcinoma in three mares. *Vet. Rec.* 144 (26): 731–732.

53 Hirayama, K., Honda, Y., Sako, T. et al. (2003). Invasive ductal carcinoma of the mammary gland in a mare. *Vet. Pathol.* 40 (1): 86–91.

54 Bussche, L., Harms, C., Buckles, E.L. et al. (2017). Carcinoma of the mammary gland in a mare. *Equine Vet. Educ.* 29 (7): 370–375.

55 Reesink, H.L., Parente, E.J., Sertich, P.L. et al. (2009). Malignant fibrous histiocytoma of the mammary gland in a mare. *Equine Vet. Educ.* 21 (9): 467–472.

56 MacEachern, K.E., McKay, J.S., and Hewicker-Trautwein, M. (2001). Malignant mammary melanoma in a young mature thoroughbred mare. *Equine Vet. Educ.* 13 (2): 68–71.

57 Spadari, A., Valentini, G., Sarli, G. et al. (2008). Mammary adenoma in a mare: clinical, histological and immunohistochemical findings. *Equine Vet. Educ.* 20 (1): 4–7.

58 Shank, A.M. (2009). Mare mammary neoplasia. Difficulties in diagnosis and treatment. *Equine Vet. Educ.* 21 (9): 475–477.

59 Hughes, K., Scase, T.J., and Foote, A.K. (2015). Estrogen receptor and signal transducer and activator of transcription 3 expression in equine mammary tumors. *Vet. Pathol.* 52 (4): 631–634.

60 Sponseller, B.A., Caston, S.S., Winter, M.D. et al. (2006). What's your diagnosis? Chronic ossifying juvenile fibroma. *J. Am. Vet. Med. Assoc.* 229 (11): 1727–1728.

61 Kodaira, K., Muranaka, M., Naito, H. et al. (2010). Histopathological characteristics of an ossifying fibroma formed in the maxilla of a racehorse. *J. Equine Sci.* 21 (1): 7–10.

62 Colitz, C.M., Gilger, B.C., Davidson, C.P. et al. (2000). Orbital fibroma in a horse. *Vet. Ophthalmol.* 3 (2–3): 213–216.

63 Poore, L.A., Duncan, N., and Williams, J. (2018). Unilateral subcutaneous fibroma in the distal femoral region of a 5-year-old Nooitgedacht mare. *J. S. Afr. Vet. Assoc.* 89 (0): e1–e4.

64 Schumacher, J., Watkins, J.P., Wilson, S.R. et al. (1986). Burn-induced neoplasia in two horses. *Equine Vet. J.* 18 (5): 410–412.

65 Kannegieter, N.J., Schaaf, K.L., Lovell, D.K. et al. (2010). Myofibroblastic fibrosarcoma with multifocal osseous metaplasia at the site of equine influenza vaccination. *Aust. Vet. J.* 88 (4): 132–136.

66 Reinertson, E.L. (1974). Fibrosarcoma in a horse. *Cornell Vet.* 64: 617–621.

67 Schaffer, P.A., Wobeser, B., Weiss, C. et al. (2013). Cutaneous neoplastic lesions of equids in the Central United States and Canada: 3351 biopsy specimens from 3272 equids (2000–2010). *J. Am. Vet. Med. Assoc.* 242 (1): 99–104.

68 Knowles, E.J., Tremaine, W.H., Pearson, G.R. et al. A database survey of equine tumors in the United Kingdom. *Equine Vet. J.* 48 (3): 280–284.

69 Potocki, L., Lewinska, A., Klukowska-Rötzler, J. et al. (2012). DNA hypomethylation and oxidative stress-mediated increase in genomic instability in equine sarcoid-derived fibroblasts. *Biochemie* 94 (9): 2013–2024.

70 Semik, E., Ząbek, T., Gurgul, A. et al. (2018). Comparative analysis of DNA methylation patterns of equine sarcoid and healthy skin samples. *Vet. Comp. Oncol.* 16 (1): 37–46.

71 Mohammad, H.O., Rebhun, W.C., and Antczak, D.F. (1992). Factors associated with the risk of developing sarcoid tumors in horses. *Equine Vet. J.* 24 (3): 165–168.

72 Davis, C.R., Valentine, B.A., Gordon, E. et al. (2016). Neoplasia in 125 donkeys (Equus asinus): literature review and survey of five veterinary schools in the United States and Canada. *J. Vet. Diagn. Invest.* 28 (6): 662–670.

73 Meredith, D., Elser, A.H., Wolf, B. et al. (1986). Equine leukocyte antigens: relationships with sarcoid tumors and laminitis in two pure breeds. *Immunogenetics* 23 (4): 221–225.

74 Knottenbelt, D.C. (2005). A suggested clinical classification for the equine sarcoid. *Clin. Tech. Equine Pract.* 4 (4): 278–295.

75 Priester, W.A. and McKay, F.W. (1980). The occurrence of tumors in domestic animals. *Natl. Cancer Inst. Monogr.* 54: 1–120.

76 Pascoe, R.R. and Summers, P.M. (1981). Clinical survey of tumors and tumor-like lesions in horses in south east Queensland. *Equine Vet. J.* 13 (4): 235–239.

77 Bristol, D.G. and Fubini, S.L. (1984). External lipomas in three horses. *J. Am. Vet. Med. Assoc.* 185 (7): 791–792.

78 Erkert, R.S., Moll, H.D., MacAllister, C.G. et al. (2007). Infiltrative lipoma in an American Quarter Horse gelding. *Equine Vet. Educ.* 19 (7): 380–383.

79 Pérez-Écija, A., Estepa, J.C., Barranco, I. et al. (2014). Verrucous hemangioma with pseudoepitheliomatous epidermal hyperplasia in an adult horse. *Vet. Pathol.* 51 (5): 992–995.

80 Johnson, G.C., Miller, M.A., Floss, J.L. et al. (1996). Histologic and immunohistochemical characterization of hemangiomas in the skin of seven young horses. *Vet. Pathol.* 33 (2): 142–149.

81 Hargis, A.M. and McElwain, T.F. (1984). Vascular neoplasia in the skin of horses. *J. Am. Vet. Med. Assoc.* 184 (9): 1121–1124.

82 Dunkel, B.M., del Piero, E., Kraus, B.M. et al. (2004). Congenital, cutaneous, oral and periarticular hemangiosarcoma in a 9-day-old Rocky Mountain horse. *J. Vet. Intern. Med.* 18 (2): 252–255.

83 Scherrer, N.M., Lassaline, M., and Engiles, J. (2018). Ocular and periocular hemangiosarcoma in six horses. *Vet. Ophthalmol.* 21 (4): 432–437.

84 Schöniger, S., Valentine, B.A., Fernandez, C.J., and Summers, B.A. (2011). Cutaneous schwannomas in 22 horses. *Vet. Pathol.* 48 (2): 433–442.

85 Strubbe, D.T. (2001). Periocular neurofibrosarcoma in a horse. *Vet. Ophthalmol.* 4 (4): 237–241.

86 Kappe, E.C., Köhler, K., Felbert, I.V. et al. (2009). Pleomorphic corneal sarcoma resembling malignant peripheral nerve sheath tumor in a horse. *Vet. Pathol.* 46 (3): 444–448.

87 Bush, J.M. and Powers, B.E. (2008). Equine giant cell tumor of soft parts: a series of 21 cases (2000–2007). *J. Vet. Diagn. Invest.* 20 (4): 513–516.

88 Cian, F., Whiteoak, S., and Stewart, J. (2016). A case of giant cell tumor of soft parts in a horse. *Vet. Clin. Pathol.* 45 (3): 501–504.

89 Valentine, B.A. (1995). Equine melanocytic tumors: a retrospective study of 53 horses (1988 to 1991). *J. Vet. Intern. Med.* 9 (5): 291–297.

90 Fleury, C., Berard, F., Balme, B. et al. (2000). The study of cutaneous melanomas in Camargue-type gray-skinned horses (1): clinical-pathological characterization. *Pigment Cell Res.* 13 (1): 39–46.

91 Ramos-Vara, J.A., Frank, C.B., DuSold, D. et al. (2014). Immunohistochemical expression of melanocytic antigen PNL2, Melan A, S100, and PGP 9.5 in equine melanocytic neoplasms. *Vet. Pathol.* 51 (1): 161–166.

92 Ginel, P.J., Zafra, R., Lucena, R. et al. (2007). Multiple generalized follicular cysts in a stallion. *Vet. Dermatol.* 18 (6): 456–459.

93 Tanner, R.B. and Hubbell, J.A.E. (2019). A retrospective study of the incidence and management of complications associated with regional nerve blocks in equine dental patients. *J. Vet. Dent.* 36 (1): 40–45.

94 Sato, F., Shibata, R., Shikichi, M. et al. (2014). Rupture of the gastrocnemius muscle in neonatal thoroughbred foals: a report of three cases. *J. Equine Sci.* 25 (3): 61–64.

95 Rosanowski, S.M., MacEoin, F., Graham, R.J.T.Y. et al. (2018). Open standing castration in thoroughbred racehorses in Hong Kong: prevalence and severity of complications 30 days post-castration. *Equine Vet. J.* 50 (3): 327–332.

96 van Veenendaal, J.C., Speirs, V.C., and Harrison, I. (1981). Treatment of hygromata in horses. *Aust. Vet. J.* 57 (11): 513–514.

97 Schwarz, B., Burford, J., and Knottenbelt, D. (2009). Cutaneous fungal granuloma in a horse. *Vet. Dermatol.* 20 (2): 131–134.

13

Cytology of the Eyes and Associated Structures

Julie Piccione[1] *and Lucien Vallone*[2]

[1] *Texas A&M Veterinary Medical Diagnostic Laboratory, College Station, TX, USA*
[2] *Department of Small Animal Clinical Sciences, College of Veterinary Medicine, Texas A&M University, College Station, TX, USA*

13.1 Introduction

Cytological specimens can be collected with minimally invasive techniques that are often inexpensive in comparison to other procedures and tests. Cytological evaluation can provide valuable information on the etiology of a lesion and guide the ordering of ancillary tests such as biopsy with histological examination, culture, polymerase chain reaction (PCR), etc. These benefits are especially useful in the equine eye, where disease is common and collection of biopsy specimens can be challenging.

Ideally, cytological evaluation and ancillary tests (e.g., bacterial and fungal cultures) should be performed together whenever possible for ocular lesions. Cytological examination provides information on the presence or absence of inflammation, which may aid in the interpretation of any bacterial or fungal growth as true infectious agents versus normal flora or contaminants. Additionally, cytological evaluation is more rapid than culture and provides general information on the size, shape, number, and gram-staining properties of any bacteria present.

Periocular and ocular masses represent approximately 10% of all equine neoplasms [1]. Nonneoplastic conditions such as abscesses, habronemiasis, conjunctival pseudotumors, and fungal granulomas can mimic tumors grossly [2–4]. Cytological evaluation can help characterize lesions as inflammatory or neoplastic and guide future diagnostic tests and therapeutics before more invasive techniques are used. However, surgical excision and histological examination with or without adjunctive therapy (radiation, chemotherapy, cryotherapy) are indicated for most ocular tumors [5].

Whilst cytological evaluation has many benefits, there are limitations that must be considered. Given the small size of cytological specimens, they may not be representative of the entire lesion. Therefore, whilst confident diagnoses can be made when certain infections agents or neoplastic populations are seen, many diseases cannot be ruled out with cytological evaluation alone. Additionally, without tissue architecture, some populations of cells can be difficult to classify as reactive (nonneoplastic) or neoplastic. Concurrent inflammation can cause dysplastic changes in cells (e.g., mesenchymal cells and squamous epithelial cells) that can mimic neoplasia cytologically. Lastly, there are many structures that can mimic infections agents to a novice microscopist (Figure 13.1).

13.2 Collection of Cytology Samples

13.2.1 Precollection Considerations

A diagnostic cytology sample should provide large numbers of intact cells in a monolayer, be free of contaminating materials (e.g., infectious agents, mucus, plant material), and representative of the sampled lesion. An ideal collection method would utilize readily available affordable materials, cause minimal discomfort for the patient, and limit artefacts in the cytological specimen. There are several methods for collecting cytological specimens of ocular lesions and the gold standard method may vary depending on the exact anatomical location and the suspected etiology.

There are several methods that can be used for restraint and to minimize discomfort for the horse during the ophthalmic examination and for collection of cytological samples. An ear or nose twitch can be used for minor, minimally uncomfortable procedures such as applying anesthetic or examining the eye. More often, chemical sedation and

Equine Hematology, Cytology, and Clinical Chemistry, Second Edition.
Edited by Raquel M. Walton, Rick L. Cowell, and Amy C. Valenciano.

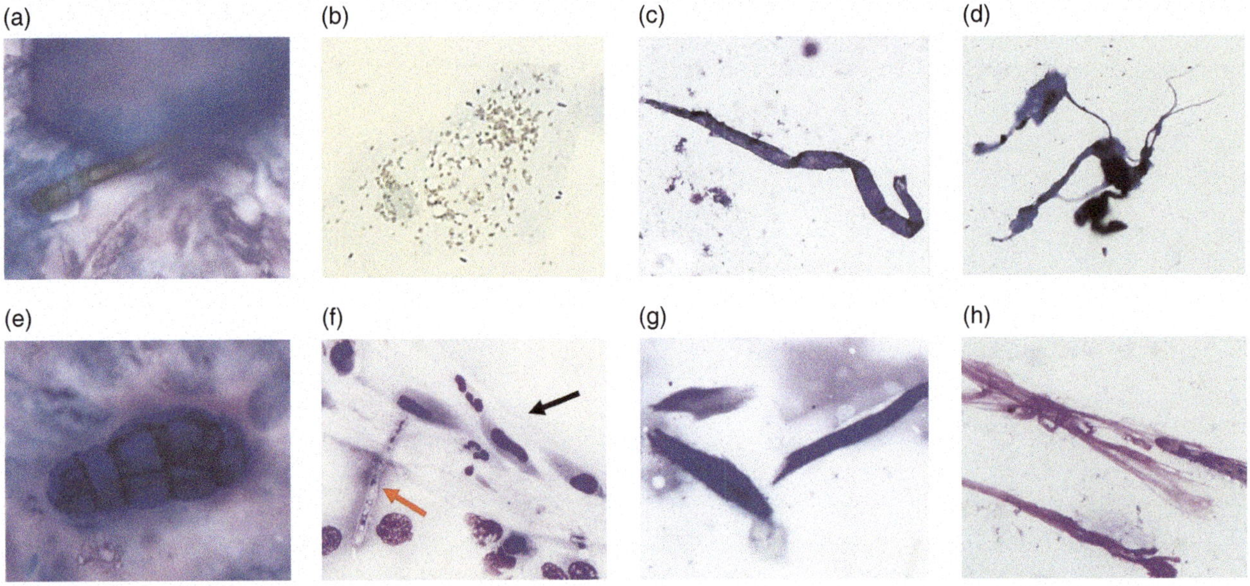

Figure 13.1 (a) Environmental plant material found in a corneal scraping can mimic fungal hyphae. (b) Orange-green melanin granules can mimic bacteria. Few basophilic, small, rod-shaped bacteria are present. (c,d) Fibers can mimic fungal hyphae. (e) *Alternaria* sp., most commonly a saprophytic contaminant. (f) Streaming mucus (*black arrow*) can be mistaken for fungal hyphae (*red arrow*) when present alone. (g) Keratin scrolls are rolled-up superficial squamous epithelial cells that can mimic fungal hyphae to novice microscopists. (h) Streaming nuclear material and proteinaceous debris should not be mistaken for fungal hyphae. *Source:* Images (a) and (e) courtesy of Dr Samantha Schlemmer.

periocular nerve blocks are required to facilitate a thorough ophthalmic examination and subsequent cytology collection. Finally, topical and/or local anesthesia is frequently needed before cytological samples can be obtained from the ocular surface or periocular tissues. These examination and restraint techniques are briefly summarized below and are reviewed more fully elsewhere [2, 6–9].

For short standing procedures, a single intravenous injection of an alpha-2 agonist such as xylazine, detomidine, or romifidine (following labeled dosing instructions) is usually sufficient. Adjunctive sedatives may be required for some patients, including the opioid butorphanol or the phenothiazine tranquilizer acepromazine.

Periocular nerve blocks are easier to perform in a sedated patient and are often needed to overcome the strength of muscle contraction within the equine eyelid, especially in circumstances where there is ocular pain. The auriculopalpebral nerve is a branch of the facial nerve and provides motor innervation to the orbicularis oculi muscle. The palpebral branch of this nerve can be palpated and blocked at multiple locations along the zygomatic arch providing akinesia to the eyelids. The supraorbital or frontal nerve is a branch of the ophthalmic branch of the trigeminal nerve, arises from the supraorbital foramen located at the dorsomedial aspect of the bony orbit, and provides sensory innervation to the upper eyelid. This nerve is blocked at the site of the supraorbital foramen to improve comfort as the patient's upper eyelid is manipulated. Common local anesthetic protocols utilize either mepivacaine or lidocaine by injecting 2–3 mL subcutaneously over each nerve and then massaging the injection site. Periocular nerve blocks should be performed away from the actual lesion of collection, limiting any interference in collection or results.

The use of topical anesthesia in ocular lesions sampled for cytology is slightly debated, the concern being that it could decrease cellular collection and alter the morphology of cells. Some studies describe absorbing excessive amounts of fluid before collecting and reported no overt abnormalities from the use of topical anesthetic [10]. Some studies in other species have shown better sample collection with the use of topical anesthetics, likely due to increased patient compliance [11]. Topical anesthesia can be obtained with tetracaine, proparacaine, lidocaine, mepivacaine, or oxybuprocaine solutions [2, 10, 12–16]. The topical anesthetics morphine and nalbuphine appear to be ineffective in the horse [17, 18]. It is typically recommended to collect samples destined for bacterial culture before the administration of any topical anesthetic; however, the use of topical proparacaine HCl does not appear to significantly affect the numbers and types of organisms cultured from the cornea or conjunctiva [19, 20]. Finally, the use of subconjunctival local anesthetics has been reported recently to provide a safe and effective means of ocular surface anesthesia for procedures lasting up to two hours [7].

There is some debate on whether to clean the surface of ocular lesions before collection of cytological samples.

Many ocular lesions can lead to excessive tearing and collection of exudate. These secretions can then become admixed with environmental debris (e.g., plant material, fungus), normal flora bacteria, and degenerative cellular debris (Figure 13.1). Ideally, collection of samples before and after cleaning would provide the most information. However, samples/slides would need to be clearly labeled as before and after cleaning. Gentle cleaning with a moistened cotton swab or flushing with sterile eyewash should aid in removing excess mucus and surface contaminants. Excess eyewash can be collected from the medial canthus with a cotton swab or gauze.

13.2.2 Collection Techniques

13.2.2.1 Periocular and Retrobulbar Lesions

Cytological evaluation of lesions associated with the dermal and subcutaneous tissues surrounding the eye can provide valuable diagnostic information. Impression smear cytology (pressing a glass slide to a lesion) should be accompanied by fine needle aspiration or scraping, as impression smears only represent the superficial surface of the lesion. Neoplastic cells may not be present superficially. Additionally, when ulceration is present, secondary infections are common which can lead to insufficient treatment. Lastly, in ulcerated lesions, atypical squamous epithelial cells are common, representing dysplastic and hyperplastic populations. However, these cells can mimic neoplastic populations, resulting in misdiagnoses, especially with novice microscopists.

Fine needle aspiration of retrobulbar lesions has the benefit of being minimally invasive and providing rapid information. However, not all neoplasms and pathological processes can be diagnosed with cytological evaluation. Some lesions are poorly cellular or poorly exfoliative, providing only small number of cells for cytological evaluation (e.g., hemangioma, certain sarcomas). Therefore, additional diagnostic tests such as advanced imaging and biopsy with histologic examination may be warranted.

13.2.2.2 Cornea and Conjunctiva

There are several methods for collecting cytological specimens from the conjunctiva and cornea which can be broadly divided into debridement and impression techniques. Debridement involves scraping, swabbing, or brushing and recommended techniques vary according to anatomical location (cornea versus conjunctiva) and disease. Debridement instruments include the following: sterile cotton-tip applicator swab or calcium alginate swab, Kimura spatula, handle edge of a disposable scalpel blade, and cytobrush (Figure 13.2a,b). Impression cytology can be performed using a glass slide or, preferably, a cellulose filter. In general, collecting samples with a cotton-tip applicator swab or directly with a glass microscope slide is not recommended if other collection methods are available. Collection with cotton-tip applicators results in poor cytological specimens due to poor cellularity and occasional contaminating fibers. Scraping (Kimura spatula or handle edge of a disposable scalpel blade) and brushing (cytobrush) collection methods are most common in the horse, though methods involving impression cytology have been reported [10, 21–23].

Scraping of corneal ulcers and other corneal lesions should be taken at the margin of the lesion to prevent further damage to the cornea and to limit necrotic cellular debris. When scraping, gentle pressure should be applied whilst scraping several times in the same direction (not back and forth) until material is collected on the end of the collection device [24]. The material can then be gently applied to the center of a clean glass slide, spreading the material thin. Cytobrush samples are collected by turning the bristled tip 3–4 times over the margin of the lesion. The cytobrush is then gently rolled onto a microscope slide. It is important to note that fungal organisms are often found in the deeper corneal layers [25] so when keratomycosis is suspected, aggressive scraping may be warranted. Care should be taken in circumstances in which stromal loss is present, as inadvertent corneal perforation can occur. Additionally, if the ulcer has started to epithelialize, it may be necessary to gently remove the superficial epithelium before collection to allow for diagnostic samples [24].

A recent study compared three common debridement methods for collecting corneal samples in horses with ulcerative keratitis: cytobrush, Kimura platinum spatula, and the handle edge of a scalpel blade [23]. All three techniques provided clinically useful samples and results; however, using the handle edge of a scalpel blade provided the most intact cells and diagnostic samples [23]. This method is also practical as scalpel blades are easily available, sterile, and affordable [23].

Impression cytology most often refers to the use of a cellulose filter, typically applied to the cornea (or conjunctiva) to collect cytological specimens [26]. This method removes the most superficial layers of cells, which can then be stained and examined microscopically or used for molecular analysis (PCR) [26, 27]. The method is increasing in popularity in human ophthalmic centers, and in veterinary research and academic settings [10, 21, 22, 26]. In brief, cellulose filters are applied directly to the area of interest either alone or attached to a plastic tube to ease application [10, 22, 26]. During collection, the eyelids must be held open to avoid introducing tear fluid, which will inhibit cell collection [26]. The filter is left in place for 5–10 seconds and then removed. The cellulose filters can then be stained with various methods and mounted onto

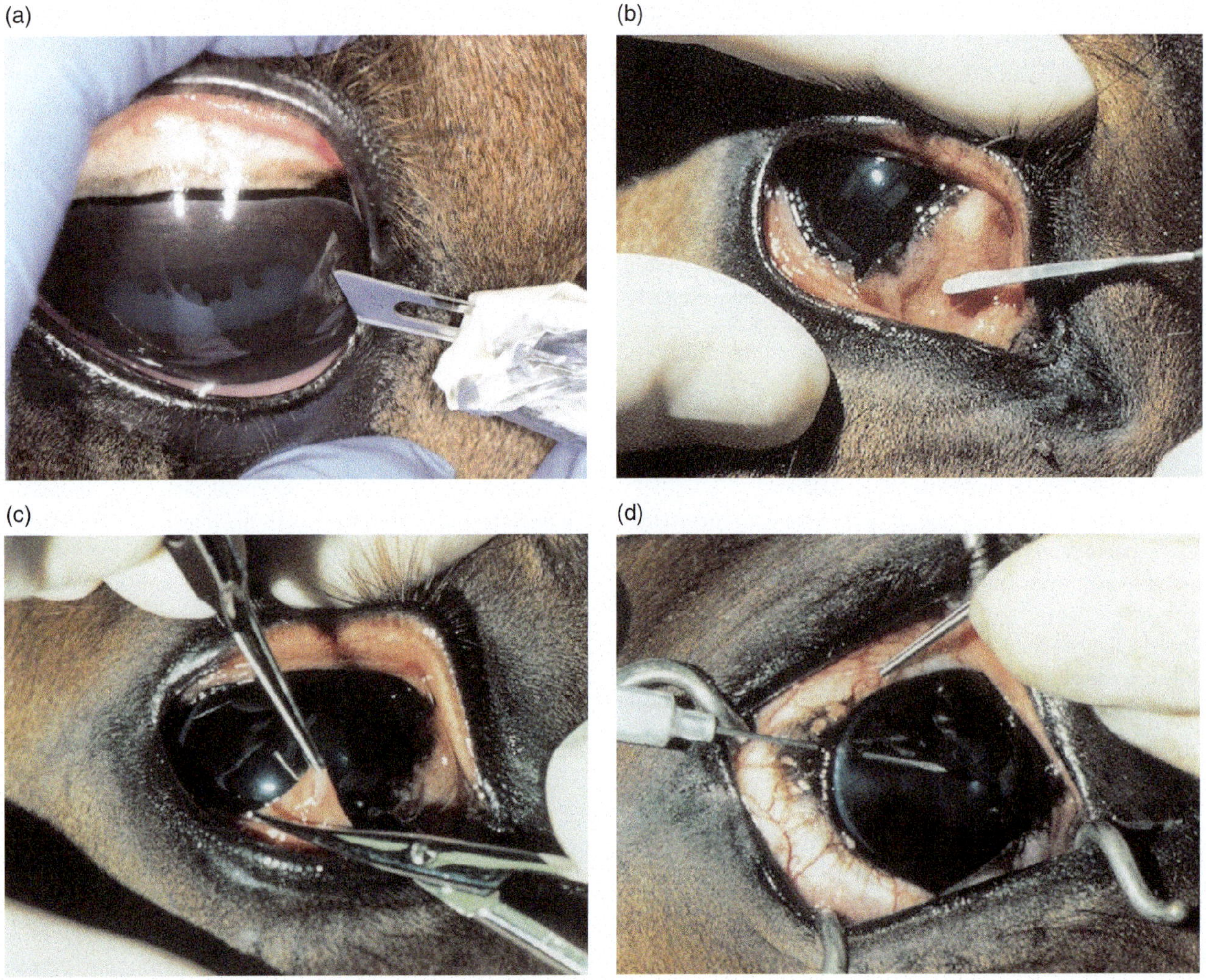

Figure 13.2 (a) Collection of cytological samples with the handle of a single-use scalpel blade. (b) Collection of cytological samples with Kimura spatula. (c) Conjunctival biopsy. Small scissors are used to excise a portion of conjunctiva. (d) Anterior chamber paracentesis. A 25 or 22 gauge needle attached to a 1 mL syringe is inserted into the bulbar conjunctiva, 3–4 mm from the limbus. The needle is threaded deep to the conjunctiva towards the limbus and enters the anterior chamber parallel to the surface of the iris. *Source:* Images (b), (c) and (d) courtesy of Drs Elizabeth A. Giuliano and Cecil P. Moore.

slides and coverslipped. Details of this collection method are described elsewhere [10, 21, 22, 26].

There are several benefits of the impression cytology technique. Several studies show that impression cytology of healthy and diseased cornea (and conjunctiva) provides sufficient numbers of well-preserved cells for cytological evaluation, similarly to cytobrush samples [10, 22]. The method appears to be more comfortable for the patient and causes less irritation and epithelial cell damage when compared to the cytobrush method [22]. Therefore, impression cytology technique may be useful for fragile or deep corneal lesions or for sensitive horses. Impression cytology also maintains cellular/tissue architecture and can better demonstrate the proportion of goblet cells, and therefore may be preferred in research settings or for goblet cell quantification [10, 21].

There are also several limitations to impression cytology, especially in a clinical setting. To begin, the collection materials may not be readily available to practitioners because they are not kept in stock for other diagnostic and treatment protocols (versus scalpel blades). The collection process may also be difficult because the eyelids must be kept open [10]. Staining and processing of the membrane can be technically demanding and may not allow for long-term storage or easy transport to a diagnostic laboratory. Additionally, impression cytology samples limit evaluation of fine cellular detail and small infectious agents due to the thicker preparations [21, 22]. Therefore, when neoplasia or bacterial etiologies are suspected, impression cytology may not be the ideal collection method [21].

Samples of the conjunctiva can be collected similarly to corneal lesions (Figure 13.2a,b). When diffuse conjunctival disease is present, the lower palpebral conjunctiva is the preferred collection site [24]. When conjunctival lesions are scraped with a scalpel handle edge or Kimura spatula, it is important to avoid the lid margin [24]. Conjunctival cytobrush samples are also collected from the lower palpebral conjunctiva and fornix in a manner similar to corneal sample collection (described above) and this method yields samples of high cellularity [28]. Larger conjunctival biopsy samples can be taken by grasping tissue adjacent to the lesion of interest and using scissors or a scalpel to excise the lesion (Figure 13.2c) [24]. Before placing the tissue sample into formalin, impression smears can be made for cytological evaluation. The tissue should be gently pressed onto a clean glass slide in several separate places make several imprints of the specimen. This sample can then be evaluated for rapid information as well as to complement histological examination of the formalin fixed tissue. Additionally, these tissue samples can be used to detect *Onchocerca* microfilaria (described below) [24].

13.2.2.3 Aqueous and Vitreous Humor

Ocular paracentesis refers to the sampling of aqueous and vitreous fluid and usually requires general anesthesia [24]. Ocular paracentesis is rarely performed in the field, as there are many associated risks, including but not limited to hemorrhage, lens perforation, endothelial damage, corneal edema, retinal detachment, and introduction of microorganisms. Where required, the procedure may be performed in standing horses with the use of deep sedation, periocular nerve blocks (including retrobulbar block), and topical corneal anesthesia [29–31].

The most common indication for ocular paracentesis is to determine an underlying etiology for uveitis. Sampling of the aqueous and/or vitreous is performed only after other less invasive diagnostic methods (e.g., complete blood count [CBC], blood culture, serology) have failed to yield a diagnosis and when inflammation is not resolving with supportive care. Vitreous paracentesis, specifically, may be considered in horses with marked vitreous opacification, exudative retinal separations, or suspected infectious endophthalmitis [24].

Aqueous humor paracentesis is performed by approaching the anterior chamber through the dorsotemporal limbus (Figure 13.2d). The conjunctiva and cornea should be cleaned with 5% aqueous povidone-iodine solution and rinsed with sterile 0.9% saline [24]. The eyelids should be retracted using a speculum. Thumb forceps are used to grasp the bulbar conjunctiva near the point of entry. A 27 or 30 gauge needle attached to a 1 mL syringe (with the plunger seal already broken) is inserted into the bulbar conjunctiva approximately 3–4 mm away from the limbus [24]. The needle is gently threaded under the conjunctiva towards the limbus until it enters the anterior chamber parallel to the surface of the iris. Then 0.2–0.5 mL of aqueous humor is gently and slowly aspirated [24]. The needle is then slowly withdrawn and gentle pressure is applied over the exit wound [24, 29]. After collection, a freshly prepared smear should be made on a glass slide in a blood smear fashion. The remaining fluid should be stored in a nonadditive sterile tube for potential culture.

Vitreous paracentesis is performed through a pars plana approach [24]. The ocular surface should be prepared as described for aqueous humor collection. A 23–25 gauge needle attached to a 1 mL syringe (with the plunger seal already broken) is inserted in the dorsolateral quadrant of the eye approximately 10–12 mm behind the limbus [32, 33]. A small amount (typically no more than 0.2 mL) of vitreous humor is gently and slowly aspirated [24]. The needle is then slowly withdrawn and gentle pressure is applied over the exit wound [24]. Slide preparation and submission of remaining fluid are the same as for sampling of aqueous humor.

In addition to cytological evaluation, fluid collected from the aqueous or vitreous can be analyzed for bacterial and fungal culture and susceptibility, protein measurement, antibody titers (e.g., *Borrelia* and *Leptospira* spp.), and PCR (e.g., *Borrelia* and *Leptospira* spp., equine herpesvirus [EHV], antigen receptor rearrangement for lymphoid neoplasms) [30, 34–40]. Diagnostic laboratories should be contacted ahead of collection to ensure proper sample collection, handling, and shipping, especially for specialized diagnostic tests such as PCR and immunofluorescence assay. For cytological evaluation, submission of both freshly prepared slides and collected fluid in nonadditive tubes is preferred. This allows pathologists to evaluate the gross appearance of the fluid, perform cell counts or access cellularity, determine total protein, and prepare concentrated slides.

13.2.3 Slide Preparation and Utilizing a Diagnostic Laboratory

Infectious agents are a major cause of ocular lesions and some special considerations are required. In-clinic stains may be prone to contamination with plant material, bacteria, fungi, and other miscellaneous debris (Figure 13.1). This material can obviously confound cytological evaluation. Therefore, thorough cleaning of stain containers and frequent replacement and monitoring of stains are recommended. Additionally, normal flora bacteria and plant material can occasionally be observed in cytological specimens from apparently healthy animals. When infectious agents are seen, evidence of a corresponding inflammatory response may increase confidence in the infectious etiology.

Although there are several limitations to cytological evaluation, there are several steps that can be taken to improve cytological conclusions, especially when using a diagnostic laboratory. To begin, providing a thorough clinical description of the lesion is paramount. Since cytological evaluation does not involve tissue architecture, providing a basic description of the lesion can often clarify cytological findings. A basic gross description would include size, shape, color, dermal versus subcutaneous localization (where applicable), duration, haired or hair loss, etc. Submission of a gross image of the lesion may improve cytological interpretation and save the time of writing out a lengthy description. Pertinent clinical history (e.g., history of neoplasms, medications used on this lesion) should also be provided. Lastly, it is important to submit at least one unstained slide when possible. This allows pathologists to use high-quality, clean stains that they are familiar with, allowing for quick and accurate scanning of the cytological specimen. Additionally, special stains can be performed, where indicated: gram stain for bacteria; Gomori methenamine silver (GMS) and periodic acid–Schiff (PAS) for fungal organisms; T-Blue and Giemsa for questionable mast cell tumors, etc.

13.3 Cytological and Clinical Findings

13.3.1 Eyelids

13.3.1.1 Normal Anatomy and Cytological Findings

The outermost portion of the eyelids and normal cytology are similar to haired skin in other anatomical locations (see Chapter 12). The innermost aspect of the eyelid is lined with palpebral conjunctiva (see normal conjunctival cytology features below). At the eyelid margin, Meibomian gland orifices can be seen with the aid of magnification. These glands are numerous and extend 5–7 mm into the eyelid and are surrounded by fibrous connective tissue, giving the eyelid structural support. Meibomian glands are sebaceous, producing the outermost lipid component of the tear film [28].

13.3.1.2 Inflammatory Lesions

Blepharitis can be caused by infectious and noninfectious etiologies. When an etiological agent is not identified cytologically but there are large numbers of inflammatory cells, bacterial and fungal cultures may be warranted. If the lesion does not resolve with supportive treatment for the inflammation, biopsy with histological examination may also be indicated. Differential diagnoses for inflammation in the eyelids and periocular regions may be similar to those described in Chapter 12, with a few conditions unique to the eyelids. Inflammatory lesions are most commonly categorized by the predominant inflammatory cell. Mixed cell inflammation with no apparent predominant cell type can be more difficult to characterize cytologically due to the variety of differential diagnoses.

13.3.1.2.1 Neutrophilic Inflammation Neutrophil-predominant inflammation in the eyelids and periocular lesions is most commonly caused by bacterial infections, whether primary or secondary to another etiology (e.g., contaminated foreign body or ulcerated neoplasm). Additional considerations for significant neutrophilic inflammation include, but are not limited to, fungal infections, trauma, sterile foreign body reactions, Meibomian cysts, and pemphigus foliaceus.

Bacterial infections in the eyelid usually occur secondary to trauma or foreign body reactions, ulcerated neoplasms, and occasionally following placement of subpalpebral lavage (SPL) systems (Figure 13.3a). Cytologically, bacterial infections typically exfoliate large numbers of nondegenerate to degenerate neutrophils (Figure 13.3b). Degenerate neutrophils are intact cells with swollen, pale nuclei. It is important not to mistake lyzed cells (which will have swollen, pale nuclei) with degenerate neutrophils. Degenerate neutrophils occur with certain bacterial infections but the lack of degenerate neutrophils does not rule out bacterial infections. Finding intracellular bacteria confirms a bacterial infection. However, cytology cannot always determine if a bacterial infection is a primary or secondary process. When there are large numbers of neutrophils present but no bacteria are found, bacterial culture is indicated as a more sensitive detection method.

Fungal infections affecting the eyelids can include opportunistic and systemic fungi [24]. Dermatophytosis in horses can be caused by *Trichophyton* or *Microsporum* spp., and lesions can be observed on the eyelids. Grossly, the lesions are often alopecic, dry to exudative, with marginal crusting. In some cases, small masses may develop. Fungal organisms can be identified with cytological examination of samples with impression smears, skin scrapings, or fine needle aspirate of masses. Cytological examination of stained specimens from dermatophytosis lesions reveals mixed cell inflammation, typically predominated by neutrophils with fewer macrophages, multinucleated giant cells, and possibly eosinophils (Figure 13.4). Arthrospores (arthroconidia) and fungal hyphae are occasionally seen (Figure 13.4a–c). Arthrospores are smaller than red blood cells (approximately $2 \times 4\,\mu m$), round to slightly elongate, and deeply basophilic with a thin nonstaining border. Unstained wet mounts of hair shafts in mineral oil or saline can also be examined for arthrospores or fungal hyphae [24].

Meibomian cyst, or chalazion, develops when there is blockage of the Meibomian glands. These are typically

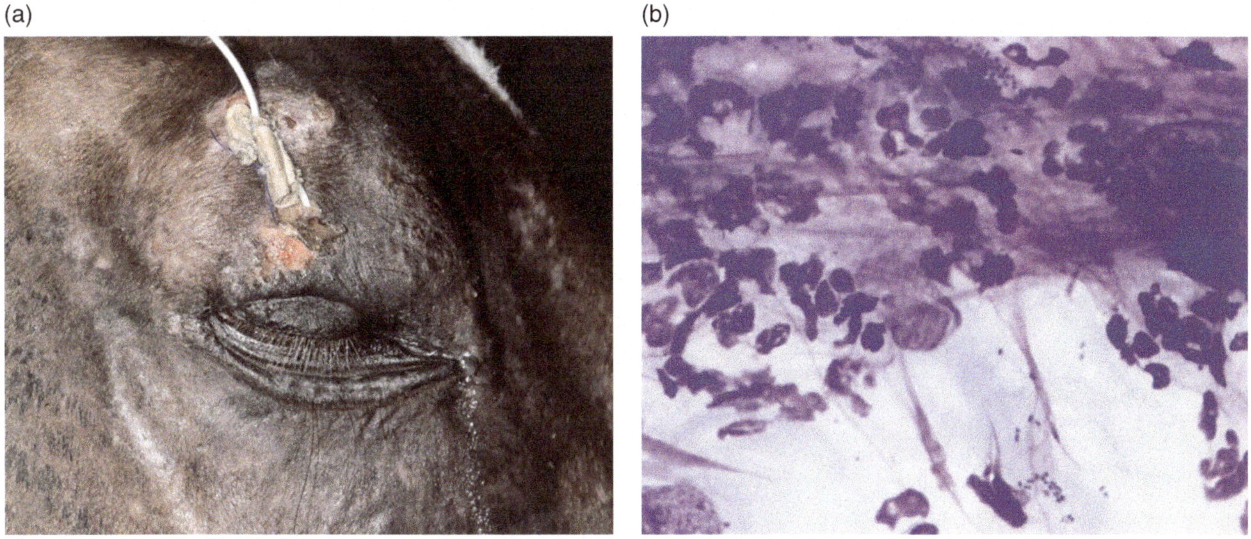

Figure 13.3 (a) Subpalpebral lavage systems can cause local cellulitis and occasionally abscessation in horses. The tape and suture were placed too close to the SPL exit site in this case, inducing local irritation and trapping debris. (b) Separate case of bacterial blepharitis. Cytological examination reveals numerous degenerate neutrophils and diplococci bacteria. Wright–Giemsa, 100× objective.

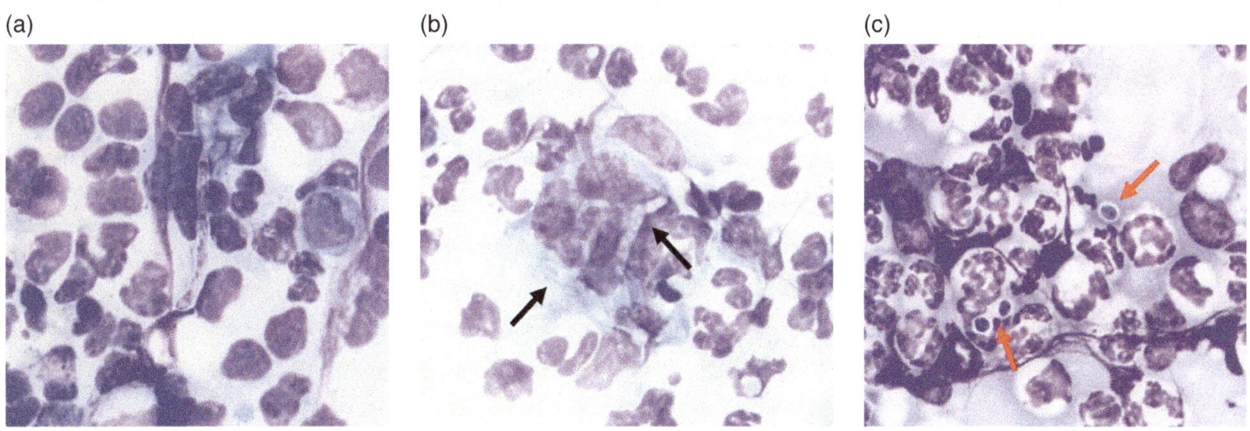

Figure 13.4 Fine needle aspirate sample collected from several small eyelid masses in a foal. Many degenerate neutrophils with rare macrophages and multinucleated giant cells are seen. (a) Basophilic staining fungal hyphae. (b) Nonstaining fungal hyphae within a multinucleated giant cell (*black arrows*). (c) Three arthrospores (*red arrows*). Fungal culture later confirmed as *Trichophyton* sp. Wright–Giemsa, 100× objective.

noninfectious but secondary infections may occur. Grossly, the lesions are on the edge of the eyelid, small, yellow to white, and often painful. On cytological examination, there are numerous nondegenerate neutrophils and macrophages (Figure 13.5). Some Meibomian gland epithelial cells may be seen but can be difficult to differentiate from macrophages.

Demodex spp. are presumed to inhabit the hair follicles and Meibomian glands of the eyelids and rarely may cause mild blepharitis [41]. Microscopic evaluation of Meibomian gland secretions (by gentle expression) or alopecic areas of the eyelid (via skin scraping) can reveal *Demodex* mites, which are species specific. Inflammation may be mild but predominated by neutrophils. Additionally, these mites may be incidental findings in samples collected from the eyelid or cornea (Figure 13.6).

Pemphigus foliaceus is another consideration for pustules on the eyelid with marked neutrophilic inflammation and no apparent bacteria. Cytological examination may reveal large numbers of nondegenerate neutrophils and acantholytic cells. Acantholytic cells are squamous epithelial cells that have lost intercellular connections to other cells and appear cytologically as densely basophilic, individual, round to oval cells. Small numbers of acantholytic cells can be seen with a variety of etiologies (e.g., bacterial dermatitis, dermatophytosis). Increased numbers of these

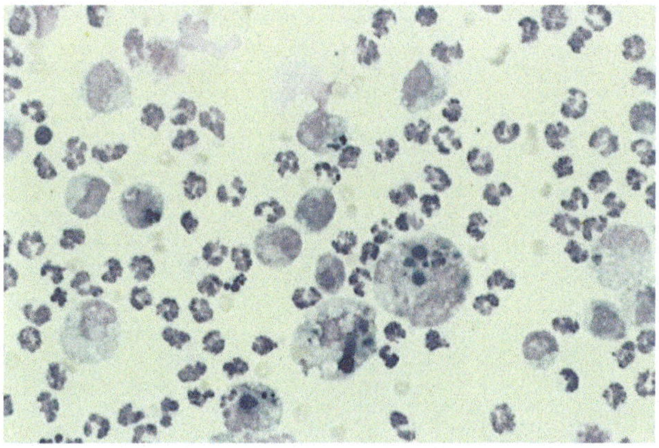

Figure 13.5 Fine needle aspirate sample from a chalazion. Many nondegenerate neutrophils with fewer foamy macrophages are seen. *Source:* Image provided by Drs Elizabeth A. Giuliano and Cecil P. Moore.

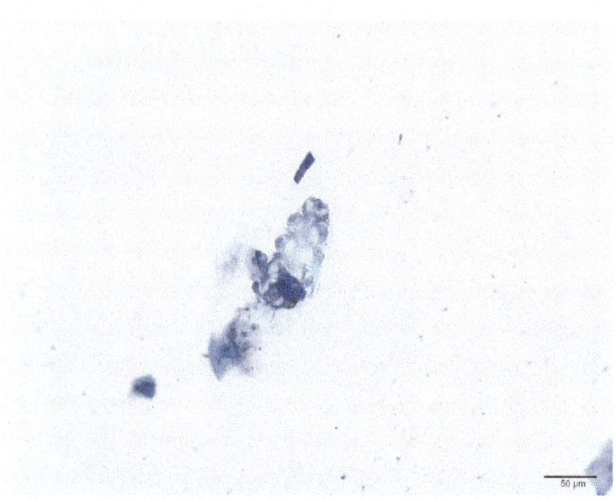

Figure 13.6 Corneal scraping from an adult horse with a history of corneal squamous cell carcinoma. One *Demodex* mite is depicted as an incidental finding from the neighboring Meibomian glands or hair follicles. Modified Wright. *Source:* Image courtesy of Dr Alexandra Myers.

cells can be suggestive of an immune-mediated process such as pemphigus foliaceus; however, the diagnosis of pemphigus foliaceus requires multiple biopsies of intact pustules and histological examination.

13.3.1.2.2 Eosinophilic Inflammation Eosinophil-predominant inflammation can be seen with habronemiasis, eosinophilic granuloma, and less commonly with fungal infections. Additionally, large numbers of eosinophils can be observed with mast cell tumors in horses. Mast cell tumors are discussed in further detail below.

Habronemiasis is caused by the larva of the nematodes *Habronema muscae*, *H. microstoma*, and *Draschia megastoma* [41]. When house and stable flies deposit larva around the eye, severe granulomatous inflammation occurs. Common locations for ocular granulomas include eyelids, third eyelid, medial canthus, and conjunctiva. The granulomas are often proliferative, ulcerated, exudative, pruritic, and painful (Figure 13.7a) [42, 43]. Fine needle aspiration, conjunctival scraping, or impression smears with cytological evaluation of these granulomas would reveal mixed cell inflammation with a predominance of eosinophils, neutrophils, and mast cells (Figure 13.7b) [43]. Biopsy with histological examination is more likely to reveal parasitic larva (Figure 13.7c) [42].

Eosinophilic granulomas are rare, typically firm, well-demarcated, round nodules with no ulceration or hair loss [24]. Fine needle aspirations typically reveal large numbers of eosinophils with fewer macrophages, mast cells, and reactive fibroblasts. This cytological appearance can be similar to habronemiasis but the gross appearance can typically differentiate habronemiasis from eosinophilic granulomas [24].

13.3.1.3 Neoplastic Lesions

Common eyelid tumors in the horse include squamous cell carcinoma (SCC) and sarcoid [5, 29, 44, 45]. Less common eyelid tumors include papilloma, melanoma, lymphosarcoma,

(a) (b) (c)

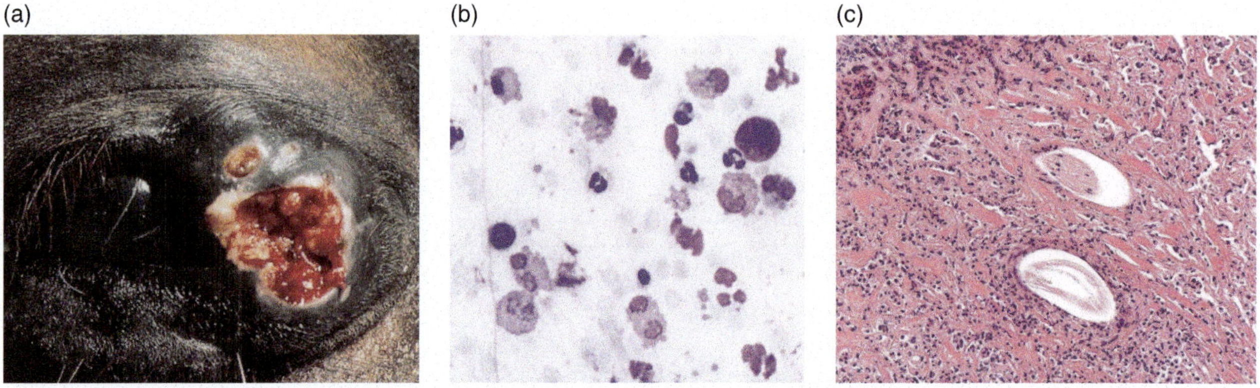

Figure 13.7 (a) Habronemiasis is characterized by nonhealing, raised, ulcerated lesions containing yellow, caseous, gritty nodules. *Source:* Image courtesy of Drs Elizabeth A. Giuliano and Cecil P. Moore. (b) Fine needle aspiration of these lesions will exfoliate eosinophils, neutrophils, and well-granulated mast cells (separate case). (c) H&E histopathology sample of an eosinophilic granuloma. Cross-sections of *Habronema* nematodes surrounded by lakes of degranulated eosinophils (separate case). *Source:* Image courtesy of Dr Andrés de la Concha-Bermejillo.

hemangioma, hemangiosarcoma, perivascular wall tumors (e.g., hemangiopericytoma), fibroma, fibrosarcoma, mast cell tumor, adenoma, myxosarcoma, and basal cell carcinoma [5, 44, 46, 47]. When neoplastic lesions are suspected in the ocular and periocular tissues, thorough palpation of regional lymph nodes and cytological evaluation may be indicated.

13.3.1.3.1 Squamous Cell Carcinoma Horses at higher risk for SCC are Paints, Appaloosas, Haflingers, quarter horses, Thoroughbreds, Belgian draft horses, and any horses with poorly pigmented eyelid margins [2, 5, 48–50]. SCCs can have varying gross appearances depending on the duration and progression of the neoplasm (Figure 13.8a). They can be small, white, elevated plaques or exophytic masses with distinct margins, or they can be larger, pink, ulcerated masses with irregular margins. Ocular SCCs are locally invasive and can have a high recurrence rate after treatment (~42%) [5, 51]. Metastasis is rare with reports ranging from 6% to 15% but can occur to the lung or regional lymph nodes [51].

Squamous cell carcinomas tend to be highly exfoliative with fine needle aspiration, providing modest to large numbers of cells for cytological evaluation (Figure 13.8b). Cells are most commonly arranged as single cells but variably sized, cohesive, sometimes disorganized clusters are also seen. Cell borders are variably distinct. The presence of elongated squamous cells, or tadpole cells, may increase suspicion for SCC but nuclear atypia is still required to diagnose malignancy [52].

The amount of cytoplasm present may vary depending on the degree of differentiation of the neoplasm [52]. More well-differentiated tumours will have many angular cells with lower N:C ratios; however, the N:C ratio is still increased compared to normal squamous cells and rounded squamous epithelial cells are still present. Poorly differentiated tumors will have increased round cells with higher N:C ratios [52]. Marked anisocytosis (variation in cell size) is typically common. Colorless refractile perinuclear cytoplasmic granules are commonly observed and may be increased in SCCs compared to reactive (nonneoplastic) populations. Dyskeratosis (dark staining cytoplasmic rings encircling the nucleus) may be observed [52]. Emperipolesis, the presence of intact cells (typically neutrophils) within the cytoplasm, may be seen. Anisokaryosis (variation in nuclear size) is common and multinucleation may be observed. Rounded squamous epithelial cell nuclei will typically have coarse chromatin and multiple prominent nucleoli. Macronuclei (>5 μm) may also be observed. Mitotic figures may or may not be present (Figure 13.8c). Secondary neutrophilic inflammation is commonly observed with SCCs, especially with concurrent ulceration and secondary bacterial infections. Although the general guidelines are to have at least five criteria of malignancy before making a diagnosis of malignant neoplasia, the overall cytological and clinical findings need to be considered.

Most of the cytological findings described above (emperipolesis, tadpole cells, dyskeratosis) are not pathognomonic for SCC and can be seen with reactive populations as well. Squamous epithelial cells can display significant cytological atypia due to benign hyperplasia and dysplasia secondary to inflammation. Therefore, a cytological diagnosis of SCC should only be made by an experienced pathologist when there is significant cellular atypia and a compatible clinical presentation. Other lesions that may exfoliate squamous epithelial cells include benign hyperplastic lesions, keratinizing cysts and neoplasms, papillomas, and carcinomas with squamous differentiation. With the exception of carcinomas with squamous differentiation, the remainder of these lesions should contain squamous epithelial cells with minimal nuclear atypia [52]. Distinguishing SCC from

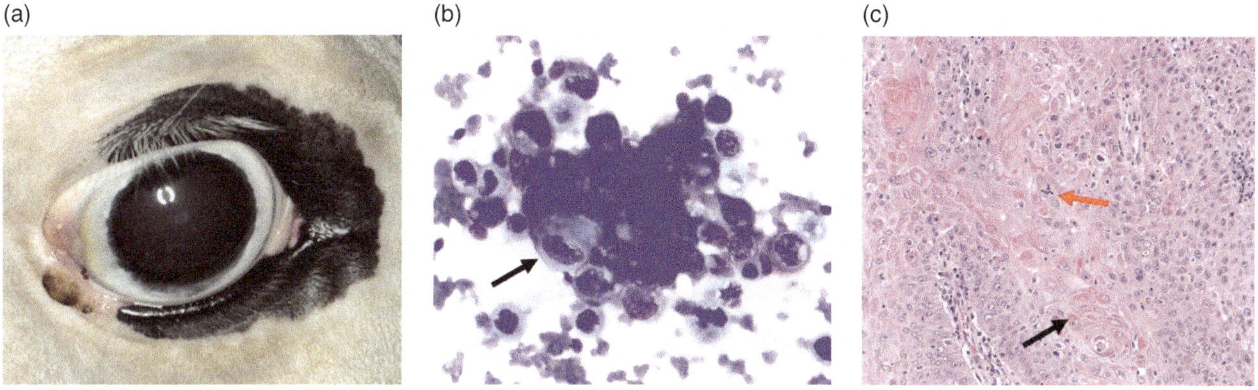

Figure 13.8 Squamous cell carcinoma. (a) SCC affecting the lower eyelid and bulbar conjunctiva of a paint horse. The lower eyelid lesion is slightly raised and is erosive, forming crusts. The conjunctival lesion is raised and vascular. Both presentations are common. (b) Fine needle aspiration of a separate eyelid SCC. Disorganized cluster of epithelial cells with anisocytosis, anisokaryosis, high N:C ratio cells, keratinization (*black arrow*), and perinuclear granulation. Wright–Giemsa, 50× objective. (c) H&E biopsy sample. Numerous neoplastic squamous cells with keratinization (*black arrow*), disorganization, and large mitoses (*red arrow*). *Source:* Image courtesy of Dr Andrés de la Concha-Bermejillo.

carcinomas with squamous differentiation can sometimes be difficult even with biopsy and histological examination, depending on the sample type, quality of the specimen, and morphology of the neoplastic cells.

When a diagnosis of SCC is made, evaluation of regional lymph nodes may be warranted. Studies in other species have shown that bilateral lymph node removal and histopathology are required to rule out metastasis [53]. However, this aggressive work-up is not always clinically and financially feasible. Cytological examination of regional lymph nodes may provide some valuable diagnostic information with minimally invasive methods, especially if regional lymph nodes are enlarged or firm.

13.3.1.3.2 Sarcoid Sarcoids are common in the eyelids and periocular regions (Figure 13.9a). These are cutaneous tumors of fibroblastic origin [5, 44]. They can have a wide range of gross appearances but alopecia and secondary ulcerations and surface infections are common. Sarcoids are considered locally invasive but do not metastasize [5, 44]. Biopsy with histological examination is required for definitive characterization of mesenchymal cell lesions; however, cytological evaluation can provide preliminary information and rule out other processes.

Aspiration of sarcoids typically provides low to modest numbers of spindled mesenchymal cells (Figure 13.9b). The mesenchymal cells are spindled to rarely plump and contain a small to rarely moderate amount of light blue cytoplasm. Cells most commonly contain a single, centrally located oval nucleus but binucleation may be seen. Concurrent mixed cell inflammation may be observed, especially with ulcerated lesions. It should be noted that mesenchymal cells from various types of lesions (benign reactive fibroplasia, peripheral nerve sheath tumors, fibroma, sarcoids, etc.) can appear similar cytologically. Characterization of mesenchymal cell populations is a major challenge of cytological examination and misdiagnoses can be common with both novice and experienced microscopists.

13.3.1.3.3 Other Eyelid Neoplasms Lymphoma of the eyelid most often presents clinically as a nonpainful, diffuse thickening of the eyelid and palpebral conjunctiva (Figure 13.10a) [54]. This form of lymphoma is often associated with high rates of mortality relative to horses with other forms of extraocular lymphoma (e.g., lymphoma of the cornea, third eyelid, or nodular forms of conjunctival lymphoma), which all seem to be more amenable to excision [54–58].

Cytologically, a normal lymphoid population should be heterogeneous with a predominance of small, well-differentiated lymphocytes. Lymphocyte size can be determined by comparing lymphocytes to neighboring red blood cells (RBCs) and neutrophils. Small lymphocytes will typically have a nucleus about the size of 1–1.5 equine RBCs. The equine neutrophil is approximately 12 μm in diameter. Immature lymphocytes are typically 12–15 μm in diameter. Unlike other neoplasms, the cytological diagnosis of lymphoma is often based on the size of lymphocytes and not on standard criteria of malignancy. A predominance of immature lymphocytes (>50%) in multiple areas of (preferably) multiple slides and sources is consistent with lymphoma.

(a) (b)

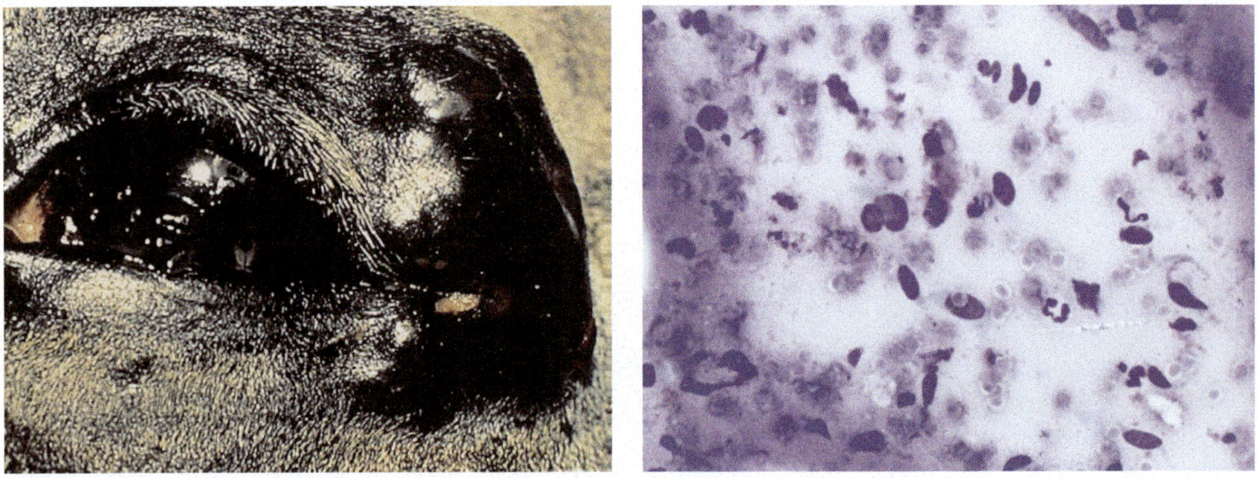

Figure 13.9 Equine sarcoid. (a) Sarcoids can present as darkly pigmented masses and should not be assumed to be melanomas. *Source:* Image courtesy of Drs Elizabeth A. Giuliano and Cecil P. Moore. (b) Fine needle aspirate sample from a periocular sarcoid in a different patient. Cytological examination reveals many poorly preserved but mildly atypical mesenchymal cells. Biopsy with histological examination was performed to confirm the diagnosis since many mesenchymal cell lesions can appear similar on fine needle aspiration samples. Wright–Giemsa, 50× objective.

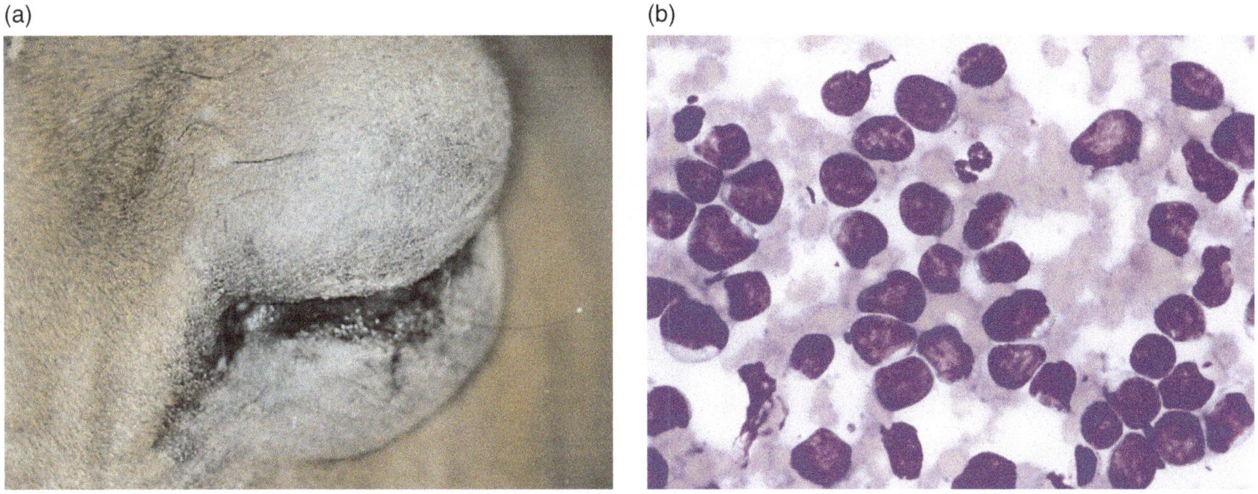

Figure 13.10 Representative images of two separate horses with eyelid swellings from lymphoma. (a) Gross appearance of eyelid swelling attributable to lymphoma. *Source:* Image courtesy of Dr Christopher Murphy. (b) Cytological appearance of lymphoma. Note the vast majority of immature lymphocytes that are larger than the neutrophil. Diff-Quik® stain, 100× objective.

In horses, some lymphomas may be more heterogeneous, limiting the cytological diagnosis. However, when intermediate to large cells predominate, a confident diagnosis can be made on cytological specimens (Figure 13.10b). Additional information on lymphoma in horses can be found in Chapter 15.

Melanomas are typically slowly progressive, pigmented, hemispheric eyelid masses, more commonly observed in older or gray horses (Figure 13.11a) [5]. Melanocytic tumors limited to the dermis in horses are typically benign but local or deep invasion or malignant melanomas may occur. Excisional removal of the mass is typically curative. Fine needle aspirations of melanocytic tumors typically provide large numbers of neoplastic cells (Figure 13.11b). The cells are typically round to oval to pleomorphic and are arranged as single cells with fewer dense aggregates. Well-differentiated melanocytes contain numerous dark green to black cytoplasmic melanin granules. These granules may limit evaluation of cellular and nuclear detail (Figure 13.11c). The absence of cytological atypia does not rule out a malignant process. Cytological features of malignant melanomas may include frequent mitotic figures, marked anisokaryosis, coarse chromatin, and one or multiple prominent nucleoli. With standard cytology slide preparation, these characteristics would only be detectable in specimens that contain poorly pigmented melanocytes.

Papillomas (warts) are the main viral-induced lesions of the eyelid and are most commonly seen in young horses. Papillomas are typically small, exophytic dermal growths that may regress within a few months [24]. Cytologically, papillomas exfoliate uniform, squamous epithelial cells with occasional mild mixed cell inflammation. Squamous

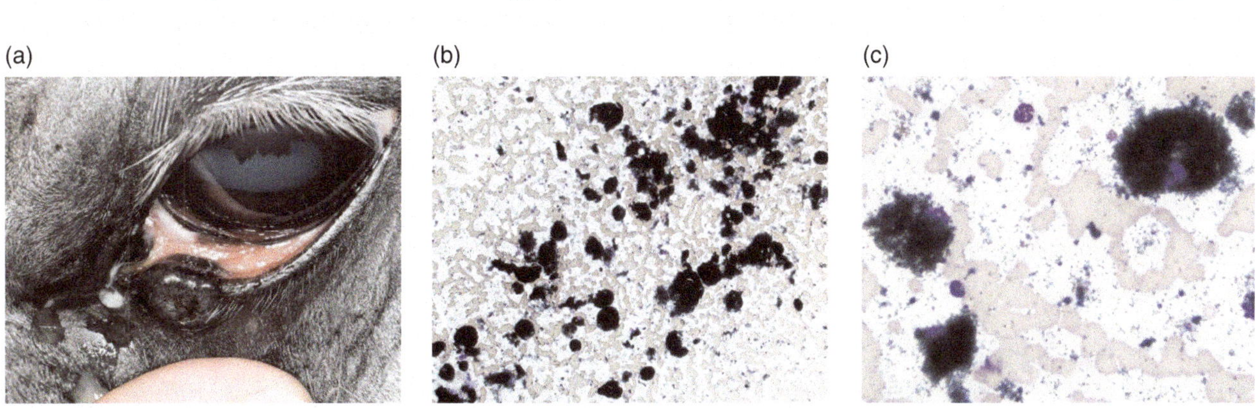

Figure 13.11 Melanoma of the eyelid. (a) The melanoma shown here is invading the lower canaliculus and puncta, blocking the nasolacrimal duct. *Source:* Image courtesy of Dr Erin Scott. (b,c) Same case. Fine needle aspirate from a melanocytic tumor on the eyelid. Wright-Giemsa stain. (b) Low magnification (20× objective) shows numerous, heavily pigmented melanocytes. (c) Higher magnification (100× objective) shows three variably sized melanocytes. Nuclear detail cannot be evaluated due to the abundance of granules, which is a common finding. There are numerous free melanin granules throughout the background.

(a) (b)

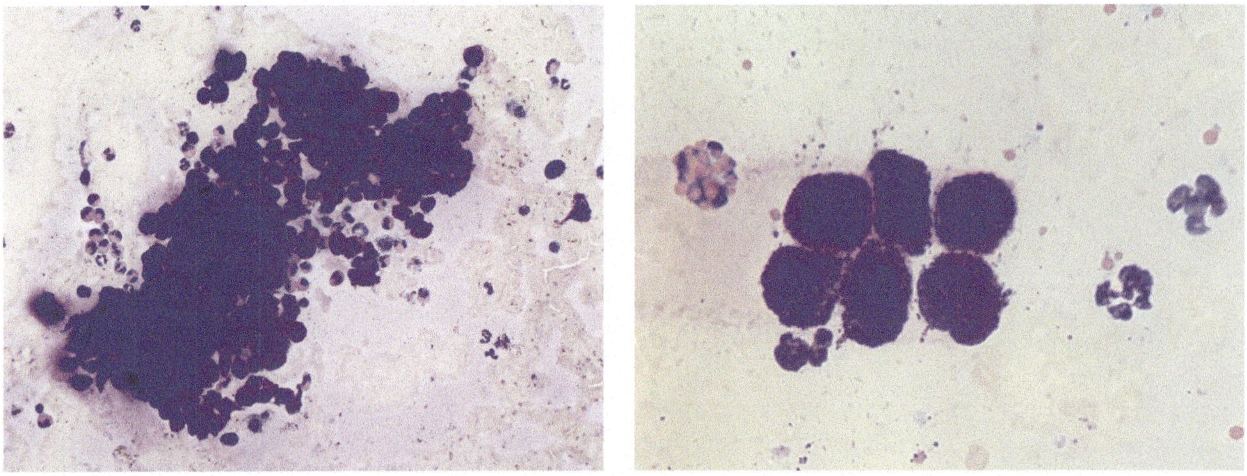

Figure 13.12 Periocular mast cell tumor in a horse. (a) Low magnification (20× objective) demonstrates large dense aggregates of highly granulated mast cells (dark magenta with round central nucleus) and eosinophils (pink with lobulated nucleus). (b) Higher magnification (100× objective) shows an aggregate of six well-granulated mast cells with fewer nondegenerate neutrophils and one eosinophil. Wright–Giemsa stain.

epithelial cells may contain a larger, round nucleus and a large amount of eosinophilic cytoplasm with peripheralized, sometimes concentric eosinophilic material.

A diagnosis of hemangioma cannot be made cytologically. The gross appearance of the mass may suggest a benign tumor of vascular origin (small, raised, red, well demarcated, and slowly growing). Cytological examination can support the clinical suspicion when there is hemodilution (without evidence of platelets to suggest iatrogenic hemorrhage) and no evidence of inflammation or atypical cells. The diagnosis of hemangioma or hemangiosarcoma is often made histologically [59–62]. However, cytological evaluation may reveal increased numbers of large basophilic atypical mesenchymal cells, hemodilution, and neutrophil pooling to support a diagnosis of hemangiosarcoma. Periocular superficial vascular malformations (e.g., orbital varices) resembling vascular eyelid tumors have been reported in the horse presenting as eyelid masses [63].

Soft tissue sarcomas such as peripheral nerve sheath tumors (e.g., schwannoma) and perivascular wall tumors (e.g., hemangiopericytomas) have been reported in the eyelids of horses [47, 64]. Although the cytological appearance of these tumors has not yet been described in this species, histological findings (and presumably, cytological findings) are similar to those described in dogs [47]. Cytologically, peripheral nerve sheath tumors and perivascular wall tumors are exfoliative, resulting in large numbers of mildly to moderately atypical mesenchymal cells with veil-like cytoplasm and occasional crown cells.

Mast cell tumors limited to the dermis or subcutaneous tissues are considered benign in horses, with surgical excision being curative. Spontaneous regression may also rarely occur [65]. Mast cells have round nuclei (versus basophils or eosinophils) and typically contain many magenta cytoplasmic granules, which may obscure the nucleus (Figure 13.12a,b). However, poorly granulated mast cell tumors do occur and granules do not always stain with in-clinic staining methods. When utilizing a diagnostic laboratory, submission of an unstained preparation is always helpful, especially if there is clinical concern for a mast cell tumor. Mast cell tumors in horses typically have infiltrates of few to many eosinophils. The predominance of eosinophils and rarity of mast cells may limit cytological diagnosis of mast cell neoplasia in some cases. When mast cells predominate, or when they are commonly observed in dense aggregates, a confident cytological diagnosis can be made. At that point, excisional biopsy with histological examination can be performed for curative intent and for further diagnostic information (e.g., infiltration).

13.4 Conjunctiva

13.4.1 Normal Anatomy and Cytological Findings

Nearly the entire surface of the equine conjunctiva is stratified columnar to cuboidal epithelium [28]. The palpebral and bulbar edges have more stratified squamous epithelium [28]. Cytobrush sampling of the conjunctiva of healthy horses provides mostly deep and intermediate epithelial cells with fewer superficial (squamous) cells and rare goblet cells and inflammatory cells [28].

Superficial cells from the stratified columnar to cuboidal epithelium (most of the conjunctiva) will appear polygonal to cuboidal on cytological preparations with a modest to large amount of pale basophilic cytoplasm and a centrally to eccentrically located nucleus (Figure 13.13a) [24, 28]. In comparison to superficial cells, intermediate cells have less cytoplasm, increased cytoplasmic basophilia, and an increased nucleus:cytoplasm (N:C) ratio. Deep conjunctival epithelial cells are round to slightly cuboidal and have a high N:C ratio with a scant amount of medium basophilic cytoplasm (Figure 13.13b). Melanin granules are occasionally observed in the cytoplasm of conjunctival epithelial cells [28].

In horses, goblet cells of the conjunctiva are in highest concentration from the nasal to the temporal edge of the inferior conjunctiva in the upper palpebral segment near the fornix (where the palpebral and bulbar conjunctivas meet) and in a part of the nasal fornix [28]. Goblet cells can be better identified with impression cytology using a cellulose filter in horses [10, 22]. Cytologically, goblet cells appear as large round to oval cells with many cytoplasmic vacuoles or blue to red granules (depending on quantity and stain), which often displace the nucleus [24]. Clinically, the enumeration of goblet cells is most important for evaluation of keratoconjunctivitis sicca, which is very rare in horses and can often be diagnosed with other means (e.g., Schirmer tear test).

Individual types of white blood cells (WBCs) typically make up less than 1% of the nucleated cell population in cytological preparations [10, 28]. As in other species, the conjunctiva demonstrates an arrangement of lymphoid cells that mirrors mucosa-associated lymphoid tissue (MALT) in other tissues (e.g., gastrointestinal, oropharyngeal, bronchial tissues). As such, the conjunctiva-associated lymphoid tissue (CALT) is arranged into two distinct patterns: diffuse lymphoepithelial and follicular arrangements. Follicles and crypt-like structures (capable of trapping debris/foreign bodies) are present within the ventral conjunctival fornix, but are arranged most densely within a patch of lymphoid tissue that can be viewed macroscopically on the bulbar surface of the third eyelid. Lymphocytes are thus expected in cytological preparations of any normal conjunctiva and are expected to vary in density according to the location of sample collection [28, 66]. The number and proportion of WBCs in cytological specimens should always be considered in light of the amount of hemodilution (blood) present.

Normal equine conjunctiva contains normal flora such as predominantly gram-positive bacterial and fungal organisms [67, 68]. Therefore, very rare bacterial and fungal organisms could be observed if cytological evaluation was performed on normal tissue from this area or in noninflammatory or infectious lesions. Due to the environment of horses, plant material is also occasionally observed (Figure 13.1a,b). Several studies have evaluated conjunctival normal flora in horses from various areas around the world [69–74].

13.4.2 Inflammatory Lesions

13.4.2.1 Neutrophilic Inflammation

Neutrophil-predominant inflammation is most commonly observed with bacterial infections, typically secondary to another disease process (Figure 13.14). The most common bacteria identified in cases of conjunctivitis and keratitis in horses are presented in Table 13.1. Primary conjunctivitis has been reported to occur with *Moraxella equi*, short

(a) (b)

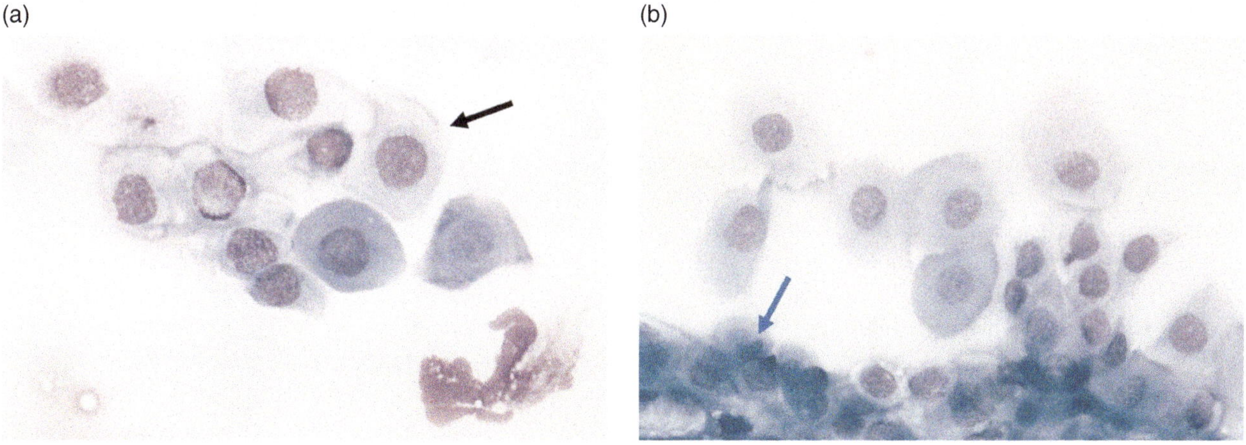

Figure 13.13 Normal conjunctival scrape. (a) Superficial epithelial cells (*black arrow*) are polygonal to irregularly shaped, have a low N:C ratio with a moderate to large amount of pale basophilic cytoplasm and a centrally located round nucleus. (b) Basal or parabasal cells (*blue arrow*) are epithelial cells from the deeper layers. These cells are more round, with deeper basophilic cytoplasm, and a higher N:C ratio. Note the lack of inflammatory cells. *Source:* Images courtesy of Drs Elizabeth A. Giuliano and Cecil P. Moore.

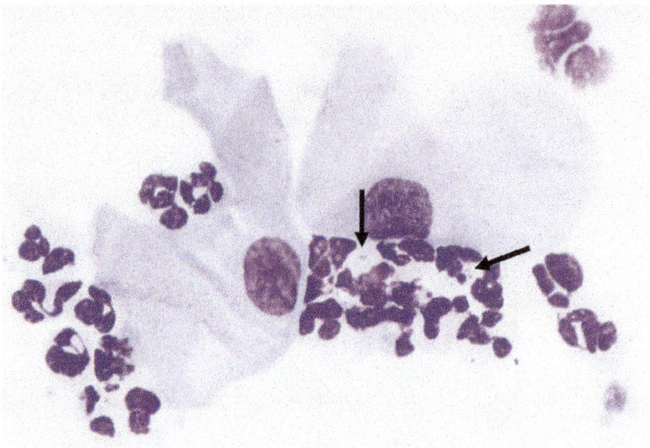

Figure 13.14 Septic conjunctivitis. Many degenerate neutrophils with degraded intracellular bacteria (*black arrows*) and two uniform superficial squamous epithelial cells. Wright–Giemsa, 100× objective.

Table 13.1 Gram staining reactions in bacterial conjunctivitis and keratitis.

Staining and morphological characteristics	Most probable causative agent
Gram-positive	
Cocci – singly or in clusters	*Staphylococcus* spp.
Cocci – in chains	*Streptococcus* spp.
Rod-shaped	*Bacillus* spp.
Filamentous/branching	*Actinomyces spp.*
Gram-negative	
Cocci – diplococci or coccobacilli	*Moraxella* spp.
Rod-shaped	*Pseudomonas aeruginosa*, *E. coli*, *Enterobacter* spp.

gram-negative coccobacilli typically seen in pairs or short chains on cytological preparations [24]. *Chlamydia* spp. can also cause conjunctivitis and has a unique cytological morphology of mostly perinuclear structures in the cytoplasm of conjunctival epithelial cells, which has been described in other species [24, 75]. Structures begin as a few solitary discrete basophilic to magenta elementary bodies (~0.5 µm) and eventually aggregate into larger bodies (~3 µm) [75].

13.4.2.2 Lymphocytic Inflammation

Conjunctivitis with a substantial lymphocyte component can be seen with a variety of etiologies such as pseudotumors, foreign body granulomas, chronic irritation/trauma, thelaziasis, and viral disease (e.g., adenovirus, equine herpesvirus) [3, 4, 76]. Lymphocytic infiltrates can also be observed in certain neoplasms such as angiosarcomas/lymphangiosarcomas [46]. Additionally, there can be

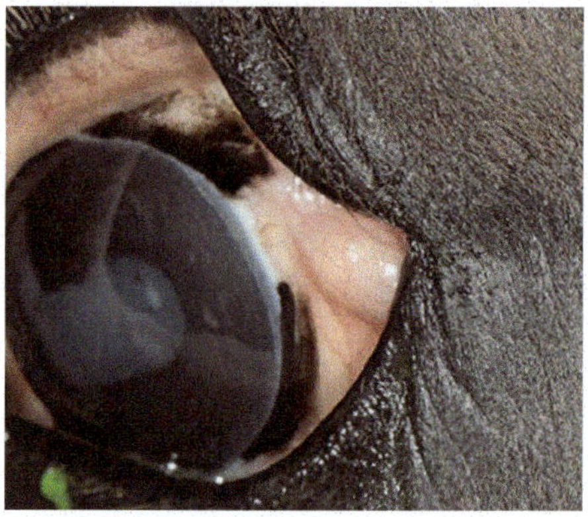

Figure 13.15 Pseudotumor, also known as nodular lymphoid hyperplasia, of the bulbar conjunctiva. This lesion is raised and partially obscured by the lateral canthus. These lesions can resemble nodular forms of conjunctival lymphoma in the horse.

aggregates of lymphocytes in the lamina propria near the fornix in apparently healthy equine eyes [28]. Therefore, low numbers of lymphocytes in cytological specimens collection from this area should not be overinterpreted.

Conjunctival pseudotumors have been described in horses. Ocular pseudotumors are proliferative inflammatory lesions involving the eye, adnexa, or orbit that grossly mimic neoplasms (Figure 13.15) [3]. Pseudotumors can be unilateral or bilateral [4]. Although the cytological features have not yet been characterized, based on the histological findings, cytological evaluation could lessen the suspicion for neoplasia as the lesions are composed predominantly of small lymphocytes with occasional macrophages, immature lymphocytes, and plasma cells.

Adenovirus infections in immunodeficient Arabian foals can cause mucopurulent rhinitis and conjunctivitis [77]. Intranuclear inclusion bodies may be observed microscopically as deep red-purple structures that marginate chromatin [24]. Macrophagic, lymphocytic, and neutrophilic inflammation are common.

Equine herpesvirus 2 and 5 (EHV-2, EHV-5) are common in all horses and may contribute to keratoconjunctivitis, especially in young horses [76, 78]. This viral infection may be considered in young horses with conjunctivitis predominated by small lymphocytes. PCR can be used to detect the presence of the virus. However, EHV-2 and EHV-5 can be detected by PCR on ocular tissue samples in clinically healthy horses and efforts to correlate this viral infection with specific ocular disease have not been demonstrated [76, 78, 79]. Therefore, the diagnosis should not be made on a positive PCR sample alone.

13.4.2.3 Eosinophilic Inflammation

Causes of conjunctival lesions that typically have substantial numbers of eosinophils include onchocerciasis, habronemiasis, thelaziasis, mast cell tumors, eosinophilic granuloma, hypersensitivity reactions, fungal infections, and eosinophilic keratoconjunctivitis. Habronemiasis, mast cell tumors, and eosinophilic granulomas are described in the eyelid section and cytological findings would be similar with conjunctival samples. Eosinophilic keratoconjunctivitis is discussed in the cornea section.

Onchocerca cervicalis microfilaria may be found in the eyelid, perilimbal cornea, palpebral conjunctiva, and anterior chamber (Figure 13.16a). Onchocerciasis is common and can be seen in horses throughout most of the United States [41]. Interestingly, clinically normal animals may have ocular microfilaria, and the presence of microfilaria is not always associated with an inflammatory response [41]. Clinical findings associated with onchocerciasis may include chemotic and hyperemic conjunctiva, follicular conjunctivitis, corneal opacities and keratitis, and uveitis [41]. Raised whited nodules in the pigmented conjunctiva next to the temporal limbus and depigmented areas in the bulbar conjunctiva near the temporal limbus are suggestive of microfilaria [24, 80].

Cytological evaluation of infected tissue may confirm the presence of microfilaria. Standard cytological preparations (dried and stained) will reveal mixed cell inflammation, typically with an eosinophil and mast cell component. Microfilaria can be rarely observed in standard cytological specimens. When onchocerciasis is suspected, a wet mount preparation may increase the odds of visualizing microfilaria. A small piece of conjunctiva tissue (procedure described above in sample collection) can be placed on a glass slide with a drop or two of warm saline. The specimen should be kept warm and examined on low magnification periodically for up to one hour (Figure 13.16b) [80]. *O. cervicalis* microfilaria are unsheathed, 200–240 μm in length and 4–5 μm in diameter, and have short tails [24].

Thelaziasis is caused by the nematode *Thelazia lacrymalis*. This nematode can be found in the conjunctival fornix of horses and is mostly considered a commensal organism [41]. Although most horses are asymptomatic, blepharitis, conjunctivitis, and keratitis can occur. Whilst diagnosis typically involves macroscopic visualization of the parasite, cytological preparations of associated lesions may demonstrate lymphocytic and eosinophilic inflammation.

Fungal infections limited to the conjunctiva are very rare and fungal conjunctivitis is typically observed with fungal keratitis or with systemic fungal infections. Cytological findings may include marked mixed cell inflammation with neutrophils, macrophages, and eosinophils. *Blastomyces*, *Cryptococcus*, and *Histoplasma* spp. may infect the conjunctiva and nasolacrimal system but these infections are quite rare and more often reported outside the United States [24]. A variety of opportunistic fungi have the potential to cause conjunctivitis.

Fungal organisms are also considered normal flora or transient inhabitants of the equine eye. In one study, fungal organisms were isolated from the conjunctiva in 94% of clinically normal horses from Florida [67]. The most common fungal organisms isolated from these animals were *Aspergillus*, *Fusarium*, *Penicillium*, *Alternaria*, and *Cladosporium* spp. [67] Therefore, fungal cultures are best performed in conjunction with cytological examination to ensure compatible inflammation and potentially intracellular fungal organisms. Fungal infections are discussed in more detail in the cornea section.

13.4.3 Neoplasia

Primary conjunctival tumors are uncommon but can include SCC, melanoma, lymphoma, papilloma, hemangioma, hemangiosarcoma, and angiosarcomas [24, 46, 81–83].

(a)

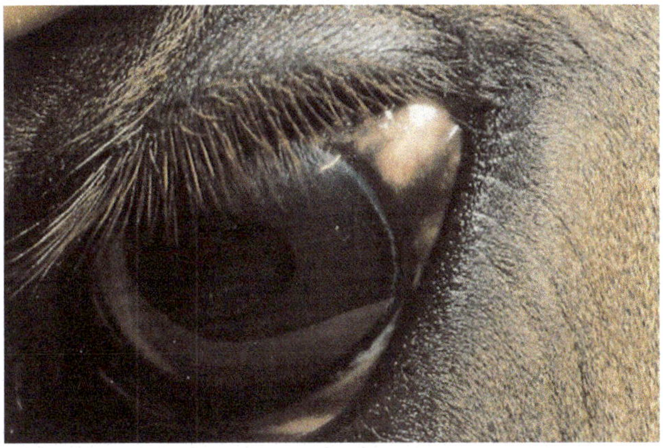

(b)

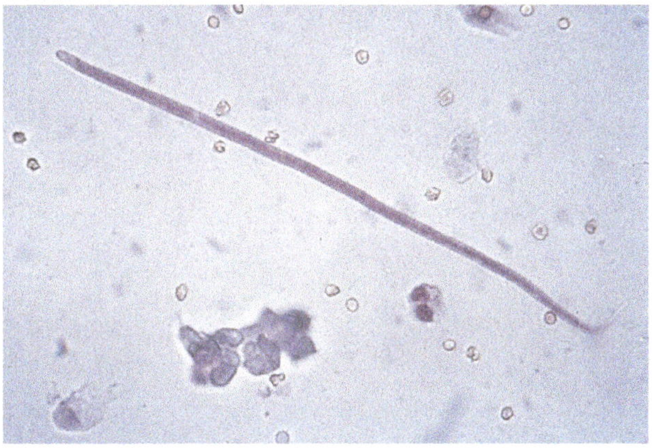

Figure 13.16 Onchocerciasis. (a) Onchocercal hypersensitivity reaction in the perilimbal bulbar conjunctiva. (b) *Onchocerca* microfilaria observed in minced conjunctival specimen. *Source:* Images courtesy of Drs Elizabeth A. Giuliano and Cecil P. Moore.

The cytological appearance of these tumors would be like those described in the eyelid section above.

In contrast to the relatively benign behavior of melanomas in the eyelid and limbus, conjunctival melanomas tend to be more aggressive in other species, and in one reported case in a horse [81]. Therefore, more aggressive clinical work-up may be warranted, such as aspiration of regional lymph nodes and rapid, wide excisional removal [81]. Although the cytological appearance of aggressive conjunctival melanomas has not been described, the histopathological findings have included marked pleomorphic cells, with high N:C ratios, multinucleation, and variable amounts of cytoplasmic melanin. These features would be recognizable cytologically in poorly granulated cells and may allow for cytological characterization of these more aggressive neoplasms. In highly pigmented specimens, a cytological diagnosis of melanocytic neoplasm can be made and excisional biopsy with histological examination can then be performed for further diagnostic information and for curative intent.

Melanin granules are occasionally observed in the cytoplasm of normal conjunctival epithelial cells [28]. Additionally, pigmented SCCs have been reported in the equine conjunctiva [84]. Therefore, the diagnosis of melanoma should not be based solely on the presence of a grossly pigmented tumur or only on the microscopic identification of melanin pigment. Fine needle aspiration of pigmented masses can provide rapid information and can support or lessen the suspicion for a true melanoma.

Conjunctival angiosarcoma (malignant endothelial cell neoplasm with unknown origin) has been described cytologically [82]. The lesion was exfoliative, providing large numbers of pleomorphic spindled to polygonal mesenchymal cells with round to oval nuclei with fibrous chromatin and one to three large nucleoli. Cells contained a variable amount of basophilic cytoplasm, with phagocytosis or emperipolesis of RBCs or lymphocytes.

13.5 Nictitating Membrane

13.5.1 Normal Anatomy and Cytological Findings

The nictitating membrane arises from the medial canthus and is composed of cartilage surrounded by conjunctiva. The cytological findings from the normal nictitating membrane would be like those described in the conjunctival section. The free margin of the nictitating membrane may be pigmented so melanin pigment may be observed in cytological specimens collected from this area. The bulbar surface typically contains lymphoid follicles so lymphocytes and some plasma cells are not unexpected in cytological specimens [24, 66].

13.5.2 Inflammation

Inflammatory lesions of the nictitating membrane are typically observed with conjunctivitis (considerations described above).

13.5.3 Neoplasia

Common tumors of the nictitating membrane include SCC and lymphoma [5, 51]. Other reported neoplasms include mast cell tumors, hemangiosarcoma, lymphangiosarcoma, and lacrimal gland adenocarcinomas [5, 46, 62, 85]. The cytological appearance of most neoplasms of the nictitating membrane would be similar to that described above (see eyelid neoplasia). Tumors on the nictitating membrane can often be surgically excised for curative intent with minimal consequences. Cytological evaluation may provide valuable information about the lesion before surgical excision, such as the need for lymph node evaluation, ideal surgical margins, premedications (e.g., diphenhydramine for mast cell tumors), etc.

Lymphoma involving the nictitating membrane can appear as a discrete nodule or as a diffuse swelling of periocular tissues (e.g., conjunctiva and eyelids) [5]. Horses with discrete nodular lymphoma in the nictitating membrane can have a good prognosis with surgical resection [55, 58].

13.6 Cornea and Sclera

13.6.1 Normal Anatomy and Cytological Findings

The superficial cornea is composed of stratified squamous epithelial cells. The intermediate layer is the stromal layer, which is composed of collagen. The deepest layer of the cornea is Desçemet's membrane, which is composed of collagen and a deep layer of endothelial cells.

Normal superficial corneal epithelial cells are large polygonal cells with distinct borders and contain a large amount of pale basophilic cytoplasm surrounding a centrally located, small round nucleus with finely stippled chromatin and indistinct nucleoli (Figure 13.17a). These cells are typically observed in large sheets when collected with debridement techniques (see section 13.2.2). Deep (e.g., basal) corneal epithelial cells are round and have a high N:C ratio with a scant amount of medium basophilic cytoplasm (Figure 13.17b). Deep corneal epithelial cells are

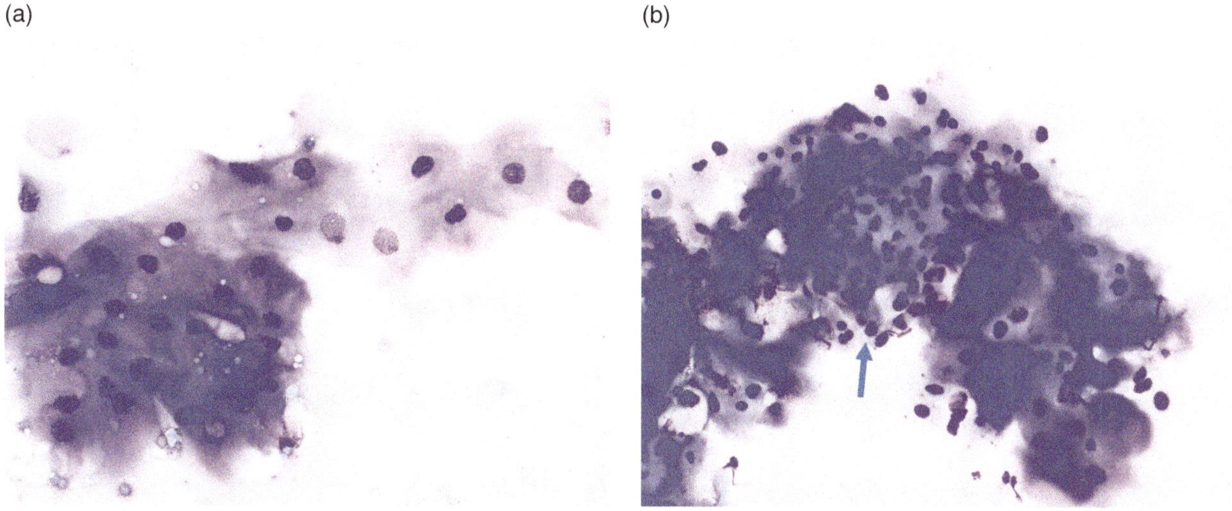

Figure 13.17 Normal cornea. Scrapings of a normal cornea may reveal only low numbers of uniform squamous epithelial cells. (a) Superficial cells are polygonal to irregularly shaped, have a low N:C ratio, and a moderate to large amount of pale basophilic cytoplasm and a centrally located round nucleus. (b) Basal and parabasal cells from the deeper layers (*blue arrow*) would be more round with a higher N:C ratio and typically more basophilic cytoplasm. However, these cells are still uniform. Note the lack of inflammatory cells. Wright–Giemsa, 50× objective.

expected to be observed with deep debridement collection and should be interpreted as dysplastic or neoplastic populations in the absence of nuclear atypia. Pigmented epithelial cells may be observed in corneal epithelial cells from the limbus or with chronic inflammation/irritation (Figure 13.18d). Low numbers of bacteria, fungi, and plant material would be expected as transient inhabitants of the healthy equine precorneal tear film (Figure 13.1a–e).

13.6.2 Inflammatory Lesions

There are a variety of cytological changes that can occur with chronic corneal inflammation or irritation. Corneal epithelial cells can display mild to moderate atypia with chronic irritation/ulceration and with attempted healing (Figure 13.18a,b). Additionally, mineralization or pigmentation of the cornea may occur, and these changes can be seen cytologically (Figure 13.18c,d). It is important to recognize that these changes occur with inflammation, and not only with neoplastic processes.

13.6.2.1 Neutrophilic Inflammation

Corneal damage can occur with a variety of etiologies, from trauma to keratoconjunctivitis sicca. Damage to the cornea allows infections from normal flora or environmental bacteria or fungus. Infectious agents can exacerbate the severity of ulcerative keratitis or form stromal abscesses. In horses with ulcerative keratitis, infectious agents were more readily identified in cytology samples collected with the handle edge of a scalpel blade than in samples collected with the Kimura spatula or cytobrush techniques [23].

Cytological examination in conjunction with bacterial culture can provide valuable information for the treatment and management of bacterial keratitis. Cytological examination should reveal numerous neutrophils with some intracellular bacteria (Figure 13.19). This supports the diagnosis of a true bacterial infection versus culture growth of normal flora or contaminants. Additionally, gram staining can be used to retrieve rapid information to aid in the identification of the bacterial populations present. Bacterial keratitis is most commonly caused by the bacteria listed in Table 13.1. However, many additional bacteria can cause keratitis in horses (e.g., *Clostridium*, *Corynebacterium* spp., *Klebsiella* spp., *Listeria monocytogenes*) [29, 86, 87].

When using cytology as a predictor of bacterial culture results, the sensitivity can be low (approximately 50% in one study) [88]. In other words, the lack of detectable bacteria in a cytological preparation does not rule out bacterial growth in a culture. This is somewhat expected as culture is considered a more sensitive test, as a larger number of bacteria need to be present for cytological detection. The specificity of cytological examination as a predictor of culture results is improved at 80% [88], meaning that, when bacteria are found in cytological specimens, bacterial growth is more likely to occur.

There are several situations that can result in a negative culture even though bacteria are seen in cytological specimens. First, there are many structures that can mimic bacteria to novice microscopists such as melanin granules, stain precipitate, proteinaceous debris, ultrasound gel, and medicinal residues (Figure 13.1b). Additionally, negative cultures can occur with preanalytical error (e.g., poor

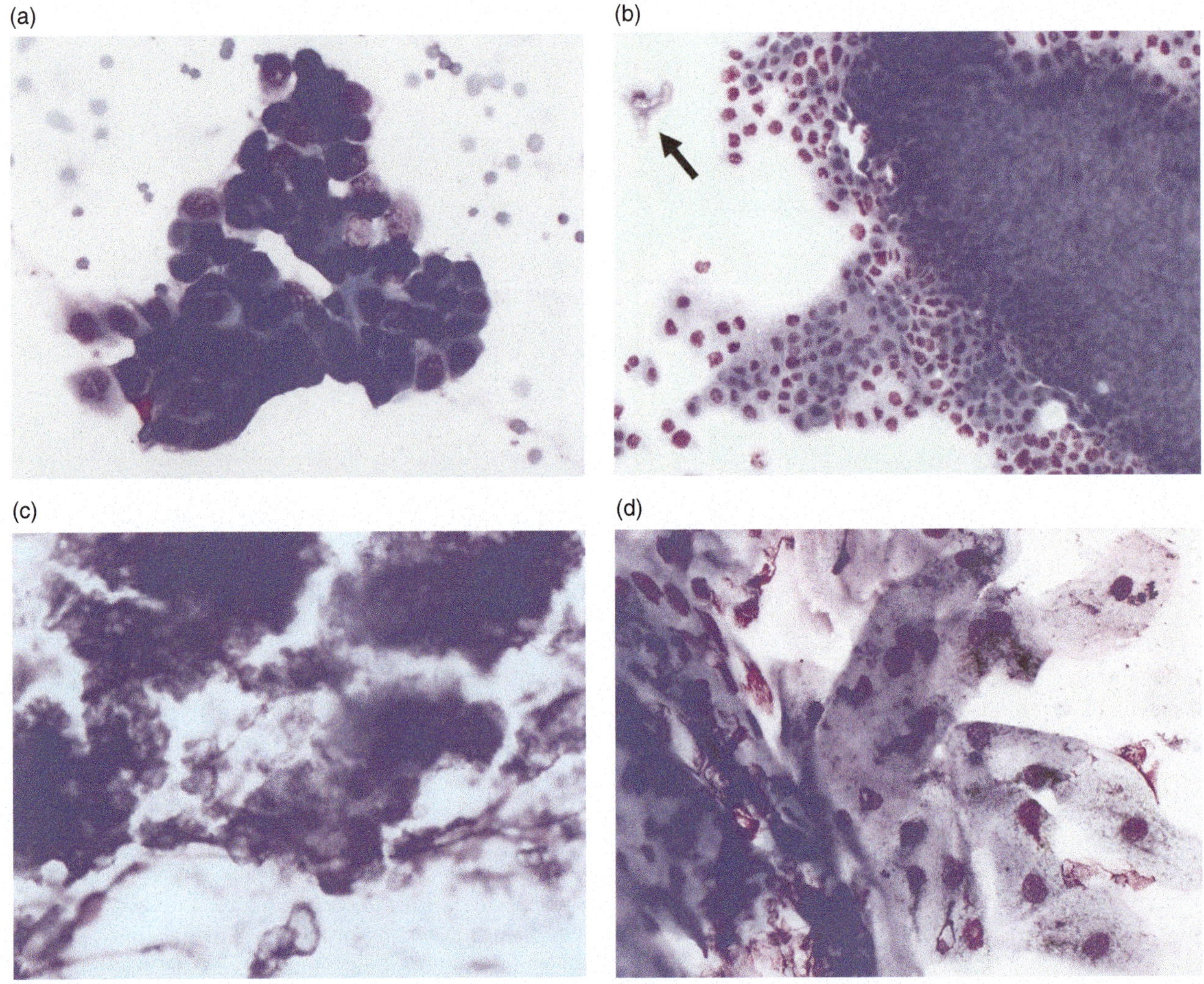

Figure 13.18 Changes to cornea with chronic inflammation or irritation. (a,b) Increased numbers of basal cells and mild atypia secondary to hyperplasia and dysplasia from chronic corneal ulceration. Note fungal hyphae (*black arrow*). (c) Mineralized debris. Chronic inflammation can lead to mineral keratopathy, where mineral builds up in the cornea. (d) Squamous epithelial cells with cytoplasmic melanin pigment. Pigmentation can also occur with chronic irritation. Additionally, the squamous epithelial cells near the limbus may contain some pigment normally. These cells should not be mistaken for a melanocytic neoplasm. Wright–Giemsa.

sample quality, inappropriate shipping or handling, nonviable bacteria) or analytical (laboratory) error. Lastly, some bacteria are fastidious and difficult to grow on cytological specimens.

On the other hand, bacteria may be cultured when no bacteria were reported on cytological examination. This can occur when only small numbers of bacteria are present (below the detection limit of cytology), either normal flora or pathogenic bacteria. When significant neutrophilic inflammation is present in cytological specimens, this supports a bacterial etiology. However, differentiation between primary and secondary bacterial infections cannot always be achieved.

Fungal keratitis is most common in warm, humid regions of the United States and is typically diagnosed with cytology, fungal culture, or, more recently, fungal PCR [89, 90]. Fungal organisms are considered normal flora of the equine eye [67]. Therefore, fungal cultures and/or PCR are best performed in conjunction with cytological examination. This will ensure there is compatible inflammation, potentially intracellular fungal organisms, and no other etiological agents or atypical cells. Additionally, fungus can be difficult to culture and fungal cultures can be negative even when fungal organisms are seen on cytological or histological examination [86].

Ulcerative fungal keratitis occasionally demonstrates highly specific clinical characteristics that should prompt collection of samples for cytology, fungal culture, and PCR. Diatomaceous fungal species are capable of elaborating pigment within fungal plaques (e.g., biofilms), which can present with marked

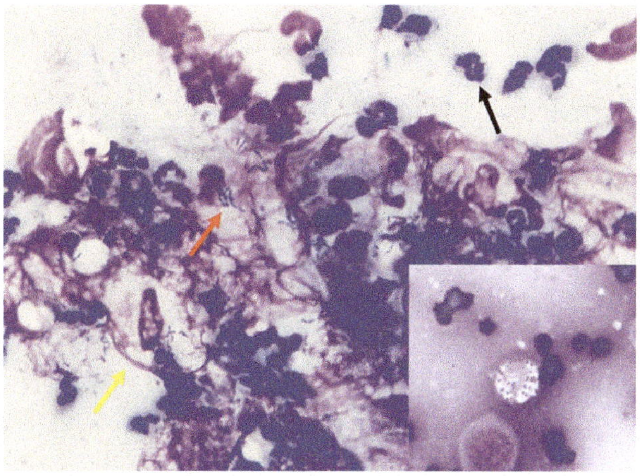

Figure 13.19 Bacterial keratitis. Numerous short rod-shaped bacteria (*red arrow*) and degenerate neutrophils (*black arrow*). Note streaming nuclear material from lyzed cells (*yellow arrow*), not to be confused with fungal hyphae. One degenerate neutrophil with many intracellular diplococci bacteria and one rod-shaped bacterium (*inset image*). Wright–Giemsa.

variation, but are easily recognized whenever brown pigment is associated with corneal ulceration (not to be confused with corneal perforation and secondary iris prolapse) (Figure 13.20a,b). Fungal organisms are known to migrate away from the site of corneal ulceration, often forming discrete white foci of infection/abscessation that are termed "satellite lesions" (Figure 13.20c). A third pattern of fungal keratitis is known specifically as subepithelial keratomycosis, which demonstrates a subtle, stippled, white appearance over the cornea regionally or diffusely (Figure 13.20d) [91, 92].

Fungal keratitis can be caused by opportunistic infections of normal flora (e.g., corneal trauma) or from contaminated foreign bodies [86]. Cytological findings include marked neutrophilic inflammation and fungal organisms, which are often observed in thick areas of inflammatory cells (Figure 13.21a,b). It is important to scan on both low and high magnification when searching for fungal organisms. The most common organisms to cause fungal keratitis in horses (e.g., *Aspergillus* spp.) are typically filamentous, branching, septated hyphae which may be basophilic or nonstaining. The exact genus of fungi cannot be determined with cytology alone.

If fungal organisms are not observed on cytological specimens but fungal keratitis is a concern, additional diagnostic tests can include GMS stains or fungal culture. GMS preparations can work well on previously stained slides with proper destaining and processing techniques. Additionally, fungal organisms are often found within the deepest layer of the cornea (Desçemet's membrane) and therefore, repeat collection may be needed [25, 89].

The most commonly isolated fungi in horses with fungal keratitis in the United States have been reported as *Aspergillus* and *Fusarium* spp. [89, 93, 94] Similar fungal organisms are observed most commonly in Texas. Other fungi reported to cause fungal keratitis in horses include, but are not limited to, *Mortierella wolfii*, *Candida*, *Cylindrocarpon*, *Curvularia*, *Cystodendron*, *Penicillium*, *Pseudallescheria*, *Mucor*, and *Histoplasma* spp. [89, 95–99]

Fungal keratitis caused by *M. wolfii* has been reported in Japan [99]. On cytological evaluation, these organisms were nonseptated hyphae, making them distinct from some of the more common causes of fungal keratitis (e.g., *Aspergillus* and *Fusarium* spp.) [99]. Outside the United States, histoplasmosis has rarely been reported as a cause of keratitis in horses [98]. Due to the unique morphology, histoplasmosis can often be confidently identified with cytological evaluation alone (see Chapter 12).

13.6.2.2 Eosinophilic Inflammation

Eosinophilic keratitis is diagnosed when there are compatible clinical signs and cytological findings [100–102]. The exact cause of eosinophilic keratitis is unknown but a hypersensitivity reaction is presumed. The disease is more commonly diagnosed in the summer [100, 101]. Common clinical signs of eosinophilic keratitis include blepharospasm, conjunctival hyperemia, chemosis, and proliferative yellow to white corneal opacities with associated mucoid discharge (Figure 13.22a) [100–102]. Secondary corneal ulcers, fungal and bacterial infections may also occur [100, 102]. Cytological evaluation of corneal samples reveals inflammatory cells, predominantly eosinophils or approximate equal proportions of eosinophils and neutrophils (Figure 13.22b) [100]. Other nucleated cells may also be observed such as mast cells, macrophages, and epithelial cells.

Parasitic diseases that can cause primary or secondary corneal lesions include onchocerciasis, thelaziasis, and habronemiasis. Corneal opacities and keratitis can be seen with onchocerciasis, and corneal scrapings may reveal mixed cell, eosinophilic inflammation and possible microfilaria [24, 41]. Habronemiasis can result in large granulomas of the eyelids, third eyelid, and conjunctiva, mutating the normal conformation of the eye, and may result in secondary corneal lesions (e.g., ulceration, dry eye). Additionally, *Habronema* sp. granulomas can be quite pruritic, potentially resulting in trauma and corneal ulceration. Additional information on these parasitic organisms are found in the eyelid and conjunctiva sections above.

13.6.3 Neoplasia

The most common corneal tumor in horses is SCC, which typically arises at the limbus and grows across the cornea (Figure 13.23a,b) [5, 24]. Grossly, the tumors typically appear as sessile, raised, pale pink masses with a

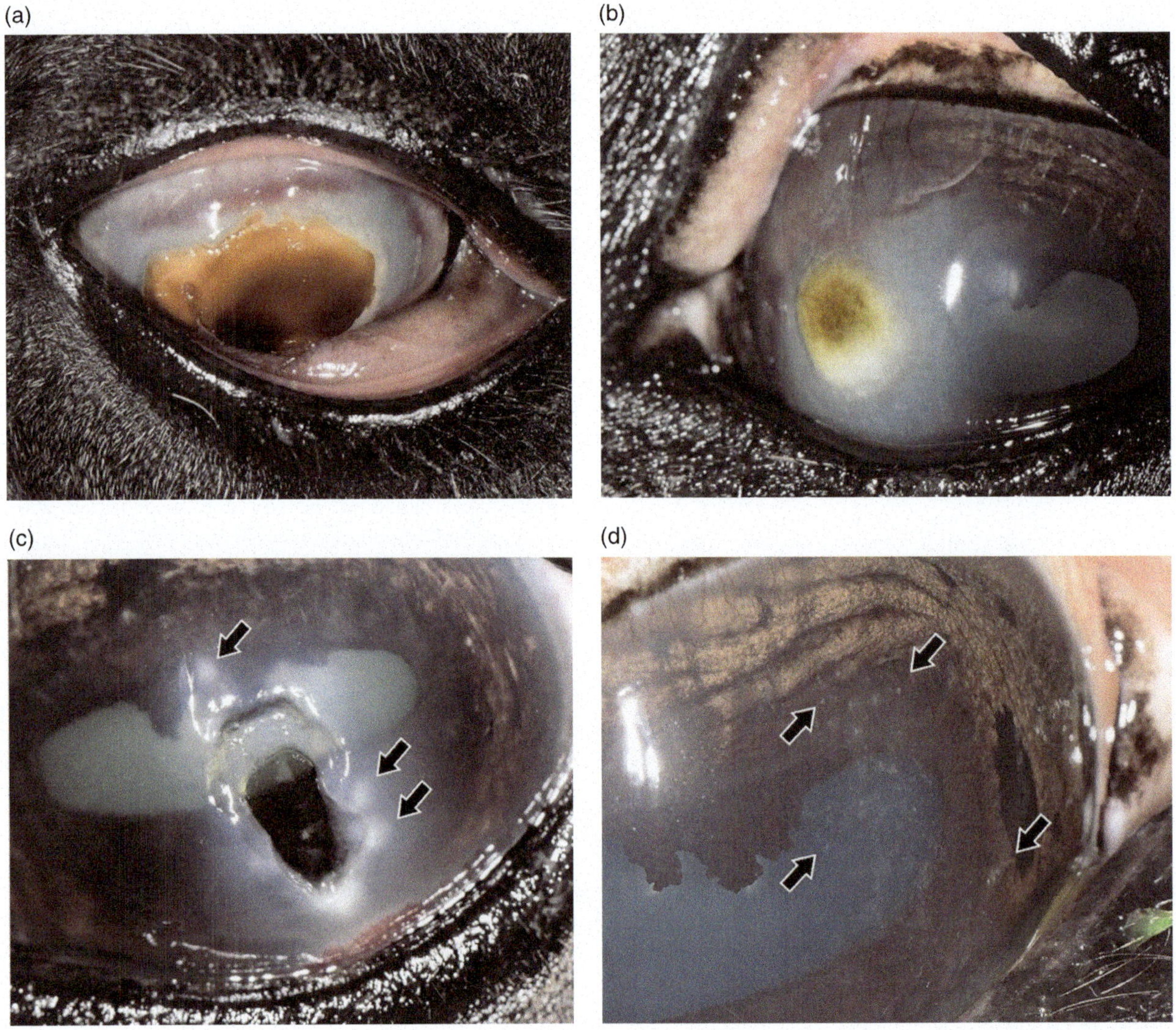

Figure 13.20 Fungal keratitis. Fungal infection of the cornea can produce several patterns of disease that should prompt collection of corneal cytology and culture. (a,b) For instance, certain types of fungi (i.e., diatomaceous species.) can elaborate pigment within dense, raised fungal plaques. (c) Fluffy white corneal opacities (*arrows*), known as satellite lesions, surround a descemetocele in which *Aspergillus* sp. was cultured. (d) Subepithelial keratomycosis is a more subtle form of fungal keratitis in which faint white opacities (*arrows*) are present within or below the corneal epithelium.

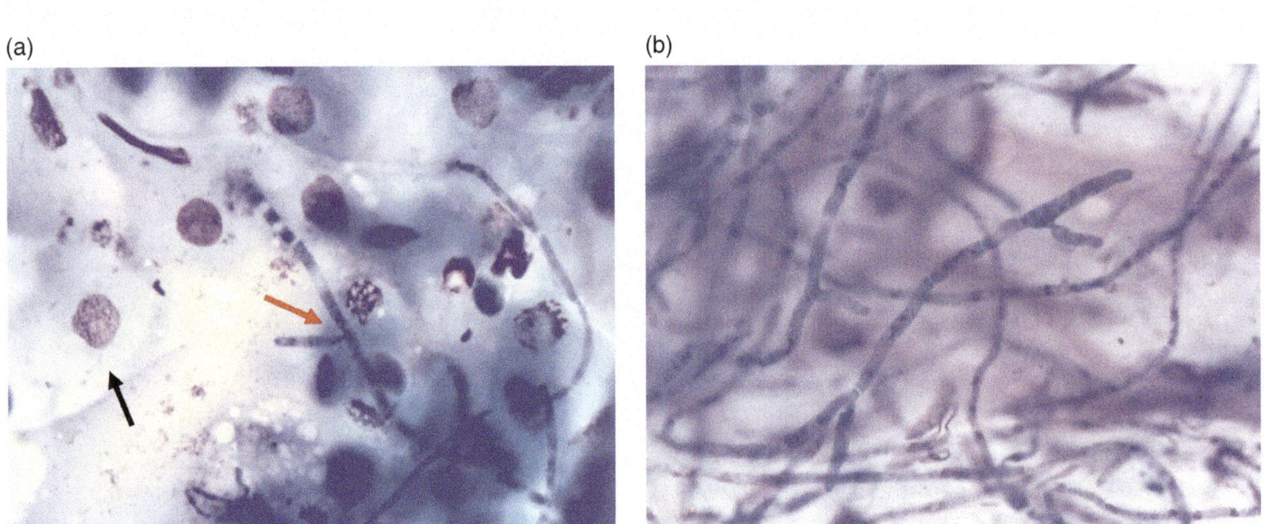

Figure 13.21 Cytological findings of fungal keratitis. (a) Basophilic staining, septate, fungal hyphae with occasional branching (*red arrow*) admixed with normal cornea squamous epithelial cells (*black arrow*). Wright–Giemsa. (b) Large mat of fungal hyphae with similar branching and septation. Modified Wright. *Source:* Image courtesy of Dr Samantha Schlemmer.

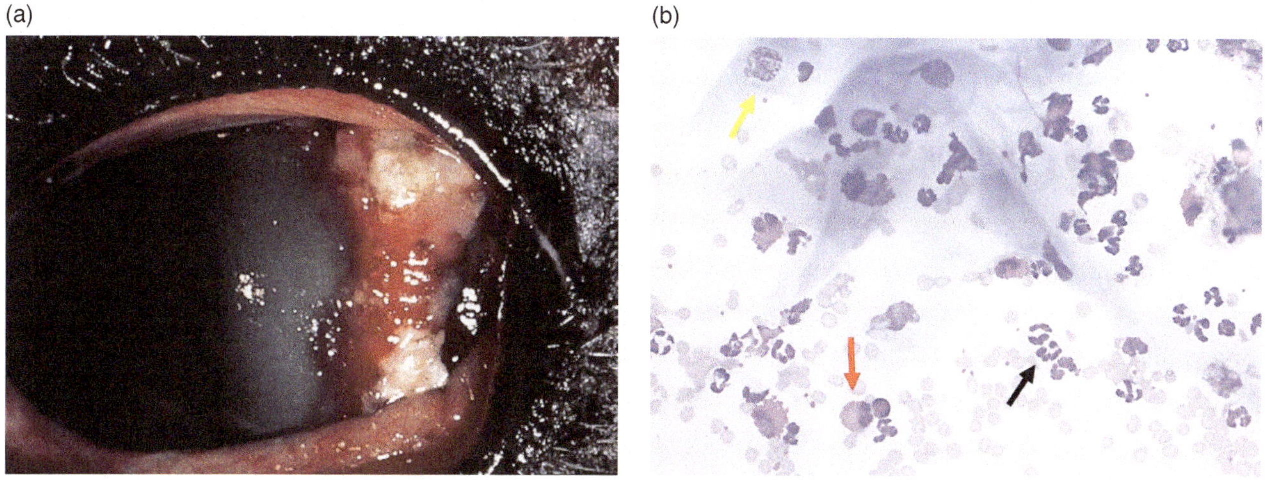

Figure 13.22 Two cases of eosinophilic keratitis. (a) Gross image of equine eosinophilic keratitis at the temporal limbus with characteristic white surface plaques. *Source:* Image courtesy of Drs Elizabeth A. Giuliano and Cecil P. Moore. (b) Cytological findings of eosinophilic keratitis. Increased numbers of eosinophils (*red arrow*) and neutrophils (*black arrow*) with fairly unremarkable squamous epithelial cells (*yellow arrow*). *Source:* Image courtesy of Dr Kathryn Jacocks.

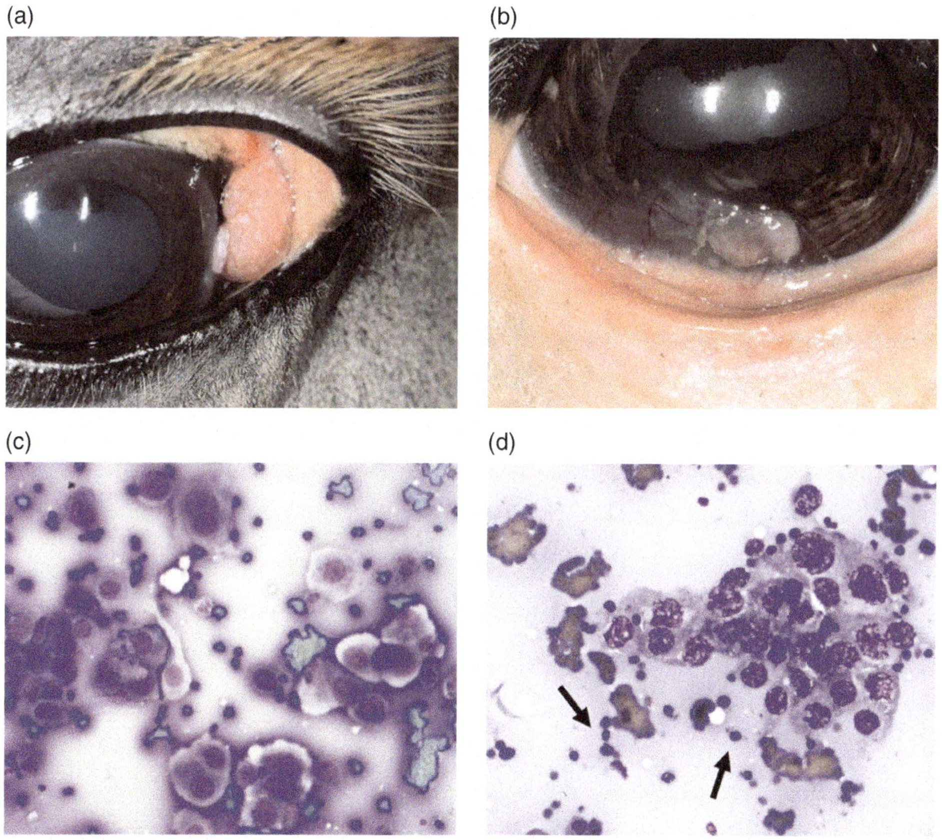

Figure 13.23 Corneal squamous cell carcinoma. (a,b) Temporal and ventral limbus SCC. *Source:* Images courtesy of Dr Erin Scott. (c) Cytological findings from a biopsy-confirmed case of corneal SCC. Note the variation in cell sizes, tadpole/elongated cell, binucleated cells, variation in nuclear sizes, prominent nucleoli, and variable N:C ratios. Diff-Quik stain, 50× objective. (d) Fine needle aspirate sample of the mandibular lymph node of a different case of corneal SCC. There is a modestly sized cluster of somewhat degraded squamous epithelial cells with many small lymphocytes (*black arrows*). There were numerous clusters of epithelial cells, confirming metastasis. Wright–Giemsa.

cobblestone appearance [5]. Other lesions that can appear similar include eosinophilic keratitis, granulation tissue, and other neoplasms [5]. When adequate samples are collected, cytological evaluation can differentiate these lesions (e.g., inflammatory or neoplastic) (Figure 13.23c,d). The cytological appearance of corneal SCCs would be like that described in the eyelid above (see eyelid neoplasia).

Other tumors reported on the ocular surface (cornea, limbus, sclera, or bulbar conjunctiva) include hemangioma, hemangiosarcoma, mast cell tumors, melanoma, peripheral nerve sheath tumur, and lymphoma [5, 46, 57, 62, 103, 104]. Mast cell tumors, melanocytic tumors, and lymphoma can be diagnosed cytologically when the lesions exfoliate large numbers of cells, which they commonly do. Cytological evaluation of hemangioma, hemangiosarcoma, and peripheral nerve sheath tumors can reveal populations of mesenchymal cells but definitive diagnosis often requires biopsy with histological examination. These neoplasms are described in more detail in the eyelid section above.

13.7 Intraocular Structures, Aqueous, and Vitreous Humor

13.7.1 Normal Anatomy and Cytological Findings

Normal aqueous humor should be clear with no flocculent material. There should be low cellularity with only extremely rare small lymphocytes, macrophages, and RBCs. Occasional extracellular melanin granules or melanocytes/melanophages may be observed. The total protein concentration of aqueous humor should be very low (average of approximately 0.06 g/dL or 60 mg/dL) [105]. The rare cells present may be degraded because of the low protein concentration of the sample [105].

Normal vitreous humor should be difficult to aspirate, as collagen fibrils prevent liquefaction and form a semi-solid hydrogel. Vitreous inflammation (hyalitis) and degeneration (hyalosis) promote liquefaction and greater ease of aspiration. When samples are obtained, they should normally possess low cellularity with only rare macrophages seen on cytological evaluation. Extracellular melanin granules may also be observed in normal vitreous humor [35].

Fine needle aspirates of solid intraocular structures are rarely performed *in vivo*, but can be collected *ex vivo* after enucleation of the globe (or postmortem), prior to histopathology, in instances where there is an immediate diagnostic need or an anticipated need for parallel morphological assessment. The reader is directed to other sources for extensive descriptions of intraocular structures and ocular anatomy [29].

13.7.2 Inflammatory Lesions

Uveitis can be seen with a variety of etiologies. An in-depth discussion of equine uveitis is beyond the scope of this chapter. However, cytological evaluation of aqueous humor may provide diagnostic information when supportive care and other diagnostic tests have failed. Additionally, fine needle aspiration of intracellular lesions may be performed for surgical and therapeutic planning.

13.7.2.1 Neutrophilic Inflammation

Neutrophilic inflammation of the aqueous humor manifests clinically as hypopyon, which refers to a dependent settling of white blood cells within the ventral anterior chamber. Hypopyon is a very common inflammatory response to corneal infection known as reflex uveitis, and commonly occurs in association with equine recurrent uveitis (ERU). Neutrophilic inflammation of the vitreous creates a yellow hue within the eye and is commonly associated with ERU. Although ERU is commonly associated with *Leptospira* organisms, culture of aqueous and/or vitreous humor is most often sterile.

Bacterial causes of neutrophilic infiltration into the aqueous or vitreous are possible. Bacterial causes of uveitis are numerous and may include, but are not limited to, any etiological agent resulting in sepsis, *Borrelia burgdorferi* infections, *Rhodococcus equi*, *Streptococcus equi* subsp. *equi*, and *Leptospira* spp. [24, 34, 36, 37, 106]. Paired diagnostic tests may include bacterial culture, related serological tests, and PCR. Thorough consideration of the clinical history and physical exam findings will help guide these ancillary diagnostic tests.

Vitreous humor with neutrophil-predominant inflammation and spirochete bacteria has been reported with *B. burgdorferi* infections [37]. On cytological preparations, these spirochete bacteria were 0.2 μm wide, 10–15 μm long, fine tapered ends and 3–8 loose spirals [37]. The use of silver stain may increase the visibility of spirochete bacteria in cytological specimens. Cytological evaluation can be more sensitive than histological evaluation in the detection of spirochete bacteria in some cases [37]. PCR would be needed to definitively differentiate *B. burgdorferi* spirochetes from tick-borne relapsing fever *Borrelia* and *Leptospira* spirochetes.

Abscesses and granulomas can occur within the equine eye. Iris abscesses are uncommon in the horse but do occur [107]. Iris lesions may or may not be obviously associated with corneal lesions [107]. Fungal infections of the equine lens are rarely reported [107]. Cytological findings of these lesions have not been formally reported but would likely be similar to other samples with fungal infections.

13.7.2.2 Lymphocytic Inflammation

When inflammatory cell infiltrates are predominantly small lymphocytes, chronic inflammation (most often ERU) or viral etiologies may be considered. Viral etiologies are often accompanied by other clinical signs such as respiratory disease or neurological disease. Viral causes of uveitis include adenovirus, EHV-1, equine influenza type A2, equine infectious anemia, and West Nile virus [24, 29, 106, 108]. Cytological examination has limited diagnostic utility for the diagnosis of most viral diseases, which often relies on systemic clinical signs and serological or molecular testing.

13.7.2.3 Eosinophilic Inflammation

Intraocular parasites may include *O. cervicalis* microfilaria, adult *Setaria* spp., and adult *Dirofilaria immitis* [41]. Aspiration of lesions associated with these parasites may reveal mixed cell inflammation with eosinophils, lymphocytes, and macrophages, based on previous reports of histological findings. When parasites are found within the equine eye, consultation with a veterinary parasitologist is recommended.

13.7.2.4 Mixed Cell Inflammation

Mixed cell inflammation in aqueous or vitreous humor or in aspirated material from intraocular lesions can be seen with a variety of etiologies, including those listed above under neutrophilic, lymphocytic, and eosinophilic inflammation.

13.7.3 Neoplasia

Intraocular tumors are rare in horses. Melanoma arising from the iris or ciliary body is the most common intraocular tumor in horses [5]. Less commonly reported tumors of the anterior chamber include medulloepithelioma, metastatic carcinoma, hemangiosarcoma, and primary lymphoma [30, 62, 109–111]. Most of the tumor types found within the eyes of horses inherently exfoliate large number of cells, allowing for cytological characterization. However, obtaining cytological specimens of intraocular specimens does not come without risk, and those risks versus rewards should be considered for each individual case. Cytological evaluation can provide preliminary diagnostic information and aid in surgical planning.

Melanoma would be the primary differential for a pigmented, anterior chamber mass distorting the pupil, especially in a gray horse [5]. Commonly reported sites for intraocular melanomas include choroid, iris, and ciliary body [112]. Intraocular melanomas are mostly considered primary neoplasms with low metastatic potential [5, 112]. Cytological evaluation of these tumurs would reveal a population of cells similar to those described in eyelid melanoma (see eyelid neoplasia).

Medulloepitheliomas are primitive neuroectodermal tumors (PNETs) that arise from embryonal neural tissue and are most commonly benign [110]. They typically arise in the anterior uvea of young horses [110] but can be observed in mature horses as well. Cytologically, these tumors exfoliate well, providing large numbers of poorly differentiated, round, high N:C ratio cells, that are often in dense aggregates. The cells occasionally form pseudorosettes (Figure 13.24a–d). It is important to differentiate PNETs from lymphoma. PNETs will typically be composed of smaller cells in dense aggregates (versus individualized) and have no lymphoglandular bodies (cytoplasmic fragments) in the background.

Lymphoma can be seen as a primary ocular disease or as a multicentric process [24, 30]. Cytological evaluation of aqueous humor may provide a diagnosis of lymphoma as cells commonly exfoliate into neighboring fluid [30]. The cytological appearance of lymphoma would be similar to that described above in the eyelid section. Prolonged contact with fluid can cause cells to swell and nucleoli to become falsely prominent, mimicking a neoplastic or blast population. Therefore, when evaluating fluid samples, it is important to ensure only fresh, intact cells are used to make a diagnosis.

Neoplasms of the posterior segment of the eye include retinoblastoma, choroidal melanoma, astrocytoma, glioma, and oligodendrocytoma [5]. Cytological evaluation of these types of tumors is rare because of the difficulty in obtaining fine needle aspirates and histological examination is often required to make these specific diagnoses.

13.8 Orbital and Retrobulbar Space

Orbital and retrobulbar lesions commonly present with exophthalmos. Causes of exophthalmos can include, but are not limited to, trauma, cellulitis, abscesses, neoplasms, fungal granulomas, and hydatid cysts. In a recent study, approximately half of the cases of retrobulbar disease in horses were caused by extension of a paranasal sinus disease process [113]. Advanced imaging (e.g., ultrasound or computed tomography) is typically utilized to identify and characterize orbital lesions. Retrobulbar disease can be associated with a poor prognosis [113]. Cytological

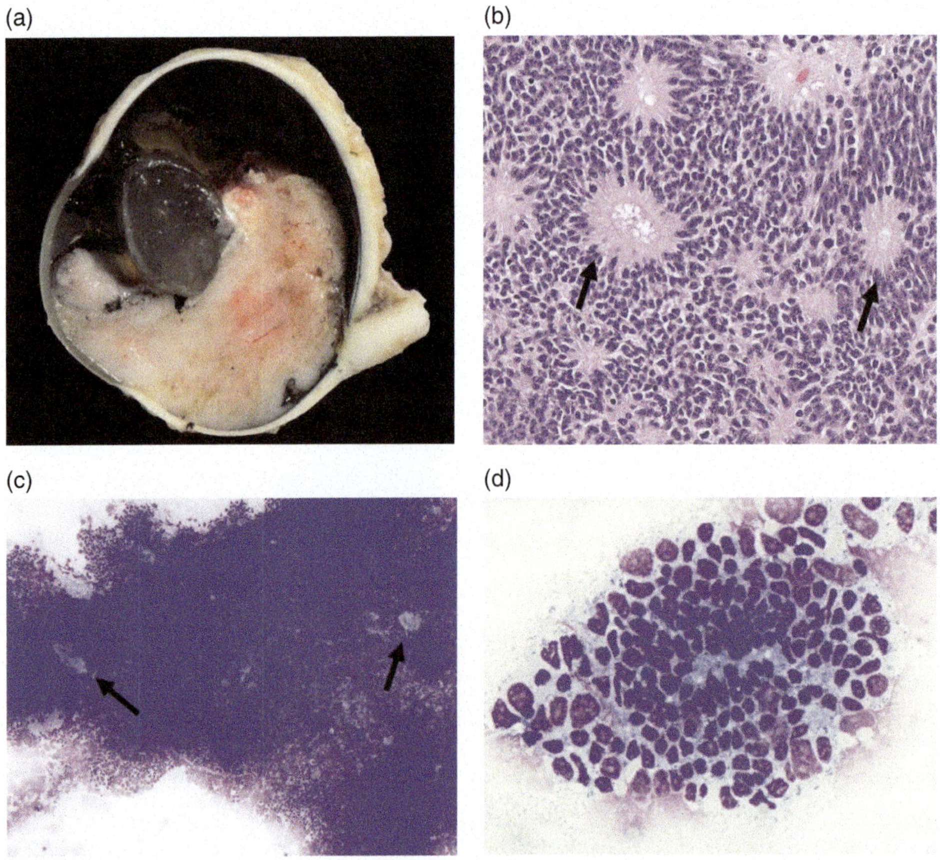

Figure 13.24 Intraocular medulloepithelioma in a 9-year-old Tennessee walking horse gelding. (a) Cross-section of the enucleated eye shows a tan mass encompassing over 50% of the globe. (b) H&E histopathology sample shows neoplastic cells forming characteristic rosettes (*black arrows*). (c,d) Fine needle aspiration of the mass was performed before enucleation for surgical planning. Cytological examination revealed numerous neoplastic cells arranged in dense aggregates with rosette-like arrangements. (*black arrows*). Wright–Giemsa. *Source:* Images courtesy of Dr Erica Beadle.

evaluation of these lesions can provide preliminary information and guide future diagnostic tests.

Clinical signs correlating with orbital or retrobulbar tumors include progressive, nonpainful exophthalmos, strabismus, raised third eyelid, and periorbital swelling [5, 114]. Nonneoplastic orbital masses such as granulomas, hematomas, cysts, and parasitic hydatid cysts must also be considered. Advanced imaging may be required to evaluate growths within the globe or periocular space [2]. Cytological evaluation of orbital masses may provide valuable information before pursuing enucleation.

13.8.1 Noninflammatory Lesions

When an fine needle aspirate of a retrobulbar mass yields no or few nucleated cells, it could indicate a nonrepresentative aspirate, poorly exfoliative lesion, or aspiration of a lipoma or cyst. Lacrimal gland cystic hamartoma and dermoid cysts are rare causes of retrobulbar masses [113, 115]. Cytological evaluation of a retrobulbar dermoid cyst revealed no nucleated cells but a high total protein (>7 g/dL) [115]. Retrobulbar hematomas are rare [116]. Cytological evaluation would likely only reveal blood and possibly macrophages with hemosiderin or phagocytized RBCs.

13.8.2 Inflammatory Lesions

Causes of inflammatory orbital lesions can include trauma, infectious agents (e.g., bacterial, fungal, and parasitic), sterile foreign body reactions, and necrosis. Orbital bacterial abscesses are rarely reported in horses and may occur secondary to foreign bodies or extension from neighboring locations [113, 117, 118]. Cytological evaluation of these lesions is as for abscesses observed anywhere else in the body. Fungal granulomas from *Aspergillus* and *Cryptococcus* spp. have been reported in the orbital space, extending from the sinus cavities [113, 119]. Hydatid cysts from larval forms of *Echinococcus* spp. have been reported in the equine orbit [41, 120]. Cytological evaluation of these lesions should reveal a predominance of inflammatory cells. It should be noted that the lack of neoplastic cells on cytological specimens does not completely rule out neoplasia. Large numbers of inflammatory cells and necrotic cellular debris can be observed with aspiration of large necrotic neoplasms.

13.8.3 Neoplasia

The most common orbital tumors in horses are neuroendocrine tumors, anaplastic sarcomas, and SCC [5, 113, 121]. In one small study of 10 orbital tumors in horses, all tumors were malignant and/or locally invasive [114]. Other orbital tumors are rarely reported such as hemangioma, hemangiosarcoma, fibroma, medulloepithelioma, melanoma, mast cell tumor, lipoma, adenocarcinoma, lymphoma, and malignant rhabdoid tumors [5, 113, 114, 122, 123].

The cytological appearance for equine retrobulbar neuroendocrine tumors (e.g., paraganglioma) has not been described. However, they would likely appear like other neuroendocrine neoplasms. Neuroendocrine neoplasms tend to exfoliate well, providing large numbers of cells for cytological evaluation. The cells are inherently fragile and typically appear as many lyzed nuclei (naked nuclei) on a sheet of lightly basophilic cytoplasm. Intact cells with distinct cytoplasmic margins are observed rarely. The cytological appearance of the other orbital tumors listed above is like those described in the other sections of this chapter.

Since complete surgical removal of orbital tumors can be difficult, if not impossible, cytological evaluation may provide general information to aid in palliative treatment and determine prognosis. Additionally, aspiration of bilateral regional lymph nodes (even if they don't appear enlarged) and thoracic radiographs may provide prognostic information. When neoplastic cells are seen in lymph node aspiration cytology, an abundance of information is achieved. However, the lack of neoplastic cells does not rule out early metastasis.

13.9 Nasolacrimal System

Cytological evaluation of nasolacrimal flush fluids is only rarely performed since dacryocystitis is uncommon. Causes of dacryocystitis may include bacterial, fungal, or parasitic infections, foreign body reactions, or possibly neoplasia [24]. Infections within the system may occur secondary to physical disruptions to normal anatomy (e.g., congenital atresia of duct, sinus infections, trauma, habronemiasis). Nasolacrimal flushing may be indicated when there is evidence of poor nasolacrimal flow, such as chronic epiphora, or, when accompanied by infection, mucopurulent discharge. The procedure can be both therapeutic (e.g., removal of foreign bodies and excessive exudate) and provide diagnostic information on primary or secondary infections. Ideally, 1–2 slides should be prepared directly from the recovered flush fluid and the remaining fluid should be placed in nonadditive sterile tubes. If the fluid is blood-tinged, some fluid should also be placed in EDTA (lavender top) tubes. When samples are submitted to a diagnostic laboratory, a thorough history should be provided with any specific clinical questions.

Fine needle aspirations of the lacrimal glands are rarely performed but have been reported in cases of lacrimal gland adenitis [124]. Lacrimal adenocarcinoma has been reported in the third eyelid of a horse but the cytological features have not been specifically described [85].

Acknowledgments

The authors wish to thank Drs Elizabeth A. Giuliano and Cecil P. Moore for their previous contributions to this chapter. Within the Texas A&M Veterinary Medical Diagnostic Laboratory, the authors wish to thank the administration for their support in sample processing, Dr Amy Swinford and Sonia Lingsweiler for providing microbiology expertise, Dr Erin Edwards for providing histopathology collaborations, and the clinical pathology laboratory technicians for their support in slide and image collection.

References

1 Sundberg, J.P., Burnstein, T., Page, E.H. et al. (1977). Neoplasms of equidae. *J. Am. Vet. Med. Assoc.* 170: 150–152.

2 Dwyer, A.E. (2012). Ophthalmology in equine ambulatory practice. *Vet. Clin. North Am. Equine Pract.* 28: 155–174.

3 Moore, C.P., Grevan, V.L., Champagne, E.S. et al. (2000). Equine conjunctival pseudotumors. *Vet. Ophthalmol.* 3: 57–63.

4 Stoppini, R., Gilger, B.C., Malarkey, D.E. et al. (2005). Bilateral nodular lymphocytic conjunctivitis in a horse. *Vet. Ophthalmol.* 8: 129–134.

5 Montgomery, K.W. (2014). Equine ocular neoplasia: a review. *Equine Vet. Educ.* 26: 372–380.
6 de Linde Henriksen, M. and Brooks, D.E. (2014). Standing ophthalmic surgeries in horses. *Vet. Clin. North Am. Equine Pract.* 30: 91–110.
7 Jinks, M.R., Fontenot, R.L., Wills, R.W. et al. (2018). The effects of subconjunctival bupivacaine, lidocaine, and mepivacaine on corneal sensitivity in healthy horses. *Vet. Ophthalmol.* 21: 498–506.
8 Labelle, A.L. and Clark-Price, S.C. (2013). Anesthesia for ophthalmic procedures in the standing horse. *Vet. Clin. North Am. Equine Pract.* 29: 179–191.
9 Marly, C., Bettschart-Wolfensberger, R., Nussbaumer, P. et al. (2014). Evaluation of a romifidine constant rate infusion protocol with or without butorphanol for dentistry and ophthalmologic procedures in standing horses. *Vet. Anesth. Analg.* 41: 491–497.
10 Pasolini, M.P., de Biase, D., Greco, M. et al. (2018). Impression technique for conjunctival exfoliative cytology in healthy horses. *J. Equine Vet. Sci.* 67: 75–80.
11 Eordogh, R., Schwendenwein, I., Tichy, A. et al. (2015). Impression cytology: a novel sampling technique for conjunctival cytology of the feline eye. *Vet. Ophthalmol.* 18: 276–284.
12 Little, E., Yvorchuk-St Jean, K., Little, W. et al. (2016). Degree of corneal anesthesia after topical application of 0.4% oxybuprocaine ophthalmic solution in normal equids. *Can. J. Vet. Res.* 80: 329–334.
13 Monclin, S.J., Farnir, F., and Grauwels, M. (2011). Duration of corneal anesthesia following multiple doses and two concentrations of tetracaine hydrochloride eyedrops on the normal equine cornea. *Equine Vet. J.* 43: 69–73.
14 Pucket, J.D., Allbaugh, R.A., Rankin, A.J. et al. (2013). Comparison of efficacy and duration of effect on corneal sensitivity among anesthetic agents following ocular administration in clinically normal horses. *Am. J. Vet. Res.* 74: 459–464.
15 Sharrow-Reabe, K.L. and Townsend, W.M. (2012). Effects of action of proparacaine and tetracaine topical ophthalmic formulations on corneal sensitivity in horses. *J. Am. Vet. Med. Assoc.* 241: 1645–1649.
16 Wieser, B., Tichy, A., and Nell, B. (2013). Correlation between corneal sensitivity and quantity of reflex tearing in cows, horses, goats, sheep, dogs, cats, rabbits, and guinea pigs. *Vet. Ophthalmol.* 16: 251–262.
17 Gordon, E., Sandquist, C., Cebra, C.K. et al. (2018). Esthesiometric evaluation of corneal analgesia after topical application of 1% morphine sulfate in normal horses. *Vet. Ophthalmol.* 21: 218–223.
18 Wotman, K.L. and Utter, M.E. (2010). Effect of treatment with a topical ophthalmic preparation of 1% nalbuphine solution on corneal sensitivity in clinically normal horses. *Am. J. Vet. Res.* 71: 223–228.
19 Fentiman, K.E., Rankin, A.J., Meekins, J.M. et al. (2018). Effects of topical ophthalmic application of 0.5% proparacaine hydrochloride on aerobic bacterial culture results for naturally occurring infected corneal ulcers in dogs. *J. Am. Vet. Med. Assoc.* 253: 1140–1145.
20 Pickett, J.P. and Champagne, E. (1995). The effect of topical 0.5% proparacaine HCL on corneal and conjunctival culture results. Proceedings of the 26th Annual Meeting of the American College of Veterinary Ophthalmologists, p. 144.
21 Bonsembiante, F., Perazzi, A., Deganello, A. et al. (2019). Impression cytology of the healthy equine ocular surface: inter-observer agreement, filter preservation over time and comparison with the cytobrush technique. *Vet. Clin. Pathol.* 48: 61–66.
22 Braus, B.K., Lehenauer, B., Tichy, A. et al. (2017). Impression cytology as diagnostic tool in horses with and without ocular surface disease. *Equine Vet. J.* 49: 438–444.
23 Proietto, L., Beatty, S.S., and Plummer, C.E. (2019). Comparison of 3 corneal cytology collection methods for evaluating equine ulcerative keratitis: Cytobrush, kimura platinum spatula, and handle edge of scalpel blade. *Vet. Ophthalmol.* 22: 153–160.
24 Giuliano, E.A. and Moore, C.P. (2002). Eyes and ocular adnexa. In: *Diagnostic Cytology and Hematology of the Horse*, 2e (eds. R.L. Cowell and R.D. Tyler), 43–64. St Louis: Mosby.
25 Ishibashi, Y. and Kaufman, H.E. (1986). Corneal biopsy in the diagnosis of keratomycosis. *Am J. Ophthalmol.* 101: 288–293.
26 Singh, R., Joseph, A., Umapathy, T. et al. (2005). Impression cytology of the ocular surface. *Br. J. Ophthalmol.* 89: 1655–1659.
27 Calonge, M., Diebold, Y., Saez, V. et al. (2004). Impression cytology of the ocular surface: a review. *Exp. Eye Res.* 78: 457–472.
28 Bourges-Abella, N., Raymond-Letron, I., Diquelou, A. et al. (2007). Comparison of cytological and histologic evaluations of the conjunctiva in the normal equine eye. *Vet. Ophthalmol.* 10: 12–18.
29 Gilger, B.C. (2017). *Equine Ophthalmology*, 3e. Ames: Wiley.
30 Trope, G.D., McCowan, C.I., Tyrrell, D. et al. (2014). Solitary (primary) uveal T-cell lymphoma in a horse. *Vet. Ophthalmol.* 17: 139–145.
31 Featherstone, H.J. and Heinrich, C.L. (2013). Ophthalmic examination and diagnostics. Part 1: the eye examination and diagnostic procedures. In: *Veterinary Ophthalmology*, 5e (eds. K.N. Gelatt, B.C. Gilger and T.J. Kern), 533–613. Ames: Wiley Blackwell.

32 Miller, T.L., Willis, A.M., Wilkie, D.A. et al. (2001). Description of ciliary body anatomy and identification of sites for transscleral cyclophotocoagulation in the equine eye. *Vet. Ophthalmol.* 4: 183–190.

33 Gemensky-Metzler, A.J., Wilkie, D.A., Weisbrode, S.E. et al. (2014). The location of sites and effect of semiconductor diode trans-scleral cyclophotocoagulation on the buphthalmic equine globe. *Vet. Ophthalmol.* 17 (Suppl 1): 107–116.

34 Malalana, F., Blundell, R.J., Pinchbeck, G.L. et al. (2017). The role of Leptospira spp. in horses affected with recurrent uveitis in the UK. *Equine Vet. J.* 49: 706–709.

35 McLaughlin, B.G. and McLaughlin, P.S. (1988). Equine vitreous humor chemical concentrations: correlation with serum concentrations, and postmortem changes with time and temperature. *Can. J. Vet. Res.* 52: 476–480.

36 Polle, F., Storey, E., Eades, S. et al. (2014). Role of intraocular Leptospira infections in the pathogenesis of equine recurrent uveitis in the southern United States. *J. Equine Vet. Sci.* 34: 1300–1306.

37 Priest, H.L., Irby, N.L., Schlafer, D.H. et al. (2012). Diagnosis of Borrelia-associated uveitis in two horses. *Vet. Ophthalmol.* 15: 398–405.

38 Wollanke, B., Rohrbach, B.W., and Gerhards, H. (2001). Serum and vitreous humor antibody titers in and isolation of Leptospira interrogans from horses with recurrent uveitis. *J. Am. Vet. Med. Assoc.* 219: 795–800.

39 Blogg, J.R., Barton, M.D., Graydon, R. et al. (1983). Blindness caused by Rhodococcus equi infection in a foal. *Equine Vet. J.* 15: 25–26.

40 Giguere, S., Cohen, N.D., Chaffin, M.K. et al. (2011). Diagnosis, treatment, control, and prevention of infections caused by Rhodococcus equi in foals. *J. Vet. Intern. Med.* 25: 1209–1220.

41 Moore, C.P., Sarazan, R., Whitley, R.D. et al. (1983). Equine ocular parasites: a review. *Equine Vet. J. Suppl.* 2: 76–85.

42 Rebhun, W.C., Mirro, E.J., Georgi, M.E. et al. (1981). Habronemic blepharoconjunctivitis in horses. *J. Am. Vet. Med. Assoc.* 179: 469–472.

43 Verhaar, N., Hermans, H., van Rooij, E. et al. (2018). Case series: periocular habronemiasis in five horses in the Netherlands. *Vet. Rec.* 182: 746.

44 Giuliano, E.A. (2010). Equine periocular neoplasia: current concepts in aetiopathogenesis and emerging treatment modalities. *Equine Vet. J. Suppl.*: 9–18.

45 Komaromy, A.M., Andrew, S.E., Brooks, D.E. et al. (2004). Periocular sarcoid in a horse. *Vet. Ophthalmol.* 7: 141–146.

46 Hacker, D.V., Moore, P.F., and Buyukmihci, N.C. (1986). Ocular angiosarcoma in four horses. *J. Am. Vet. Med. Assoc.* 189: 200–203.

47 Serena, A., Joiner, K.S., and Schumacher, J. (2006). Hemangiopericytoma in the eyelid of a horse. *Vet. Pathol.* 43: 576–578.

48 Bellone, R.R. (2017). Genetic testing as a tool to identify horses with or at risk for ocular disorders. *Vet. Clin. North Am. Equine Pract.* 33: 627–645.

49 Dugan, S.J., Curtis, C.R., Roberts, S.M. et al. (1991). Epidemiologic study of ocular/adnexal squamous cell carcinoma in horses. *J. Am. Vet. Med. Assoc.* 198: 251–256.

50 Estell, K. (2017). Periocular neoplasia in the horse. *Vet. Clin. North Am. Equine Pract.* 33: 551–562.

51 Schwink, K. (1987). Factors influencing morbidity and outcome of equine ocular squamous cell carcinoma. *Equine Vet. J.* 19: 198–200.

52 Garma-Avina, A. (1994). The cytology of squamous cell carcinomas in domestic animals. *J. Vet. Diagn. Invest.* 6: 238–246.

53 Grimes, J.A., Mestrinho, L.A., Berg, J. et al. (2019). Histologic evaluation of mandibular and medial retropharyngeal lymph nodes during staging of oral malignant melanoma and squamous cell carcinoma in dogs. *J. Am. Vet. Med. Assoc.* 254: 938–943.

54 Rebhun, W.C. and del Piero, F. (1998). Ocular lesions in horses with lymphosarcoma: 21 cases (1977–1997). *J. Am. Vet. Med. Assoc.* 212: 852–854.

55 Glaze, M.B., Gossett, K.A., McCoy, D.J. et al. (1990). A case of equine adnexal lymphosarcoma. *Equine Vet. J. Suppl.* 10: 83–84.

56 Murphy, C.J., Lavoie, J.P., Groff, J. et al. (1989). Bilateral eyelid swelling attributable to lymphosarcoma in a horse. *J. Am. Vet. Med. Assoc.* 194: 939–942.

57 Vallone, L.V., Neaderland, M.H., Ledbetter, E.C. et al. (2016). Suspected malignant transformation of B lymphocytes in the equine cornea from immune-mediated keratitis. *Vet. Ophthalmol.* 19: 172–179.

58 Schnoke, A.T., Brooks, D.E., Wilkie, D.A. et al. (2013). Extraocular lymphoma in the horse. *Vet. Ophthalmol.* 16: 35–42.

59 Arenas-Gamboa, A.M. and Mansell, J. (2011). Epithelioid haemangiosarcoma in the ocular tissue of horses. *J. Comp. Pathol.* 144: 328–333.

60 Bolton, J.R., Lees, M.J., Robinson, W.F. et al. (1990). Ocular neoplasms of vascular origin in the horse. *Equine Vet. J. Suppl.*: 73–75.

61 Moore, P.F., Hacker, D.V., and Buyukmihci, N.C. (1986). Ocular angiosarcoma in the horse: morphological and immunohistochemical studies. *Vet. Pathol.* 23: 240–244.

62 Scherrer, N.M., Lassaline, M., and Engiles, J. (2018). Ocular and periocular hemangiosarcoma in six horses. *Vet. Ophthalmol.* 21: 432–437.

63 Trope, G.D., Steel, C.M., Bowers, J.R. et al. (2010). Distensible superficial venous orbital malformations

involving the lower eyelid in two horses. *J. Am. Vet. Med. Assoc.* 237: 943–948.

64 Lavach, J.D. and Severin, G.A. (1977). Neoplasia of the equine eye, adnexa, and orbit: a review of 68 cases. *J. Am. Vet. Med. Assoc.* 170: 202–203.

65 McEntee, M.F. (1991). Equine cutaneous mastocytoma: morphology, biological behaviour and evolution of the lesion. *J. Comp. Pathol.* 104: 171–178.

66 Vallone, L., Scott, E., and Irby, N. (2019). The conjunctival crypt of the equine third eyelid. *Equine Vet. Educ.* 31: 491–495.

67 Samuelson, D.A., Andresen, T.L., and Gwin, R.M. (1984). Conjunctival fungal flora in horses, cattle, dogs, and cats. *J. Am. Vet. Med. Assoc.* 184: 1240–1242.

68 Whitley, R.D., Burgess, E.C., and Moore, C.P. (1983). Microbial isolates of the normal equine eye. *Equine. Vet. J. Suppl.* 15: 138–140.

69 Hampson, E., Gibson, J.S., Barot, M. et al. (2019). Identification of bacteria and fungi sampled from the conjunctival surface of normal horses in South-East Queensland, Australia. *Vet. Ophthalmol.* 22: 265–275.

70 Johns, I.C., Baxter, K., Booler, H. et al. (2011). Conjunctival bacterial and fungal flora in healthy horses in the UK. *Vet. Ophthalmol.* 14: 195–199.

71 Khosravi, A.R., Nikaein, D., Sharifzadeh, A. et al. (2014). Ocular fungal flora from healthy horses in Iran. *J. Mycol. Med.* 24: 29–33.

72 Voelter-Ratson, K., Monod, M., Unger, L. et al. (2014). Evaluation of the conjunctival fungal flora and its susceptibility to antifungal agents in healthy horses in Switzerland. *Vet. Ophthalmol.* 17 (Suppl 1): 31–36.

73 Zak, A., Siwinska, N., Slowikowska, M. et al. (2018). Conjunctival aerobic bacterial flora in healthy Silesian foals and adult horses in Poland. *BMC Vet. Res.* 14: 261.

74 Scott, E.M., Arnold, C., Dowell, S. et al. (2019). Evaluation of the bacterial ocular surface microbiome in clinically normal horses before and after treatment with topical neomycin-polymyxin-bacitracin. *PLoS One* 14: e0214877.

75 Hillstrom, A., Tvedten, H., Kallberg, M. et al. (2012). Evaluation of cytological findings in feline conjunctivitis. *Vet. Clin. Pathol.* 41: 283–290.

76 Borchers, K., Ebert, M., Fetsch, A. et al. (2006). Prevalence of equine herpesvirus type 2 (EHV-2) DNA in ocular swabs and its cell tropism in equine conjunctiva. *Vet. Microbiol.* 118: 260–266.

77 McChesney, A.E., England, J.J., and Rich, L.J. (1973). Adenoviral infection in foals. *J. Am. Vet. Med. Assoc.* 162: 545–549.

78 Rushton, J.O., Kolodziejek, J., Tichy, A. et al. (2013). Detection of equid herpesviruses 2 and 5 in a herd of 266 Lipizzaners in association with ocular findings. *Vet. Microbiol.* 164: 139–144.

79 Hollingsworth, S.R., Pusterla, N., Kass, P.H. et al. (2015). Detection of equine herpesvirus in horses with idiopathic keratoconjunctivitis and comparison of three sampling techniques. *Vet. Ophthalmol.* 18: 416–421.

80 Cello, R.M. (1971). Ocular onchocerciasis in the horse. *Equine Vet. J.* 3: 148–154.

81 Moore, C.P., Collins, B.K., Linton, L.L. et al. (2000). Conjunctival malignant melanoma in a horse. *Vet. Ophthalmol.* 3: 201–206.

82 Schultze, A.E., Morgan, R.V., and Patton, C.S. (1996). What is your diagnosis? Conjunctival mass from a 9-year-old American paint horse. *Vet. Clin. Pathol.* 25: 79.

83 Vestre, W.A., Turner, T.A., and Carlton, W.W. (1982). Conjunctival hemangioma in a horse. *J. Am. Vet. Med. Assoc.* 180: 1481–1482.

84 McCowan, C. and Stanley, R.G. (2004). Pigmented squamous cell carcinoma of the conjunctiva of a horse. *Vet. Ophthalmol.* 7: 421–423.

85 Mathes, R.L., Paige Carmichael, K., Peroni, J. et al. (2011). Primary lacrimal gland adenocarcinoma of the third eyelid in a horse. *Vet. Ophthalmol.* 14: 48–54.

86 Andrew, S.E. (1999). Corneal stromal abscess in a horse. *Vet. Ophthalmol.* 2: 207–211.

87 Sanchez, S., Studer, M., Currin, P. et al. (2001). Listeria keratitis in a horse. *Vet. Ophthalmol.* 4: 217–219.

88 Jeffery, U., Gervais, K., Mowat, F. et al. (2012). Ability of corneal cytology to predict bacterial culture results. Annual Meeting of the American Society for Veterinary Clinical Pathology (ASVCP), Seattle, WA.

89 Andrew, S.E., Brooks, D.E., Smith, P.J. et al. (1998). Equine ulcerative keratomycosis: visual outcome and ocular survival in 39 cases (1987–1996). *Equine Vet. J.* 30: 109–116.

90 Zeiss, C., Neaderland, M., Yang, F.C. et al. (2013). Fungal polymerase chain reaction testing in equine ulcerative keratitis. *Vet. Ophthalmol.* 16: 341–351.

91 Brooks, D.E., Plummer, C.E., Mangan, B.G. et al. (2013). Equine subepithelial keratomycosis. *Vet. Ophthalmol.* 16: 93–96.

92 Ledbetter, E.C., Irby, N.L., and Kim, S.G. (2011). In vivo confocal microscopy of equine fungal keratitis. *Vet. Ophthalmol.* 14: 1–9.

93 Pearce, J.W., Giuliano, E.A., and Moore, C.P. (2009). In vitro susceptibility patterns of Aspergillus and Fusarium species isolated from equine ulcerative keratomycosis cases in the midwestern and southern United States with inclusion of the new antifungal agent voriconazole. *Vet. Ophthalmol.* 12: 318–324.

94 Sherman, A.B., Clode, A.B., and Gilger, B.C. (2017). Impact of fungal species cultured on outcome in horses with fungal keratitis. *Vet. Ophthalmol.* 20: 140–146.

95 Brilhante, R.S.N., Bittencourt, P.V., de Souza Collares Castelo-Branco, D. et al. (2017). Biofilms of Candida spp. from the ocular conjunctiva of horses with reduced azole susceptibility: a complicating factor for the treatment of keratomycosis? *Vet. Ophthalmol.* 20: 539–546.

96 Friedman, D.S., Schoster, J.V., Pickett, J.P. et al. (1989). Pseudallescheria boydii keratomycosis in a horse. *J. Am. Vet. Med. Assoc.* 195: 616–618.

97 Reed, Z., Thomasy, S.M., Good, K.L. et al. (2013). Equine keratomycoses in California from 1987 to 2010 (47 cases). *Equine Vet. J.* 45: 361–366.

98 Richter, M., Hauser, B., Kaps, S. et al. (2003). Keratitis due to Histoplasma spp. in a horse. *Vet. Ophthalmol.* 6: 99–103.

99 Wada, S., Ode, H., Hobo, S. et al. (2011). Mortierella wolfii keratomycosis in a horse. *Vet. Ophthalmol.* 14: 267–270.

100 Edwards, S., Clode, A.B., and Gilger, B.C. (2015). Equine eosinophilic keratitis in horses: 28 cases (2003–2013). *Clin. Case Rep.* 3: 1000–1006.

101 Lassaline-Utter, M., Miller, C., and Wotman, K.L. (2014). Eosinophilic keratitis in 46 eyes of 27 horses in the mid-Atlantic United States (2008–2012). *Vet. Ophthalmol.* 17: 311–320.

102 Yamagata, M., Wilkie, D.A., and Gilger, B.C. (1996). Eosinophilic keratoconjunctivitis in seven horses. *J. Am. Vet. Med. Assoc.* 209: 1283–1286.

103 Halse, S., Pizzirani, S., Parry, N.M. et al. (2014). Mast cell tumor invading the cornea in a horse. *Vet. Ophthalmol.* 17: 221–227.

104 Ramadan, R.O. (1975). Primary ocular melanoma in a young horse. *Equine Vet. J.* 7: 49–50.

105 Hazel, S.J., Thrall, M.A., Severin, G.A. et al. (1985). Laboratory evaluation of aqueous humor in the healthy dog, cat, horse, and cow. *Am. J. Vet. Res.* 46: 657–659.

106 Hughes, K.J. (2010). Ocular manifestations of systemic disease in horses. *Equine Vet. J. Suppl.* 42: 89–96.

107 Brooks, D.E., Taylor, D.P., Plummer, C.E. et al. (2009). Iris abscesses with and without intralenticular fungal invasion in the horse. *Vet. Ophthalmol.* 12: 306–312.

108 Hussey, G.S., Goehring, L.S., Lunn, D.P. et al. (2013). Experimental infection with equine herpesvirus type 1 (EHV-1) induces chorioretinal lesions. *Vet. Res.* 44: 118.

109 Bradley, A.E., Pries, R.S., and MacIntyre, N. (2000). Thyroid carcinoma with multiple metastases in a horse. *Equine Vet. Educ.* 12: 170–174.

110 Dubielzig, R. (2017). Tumors of the eye. In: *Tumors in Domestic Animals*, 5e (ed. D. Meuten), 892–922. Ames: Wiley.

111 Matheis, F.L., Birkmann, K., Ruetten, M. et al. (2013). Ocular manifestations of a metastatic adenocarcinoma in a horse. *Vet. Ophthalmol.* 16: 214–218.

112 Barnett, K.C. and Platt, H. (1990). Intraocular melanomata in the horse. *Equine Vet. J. Suppl.* 10: 76–82.

113 Knickelbein, K.E., Holmberg, B.J., and Lassaline, M.E. (2019). Equine retrobulbar disease: diagnoses and outcomes of 15 horses with exophthalmos (1988–2017). *Equine Vet. Educ.* 31: 601–608.

114 Baptiste, K.E. and Grahn, B.H. (2000). Equine orbital neoplasia: a review of 10 cases (1983–1998). *Can. Vet. J.* 41: 291–295.

115 Munoz, E., Leiva, M., Naranjo, C. et al. (2007). Retrobulbar dermoid cyst in a horse: a case report. *Vet. Ophthalmol.* 10: 394–397.

116 Boroffka, S.A.E.B. and vandenBelt, A.J.M. (1996). CT/ultrasound diagnosis – retrobulbar hematoma in a horse. *Vet. Radiol. Ultrasound* 37: 441–443.

117 van den Top, J.G.B., Schaafsma, I.A., Boswinkel, M. et al. (2007). A retrobulbar abscess as an uncommon cause of exophthalmos in a horse. *Equine Vet. Educ.* 19: 579–583.

118 Hubert, J., Williams, J., Hamilton, H.L. et al. (1996). What is your diagnosis? Chronic retrobulbar abscess in a horse. *J. Am. Vet. Med. Assoc.* 209: 1703–1704.

119 Scott, E.A., Duncan, J.R., and McCormack, J.E. (1974). Cryptococcosis involving the postorbital area and frontal sinus in a horse. *J. Am. Vet. Med. Assoc.* 165: 626–627.

120 Barnett, K.C., Cottrell, B.D., and Rest, J.R. (1988). Retrobulbar hydatid cyst in the horse. *Equine Vet. J.* 20: 136–138.

121 Miesner, T., Wilkie, D., Gemensky-Metzler, A. et al. (2009). Extra-adrenal paraganglioma of the equine orbit: six cases. *Vet. Ophthalmol.* 12: 263–268.

122 Colitz, C.M., Gilger, B.C., Davidson, C.P. et al. (2000). Orbital fibroma in a horse. *Vet. Ophthalmol.* 3: 213–216.

123 Ueda, Y., Senba, H., Nishimura, T. et al. (1993). Ocular medulloepithelioma in a thoroughbred. *Equine Vet. J.* 25: 558–561.

124 Reimer, J.M. and Latimer, C.S. (2011). Ultrasound findings in horses with severe eyelid swelling, and recognition of acute dacryoadenitis: 10 cases (2004–2010). *Vet. Ophthalmol.* 14: 86–92.

14

Cytology of the Oral and Nasal Cavities, Pharynx, Guttural Pouches, and Paranasal Sinuses

Susan E. Fielder and Maggie R. McCourt

Department of Veterinary Pathobiology, College of Veterinary Medicine, Oklahoma State University, Stillwater, OK, USA

14.1 Indications for Cytological Examination

14.1.1 Oral Cavity, Nasal Cavity, and Paranasal Sinuses

Clinical signs associated with pathological conditions of the oral cavity include ptyalism, quidding, foul odor, dysphagia, depression, nasal discharge, lymphadenopathy, and weight loss [1].

Conditions of the nasal passages may result in nasal discharge, epistaxis, dyspnea, nasal stertor, reduced air flow, facial distortion, facial swelling, and foul breath. Involvement of the nasopharynx can be associated with dysphagia, dyspnea, abnormal respiratory noise, and exercise intolerance [2].

Horses have seven pairs of paranasal sinuses: frontal, dorsal conchal, middle conchal (ethmoidal), ventral conchal, caudal maxillary, rostral maxillary, and sphenopalatine sinuses. Pathological conditions of the paranasal sinuses may result in unilateral purulent nasal discharge, facial distortion, facial swelling, decreased air flow, foul breath, nasal stertor, dullness on percussion of the involved sinus, and formation of a chronic fistula [2].

14.1.2 Guttural Pouches

The guttural pouches are extensions of the Eustachian tubes that connect the pharynx to the middle ear. Anatomically, they are near the basisphenoid bone, retropharyngeal lymph nodes, pharynx, esophagus, atlantooccipital joint, parotid and mandibular salivary glands, petrous temporal bone, tympanic bulla, and auditory meatus.

Clinical signs of guttural pouch disease can be attributed to the specific nerves and arteries associated with the guttural pouch and the auditory system if involved. The internal and external carotid arteries, cranial cervical ganglion, cervical sympathetic trunk and the vagus, glossopharyngeal, hypoglossal, spinal accessory, cranial laryngeal, facial, vestibulocochlear, and mandibular nerves are associated with the guttural pouches. Clinical signs associated with guttural pouch disease include nasal discharge (usually unilateral), unilateral epistaxis, and swelling and/or pain in the area of the parotid salivary gland. The amount of nasal discharge often increases when the head is lowered. Neurological signs (i.e., Horner syndrome) may be present [3].

14.2 Examination

If disease of the oral cavity is suspected, a thorough examination can usually be conducted in the standing animal with the use of sedation. Food material in the oral cavity may conceal lesions and should be removed by flushing with water or 0.1% chlorhexidine solution before examination. A mouth speculum, headlight, mirror, or oral endoscope may facilitate visualization. Lesions near the base of the tongue are often difficult to visualize and careful digital palpation may be necessary. Radiographic evaluation is sometimes helpful, especially if teeth or bony structures are involved [1].

Diseases of the nasal passages and nasopharynx often require endoscopic examination for adequate visualization. Sedation may distort the nasopharynx by relaxation of the soft tissues. Therefore, if pharyngeal involvement is suspected, initial endoscopic examination of this area should be conducted without the aid of sedation, if possible. Imaging including radiography, computed tomography (CT), or magnetic resonance imaging (MRI) may also help define the extent of lesions in this area [2, 4].

Equine Hematology, Cytology, and Clinical Chemistry, Second Edition.
Edited by Raquel M. Walton, Rick L. Cowell, and Amy C. Valenciano.

Examination of the paranasal sinuses includes percussion of the sinuses as well as a thorough oral examination. Endoscopy is important in determining the origin of nasal discharge and radiographic evaluation can establish the location and extent of sinus disease. Once sinus involvement is confirmed, the involved sinus can be aspirated for culture and cytological evaluation [2].

The guttural pouches can be evaluated by palpation, endoscopy, and imaging including radiography, CT, and MRI. Endoscopy provides the most information regarding guttural pouch disease and is done under sedation. One method used to enter the guttural pouch is to place a biopsy instrument in the biopsy channel of the endoscope and extend it 2 or 3 cm past the end of the endoscope. Then the biopsy instrument is inserted into the guttural pouch opening and the endoscope rotated to open the guttural pouch flap. Then the endoscope is advanced into the guttural pouch. Another method uses a Chambers mare catheter to rotate and open the flap, allowing the endoscope to enter the guttural pouch (Figure 14.1). The flexible endoscope is passed dorsal or ventral to the catheter and into the pouch as the Chambers catheter is withdrawn [3].

14.3 Sample Collection

Lesions in the oral cavity, nasal passages, nasopharynx, paranasal sinuses, and guttural pouches may be evaluated by cytological or histopathological examination, and/or culture (bacterial, fungal).

14.3.1 Oral Cavity

Cytological samples from the oral cavity are usually limited to fine needle aspirates of masses or impression smears from excised tissues. Cytological preparations from ulcerative lesions may be collected by imprinting, swabbing, or scraping (see Chapter 12).

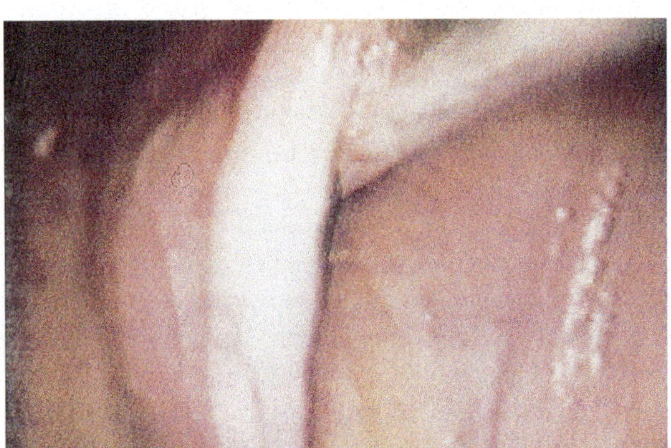

Figure 14.1 Endoscopic view of the opening of the guttural pouch. A Chambers mare catheter is placed through the opening. Note the yellowish exudate draining from the guttural pouch. *Source:* Courtesy of Dr C.G. MacAllister.

14.3.2 Nasal Passages and Nasopharynx

Cytological samples from nasal passages and the nasopharynx are collected directly via the external nares or with a flexible endoscope. Atheromas are accessible for percutaneous aspiration and fungal polyps often are close enough to the external nares to make direct imprints or collect fine needle aspirate or biopsy specimens. Samples of exudates in nasal passages can be collected via polyethylene tubing passed through the biopsy port of a flexible endoscope. Masses and fungal plaques can be sampled with an endoscopic biopsy instrument.

14.3.3 Paranasal Sinuses

Though exudate from paranasal sinuses can be collected endoscopically, samples for cytological evaluation and culture should be taken directly from the involved sinus. Sinus aspiration (sinocentesis) is usually possible in a standing horse using sedation and local anesthesia. After surgical preparation and local anesthetic infiltration, a stab incision is made in the skin and a small Steinmann pin is used to drill into the sinus. Exudate is retrieved by aspiration using an indwelling or rigid catheter. If exudate is not easily obtained, infuse and aspirate 20–30 mL of warm saline. Alternatively, the sinus can be lavaged with 500 mL of warm saline and the nasal discharge examined. If sinus contents are too thick for aspiration, use the eyed end of a large suture needle for sample collection [2].

14.3.4 Guttural Pouches

To collect cytological samples from the guttural pouch, pass polyethylene tubing through the biopsy port of the endoscope and into the guttural pouch. In most instances, exudate is present on the floor of the pouch and is easily aspirated into the tubing. If exudate is not present, infuse 20–30 mL of physiological saline through the tubing and onto the lesion. The saline pools on the floor of the guttural pouch and is easily aspirated. A percutaneous aspiration technique through Viborg's triangle has been described for guttural pouch lavage and sample collection [5].

14.4 Sample Preparation

Swabbed samples should be gently rolled across a clean glass microscope slide and allowed to air dry. Rolling the swab avoids the rupturing of cells that often occurs if the swab is rubbed or dragged across the slide. Samples collected by brushing should be impressed on the slide. Rubbing or dragging the brush across the slide surface should be avoided to prevent excessive damage to cells.

Cells collected by washes can be harvested by centrifugation in a clinical centrifuge using the same speed as is used for urine sedimentation. The supernatant is poured off, the pelleted material is gently resuspended and a drop of the suspension is applied to a clean glass microscope slide with an applicator or pipette. The sediment is then spread using a blood smear technique and allowed to air dry.

14.5 Normal Cytological Features

The oral cavity and upper respiratory tract are composed of several mucous membrane-lined, communicating passages and cavities: the oral and nasal cavities, pharynx, guttural pouches, and paranasal sinuses. Cytological samples of the normal oral cavity or upper respiratory tract, collected by washing, swabbing, or brushing, consist of the exfoliated epithelial cells characteristic of the area sampled.

14.5.1 Oral Cavity and Nasal Passages

The epithelium of the mucous membranes lining the oral cavity and rostral portion of the nasal passages consists of keratinized and nonkeratinized stratified squamous epithelium; therefore, these surfaces exfoliate squamous epithelial cells (Figure 14.2). Squamous epithelial cells appear cytologically as large flattened cells with angular borders and abundant, pale-staining cytoplasm and a condensed to pyknotic central nucleus.

The nasal epithelium caudal to the vestibule progresses from stratified squamous epithelium to pseudostratified ciliated and nonciliated columnar epithelium with numerous goblet cells and exfoliates these various epithelial cells and goblet cells. Columnar epithelial cells appear cytologically as medium-sized, elongated cells with basophilic cytoplasm and central to basal nuclei. Ciliated cells have pink-staining, hair-like cilia extending as a fringe from one end of the cell (Figure 14.3). Goblet cells contain numerous, red to purple staining cytoplasmic mucin granules (Figure 14.4). The cytological appearance of cells from the oral cavity and upper respiratory tract can be complicated by the presence of cells from specialized structures of the mucosa, such as papillae of various types, and taste and olfactory cells.

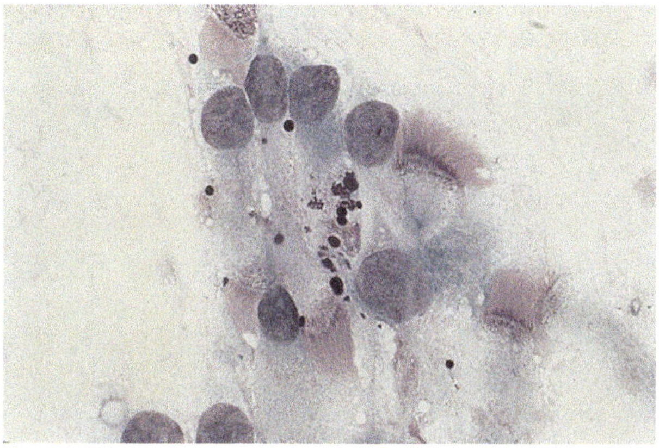

Figure 14.3 Swab smear from the nasal cavity of a normal horse. Ciliated columnar epithelial cells and goblet cells are evident. Original magnification 250×. *Source:* Courtesy of Oklahoma Veterinary Diagnostics.

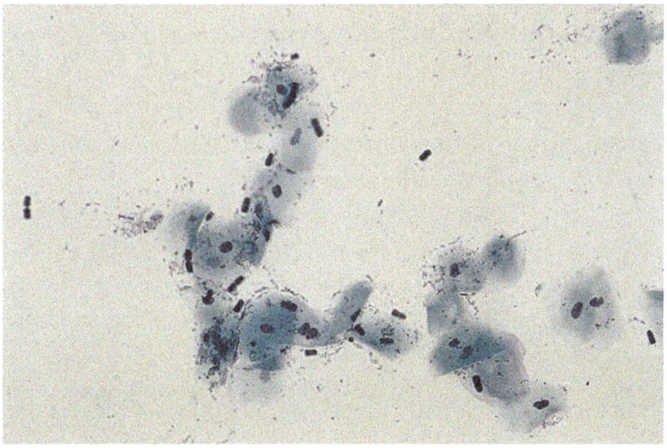

Figure 14.2 Swab smear from the oral cavity of a normal horse. Squamous epithelial cells and a multimorphic bacterial population, including *Simonsiella*, are evident. *Source:* Courtesy of Oklahoma Veterinary Diagnostics.

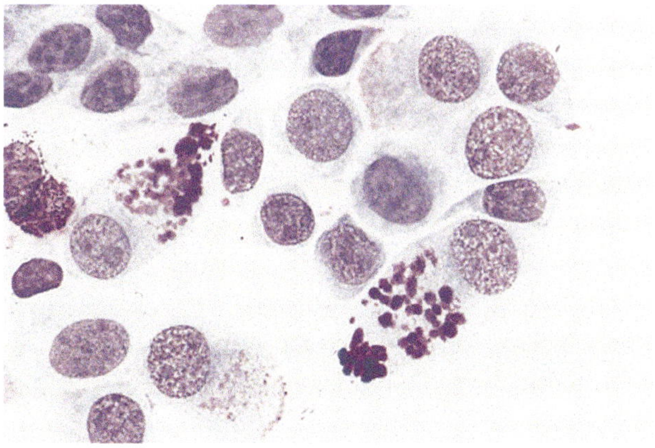

Figure 14.4 Goblet cells. Two goblet cells appear as columnar to cuboidal epithelial cells with numerous pink granules in the cytoplasm. *Source:* Courtesy of Dr R.L. Cowell.

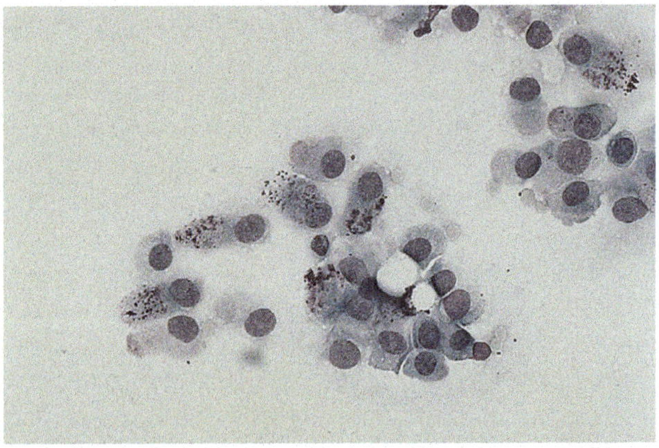

Figure 14.5 Swab smear of normal pharyngeal recess. Note cuboidal and columnar epithelial cells and goblet cells. *Source:* Courtesy of Oklahoma Veterinary Diagnostics.

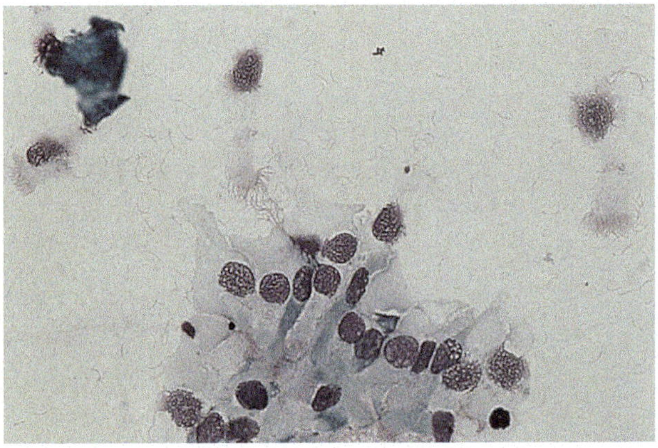

Figure 14.6 Wash sediment from normal guttural pouch. Note cuboidal and columnar epithelial cells and free cilia. *Source:* Courtesy of Oklahoma Veterinary Diagnostics.

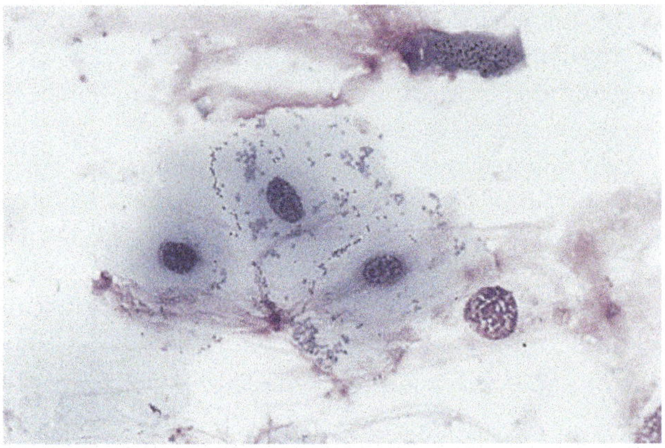

Figure 14.7 Swab smear from oral cavity. Squamous epithelial cells with commensal bacteria. *Source:* Courtesy of Dr R.L. Cowell.

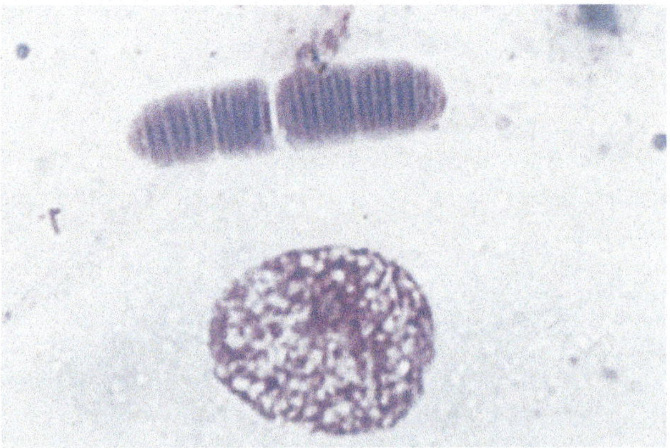

Figure 14.8 Swab smear from oral cavity. *Simonsiella* spp. is seen alongside a squamous epithelial cell (*bottom*). *Source:* Courtesy of Dr R.L. Cowell.

14.5.2 Pharynx, Guttural Pouches, and Paranasal Sinuses

The type of cells exfoliated from the pharyngeal mucosa depends on the area sampled. The pharynx is lined primarily by pseudostratified ciliated columnar epithelium, but it also has areas of stratified squamous epithelium (Figure 14.5). The mucosa of the guttural pouches and paranasal sinuses consists of transitional epithelium and simple ciliated columnar or cuboidal epithelium containing goblet cells (Figure 14.6). Cytologically, cuboidal epithelial cells of transitional epithelium appear as medium-sized, cuboidal cells with rounded borders, basophilic cytoplasm and large central nuclei composed of finely stippled chromatin with areas of condensed chromatin.

14.5.3 Microorganisms

Bacteria from numerous commensal species normally inhabit the oral cavity and upper respiratory tract in large numbers. This bacterial population is typically heterogeneous and consists of both rods and cocci (see Figure 14.2). Normal bacterial flora do not elicit a significant inflammatory response (i.e., neutrophil exudation) (Figure 14.7). Perhaps the most striking of the normal bacterial flora of the oral cavity are *Simonsiella* spp., which appear as giant rod-like structures (see Figure 14.2). These apparent giant rods are composed of multiple *Simonsiella* rods apposed side to side (Figure 14.8).

Cytological samples of the oral cavity and upper respiratory tract of horses also often contain "barn mold," that is, mycelial and fruiting bodies of saprophytic fungi commonly encountered in barn air and feed (Figure 14.9). Cytologically, these are typically large (>1–2 red blood cells [RBC] diameters in size), green- to turquoise-staining, round to elliptical structures.

14.5.4 Underlying Structures

In addition to the mucosal epithelium, numerous and varied structures underlie the mucosa of the oral and upper

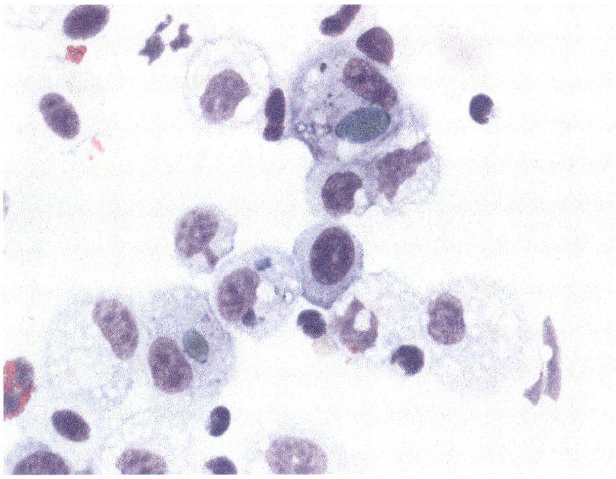

Figure 14.9 Wash from the upper respiratory tract. Vacuolated macrophages are seen with intracellular fungal elements. These structures are consistent with "barn mold" and are nonpathogenic.

respiratory tracts (cartilage, bone, adipose tissue, salivary glands, lymphoid tissue). Core biopsies, surgical biopsies, or fine needle aspirates can be used to obtain cells characteristic of these structures.

14.6 Abnormal Cytological Features

14.6.1 Irritation

Conditions that irritate the mucosal lining of the upper respiratory tract can result in increased goblet cells and production of increased amounts of mucin, which appears cytologically as mats of homogeneous, pink- to red-staining material or as a finely mottled pink background (Figure 14.10). Goblet cells are rarely seen in washes of normal oronasopharyngeal structures. Free mucin granules may also be seen in smears from irritated mucosa. These appear as small, round, rose-colored structures (1 RBC diameter) (Figure 14.11).

14.6.2 Inflammation and Infection

The cytological hallmark of inflammation is increased numbers of inflammatory cells (neutrophils, macrophages, etc.) (Figure 14.12). Noxious stimuli such as foreign bodies, trauma or infectious organisms can provoke an inflammatory response resulting in increased inflammatory cells in smears.

14.6.2.1 Bacterial Infection

Bacterial infections are readily detected by cytological examination. Typically, bacterial infection is associated with intense infiltration of neutrophils into tissues and exudation of neutrophils through the mucosa (see Figure 14.12). Because many bacteria produce toxins, neutrophils migrating

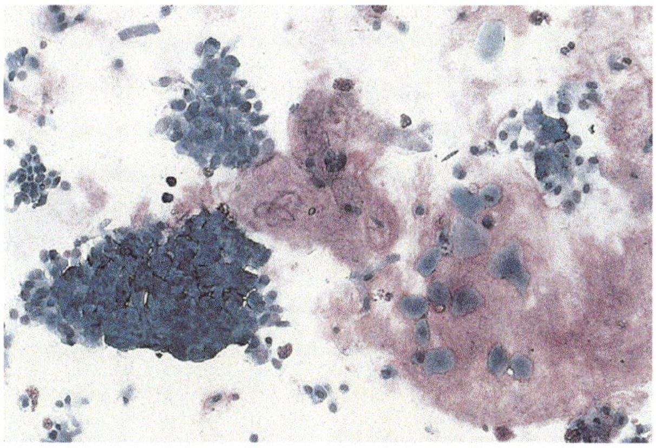

Figure 14.10 Wash sediment from a horse with guttural pouch irritation. Large amounts of amorphous pink-staining mucin are evident, with clusters of columnar epithelial cells. *Source:* Courtesy of Oklahoma Veterinary Diagnostics.

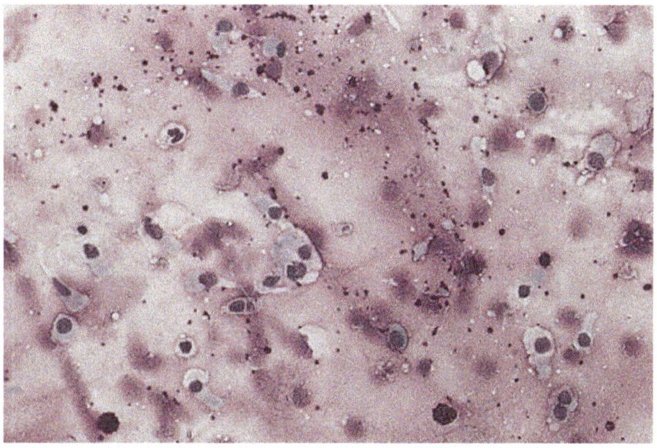

Figure 14.11 Wash sediment from a horse with guttural pouch irritation. Large amounts of mucin and free mucin granules are evident with cuboidal and columnar epithelial cells. *Source:* Courtesy Oklahoma Veterinary Diagnostics.

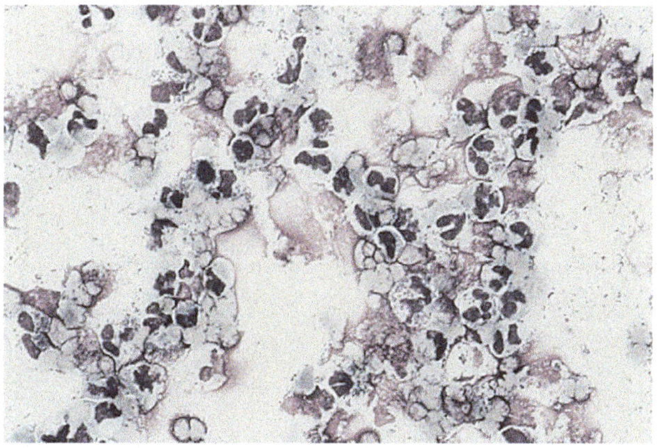

Figure 14.12 Smear of exudate from paranasal sinus. Smear contains large numbers of neutrophils and extracellular and intracellular bacteria. *Source:* Courtesy of Oklahoma Veterinary Diagnostics.

into infected sites often become degenerate. In cytological preparations, degenerate neutrophils appear swollen, lose their nuclear segmentation, and have lighter, pink-staining chromatin that gives them a monocytoid appearance (Figure 14.13). The presence of degenerate neutrophils in a neutrophilic cytological smear suggests bacterial infection, even if bacteria are not directly observed.

Cytologically, bacteria appear as collections of uniform rod-like to coccoid structures that typically stain dark blue with hematological stains (see Figure 14.12). Bacteria can be located extracellularly or intracellularly (Figures 14.14 and 14.15). If bacteria are located only extracellularly and only small numbers of neutrophils are seen, one must exercise caution in differentiating bacterial infection from normal flora or contamination of the sample. In contrast, the presence of phagocytized bacteria indicates bacterial infection (primary or secondary).

Free mucin granules (see Figure 14.11), free cilia (see Figure 14.6), stain precipitate, or necrotic debris on cytological smears can be mistaken for bacteria. As discussed before, bacterial infection is almost always associated with neutrophilic infiltration and phagocytized bacteria. Caution should be exercised in interpreting structures like bacteria if neutrophilic infiltration and phagocytized bacteria are not seen.

Bacterial infections of the upper respiratory mucosae can involve numerous bacterial species. Identification of bacterial pathogens based on their cytological appearance is not reliable so culture (and antimicrobial sensitivity testing) should be used to identify the organisms involved.

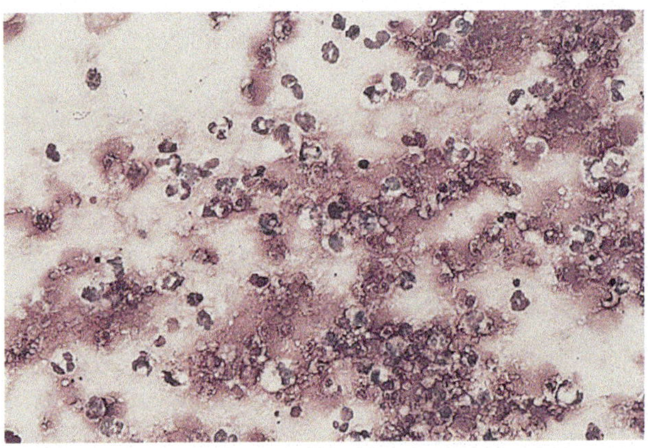

Figure 14.13 Smear of exudate from paranasal sinus. Note large numbers of degenerate neutrophils, debris from lyzed neutrophils, and small numbers of small rods in short chains. *Source:* Courtesy of Oklahoma Veterinary Diagnostics.

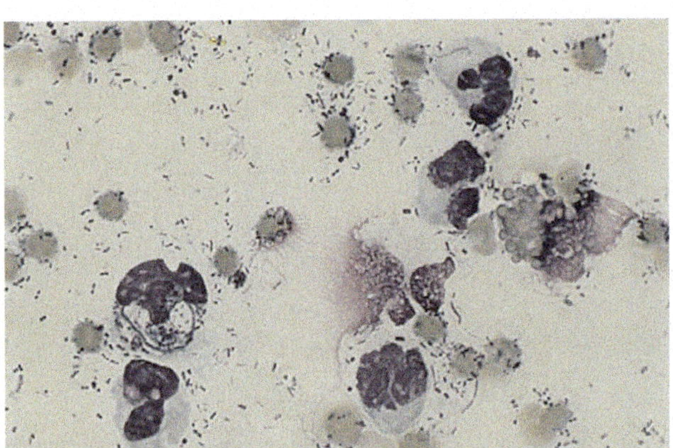

Figure 14.14 Smear of exudate from paranasal sinus. Note large multimorphic bacterial population seen extracellularly and within neutrophils. *Source:* Courtesy of Oklahoma Veterinary Diagnostics.

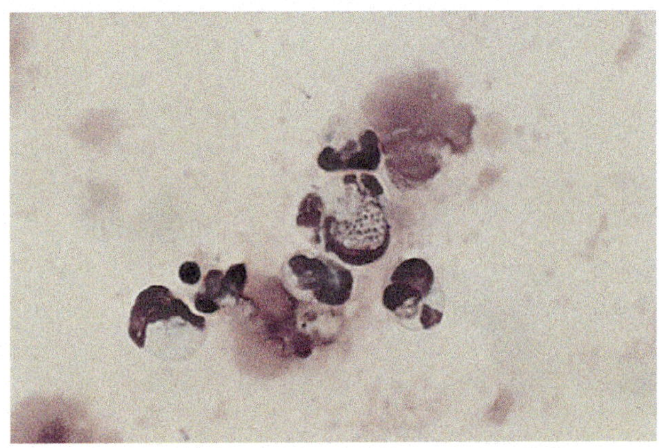

Figure 14.15 Smear of exudate from paranasal sinus. Note ruptured cells and degenerate neutrophils containing phagocytized coccobacilli. *Source:* Courtesy of Oklahoma Veterinary Diagnostics.

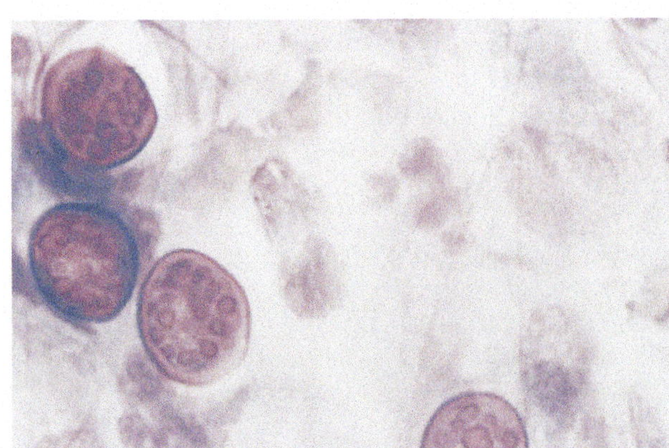

Figure 14.16 Smear from the nasal cavity. Several spherical rhinosporidia about the size of a neutrophil, with enclosed endospores, are identified. Inflammatory cells are present in the background. *Source:* Courtesy of Oklahoma Veterinary Diagnostics.

14.6.2.2 Fungal Infection

Samples from horses with mycotic rhinitis and sinusitis typically contain large numbers of neutrophils and macrophages. Multinucleated inflammatory giant cells, lymphocytes, and reactive stromal cells may also be seen. Fungal hyphae are readily recognized as filamentous structures with a width greater than 1 RBC diameter (wider than filamentous bacteria); some have septal divisions. Determining the species of fungal hyphae using cytological features is not reliable and fungal culture or molecular techniques are recommended for identification. Mycotic rhinitis is occasionally associated with infection by *Rhinosporidium seeberi* (Figure 14.16), *Cryptococcus neoformans*, *Pythium* spp., *Sporothrix schenckii*, *Prototheca* spp., and *Pithomyces chartarum* [6–8].

14.6.2.3 Parasitic Infection

The horse nasal bot (family Oestridae, subfamily Oestrinae, genus *Rhinoestrus*) can affect species of the family Equidae and infections have been documented in Africa (including Egypt, Senegal, Niger), Asia, Italy, and France [9, 10]. As is typical for parasitic infections, the associated inflammatory response is primarily eosinophilic with mast cells and lower numbers of other types of inflammatory cells [9].

14.6.2.4 Hypersensitivity Reactions

Inflammation in association with allergic disease or hypersensitivity reactions can result in increased numbers of eosinophils, basophils, or mast cells in cytological smears. Antigenic stimulation is associated with increased numbers of small lymphocytes and plasma cells.

14.7 Nasal Passage and Paranasal Sinus Disease

In two large-scale retrospective studies of equine sinonasal disease including 477 horses, the disease distribution was primary (idiopathic) sinusitis (acute or chronic; 33%), dental-associated sinusitis (21%), sinus cysts (13%), sinonasal neoplasia (7%), ethmoid hematoma (6%), sinonasal trauma (6%), mycotic lesions (4%), dental-related oromaxillary fistula (3%), nasal polyp (2%), epidermal inclusion cyst (2%), and miscellaneous causes (3%) [11, 12].

14.7.1 Empyema of the Nasal Conchal Bulla

Some cases of chronic primary sinusitis (15–23%) develop a sinonasal fistula between the dorsal or ventral conchal bullae and the nasal cavity. Within these bullae are masses of inspissated pus and, sometimes, sequestered conchal bone. Sinusitis, rhinitis, and nasal discharge do not resolve in these cases unless the inspissated pus and sequestered bone are removed [11, 13].

14.7.2 Cysts and Hematomas

Cytological examination of samples from fluid-filled structures of the dermis, mucosa, glands, or associated ducts often helps identify the process involved. Epidermal inclusion cysts (atheromas) are epidermoid cysts of the nasal diverticulum. They consist of large numbers of squamous epithelial cells (Figure 14.17) and a variable amount of sebum or cholesterol crystals [14, 15]. Paranasal sinus cysts are definitively diagnosed via histopathology where the tissue component can be visualized, but sinocentesis results in aspiration of viscous, translucent, odorless, yellow acellular fluid [16, 17].

Hematomas (i.e., ethmoid hematomas) are definitively diagnosed via histopathology but a tentative diagnosis can be made from the history, clinical signs, endoscopic, and imaging findings [2]. If fine needle aspirates for cytological evaluation are obtained, samples contain RBCs in various stages of RBC catabolism (intact RBCs, erythrophagocytosis, hematoidin crystals, hemosiderin) with few macrophages [2, 15]. Mild or chronic inflammation is often associated with cystic or hemorrhagic structures and increased neutrophils are often seen in the cytological preparations of cystic fluid [15].

14.7.3 Nasal Amyloidosis

Nasal amyloidosis is an uncommon disease of the nasal cavity in horses. In one report, out of 16,000 horses referred for examination, only six (0.04%) had nasal amyloidosis [18]. All of these horses were evaluated due to the development of epistaxis [18]. Other clinical signs associated with

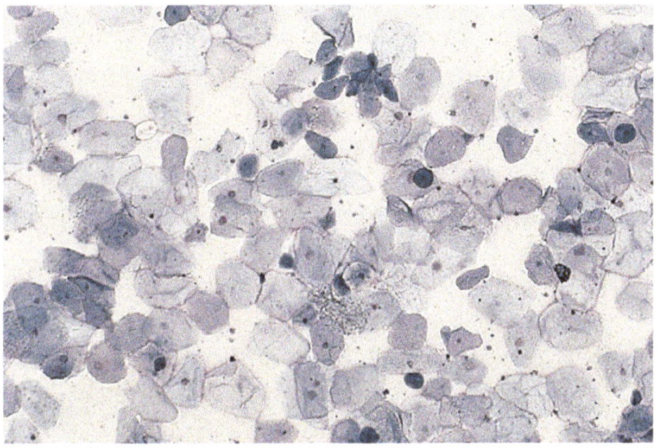

Figure 14.17 Fine needle aspirate from a cystic lesion. Note large numbers of squamous epithelial cells, many with pyknotic nuclei or no nucleus and some that are keratinized. *Source:* Courtesy of Oklahoma Veterinary Diagnostics.

nasal amyloidosis include development of mass lesions with resultant dyspnea and exercise intolerance [19–21]. Most reports of nasal amyloidosis have been diagnosed via histopathology only, with findings including large areas of hyaline eosinophilic material that, when stained with Congo red and examined with polarized light, produced apple-green birefringence [18, 21]. Recently, a report described the cytological findings of nasal amyloidosis including the presence of plasmacytic and granulomatous inflammation with macrophages and multinucleated giant cells containing intracytoplasmic granular to fibrillar, gray to brightly eosinophilic material which was presumed to be amyloid. This was confirmed with histopathology and the presence of Congo red-positive material that when examined with polarized light displayed apple-green birefringence [22].

14.7.4 Neoplasia

Neoplasms involving the upper respiratory tract consist of carcinomas arising from the mucosa and/or its associated glands, or tumors of structures underlying the mucosa, such as osteosarcoma or lymphoma. Overall, equine sinonasal tumors are infrequent and when they do occur, they are more likely to involve the paranasal sinuses (especially the caudal maxillary sinus) rather than present as a primary nasal tumor [23]. In a literature review of 50 equine sinonasal tumors, the distribution of tumor types was squamous cell carcinoma (34%), bone tumors (28%), tumors of mesenchymal origin (14%), adenocarcinoma (12%), lymphoma (8%), and dental tumors (4%) [23]. Another report of 28 equine sinonasal tumors reported a distribution including squamous cell carcinoma (25%), adenocarcinoma (18%), fibroosseous and bone tumors (18%), undifferentiated carcinoma (10%), adenoma (7%), and a single case each of ameloblastoma, fibroma, fibrosarcoma, undifferentiated sarcoma, melanoma, and lymphoma [24]. Other sinonasal tumors reported include spindle cell sarcoma, ethmoid carcinoma, hemangiosarcoma, osteoma, cementoma, ossifying oronasal carcinoma, and histiocytic sarcoma [25–30].

Squamous cell carcinoma is the most common equine sinonasal tumor. These carcinomas exfoliate moderate numbers of single or multiple cell clusters of medium-sized to large, pleomorphic epithelial cells [31]. These cells are polygonal and rounded, with distinct cell margins, abundant slightly granular blue to smooth turquoise cytoplasm, large round to oval single or double nuclei, reticulate to ropy chromatin pattern, and one or multiple nucleoli (Figure 14.18). Other carcinomas have a similar anaplastic epithelial cytological appearance [6].

Nasal polyps are usually secondary to chronic inflammation and not of neoplastic origin. They consist of a mucosal lining surrounding fibrous tissue [15].

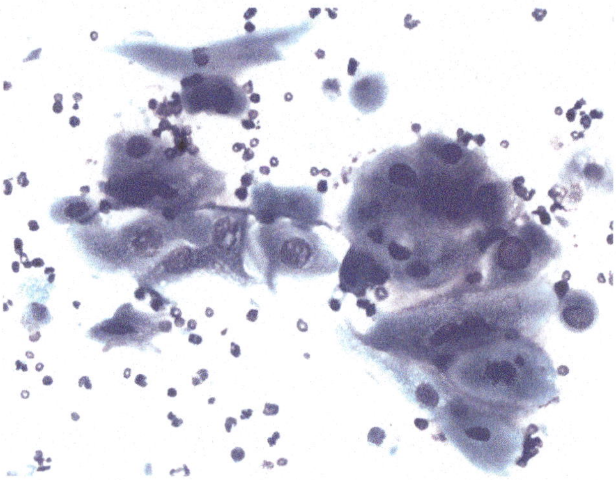

Figure 14.18 Fine needle aspirate from the oral cavity. Atypical epithelial cells with anisocytosis, anisokaryosis, and prominent nucleoli. Some cells show perinuclear vacuolation. Elongate epithelial cells are often associated with squamous cell carcinoma.

14.8 Oral Cavity and Pharyngeal Disease

14.8.1 Pharyngeal Lymphoid Hyperplasia

Horses lack structural tonsils and instead have lymphoid follicles diffusely distributed on the dorsal and lateral walls of the pharynx. Reactive hyperplasia of these follicles in response to an antigenic stimulus can result in significant edema and hyperemia [32].

14.8.2 Neoplasia

Most oral pathologies are associated with dental disease and neoplasia of the oral cavity is rare [33]. Squamous cell carcinoma is the most common oral tumor and may be associated with any mucosal surface (see Figure 14.18). Other tumors reported in the oral cavity include melanoma, fibrosarcoma, hemangiosarcoma, lymphoma, rhabdomyoma, rhabdomyosarcoma, chondrosarcoma, adenocarcinoma, and mast cell tumor [34–42].

14.9 Guttural Pouch Disease

14.9.1 Inflammation and Infection

14.9.1.1 Guttural Pouch Empyema

Bacterial infection of the guttural pouches is often secondary to an upper respiratory infection and may be associated with rupture of the retropharyngeal lymph node. Cytological examination of fluid from the guttural pouch reveals large numbers of variably degenerate neutrophils and bacteria seen both intracellularly and extracellularly. *Streptococcus equi* subsp. *equi* infection is the most common bacterium involved. Whilst bacteria can be readily identified on cytology, culture and polymerase chain reaction for *S. equi* subsp. *equi* is necessary for definitive identification. Accumulation of purulent material within the guttural pouches can lead to the formation of chondroids [43].

14.9.1.2 Guttural Pouch Mycosis

Samples from horses with guttural pouch mycosis typically contain large numbers of neutrophils and macrophages. Multinucleated inflammatory giant cells, lymphocytes, and reactive stromal cells may also be seen. Fungal hyphae are readily recognized and some have septal divisions (Figure 14.19). *Aspergillus* spp., particularly *Aspergillus fumigatus*, are the most commonly cultured organisms [44]. However, determining the species using cytological features is not reliable. Fungal culture or molecular techniques are necessary for identification.

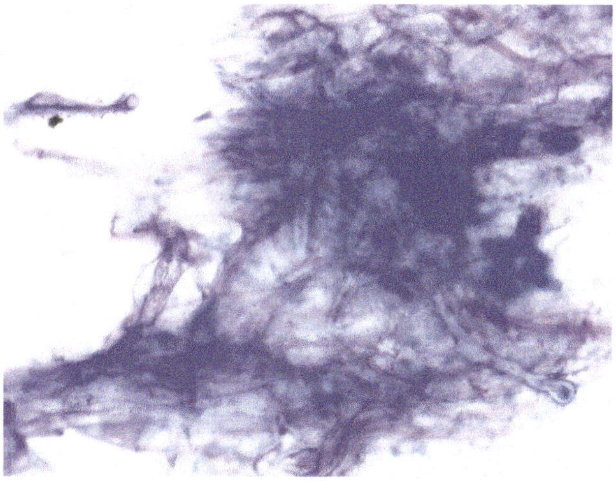

Figure 14.19 Smear of exudate from guttural pouch. Large basophilic structures are present with large numbers of nonstaining to blue-staining fungal hyphae. *Source:* Courtesy of Dr R.W. Allison.

14.9.2 Neoplasia

Neoplasia is uncommon in the guttural pouch and is rarely diagnosed on cytology. Melanocytic tumors are the most common neoplasm found in the guttural pouch and may be benign or malignant [45]. Other tumors reported in the guttural pouch include squamous cell carcinoma, leiomyosarcoma, hemangioma, hemangiosarcoma, and fibroma [46–50].

References

1 Stick, J.A. and Prange, T. (2019). Oral cavity and salivary glands. In: *Equine Surgery* (eds. J.A. Auer and J. Stick), 440–474. St Louis: Elsevier.

2 Nickels, F.A. and O'Neill, H. (2019). Nasal passages and paranasal sinuses. In: *Equine Surgery* (eds. J.A. Auer and J. Stick), 698–710. St Louis: Elsevier.

3 Freeman, D.E. (2019). Guttural pouch. In: *Equine Surgery* (eds. J.A. Auer and J. Stick), 770–796. St Louis: Elsevier.

4 Ducharme, N.G. and Cheetham, J. (2019). Pharynx. In: *Equine Surgery* (eds. J.A. Auer and J. Stick), 710–733. St Louis: Elsevier.

5 Chiesa, O.A., Lopez, C., Domingo, M. et al. (2000). A percutaneous technique for guttural pouch lavage. *Equine Pract.* 22 (3): 8–11.

6 Allison, R.W. and Ramachandran, A. (2015). What is your diagnosis? Ulcerative nasal lesion in a quarter horse. *Vet. Clin. Pathol.* 44 (3): 455–456.

7 Schoniger, S., Roschanski, N., Rosler, U. et al. (2016). Prototheca species and Pithomyces Chartarum as causative agents of rhinitis and/or sinusitis in horses. *J. Comp. Pathol.* 155 (2–3): 121–125.

8 Souto, E.P.F., Maia, L.A., Olinda, R.G. et al. (2016). Pythiosis in the nasal cavity of horses. *J. Comp. Pathol.* 155 (2–3): 126–129.

9 Angulo-Valadez, C.E., Scholl, P.J., Cepeda-Palacios, R. et al. (2010). Nasal bots...a fascinating world! *Vet. Parasitol.* 174 (1–2): 19–25.

10 Hilali, M.A., Mahdy, O.A., and Attia, M.M. (2015). Monthly variations of Rhinoestrus spp. (Diptera: Oestridae) larvae infesting donkeys in Egypt: morphological and molecular identification of third stage larvae. *J. Adv. Res.* 6 (6): 1015–1021.

11 Dixon, P.M., Parkin, T.D., Collins, N. et al. (2012). Equine paranasal sinus disease: a long-term study of 200 cases (1997–2009): ancillary diagnostic findings and involvement of the various sinus compartments. *Equine Vet. J.* 44 (3): 267–271.

12 Tremaine, W.H. and Dixon, P.M. (2001). A long-term study of 277 cases of equine sinonasal disease. Part 1: details of horses, historical, clinical and ancillary diagnostic findings. *Equine Vet. J.* 33 (3): 274–282.

13 Dixon, P.M., Froydenlund, T., Luiti, T. et al. (2015). Empyema of the nasal conchal bulla as a cause of chronic unilateral nasal discharge in the horse: 10 cases (2013–2014). *Equine Vet. J.* 47 (4): 445–449.

14 Boles, C. (1979). Abnormalities of the upper respiratory tract. *Vet. Clin. North Am. Large Anim. Pract.* 1 (1): 89–111.

15 Tremaine, W.H., Clarke, C.J., and Dixon, P.M. (1999). Histopathological findings in equine sinonasal disorders. *Equine Vet. J.* 31 (4): 296–303.
16 Fenner, M.F., Verwilghen, D., Townsend, N. et al. (2019). Paranasal sinus cysts in the horse: complications related to their presence and surgical treatment in 37 cases. *Equine Vet. J.* 51 (1): 57–63.
17 Freeman, D.E. (2003). Sinus disease. *Vet. Clin. North Am. Equine Pract.* 19 (1): 209–243. Viii.
18 Van Andel, A.C., Gruys, E., Kroneman, J. et al. (1988). Amyloid in the horse: a report of nine cases. *Equine Vet. J.* 20 (4): 277–285.
19 Nappert, G., Vrins, A., Dore, M. et al. (1988). Nasal amyloidosis in two quarter horses. *Can. Vet. J.* 29 (10): 834–835.
20 Ostevik, L., Gunnes, G., de Souza, G.A. et al. (2014). Nasal and ocular amyloidosis in a 15-year-old horse. *Acta Vet. Scand.* 56: 50.
21 Shaw, D.P., Gunson, D.E., and Evans, L.H. (1987). Nasal amyloidosis in four horses. *Vet. Pathol.* 24 (2): 183–185.
22 Leissinger, M.K., Mccauley, C., Fowlkes, N. et al. (2017). What is your diagnosis? Nasal lesion in a horse. *Vet. Clin. Pathol.* 46 (2): 361–362.
23 Head, K.W. and Dixon, P.M. (1999). Equine nasal and paranasal sinus tumours. Part 1: review of the literature and tumour classification. *Vet. J.* 157 (3): 261–278.
24 Dixon, P.M. and Head, K.W. (1999). Equine nasal and paranasal sinus tumours: part 2: a contribution of 28 case reports. *Vet. J.* 157 (3): 279–294.
25 Acland, H.M., Orsini, J.A., Elkins, S. et al. (1984). Congenital ethmoid carcinoma in a foal. *J. Am. Vet. Med. Assoc.* 184 (8): 979–981.
26 Chan, C.W. and Collins, E.A. (1985). Case of Angiosarcoma of the nasal passage of the horse – ultrastructure and differential diagnosis from progressive haematoma. *Equine Vet. J.* 17 (3): 214–218.
27 Da Silva, A.P.C., Cassou, F., Andrade, B.S.C. et al. (2012). Ossifying oronasal carcinoma in a horse. *Braz. J. Vet. Pathol.* 5 (3): 128–132.
28 Mason, B.J.E. (1975). Spindle cell sarcoma of the equine para nasal sinuses and nasal chamber. *Vet. Rec.* 96 (13): 287–288.
29 Paciello, O., Passantino, G., Costagliola, A. et al. (2013). Histiocytic sarcoma of the nasal cavity in a horse. *Res. Vet. Sci.* 94 (3): 648–650.
30 Schaaf, K.L., Kannegieter, N.J., and Lovell, D.K. (2007). Calcified tumours of the paranasal sinuses in three horses. *Aust. Vet. J.* 85 (11): 454–458.
31 Tuckey, J., Hilbert, B., Beetson, S. et al. (1995). Squamous cell carcinoma of the pharyngeal wall in a horse. *Aust. Vet. J.* 72 (6): 227.
32 Smith, B.P., van Metre, D.C., and Pusterla, N. (2019). *Large Animal Internal Medicine*, 6e. St Louis: Mosby.
33 Anthony, J., Waldner, C., Grier, C. et al. (2010). A survey of equine oral pathology. *J. Vet. Dent.* 27 (1): 12–15.
34 Castleman, W.L., Toplon, D.E., Clark, C.K. et al. (2011). Rhabdomyosarcoma in 8 horses. *Vet. Pathol.* 48 (6): 1144–1150.
35 Dixon, P.M. and Gerard, M.P. (2019). Oral cavity and salivary glands. In: *Equine Surgery* (eds. J.A. Auer and J. Stick), 440–474. St Louis: Elsevier.
36 Durham, A.C., Pillitteri, C.A., Myint, M.S. et al. (2013). Two hundred three cases of equine lymphoma classified according to the World Health Organization (WHO) classification criteria. *Vet. Pathol.* 50 (1): 86–93.
37 Fulvio, L., Giacomo, R., Emanuele, P. et al. (2014). Adenocarcinoma involving the tongue and the epiglottis in one horse. *J. Vet. Med. Sci* 76: 467–470.
38 Horbal, A. and Dixon, P.M. (2016). Gingival fibrosarcoma in a horse: a case report. *J. Vet. Dent.* 33 (4): 243–248.
39 Johns, I., Stephen, J.O., del Piero, F. et al. (2005). Hemangiosarcoma in 11 young horses. *J. Vet. Intern. Med.* 19 (4): 564–570.
40 Phillips, J.C. and Lembcke, L.M. (2013). Equine melanocytic tumors. *Vet. Clin. North Am. Equine Pract.* 29 (3): 673–687.
41 Seeliger, F., Heß, O., Pröbsting, M. et al. (2007). Confocal laser scanning analysis of an equine oral mast cell tumor with atypical expression of tyrosine kinase receptor c-kit. *Vet. Pathol.* 44 (2): 225–228.
42 Wilson, G.J. and Anthony, N.D. (2007). Chondrosarcoma of the tongue of a horse. *Aust. Vet. J.* 85 (4): 163–165.
43 Judy, C.E., Chaffin, M.K., and Cohen, N.D. (1999). Empyema of the guttural pouch (auditory tube diverticulum) in horses: 91 cases (1977–1997). *J. Am. Vet. Med. Assoc.* 215 (11): 1666–1670.
44 Ludwig, A., Gatineau, S., Reynaud, M.-C. et al. (2005). Fungal isolation and identification in 21 cases of guttural pouch mycosis in horses (1998–2002). *Vet. J.* 169 (3): 457–461.
45 Metcalfe, L.V., O'Brien, P.J., Papakonstantinou, S. et al. (2013). Malignant melanoma in a grey horse: case presentation and review of equine melanoma treatment options. *Ir. Vet. J.* 66 (1): 22.
46 Baptiste, K.E., Moll, H.D., and Robertson, J.L. (1996). Three horses with neoplasia including growth in the guttural pouch. *Can. Vet. J.* 37 (8): 499–501.
47 Drew, S., Meehan, L., Reardon, R. et al. (2018). Guttural pouch leiomyosarcoma causing nasopharyngeal compression in a pony. *Equine Vet. Educ.* 30 (2): 64–69.
48 Greene, H.J. and O'Connor, J.P. (1986). Haemangioma of the guttural pouch of a 16-year-old thoroughbred mare: clinical and pathological findings. *Vet. Rec.* 118 (16): 445–446.
49 Merriam, J.G. (1972). Guttural pouch fibroma in a mare. *J. Am. Vet. Med. Assoc.* 161 (5): 487–489.
50 Perrier, M., Schwarz, T., Gonzalez, O. et al. (2010). Squamous cell carcinoma invading the right temporomandibular joint in a Belgian mare. *Can. Vet. J.* 51 (8): 885.

15

Cytology of the Lymph Nodes

Kathryn Jacocks

IDEXX Laboratories, Inc., Dallas, TX, USA

15.1 Introduction

Lymph node samples generally exfoliate extremely well for cytological evaluation so examination of lymph node aspirates can often provide an expedient and fairly simple way to elucidate a causative pathological process for lymphadenopathy or lymph node enlargement. Cytology can frequently provide a diagnosis (i.e., lymphoma, infectious agents, metastatic neoplasia, etc.) or it may point to various disease processes (i.e., lymphadenitis, hyperplasia, etc.).

Lymphadenopathy can be localized or generalized and primary or secondary in nature. Differentials for lymphadenopathy include hyperplasia or reactive lymphadenopathy, lymphadenitis (neutrophilic, macrophagic, eosinophilic, mixed), lymphoma, and metastatic neoplasia. An algorithmic approach to lymph node aspirate evaluation and interpretation is presented in Figure 15.1.

15.2 Sample Collection and Preparation

When one is aspirating peripheral lymph nodes, the site of aspiration is prepared as for an injection. Suitable fine needle aspirate can be collected using a 21–25 gauge needle attached to a 5 mL or larger syringe or holding the hub of the needle without a syringe (nonaspiration technique). Small (5 mL) syringes can be used when aspirating lymph nodes because lymph node cells exfoliate more easily than those of many other body tissues and the cells are often fragile as well.

For collection, the lymph node is isolated between the collector's thumb and forefinger. Remember that lymphoid tissue can be fairly heterogeneous, and sampling many areas of the node is ideal [1]. Holding either the syringe with needle attached or the hub of the needle directly, insert the needle into the node and apply gentle suction (if syringe attached). Then redirect the needle inside the node without removing completely from the tissue. If using a syringe method (active suctioning technique), the plunger should be mostly pulled out before the tip of the needle exits the node. Forceful suction often lyzes the cells and may cause blood contamination or hemodilution. After collection, place a 5 mL syringe on the hub (if using non-aspiration technique) and gently expel onto the slide at a close distance. Smear the sample like a blood film or place a glider slide on top of the sample and gently pull perpendicularly to the sample. Heat fixing is not necessary and may rupture cells; air drying is the ideal method of "fixing" the cells to the slide prior to staining. If multiple lymph nodes are enlarged, collection from all affected nodes may increase the chances of a diagnosis.

15.3 Lymph Node Cell Types

Several cell types will be seen in normal lymph node aspirates: small lymphocytes, intermediate sized lymphocytes, large lymphocytes (lymphoblasts), plasma cells, and Mott cells. Inflammatory cells such as neutrophils, macrophages, eosinophils, and mast cells can be identified when the lymph node is inflamed or draining an area of inflammation. Primary and metastatic cancer cells can also populate a lymph node.

15.3.1 Small Lymphocytes

Small lymphocytes are <9 μm in diameter (smaller than a neutrophil, equal to or slightly larger than an erythrocyte) with round to oval nuclei, dense chromatin, and a scant amount of pale to mildly basophilic cytoplasm.

Equine Hematology, Cytology, and Clinical Chemistry, Second Edition.
Edited by Raquel M. Walton, Rick L. Cowell, and Amy C. Valenciano.

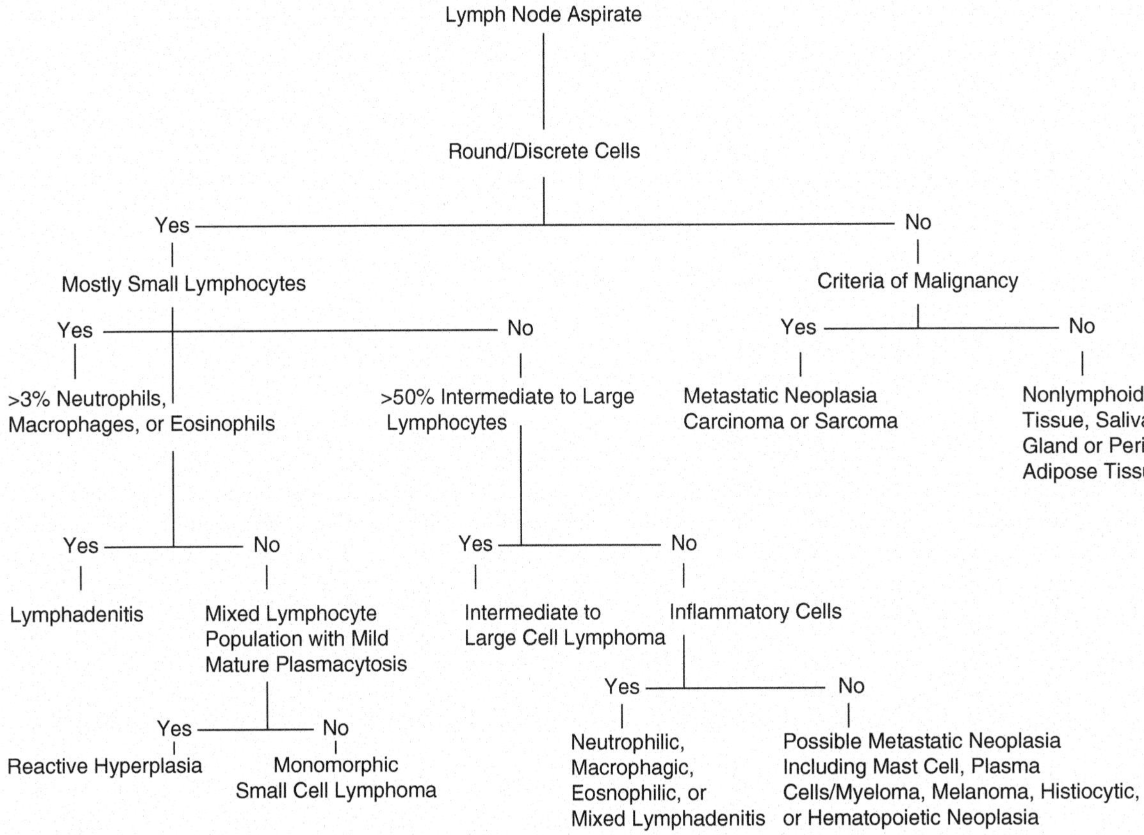

Figure 15.1 Algorithmic approach to cytological evaluation of lymph node aspirates.

15.3.2 Intermediate Lymphocytes

Intermediate lymphocytes (prolymphocytes) are 9–12 μm in diameter (about the same size as a neutrophil) with round to oval to occasionally cleaved nuclei, smooth to stippled chromatin, occasionally visible nucleoli, and a scant to mild amount of mildly basophilic cytoplasm.

15.3.3 Large Lymphocytes (Lymphoblasts)

Large lymphocytes are larger than neutrophils (>12 μm in diameter) with oval nuclei, dispersed chromatin, visible to prominent and occasional multiple nucleoli, and a mild amount of deeply basophilic and occasionally circumferential cytoplasm.

15.3.4 Plasma Cells

Plasma cells are usually the size of a small to intermediate sized lymphocyte with round, eccentric nuclei, stippled to coarse chromatin, and a moderate amount of deeply basophilic circumferential cytoplasm. Usually, the cells have a perinuclear clear zone representing the Golgi apparatus. Plasma cells whose cytoplasm is filled with clear or pale staining globules (often round but can be linear in appearance) are known as Mott cells. The globules are called Russell bodies which are dilated endoplasmic reticulum cisternae containing retained immunoglobulins.

15.3.5 Neutrophils

Neutrophils have a segmented nucleus with coarsely clumped chromatin and a mild amount of clear cytoplasm.

15.3.6 Macrophages

Macrophages are large phagocytic cells generally larger than a lymphoblast and have round to oval nuclei and a mild to abundant amount of variably basophilic cytoplasm with rounded borders. Macrophages can have an extremely variable appearance and range from vacuolated, spindloid appearing, epithelioid appearing, binucleated and multinucleated (giant cells). Frequently macrophages will have phagocytized material in their cytoplasm.

15.3.7 Eosinophils

Eosinophils are slightly larger than neutrophils and have a segmented nucleus with coarse chromatin, and numerous large, round, bright, eosinophilic cytoplasmic granules.

15.4 Metastatic Cancer Cells

Tumor metastasis to lymph nodes is identified by recognizing cell types that are not normally present in lymph node aspirates or by noting a significant increase in numbers of a cell type that is normally present in only small numbers.

Metastatic disease invading a lymph node involves the presence of mesenchymal, epithelial, or round cells. Mesenchymal neoplasms or sarcomas tend to be locally invasive and infrequently metastasize to nodes; therefore, metastatic sarcomas are rarely appreciated in lymph nodes. Malignant epithelial neoplasia (i.e., carcinoma/adenocarcinoma) is identified with some frequency. Malignant round cell tumors include lymphoma (which can be primary or metastatic), melanoma, mast cell tumors, plasma cell tumors/myeloma, and, rarely in the horse, histiocytic tumors or hematopoietic neoplasia.

15.5 Cytological Evaluation

Knowledge of normal cytological characteristics of lymph node aspirates enables the evaluator to recognize abnormal findings. Some diagnoses that can be reliably made by cytological examination of lymph node aspirates include the following.

- *Lymphoma (lymphosarcoma)*: >50% of the cells in the smear are large lymphocytes (lymphoblasts) and/or intermediate sized lymphocytes (prolymphocytes).
- *Lymphadenitis*: though lymphadenitis may be present and sometimes can be recognized by experienced cytologists when smaller numbers of inflammatory cells are present than are listed below, the cell concentrations given are suggested for novice cytologists in an effort to prevent "overdiagnosis."
  - Neutrophilic lymphadenitis: >5 neutrophils/100×
  - Purulent lymphadenitis: >20 neutrophils/100×
  - Eosinophilic lymphadenitis: >3 eosinophils/100×
  - Macrophagic lymphadenitis: >5 macrophages/100×
  - Reactive or immune stimulation: >2–3 plasma cells/100×
- *Metastatic neoplasia*: metastatic cancer cells are observed. These may be recognized as cell types not normally present in lymph node aspirates, with three or more criteria of malignancy, or as significantly increased numbers of a cell type that are normally present in lymph node aspirates in very small numbers.

As cytology collects the sample from only a few, small, discrete foci of a lymph node, recognition of one or more of the above processes does not totally rule out the possibility of other concurrent processes. However, lymphadenitis is nearly always diffuse throughout the node, and lymphoma generally is sufficiently diffuse to be reliably identified when the affected node is enlarged. Nevertheless, metastatic tumor cells may be focal or diffuse (i.e., effacing the lymph node).

15.6 Normal Lymph Nodes

Traditionally, a normal or benign lymph node may appear similar to a reactive lymph node, but lymph node enlargement is usually not appreciated with a normal node. Small lymphocytes (size of an erythrocyte or slightly larger) make up >75% of the nucleated cell population. Plasma cells, intermediate lymphocytes, and large lymphocytes (lymphoblasts) compose <25% of the lymphoid population. Often peripheral blood, associated leukocytes, and platelets can be seen. Most aspirates with lymphoid tissue have lymphoglandular bodies or basophilic cytoplasmic fragments that may form from lyzed and/or dividing cells.

15.7 Lymphoid Hyperplasia

Reactive or hyperplastic lymph nodes are dominated by small lymphocytes with dense chromatin and a scant amount of mildly basophilic cytoplasm with low numbers of plasma cells and large lymphocytes (lymphoblasts). These findings are generally consistent with a normal node except for the presence of lymphadenopathy (lymph node enlargement). Often a mild, mature plasmacytosis will be present secondary to immune stimulation. Large lymphocytes or lymphoblasts with visible to prominent nucleoli are noted but generally compose <30% of the total nucleated population (Figures 15.2 and 15.3). Localized lymphoid hyperplasia usually occurs secondary to inflammation or antigenic stimulation that drains to that node. Other inflammatory cells may be visualized in low numbers.

Generalized lymphoid hyperplasia is usually associated with systemic disease, generalized skin pathology, immune-mediated diseases, and sepsis. Viral, fungal, and rickettsial diseases can also result in a generalized reactive lymphadenopathy.

15.8 Lymphadenitis

Lymphadenitis may be neutrophilic (Figure 15.4), eosinophilic (Figures 15.5 and 15.6), macrophagic/granulomatous (Figure 15.7), or any combination of these reactions (i.e., mixed, pyogranulomatous) (Figure 15.8). Lymphadenitis may be due to inflammation or infection directly involving

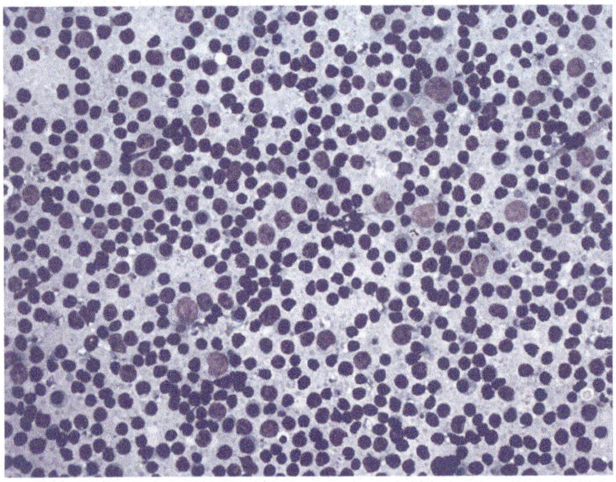

Figure 15.2 Reactive lymphoid hyperplasia in a horse. Note small lymphocytes predominate with lower numbers of plasma cells and large lymphocytes. Modified Wright–Giemsa stain, 500×.

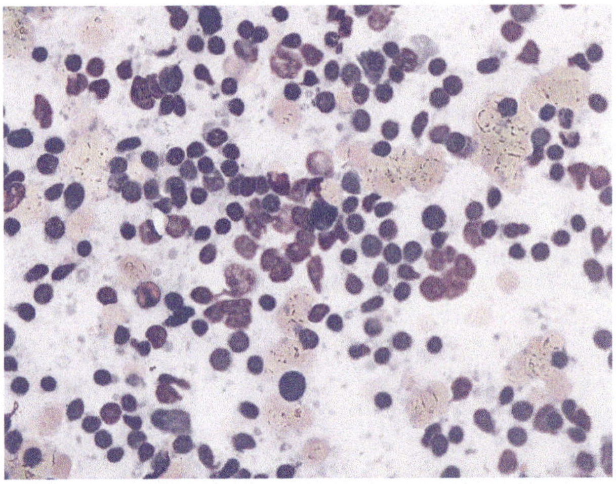

Figure 15.3 Reactive lymphoid hyperplasia in a horse. Mostly small lymphocytes with few plasma cells, large lymphocytes, and numerous small, basophilic lymphoglandular bodies with admixed peripheral blood. Modified Wright–Giemsa stain, 1000×.

the node (primary) or inflammation in the area of the node which drains to the node (secondary). The top differential for a primary lymphadenitis causing a severe neutrophilic or purulent response is strangles caused by *Streptococcus equi*. Strangles typically presents with lymphadenomegaly of the mandibular, submaxillary, and retropharyngeal lymph nodes which become markedly infiltrated with degenerate neutrophils and subsequent lymph node abscessation. Often organisms can be identified in the aspirates indicating direct infection of the nodes as well. Other less likely considerations include *Corynebacterium pseudotuberculosis* and *Actinomyces* spp. [2] which may infect the nodes and elicit a suppurative or purulent response.

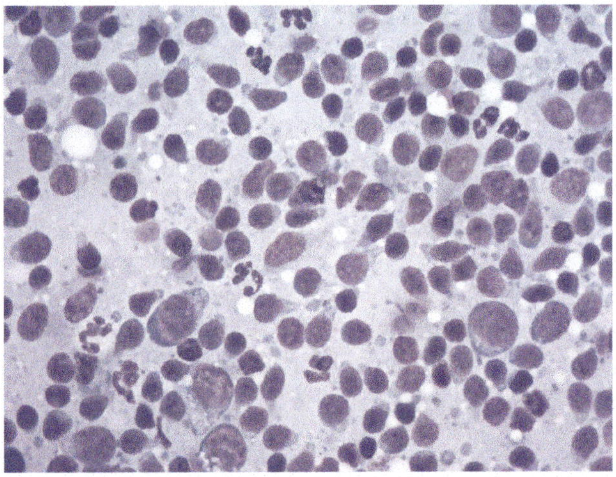

Figure 15.4 Neutrophilic lymphadenitis in a horse: >5 neutrophils/100×. Modified Wright–Giemsa stain, 1000×.

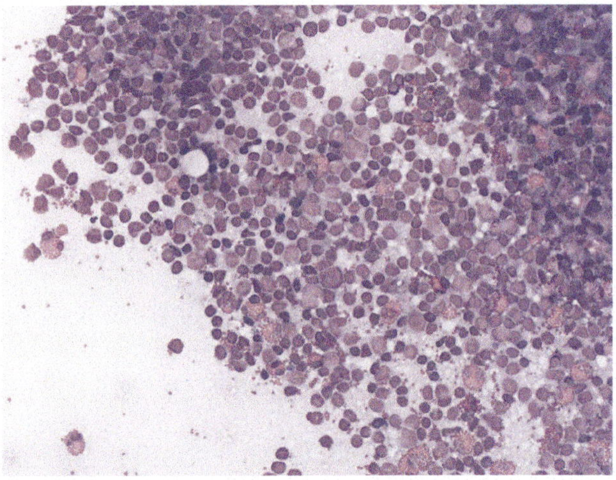

Figure 15.5 Eosinophilic lymphadenitis in a horse. Modified Wright–Giemsa stain, 500×.

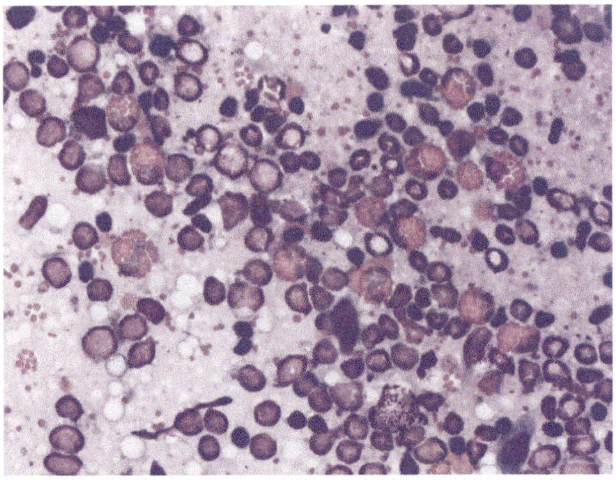

Figure 15.6 Eosinophilic lymphadenitis in a horse. Modified Wright–Giemsa stain, 1000×.

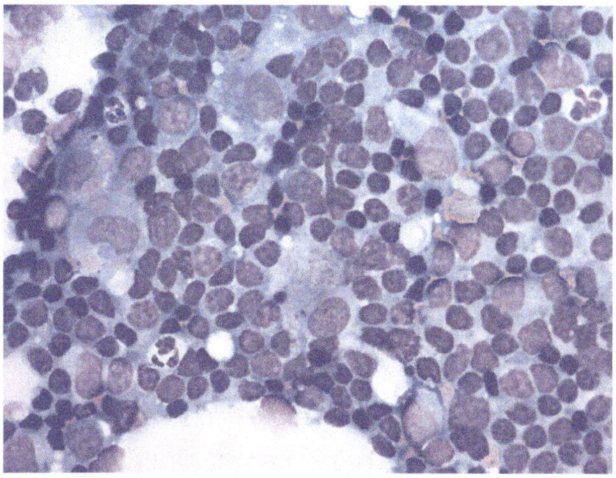

Figure 15.7 Macrophagic lymphadenitis with >5 macrophage/100×. Note erythrophagic macrophages and hemosiderophages in the sample suggestive of hemorrhage. Modified Wright-Giemsa stain, 1000×.

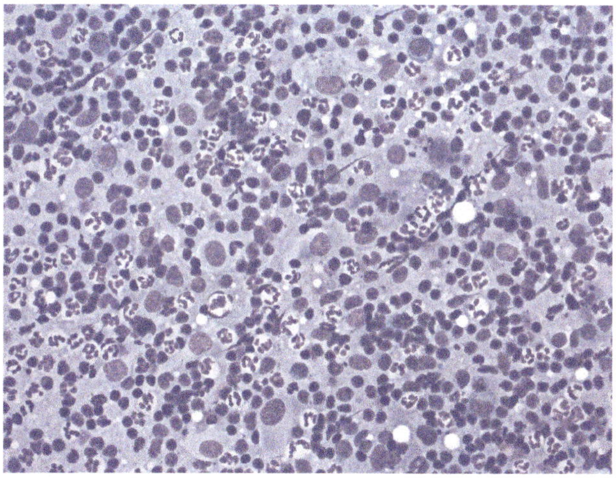

Figure 15.8 Mixed lymphadenitis or pyogranulomatous lymphadenitis with numerous neutrophils and macrophages admixed with lymphocytes. Modified Wright-Giemsa stain, 500×.

Eosinophilic lymphadenitis is most common in lymph nodes draining the skin, respiratory, or digestive tract. Any allergic or hypersensitivity (including parasitic) response which drains to the node can stimulate a secondary eosinophilic lymphadenitis. A cause for primary eosinophilic lymphadenitis is multisystemic eosinophilic epitheliotropic disease (MEED) which is a rare disease characterized by eosinophilia and eosinophilic infiltration of several organs, including lymph nodes.

Granulomatous or pyogranulomatous lymphadenitis can be associated with systemic fungi, protozoa, or algae infections. Oomycetes including *Pythium* spp. may elicit a marked macrophagic response; however, occasionally *Pythium* and some fungal infections can cause an eosinophilic infiltrate as well. Some bacterial infections including *Listeria monocytogenes*, *Salmonella typhimurium*, *Actinobacillus* spp., and *Mycobacterium* spp. can elicit a granulomatous lymphadenitis [3, 4].

15.9 Lymphoproliferative Neoplasia (Lymphoma and Plasma Cell)

In horses, lymphoma is the most common malignant neoplasm, is usually fatal, and affects equids of all ages with no gender or breed predilection. Lymphoma is usually classified based on anatomical location including a multicentric form which may involve peripheral and/or internal lymph nodes as well as variable organs. Multicentric is the most frequently occurring lymphoma followed by cutaneous and gastrointestinal [5]. Lymphoma is subtyped based on histology and immunophenotyping.

On cytology, lymphoma architecture cannot be appreciated so lymphoma is usually categorized as large cell or lymphoblastic (Figures 15.9 and 15.10), intermediate sized, or small cell (indolent) lymphoma (Figure 15.11). Intermediate or large cell lymphoma are usually characterized by >50% (of the lymphoid population) being intermediate to large lymphocytes with round to oval to cleaved nuclei, smooth to dispersed chromatin, visible or prominent nucleoli, and a mild amount of basophilic cytoplasm. T-zone small cell lymphoma as well as chronic lymphocytic leukemia with lymphoid tissue infiltration have been described in the horse [6, 7]. Small cell lymphoma is often characterized by a predominance or monomorphic population of small lymphocytes with a

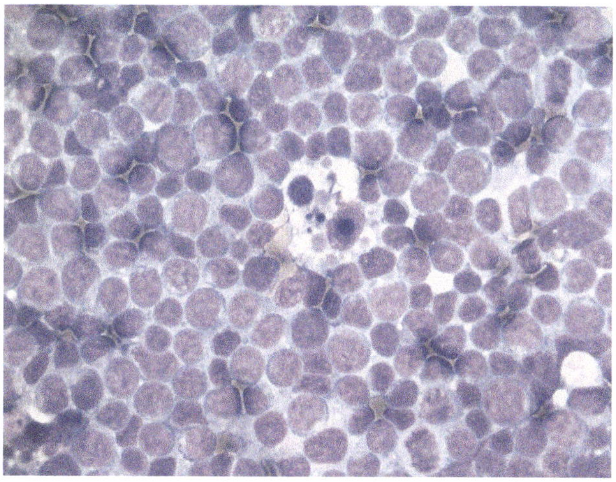

Figure 15.9 Large cell (lymphoblastic) lymphoma with >50% large lymphocytes with immature features. Tingible body macrophage in the center. Modified Wright-Giemsa stain, 1000×.

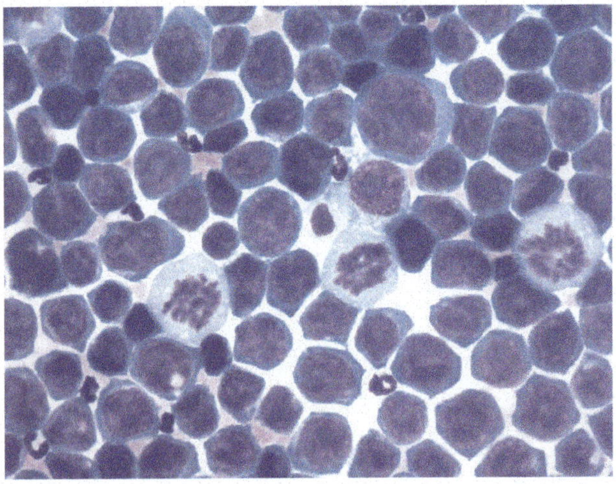

Figure 15.10 Large cell (lymphoblastic) lymphoma with a homogeneous population of large lymphocytes with prominent nucleoli. Modified Wright–Giemsa stain, 1000×.

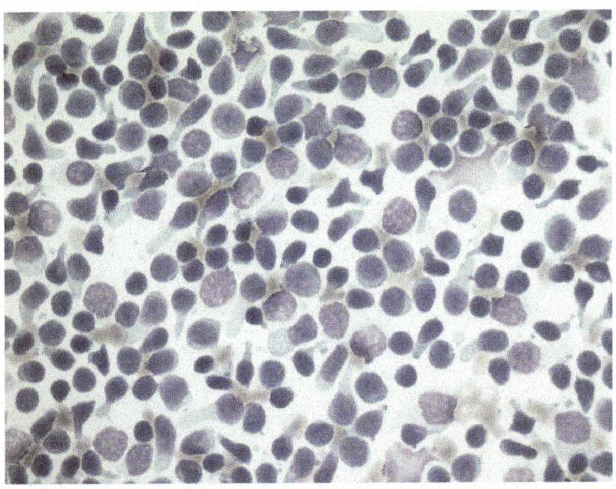

Figure 15.11 Small cell lymphoma consisting of a monomorphic population of small lymphocytes with smooth chromatin and a mild amount of basophilic cytoplasm with frequent cytoplasmic pseudopodia. Modified Wright–Giemsa stain, 1000×.

small rim of basophilic cytoplasm and occasional to frequent cytoplasm pseudopodia with round nuclei and dense chromatin. Immunophenotyping of the lymphoid cells by flow cytometry, immunocytochemistry, and immunohistochemistry is available to further characterize the neoplastic lymphocytes.

Multiple or plasma cell myeloma is also a lymphoproliferative neoplasm but is rare in the horse and primarily involves the bone marrow but may also originate from extramedullary locations (including lymph node) and occur as a solitary tumor (plasmacytoma). It is characterized by autonomously replicating neoplastic plasma cells (B-cells).

15.10 Metastatic Neoplasia

Tumor metastasis to lymph nodes is characterized by moderate to large numbers of cells that either are not normally found in lymph nodes or are typically present only in very small numbers. Squamous cell carcinoma and melanoma are the most common malignant neoplasms of the horse which potentially metastasize to lymph nodes [5]. Squamous cell carcinoma is recognized by moderately to markedly atypical squamous cells admixed with lymphocytes (Figures 15.12 and 15.13), whilst other types of metastatic

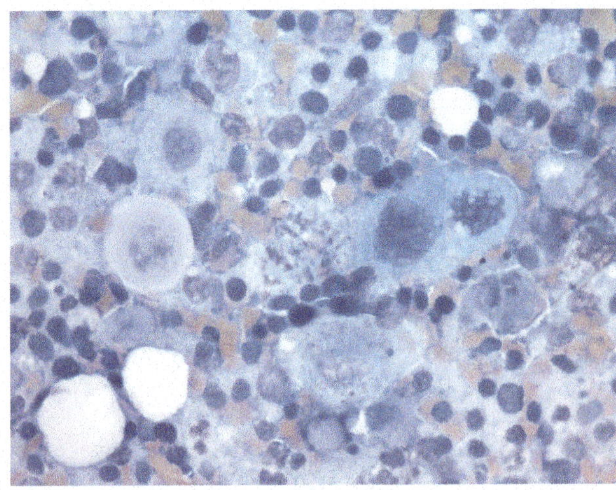

Figure 15.12 Metastatic squamous cell carcinoma involving the submandibular lymph node. Note several atypical squamous epithelial cells admixed within a reactive lymphoid population. Modified Wright–Giemsa stain, 1000×.

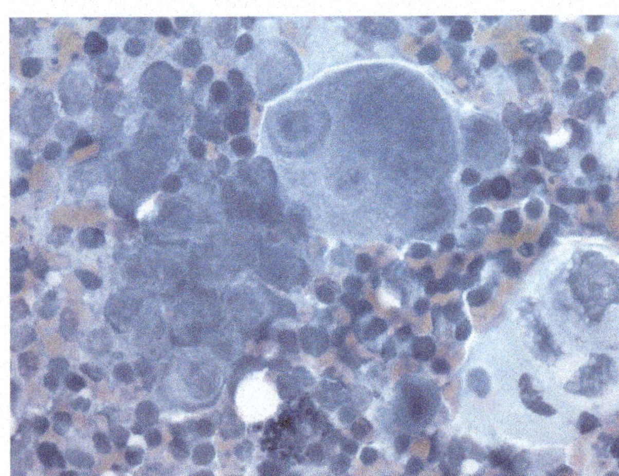

Figure 15.13 Metastatic squamous cell carcinoma involving the submandibular lymph node. Several highly atypical squamous epithelial cells with marked criteria of malignancy including the following: anisocytosis, anisokaryosis, multinucleation, prominent and multiple nucleoli and nuclear crowding. Modified Wright–Giemsa stain, 1000×.

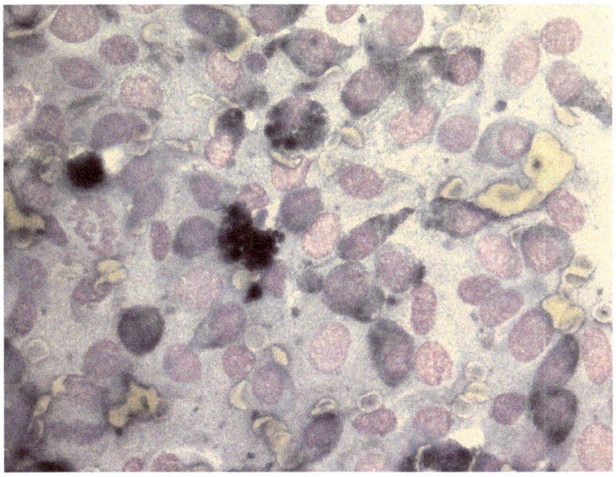

Figure 15.14 Malignant melanoma with metastases to the submandibular lymph node. The node is effaced with numerous, atypical melanocytes with moderate to marked atypia and variable cytoplasmic granulation with melanin granules. Modified Wright-Giemsa stain, 1000×.

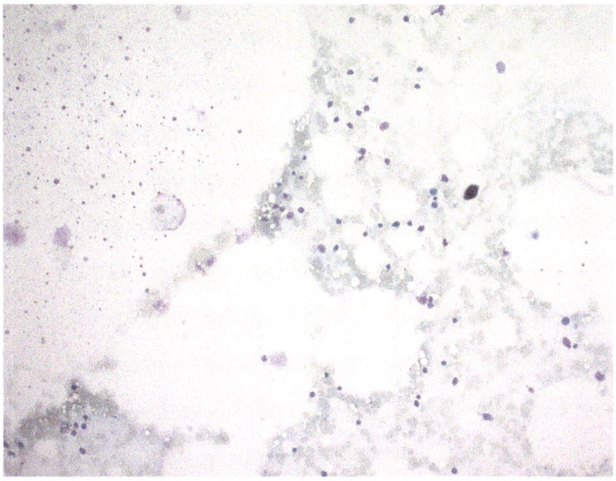

Figure 15.15 Aspiration of mostly perinodal adipose tissue with a scant amount of normal lymph node. Note numerous, variably sized lipid droplets. Modified Wright-Giemsa stain, 200×.

epithelial neoplasms (carcinoma or adenocarcinoma) may be identified by clustering of atypical epithelial cells with significant criteria of malignancy.

Malignant melanoma involving the node is usually identified by an atypical round or spindloid population of cells with variable amount of cytoplasmic melanin granules (Figure 15.14).

Rarely, malignant spindle cell tumors or sarcomas may be identified in lymph node aspirates. Large numbers of cells exhibiting cytoplasm that trails away from the nucleus in one or two directions with nuclear criteria of malignancy indicate a malignant spindle cell tumor.

Mast cell tumors rarely metastasize to the lymph nodes in horses and in those cases mast cells may exhibit atypia, are found in aggregates, or completely efface the nodes with sheets of mast cells present.

Also, myeloproliferative neoplasms such as malignant histiocytosis and myeloid leukemia may involve the node and should be considered when an atypical round cell population is present in the node in high numbers.

15.11 Aspiration of Nonlymphoid Tissue

Subcutaneous fat is the most common nonlymphoid tissue accidentally aspirated when attempting to collect cytological samples from lymph nodes. Fat is recognized grossly by its wet (oily) appearance on the slide and its occasional failure to dry (Figure 15.15).

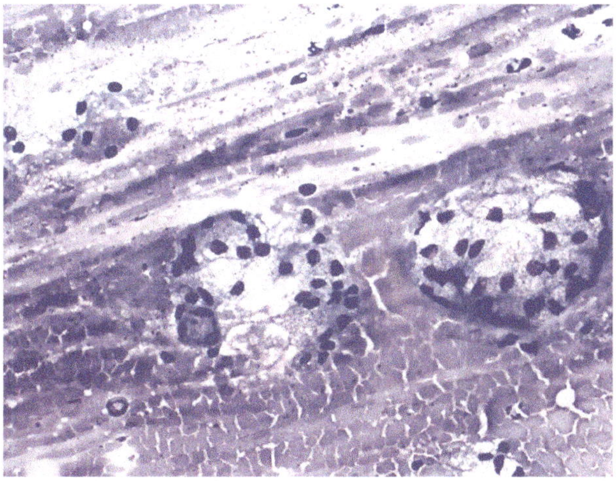

Figure 15.16 Aspiration of normal salivary gland tissue in a horse. Note numerous, uniform clusters of glandular epithelial cells in a background of mucoid material and blood. Modified Wright-Giemsa stain, 500×.

Also, salivary gland tissue may be accidentally aspirated when mandibular lymph node aspirates are attempted. Slides made from salivary gland aspirates usually consist of clusters of salivary cells in a background of mucoid material and pink mucinous granules. Salivary cells have uniform nuclei with a moderate amount of pale, foamy cytoplasm (Figure 15.16).

References

1 Blauvelt, M. and Messick, J.B. (2020). The lymph nodes. In: *Cowell and Tyler's Diagnostic Cytology and Hematology of the Dog and Cat*, 5e (eds. A.C. Valenciano and R.L. Cowell), 172. St Louis: Elsevier.

2 Beck, A., Baird, J.D., and Slavic, Đ. (2011). Submandibular lymph node abscess caused by Actinomyces denticolens in a horse in Ontario. *Can. Vet. J.* 52: 513–514.

3 Ohba, T., Shibahara, T., Kobayashi, H. et al. (2010). Granulomatous lymphadenitis associated with *Actinobacillus* pleuropneumoniae serotype 2 in slaughter barrows. *Can. Vet. J.* 51: 733–737.

4 Nemeth, N.M., Blas-Machado, U., Hopkins, B.A. et al. (2012). Granulomatous typhlocolitis, lymphangitis, and lymphadenitis in a horse infected with *Listeria monocytogenes*, *Salmonella typhimurium*, and cyathostomes. *Vet. Pathol.* 50 (2): 252–255.

5 Miller, M.A., Moore, G., Bertin, F. et al. (2016). What's new in old horses? Postmortem diagnoses in mature and aged equids. *Vet. Pathol.* 53 (2): 390–398.

6 Cian, F., Tyner, G., Martini, V. et al. (2013). Leukemic small cell lymphoma or chronic lymphocytic leukemia in a horse. *Vet. Clin. Pathol.* 42 (3): 301–306.

7 Durham, A.C., Pillitterri, C., San Myint, M. et al. (2012). Two hundred three cases of equine lymphoma classified according to the World Health Organization (WHO) classification criteria. *Vet. Pathol.* 50 (1): 86–93.

16

Cytology of the Endometrium

Luisa Ramírez-Agámez[1], Camilo Hernández-Avilés[2], and Chelsea Makloski-Cohorn[3]

[1] Animal Reproductive Services, Bogotá, Colombia
[2] Large Animal Clinical Sciences, College of Veterinary Medicine and Biomedical Sciences, Texas A&M University, College Station, TX, USA
[3] Pinnacle Equine Veterinary Services, PLLC, Whitesboro, TX, USA

As with the stallion, the evaluation of a mare's reproductive health is based on the assessment of breeding records, physical examination of the reproductive tract and the use of complementary tests to determine subclinical or clinical conditions that cannot be obviously diagnosed during the physical exam. Although a complete description of the breeding soundness examination of the mare is beyond the scope of this chapter, it is important to remember that the examination of the mare should include [1]:

- a brief general physical exam of the mare, paying special attention to musculoskeletal conformation and body condition score
- a complete examination of the mare's external genitalia, including vulvar position and labia conformation, perineum conformation, vestibule-vaginal sphincter, presence of vulvar discharge and udder
- a thorough examination of the mare's internal reproductive tract, including vestibulum, vagina, cervix, uterine body, uterine horns, and ovaries by using transrectal palpation and ultrasonography. Other diagnostic aids that can be used for evaluation of the mare's internal reproductive tract include the use of endoscopy (hysteroscopy), particularly in cases of suspected uterine disease (endometrial cysts, adhesions) or oviductal disease (blockage)
- use of complementary diagnostic aids such as endometrial culture, cytology, and biopsy. Other more advanced diagnostics that may help to determine the reproductive status of a mare or less common causes of subfertility/infertility include genetic tests (karyotyping).

In general terms, the use of endometrial cytology is less common amongst veterinary practitioners compared to the use of endometrial culture, particularly in busy private practices. This is due to inconsistent results, lack of familiarity with the technique or difficulty in the evaluation and interpretation of the cell types present [2]. However, the use of two or more diagnostic aids when performing a thorough reproductive examination is necessary to adequately determine whether or not a mare is suffering from an endometrial inflammatory process (endometritis), and to determine the course of action that should be taken [1–4]. In fact, some studies have demonstrated that the use of endometrial cytology in conjunction with endometrial culture or biopsy is related to a higher capacity to accurately detect endometritis in subfertile mares, particularly when this condition is related to the presence of bacteria such as *Streptococcus zooepidemicus*, *Staphylococcus aureus* or *Klebsiella pneumoniae* [2, 5, 6]. Thus, it is imperative that veterinarians become familiar with the adequate collection, processing, and interpretation of endometrial cytology. This chapter will focus on the most common techniques for collecting and processing samples for cytological analysis and their interpretation.

16.1 Sample Collection Techniques

Since their introduction in the early 1960s, several techniques have been reported for the collection of cytological specimens. Most of these sampling techniques have included the use of uterine culture swabs, double-guarded culture swabs, uterine cytology brushes, uterine biopsies, or specimens resulting from uterine lavage fluids. Although all these techniques have their potential advantages and disadvantages, practitioners must be aware that regardless of the technique chosen for sampling, these must (i) be harmless to the mare's endometrium, (ii) avoid the introduction of

Equine Hematology, Cytology, and Clinical Chemistry, Second Edition.
Edited by Raquel M. Walton, Rick L. Cowell, and Amy C. Valenciano.

pathogens to the uterine environment, and (iii) facilitate the collection of sufficient numbers of endometrial and other cells to allow a reliable cytological examination. The decision to use one technique or another should also depend on the preferences of the practitioner in terms of ease, associated costs, and time required.

The acquisition of cytological samples is most commonly done during midestrus, since at this stage of the cycle the cervix is open and the uterine immune mechanisms are more active [7]. Hence, the likelihood of finding inflammatory cells (neutrophils) or bacteria will be increased [8, 9]. Others have suggested that endometrial cytology should be acquired during late diestrus–early estrus, particularly if that cycle is intended to be used for breeding the mare [8]. However, the odds of producing more false-negative results, as well as the chances of inducing an iatrogenic infection of the endometrium, are higher when diestral cytology is taken [9, 10].

Prior to sampling, the mare should be placed in stocks and prepared in the same way as for artificial insemination. This implies that all feces must be removed from the rectum, and the vulva, perineum, and perianal region must be scrubbed using either a chlorhexidine- or iodine-based solution and washed with clean water. Particular care must be taken when cleaning the vulvar labia and clitoral fossa, since these places harbor several commensal and potentially pathogenic bacteria that could be accidentally infused into the mare's endometrium [11]. The practitioner must wear a sterile sleeve and place the tip of the culture device (swab or uterine catheter) into the palm of the hand, to avoid it coming into contact with lubricant, the skin or mucosa whilst passing through the vulva and vagina. Sterile, nonbacteriostatic lubricant should be placed on the top of the hand, making sure that the tip of the culture device is not contaminated with the lubricant. Then, the hand and the culture device are passed through the vulvar labia, vestibule, and vagina until reaching the external cervical os. Subsequently, a finger is used to guide the culture device through the cervical os and then into the uterine lumen.

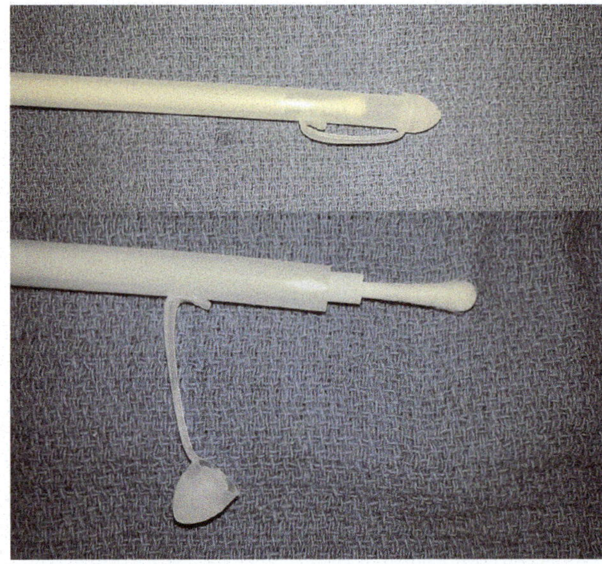

Figure 16.1 The Kalayjian single-guarded endometrial swab. Observe the cap in the outer plastic tube, which is used to collect endometrial cell samples.

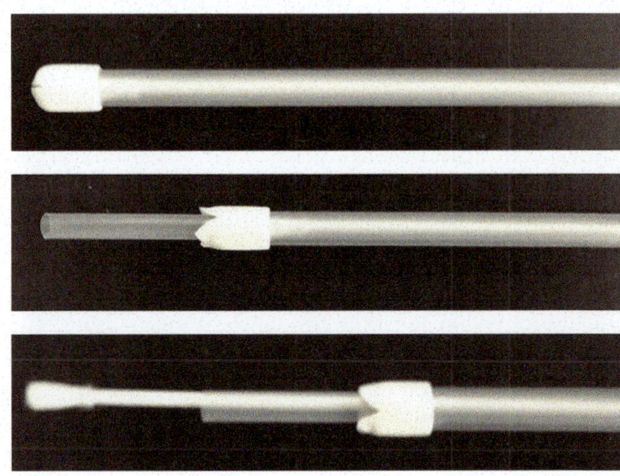

Figure 16.2 The McCullough double-guarded endometrial swab. (*Top*) Appearance of the double-guarded swab prior to passing it through the mare's reproductive tract. (*Middle*) The inner plastic tube is propelled through the tip of the culture device. (*Bottom*) The swab is propelled through the inner plastic tube to take the sample from the uterine lumen.

16.1.1 Single-Guarded and Double-Guarded Swabs and Cytological Brushes

At least three different types of culture swabs have been commonly described for cytological examination of the mare's endometrium. The Kalayjian single-guarded uterine swab (Kalayjian Industries Inc., Long Beach, CA) (Figure 16.1) and the McCullough double-guarded uterine swab (McCullough Cartwright, Barrington, IL) (Figure 16.2) are the most commonly used for this purpose, with the latter mostly preferred by the authors [2, 3, 12–14]. All of them comprise outer guarded tubes with an inner rod holding a calcium alginate swab. Calcium alginate swabs are better than cotton swabs due to the likelihood of having cotton fibers on the stained smear which may interfere with the staining process or cytology interpretation [12]. The use of double-guarded swabs is more advantageous in terms of avoiding sample contamination with cells and bacteria from the mare's vagina or cervix [13].

After passing the swab through the cervix, the swab is pushed forward from its plastic guard. It is recommended to roll the swab against the endometrium and allow contact between the swab and the uterus for at least 30 seconds (for microbiological analysis). Then, the swab is retracted back into the plastic guard and removed from the reproductive tract, in order to avoid sample contamination.

Recently, the use of cytological brushes (Minitube GmbH, Tiefenbach, Germany) (Figure 16.3) has become more popular for obtaining samples for cytological analysis, particularly in North America and Europe. The main advantage of using a cytological brush over a culture swab is the capacity to obtain a high proportion of diagnostic smears, with more cellular intactness and less chance of preparation artefacts [15–17] (Figure 16.4). The procedure for taking samples for endometrial cytology is the same as for guarded swabs.

Practitioners may also prefer to collect a sample for endometrial cytology by passing the culture swab or cytological brush through a sterile disposable vaginal speculum (Figure 16.5). Using this procedure is advantageous in mares with vulvoplasty (Caslick), to avoid inconvenience whilst passing the hand through the vulvar labia. Also, this technique has been described to reduce the incidence of sample contamination for microbiological analysis when compared to passage of the guarded swab using a sterile sleeve and the hand [18, 19].

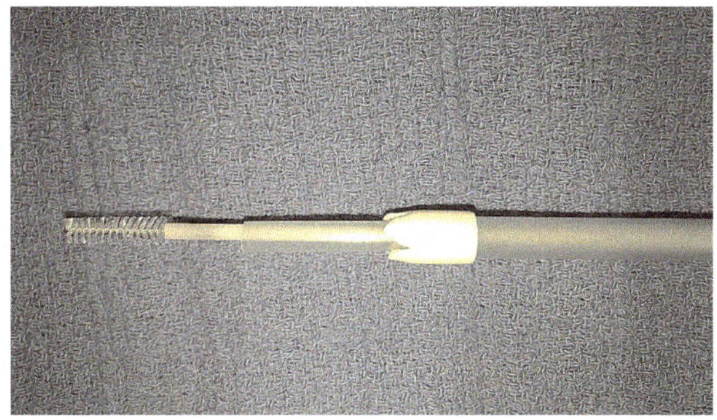

Figure 16.3 A cytological brush (Cytobrush). The system used to protect the brush from contamination is the same as for the double-guarded endometrial swab.

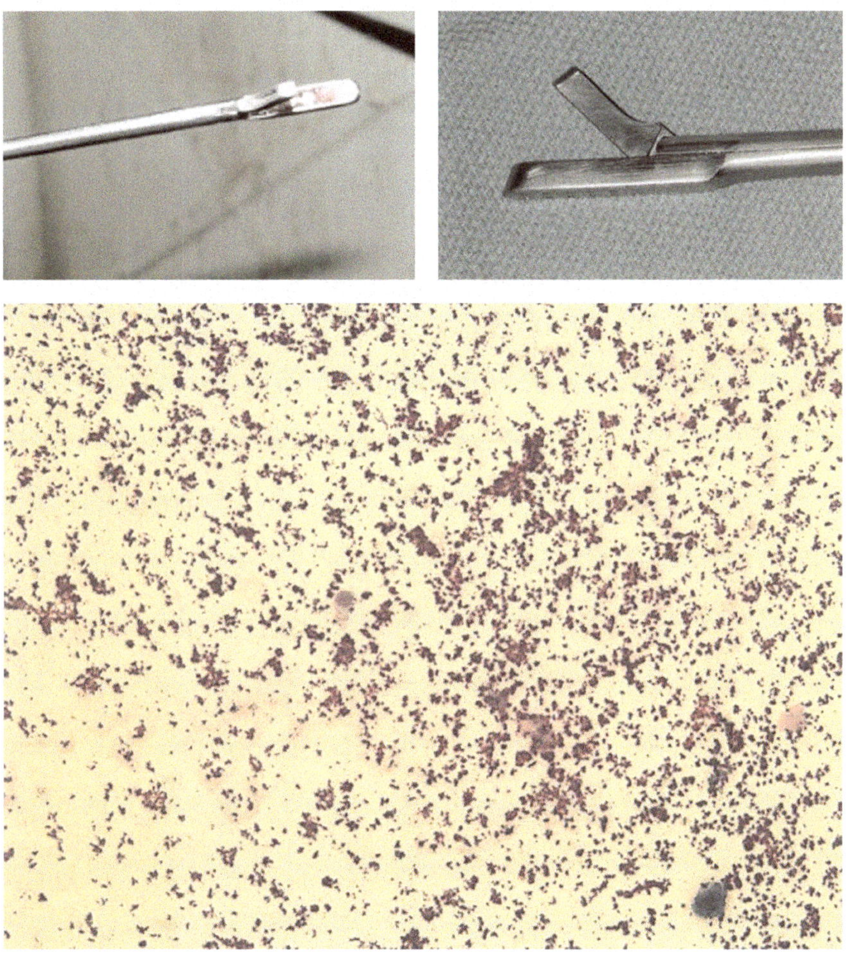

Figure 16.4 Jackson uterine biopsy forceps without (*left*) and with (*right*) sample. Cytological samples obtained from endometrial biopsies are more cellular.

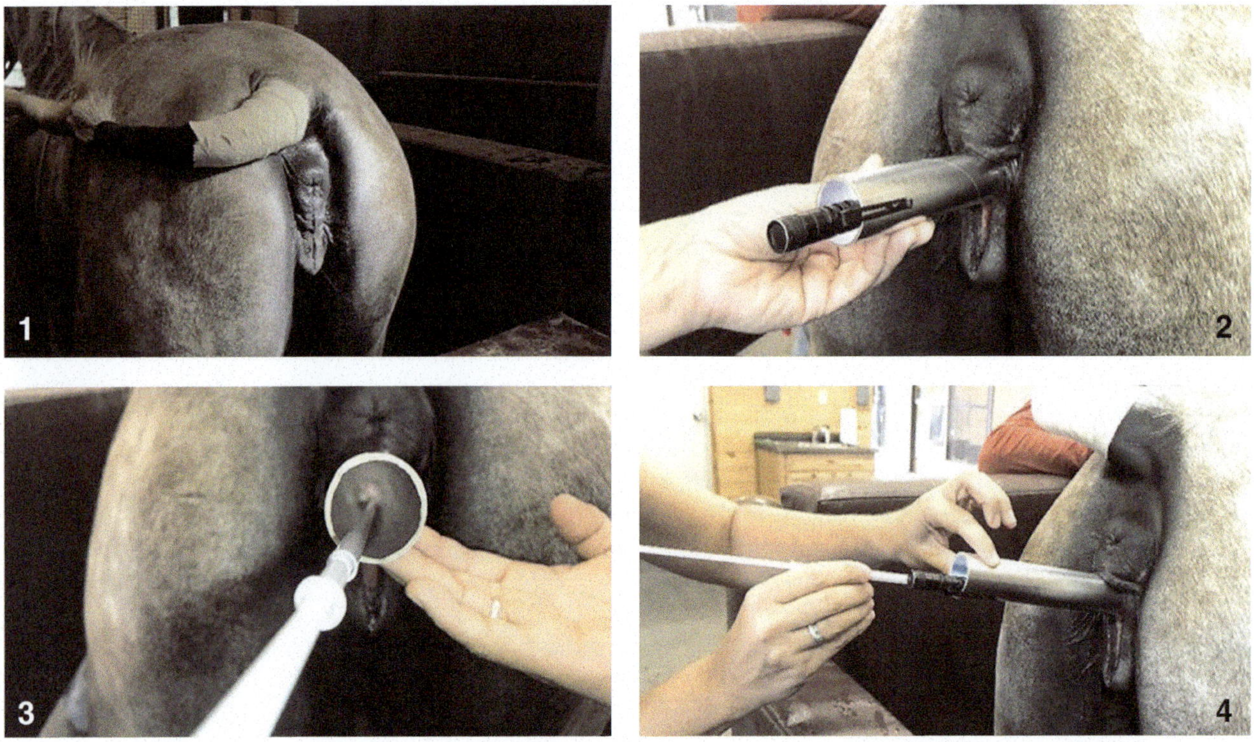

Figure 16.5 Passing an endometrial culture device through a speculum. This method is helpful in mares with Caslick suture as well as to prevent some degree of contamination, particularly when the endometrial swab is passed through the vulva and vagina.

Although both methods described above are easy to conduct and inexpensive under field conditions, disadvantages of their use are related to the fact that the samples obtained may not be completely representative of the entire endometrial surface; thus, the odds of misdiagnosing endometrial inflammation are increased. Several studies have demonstrated that the use of only guarded swabs for diagnosis of endometritis is not sufficient and may lead to false-negative results, when compared to the use of two or more diagnostic techniques, or when compared to other techniques for sample acquisition (uterine lavage or biopsy) [4, 6, 15, 17]. In the same way, it is always recommended to take samples for uterine cytology and culture, since the capacity to truly detect endometritis, particularly infectious endometritis due to *Escherichia coli* or *Pseudomonas aeruginosa*, is improved [3, 20].

16.1.2 Uterine Lavage and Low-Volume Uterine Lavage

The initial descriptions of the use of uterine lavage for recovering material intended for endometrial cytology were published in the mid-late 1980s. Ball et al. demonstrated that the infusion of 60 mL of phosphate-buffered saline (PBS) solution into the uterine body and its subsequent recovery improved the capacity to obtain microbiological and cytological samples from subfertile mares [21]. Recent studies have suggested that the use of uterine lavage is advantageous in correctly diagnosing mares that suffer from endometritis, compared to the use of swabbing techniques alone [6, 16, 17, 22]. In most of these reports, the infusion of approximately 50–60 mL of a physiological solution (PBS, lactated Ringer's or saline solution) was performed; however, the recovery rate of fluid by using this method is relatively low (30–35 mL on average).

Even when this method is superior to the use of swabs for sampling a wide area of the uterus, some authors believe that the volume infused is not enough to cover the whole surface of the endometrium [23]. Thus, other researchers have used up to 250 mL of fluid to recover endometrial cells for cytological and microbiological analysis with good results [16, 24]. In the authors' opinion, the use of 250 mL or up to 3–6 L of fluids for lavage may have not only a diagnostic but also a therapeutic benefit, particularly in mares suffering postbreeding endometritis [25]. We consider that the infusion and lavage of the uterus with large volumes of fluid may help to reduce the inflammatory response, as has been previously demonstrated, as well as helping to remove cellular debris and bacteria present in the uterus [25, 26]. After recovering the fluid from the uterus, the samples can be collected by centrifugation (200–600 g × 10 minutes) and then smeared and stained for analysis.

In order to perform a low-volume uterine lavage for endometrial cytology, the practitioner has to clean the mare's perineal region, as described above. Then, a sterile uterine catheter is passed through the vagina and cervix, as described above for taking endometrial swabs. Most practitioners use a 60–80 cm uterine lavage silicone catheter with an air cuff, in order to place the tip of the catheter inside the uterus without worrying about losing fluid through the cervix. After passing the catheter, single-line plastic tubing attached to a 150 mL sterile saline solution is connected to the end of the catheter. A syringe is connected to the cuff of the catheter and inflated with approximately 75 mL of air. Then, the cuff should be gently pulled out to verify that the catheter is correctly placed against the internal cervical os. Finally, the bag containing the sterile saline is elevated, in order to allow the flow of liquid to the uterus by gravity. The fluid is allowed to stay into the uterus for 2–3 minutes. In the meantime, the uterus may be gently massaged transrectally to ensure wide distribution of the fluid. The bag is then lowered (generally to ground level) to allow the return of the fluid by gravity (Figure 16.6). Under some circumstances, particularly in multiparous mares with a pendulous uterus, gently lifting the uterine horns and body can help to recover the infused fluid. Simultaneously, a single IV dose of oxytocin (10–20 IU) can be given to stimulate uterine contractions and increase fluid recovery [27, 28].

As mentioned above, the quantities of fluid that can be used are variable. If larger quantities of fluid are to be used, the authors recommend using either 1 L lactated Ringer's solution or sterile saline solution connected to the single-line tubing. Furthermore, a cost-effective and practical alternative is described by Brinsko [26], in which a gallon of saline solution is instilled into the uterus using a sterile sleeve attached to the end of the uterine catheter. With this method, it is recommended to allow the cells to settle by gravity before processing for cytological analysis.

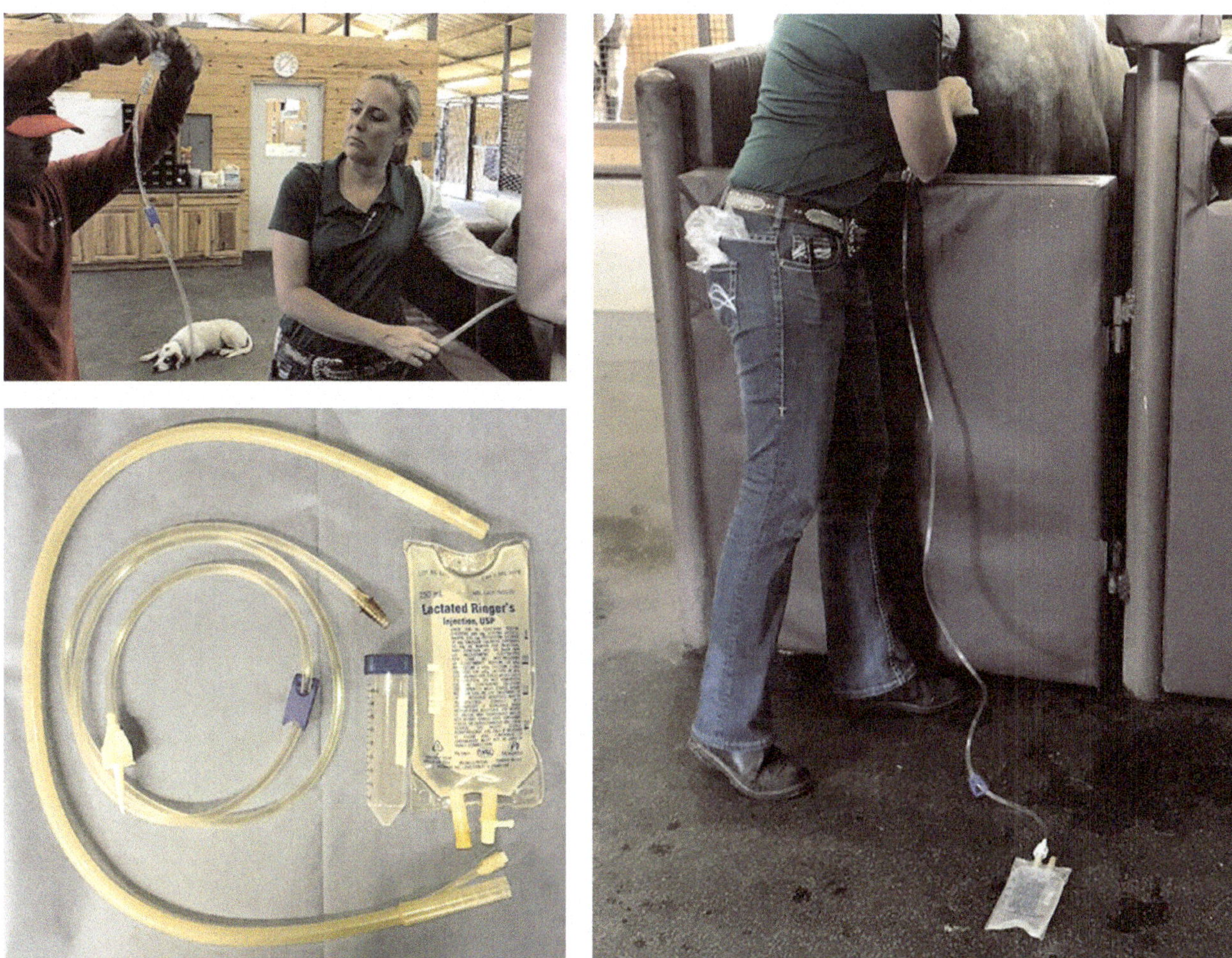

Figure 16.6 Obtaining a sample via uterine lavage. The fluid is first infused into the uterus by gravity flow. Then, the bag is lowered to the ground to recover the fluid.

16.1.3 Endometrial Biopsy

Some practitioners use impression smears of endometrial tissues obtained with the Jackson uterine biopsy forceps (Jorgensen Labs, Loveland, CO) prior to placing in fixative agents for cytology (see Figure 16.4). Such samples may be helpful in diagnosing infiltrative inflammation and infection and may be helpful in conjunction with histopathology and culture. Cytological samples obtained from such impression smears are far more cellular than the previously described procedures and a well-defined grading scale has not been established at this time to determine extent of inflammation.

16.2 Cytology Processing and Staining

Cytology samples obtained from a swab or cytology brush must be rolled immediately onto a clean glass microscope slide. It is recommended to prepare at least two slides per sample, in case of processing error or damage. The most commonly used technique for preparing cytological smears includes making two separate lines per slide by rolling the swab along the surface of the microscope slide (Figure 16.7). We prefer to air dry the slides prior to staining. This can be done by placing the slides on top of a plate warmer (37–38 °C). If endometrial cytology and culture are required, it is recommended first to streak the culture plate with the swab and then prepare the smears in the slides, to avoid contamination of the culture plate and false-positive culture results. This can be avoided by using sterile microscope slides, or two endometrial swabs when recovering samples (one for microbiological analysis and the other for cytology).

If an endometrial sample is acquired by uterine lavage, the recovered fluid can be transferred to 50 mL conical tubes (Falcon Tubes, VWR International, Radnor, PA), and centrifuged. This is commonly done when a 150 mL saline bag is used. On the other hand, if a larger volume of fluid was used for uterine lavage, the sleeve or bag containing

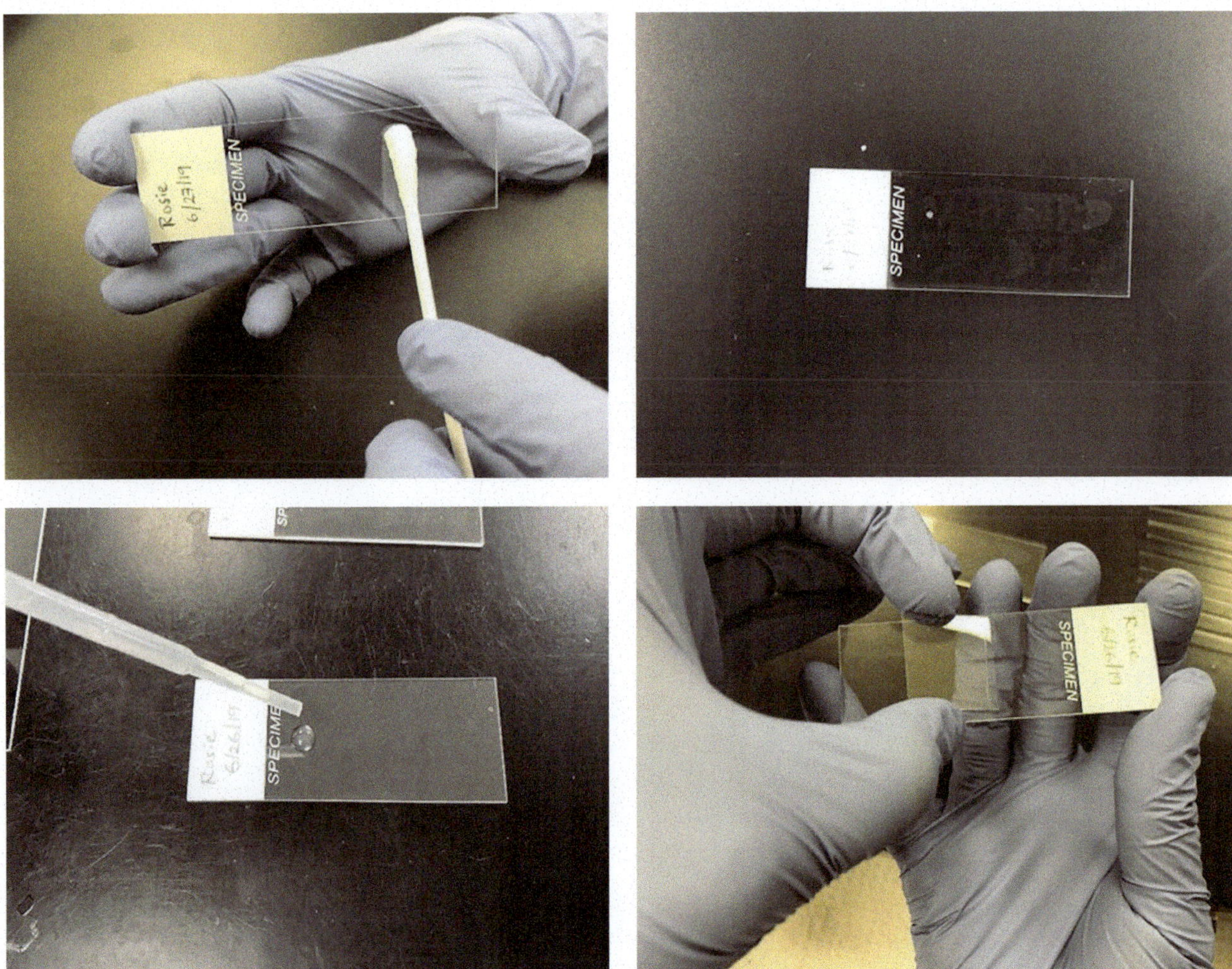

Figure 16.7 Smearing a sample onto a microscope slide. (*Top left*) Smear made using an endometrial swab. (*Top right*) Two separate lines were made on the slide for staining purposes. (*Bottom left*) Placing a drop of fluid obtained from uterine lavage. (*Bottom right*) Smearing the drop on the slide using a coverslip.

the fluid is allowed to settle (3–4 hours). Then, a small hole is punctured into the ventral part of the bag (using a new hypodermic needle) and the fluid and cells are recovered into a 50 mL conical tube. In both cases, the tubes can be centrifuged at 200–600 g × 10 minutes to concentrate all the cells in the resulting pellet [16]. After centrifugation, all but approximately 3 mL of the supernatant is discarded. Then, a small amount of the resulting pellet (20–50 μL) is loaded onto a microscope slide with a plastic transfer pipette. Conversely, a sterile swab can also be impregnated with the fluid and a smear can be prepared as described above. If the pipette method is used, then a coverslip or another slide can be used for smearing the sample.

Fixation of cytological samples can be done in two ways. Air drying slides is easy to do in the clinic or on the road in an ambulatory practice and there is greater preservation of cellular material (less loss) than wet fixation. The disadvantage of air-dry fixation is that there is less cellular detail due to mucoproteins. Wet fixation tends to float this mucoproteinaceous material off the slide, preserving cellular detail. For example, if a sample has moderate to heavy mucus on the swab, then the slides should be immediately stained with Diff-Quik rather than air dried. Alternatively, a mucus-contaminated swab can be placed in a centrifuge tube containing saline or 40% ethanol solution and centrifuged to recover cellular content.

The air-dried and ethanol-fixed slides can be stained either with modified Wright's or Diff-Quick. If Diff-Quik is used, it is important to have fresh staining solutions (refreshed monthly) and the authors prefer to dip each slide about 5–7 times into each one of the staining solutions, instead of 10 times (as recommended by the manufacturers). This avoids overstaining the cells. If the samples are not evaluated immediately after collection (<12 hours), a methanol or spray fixative can be used to preserve the cellular integrity in the sample. Other stains that can be used when analyzing an endometrial cytology include gram stains or silver stain for fungus (Grocott methenamine silver – GMS).

16.3 Evaluation and Interpretation

The main goal of endometrial cytology is to determine the presence of cellular associations indicative of an active inflammatory response in the uterus. The evaluation of endometrial cytology must be systematic, and its interpretation and the clinical decisions made after analysis have to be relevant to the history of the mare, and other clinical signs observed after the reproductive examination. Thus, it is important that practitioners do not base their clinical decisions solely on the results of endometrial cytology or culture. This is particularly true in cases where a mare has a positive culture but the cytology does not show any evidence of an inflammatory response. However, it is also important to recognize that some pathogens, such as *P. aeruginosa* or *E. coli*, may create positive culture results but negative cytology results, due to their capacity to produce biofilms, which may reduce the capacity of the inflammatory cells to migrate through the endometrium. Similarly, since not all cases of endometritis are caused by infectious agents, adequate interpretation of the results from endometrial cytology may help to reduce the indiscriminate use of antibiotics in mares which may not require them. In the authors' view, a great proportion of mares evaluated in private practice for endometritis receive antibiotic therapies for cases of endometritis which could have been solved by the use of ecbolic agents or using uterine lavages.

The first step when evaluating endometrial cytology is to determine whether or not the sample is of diagnostic quality. This means that the number of cells recovered is adequate for interpretation. When the number of cells is low, a new slide can be made. If the problem persists, a new sample should be collected. Also, the presence of cellular aggregates, extraneous materials (mucus) or foreign materials (feces, hair, cotton fibers) should be noted. Lastly, the quality of the staining must be considered. If the staining of the cells is too faint, a new smear should be prepared and stained. This initial approach to cytology is commonly done at 100× (10× objective × 10× eyepiece). If the sample is determined to be of diagnostic quality, the slide is then evaluated under a high-power field (hpf – 400×). Then, the stained cytology sample is examined for the presence and appearance of the different cellular associations, which commonly include uterine epithelial cells (endometrial cells), inflammatory cells (neutrophils, macrophages, eosinophils, lymphocytes), red blood cells (RBCs), bacteria, yeast, or fungal organisms, and debris.

16.3.1 Uterine Epithelial Cells

This cell type is the most commonly seen during examination of normal endometrial cytology smears. Depending on whether or not the mare is cycling, the shape of these cells can vary from tall columnar epithelial cells (Figures 16.8 and 16.9) in the cycling mare, to cuboidal cells when the mare is in anestrus [29]. Most of the cells found in endometrial cytology of anestrus mares have hypochromatic nuclei, whilst cells obtained during the physiological breeding season hace a uniformly stained nucleus, located in the basal portion of the cytoplasm. Other normal changes associated with cyclicity include the appearance of small vacuoles in the cytoplasm [29, 30]. Typically, uterine epithelial cells are not ciliated, but it is not uncommon to find cells with cilia in normal mares (Figures 16.10 and 16.11).

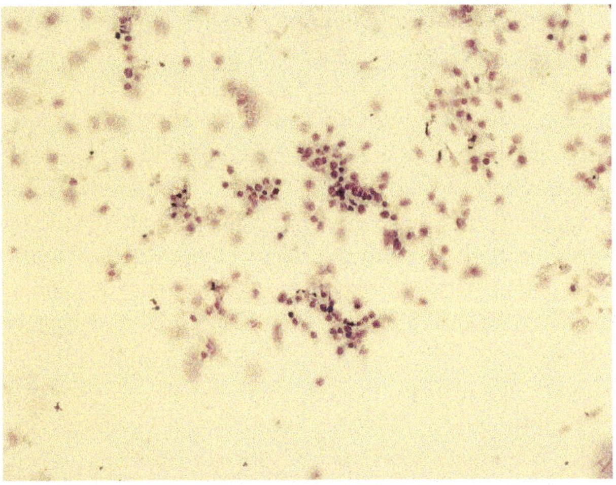

Figure 16.8 Normal uterine epithelial cells (endometrial cells). Diff-Quik, original magnification 100×.

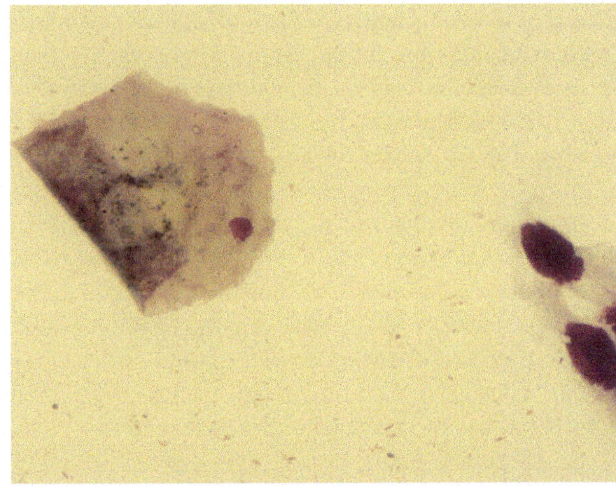

Figure 16.10 (*Right*) Uterine epithelial cells (endometrial cells) and (*left*) squamous epithelial cells from the vagina. Sample obtained by uterine lavage. Diff-Quik, original magnification 1000×.

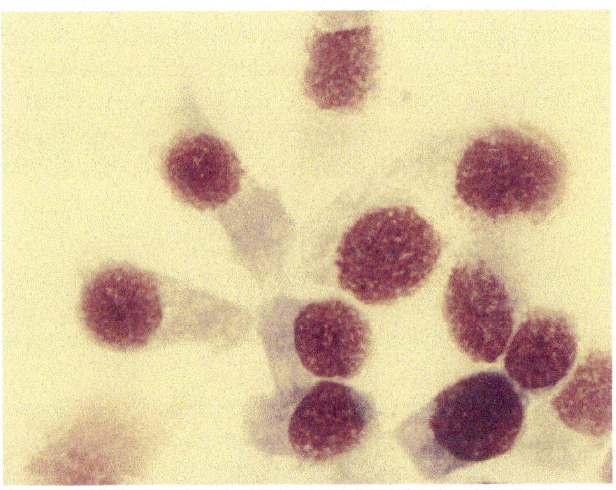

Figure 16.9 Endometrial cells from the same cytology sample as Figure 16.8. Observe the formation of small vacuoles in the cytoplasm, which is normal in cycling mares. Diff-Quik, original magnification 1000×.

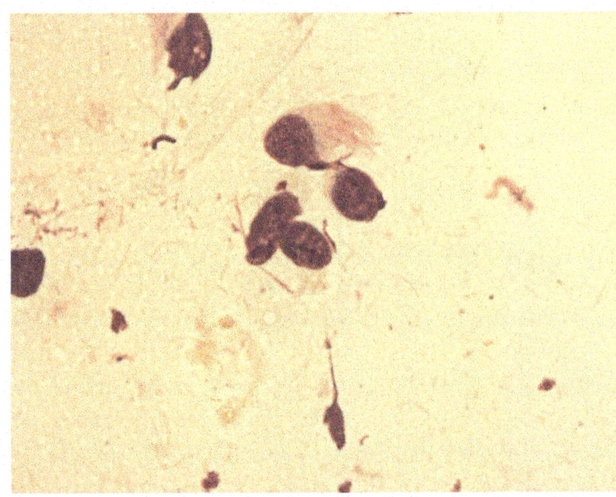

Figure 16.11 Uterine epithelial cells. Note the endometrial cell in the center has cilia. Sample obtained by endometrial cytobrush. Diff-Quik, original magnification 1000×.

Uterine epithelial cells can be observed as individual cells or as part of groups or clumps. Some atypical findings in uterine epithelial cells include increased cytoplasmic granularity, presence of large vacuoles, pyknosis (nucleus degeneration) and "giant" cell formation. Also, the presence of squamous epithelial cells (see Figure 16.10) suggests contamination of the sample with vaginal mucosa, particularly when swabbing procedures are done. Their presence has also been reported in postpartum mares, and in mares with urine reflux into the uterus [31]. Another cellular contaminant could be cervical epithelial cells. These are squamous, cuboidal, or columnar in appearance, are smaller and darker staining than endometrial cells and are often found in sheets and clumps.

16.3.2 Inflammatory Cells: Neutrophils, Macrophages, Eosinophils, Lymphocytes

Neutrophils are the predominant inflammatory cells found in mares with endometritis. Neutrophils are 10–12 μm in diameter, with a single nucleus that may be divided into 3–5 segments. In clinically normal mares, the number of neutrophils should be few to none, unless a certain degree of blood contamination is sustained during sample acquisition. On the other hand, the number of neutrophils that can be found after breeding can substantially increase, due to the normal inflammatory response of the uterus to the sperm [32, 33] (Figures 16.12 and 16.13). This transient inflammatory response is known as postbreeding endometritis, which in resistant mares is commonly cleared 12–24 hours after breeding [34]. Conversely, susceptible mares tend to develop stronger inflammatory responses post insemination; thus, the clinical signs observed in these mares, including fluid accumulation in the uterine lumen and higher number of neutrophils in cytological examinations, are more evident and do not usually resolve unless therapeutic intervention is done. It is not uncommon to observe neutrophils 2–3 days after breeding, after uterine lavage, or during the early postpartum period. In mares with an active inflammatory response, it is common to observe nuclear hypersegmentation and pyknosis. In cases of bacterial endometritis, it is common also to observe degenerated neutrophils (vacuolized cytoplasm and hypersegmented nucleus) with phagocytized bacteria (Figure 16.14).

Other inflammatory cell types are less often seen in mares unless a chronic insult to the uterine lumen (chronic endometritis) is present. Lymphocytes are small cells (7–8 μm diameter), with dark nuclei and virtually no cytoplasm. Macrophages are typically large (20 μm diameter), with an abundant, slightly blue cytoplasm and a large dark nucleus (Figure 16.15). It is common to observe vacuoles in the cytoplasm, as well as phagocytized bacteria. These two cell types can also be seen in the early postpartum period,

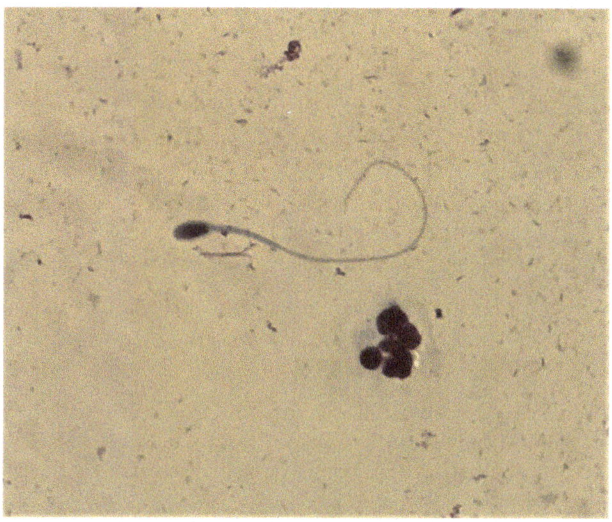

Figure 16.12 A neutrophil observed in a cytological specimen from a mare 12 hours after breeding with cool-stored semen. A spermatozoon is also observed. This mare had a small amount of fluid in the uterine lumen, as observed by ultrasonography. Diff-Quik, original magnification 1000×.

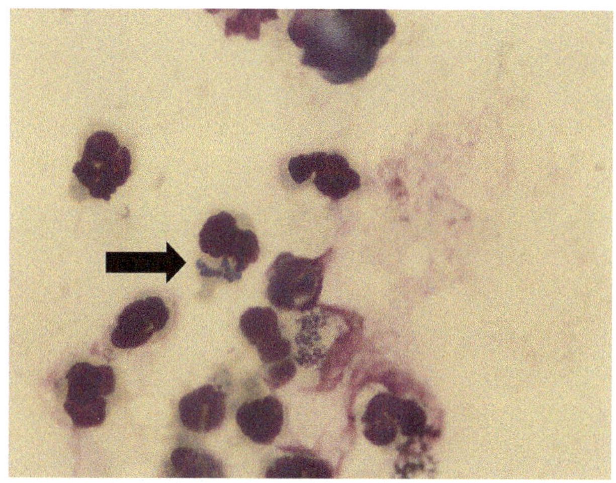

Figure 16.14 A degenerated neutrophil is observed phagocytizing bacteria (*arrow*) in an endometrial cytology from a mare with infectious endometritis due to *Streptococcus zooepidemicus*. Other neutrophils can also be appreciated in this image. Diff-Quik, original magnification 1000×.

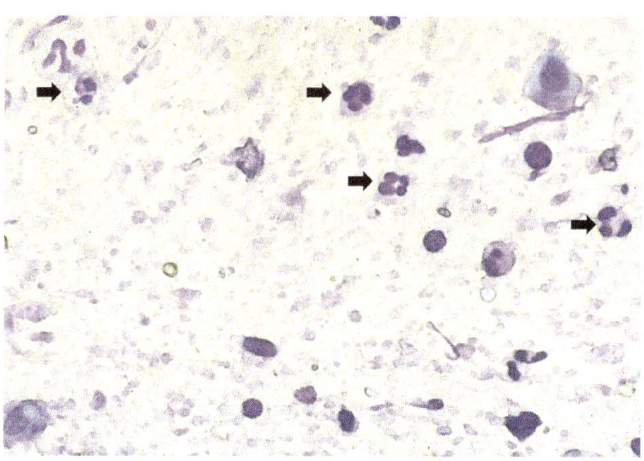

Figure 16.13 Positive endometrial cytological sample from a mare. Neutrophils (*arrows*) and endometrial cells are present. The background debris is most likely due to mucus in the uterus. This mare had greater than 1 cm of endometrial fluid in the uterus during her ultrasound examination. Sample obtained by endometrial swab. Diff-Quik, original magnification 1000×.

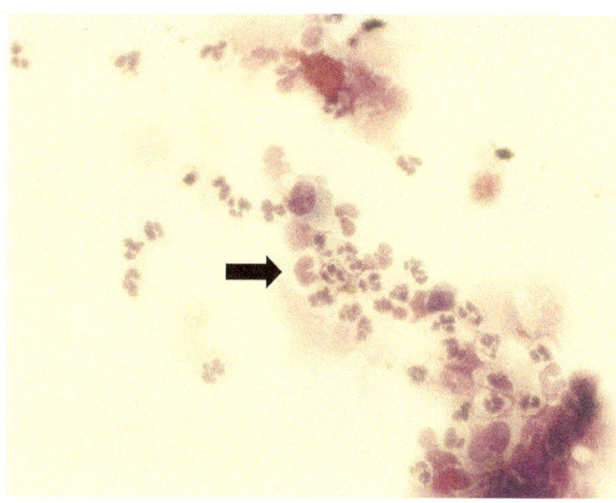

Figure 16.15 Neutrophils and macrophage (*arrow*) present in a mare with chronic endometritis due to delayed uterine clearance caused by cervical incompetence. Diff-Quik, original magnification 200×.

particularly lymphocytes, whilst macrophages are also seen in the resolution phase of endometritis, or during spring or fall transition and winter anestrus [12, 29]. Eosinophils are bigger than neutrophils but smaller than macrophages (12–15 μm diameter). These cells are characterized by a blue-stained lobulated nucleus and large, round intracytoplasmic vacuoles which commonly stain pink-red (Figure 16.16). This cell type is most commonly observed in mares with chronic yeast infections, pneumovagina, or vesicovaginal reflux (Figure 16.17) [2,35,36].

Although there is no consensus on how to classify the degree of inflammation based on cytology results, most practitioners use a classification system in which the number of white blood cells (particularly neutrophils) are counted in a high-power field (400×). This analysis is done in at least 10 fields. It is recommended that each field should contain numerous uterine epithelial cells to confirm that the sample is of high diagnostic quality. Using this system, the inflammation can be classified as normal (0–2 neutrophils/hpf), moderate (3–5 neutrophils/hpf) or severe (>5 neutrophils/hpf) (see Figure 16.13). Others also include a category between normal and moderate inflammation: mild inflammation (1–2 neutrophils/hpf) [37]. Other studies have used higher threshold values to classify the degree of endometrial inflammation: normal (0 neutrophils), mild (1–10 neutrophils/10 hpf), moderate (>10 neutrophils/10 hpf), or strong (large clumps of neutrophils) [38]. These two systems are commonly used when the endometrial cytology is acquired by swabbing methods.

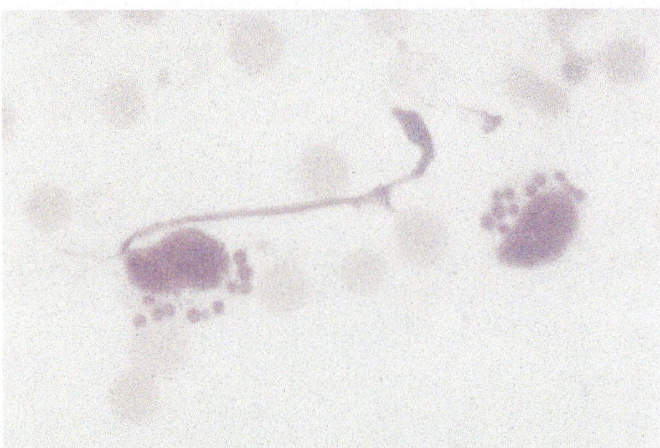

Figure 16.16 The presence of eosinophils in the endometrial cytology of a mare can be the result of poor perineal conformation, pneumovagina, or urine pooling in the vagina.

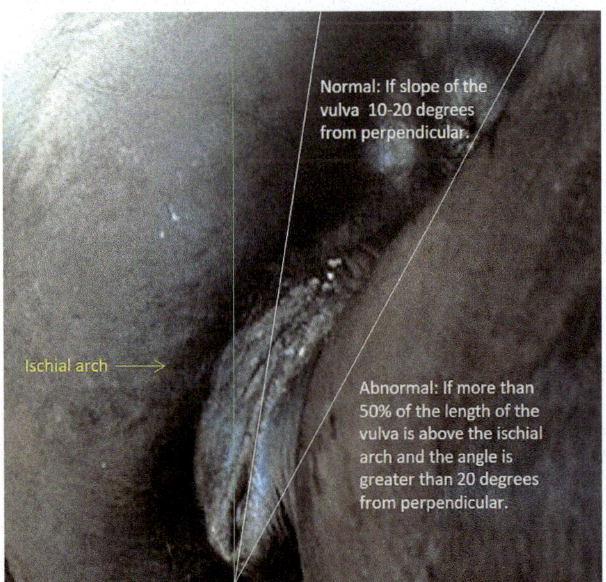

Figure 16.17 Example of poor perineal conformation in the mare that may result in urine pooling (vesiculovaginal reflux) or pneumovagina ("windsuckers").

Another proposed system for classifying the degree of endometrial inflammation involves performing a differential cell count whilst analyzing the cytology, where the number of neutrophils is counted in 10 hpf (400×), and then the value is expressed as the proportion of neutrophils per total cell count. Most laboratories using this method use a threshold value of 1 neutrophil to 40 epithelial cells (approximately 2%) as an indicator of endometrial inflammation [21, 31]. This method is most commonly used when the endometrial samples are acquired by uterine lavage, since the centrifugation process will concentrate all the cell types into the pellet; thus, a higher proportion of neutrophils will be seen in each high-power field, particularly in mares with mild inflammatory changes.

16.3.3 Red Blood Cells

Red blood cells are small (6 μm diameter) with a central pallor. This cell type is commonly found in low numbers (<4/hpf) in normal mares. However, numbers of RBC can be found in postpartum mares (in conjunction with siderophages), or in mares that have recently received an endometrial biopsy or other type of endometrial trauma. These cells are faint staining, light gray to pink, and may appear as "ghost" cells dispersed amongst the other cells in the microscope slide [12].

16.3.4 Bacteria, Yeast or Fungal Organisms

Bacteria, rods, and cocci can be observed in smears stained with Diff-Quik under oil immersion (1000×) (Figure 16.18). The presence of white blood cell-phagocytized bacteria may help to differentiate an active infectious endometritis from sample contamination [37]. The bacterial species most commonly associated with infectious endometritis in the mare are *S. zooepidemicus*, *E. coli*, *P. aeruginosa*, and *K. pneumoniae*.

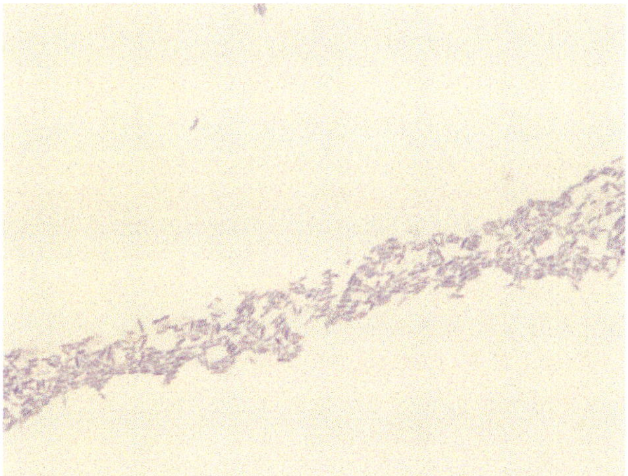

Figure 16.18 Bacteria (rod-shaped) observed in a stained smear from a mare uterus. This mare had a uterine infection associated with *Pseudomonas aeruginosa*. Diff-Quik, original magnification 1000×.

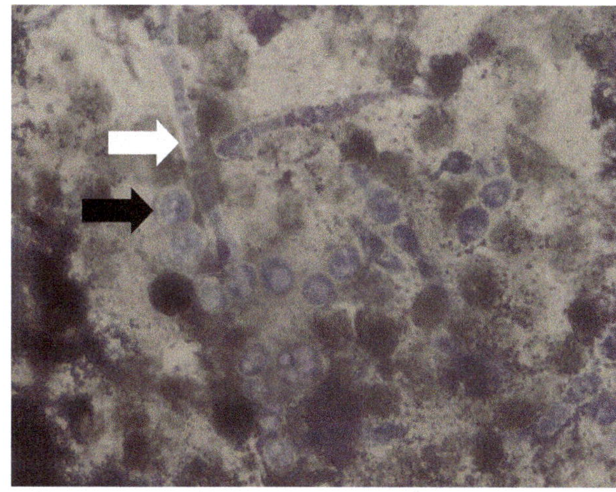

Figure 16.19 Hyphae fungal organisms in a mare suffering fungal endometritis. Observe the presence of yeast (*black arrow*) and hyphae (*white arrow*), with a distinctive clear halo around the organism (cell wall). The causative agent was not determined. Diff-Quik, original magnification 1000×. *Source:* Courtesy of Dr Steven Brinsko, College of Veterinary Medicine and Biomedical Sciences, Texas A&M University.

The first is a gram-positive coccus (approximately 1 μm diameter) that forms chains of different length, whilst the others are gram-negative rods (3–6 μm). It is important that practitioners recognize that color acquired by the bacteria after staining with modified Wright or Diff-Quik is not equivalent to the color obtained by gram staining.

Yeasts are typically 5–8 μm in size with a particular clear "halo" around the organism, whilst fungal organisms are commonly seen as long branching chains linked together, known as branching hyphae. The most common fungal and yeast organisms found in clinical cases of endometritis in mares are *Candida albicans* and *Aspergillus fumigatus* (Figure 16.19) [39]. In many instances, observation of fungal organisms during the endometrial cytology examination may be the only evidence of fungal endometritis, as these organisms require very specific culture conditions. Other methods for detection of fungal organisms include the use of endometrial biopsies or staining of fixed smears with GMS or periodic acid–Schiff (PAS) staining.

16.4 Conclusion

The advantages of conducting a cytological analysis whilst investigating reproductive failure in mares or determining the effectiveness of a therapeutic approach are related to their ability to be conducted with relatively minimal equipment, and the capacity to obtain fast results at the farm. However, endometrial cytology should not be solely relied upon when trying to define whether or not a mare is suffering an endometrial inflammatory process. Thus, practitioners are encouraged to familiarize themselves with the various methods that are available for the diagnosis of endometritis, including endometrial cytology, culture, and biopsy. The use of two or more of these diagnostic methods will promote the best therapeutic decisions and obtain the best outcome: a pregnant mare.

References

1 LeBlanc, M.M. (2008). The chronically infertile mare. *Proc. Am. Assoc. Equine Pract.* 54: 391–407.

2 Dascanio, J., Ley, W.B., and Bowen, J.M. (1997). How to perform and interpret uterine cytology. *Proc. Am. Assoc. Equine Pract.* 43: 182–186.

3 Riddle, W., LeBlanc, M.M., and Stromberg, A. (2007). Relationships between uterine culture, cytology and pregnancy rates in a thoroughbred practice. *Theriogenology* 68: 395–402.

4 Diel de Amorim, M., Gartley, C.J., Foster, R.A. et al. (2016). Comparison of clinical signs, endometrial culture, endometrial cytology, uterine low-volume lavage, and uterine biopsy and combinations in the diagnosis of equine endometritis. *J. Equine Vet. Sci.* 44: 54–61.

5 Nielsen, J.M. (2005). Endometritis in the mare: a diagnostic study comparing cultures from swab and biopsy. *Theriogenology* 64: 510–518.

6 Overbeck, W., Witte, T.S., and Heuwieser, W. (2011). Comparison of three diagnostic methods to identify subclinical endometritis in mares. *Theriogenology* 75: 1311–1318.

7 Ganjam, V.K., McLeod, C., Klesius, P.H. et al. (1984). Effect of ovarian hormones on the phagocytic response of ovariectomized mares. *J. Reprod. Fertil. (Suppl.)* 32: 169–174.

8 Allen, W.R. and Newcombe, J.R. (1979). Aspects of genital infection and swabbing techniques in the mare. *Vet. Rec.* 104: 228–231.

9 Liu, I.K.M. (1988). Uterine defense mechanisms in the mare. *Vet. Clin North Am Large Anim. Pract.* 4: 221–228.

10 Brook, D. (1993). Uterine cytology. In: *Equine Reproduction* (eds. A.O. McKinnon and J.L. Voss), 246–254. Philadelphia: Lea & Febiger.

11 Hinrichs, K., Cummings, M.R., Ser-tich, P.L., and Kenney, R.M. (1988). Clinical significance of aerobic bacterial flora of the uterus, vagina, vestibule, and clitoral fossa of clinically normal mares. *J. Am. Vet. Med. Assoc.* 193 (1): 72–75.

12 Ley, W.B., Digrassie, W.A., Holyoak, G.R., and Slusher, S.H. (2001). Endometrium. In: *Diagnostic Cytology and Hematology of the Horse*, 2e (eds. R.L. Cowell and R.D. Tyler), 180–186. St Louis: Mosby.

13 Blanchard, T.L., Cummins, M.R., Garcia, M.C. et al. (1981). Comparison between two techniques for endometrial swab culture and between biopsy and culture in barren mares. *Theriogenology* 16 (5): 541–552.

14 Aguilar, J., Hanks, M., Shaw, D. et al. (2006). Importance of using guarded techniques for the preparation of endometrial cytology smears in mares. *Theriogenology* 66: 423–430.

15 Walter, J., Neuberg, K.P., Failing, K., and Wehrend, A. (2012). Cytological diagnosis of endometritis in the mare: investigations of sampling techniques and relation to bacteriological results. *Anim. Reprod. Sci.* 132: 178–186.

16 Bohn, A.A., Ferris, R.A., and McCue, P.M. (2014). Comparison of equine endometrial cytology samples from uterine swab, uterine brush, and low volume lavage collected from healthy mares. *Vet. Clin. Pathol.* 43 (4): 594–600.

17 Cocchia, N., Paciello, O., Auletta, L. et al. (2012). Comparison of the cytobrush, cottonswab, and low-volume uterine flush techniques to evaluate endometrial cytology for diagnosing endometritis in chronically infertile mares. *Theriogenology* 77: 89–98.

18 Ricketts, S.W. (1981). Bacteriological examinations of the mare's cervix: techniques and interpretation of results. *Vet. Rec.* 108: 46–51.

19 Ricketts, S.W. and Mackintosh, M.E. (1987). Role of anaerobic bacteria in equine endometritis. *J. Reprod. Fertil. Suppl.* 35: 343–351.

20 Nielsen, J.M., Troedsson, M.H., Pedersen, M.R. et al. (2010). Diagnosis of endometritis in the mare based on bacteriological and cytological examinations of the endometrium: comparison of results obtained by swabs and biopsies. *J. Equine Vet. Sci.* 30 (1): 27–30.

21 Ball, B.A., Shin, S.J., Patten, V.H. et al. (1988). Use of a low-volume uterine flush for microbiologic and cytologic examination of the mare's endometrium. *Theriogenology* 29 (6): 1269–1283.

22 LeBlanc, M.M., Magsig, J., and Stromberg, A.J. (2007). Use of a low-volume uterine flush for diagnosing endometritis in chronically infertile mares. *Theriogenology* 68: 403–412.

23 Katila, T. (2016). Evaluation of diagnostic methods in equine endometritis. *Reprod. Biol.* 16: 189–196.

24 Christoffersen, M., Brandis, L., Samuelsson, J. et al. (2015). Diagnostic double-guarded low-volume uterine lavage in mares. *Theriogenology* 83: 222–227.

25 Brinsko, S.P., Varner, D.D., and Blanchard, T.L. (1991). The effect of uterine lavage performed four hours post insemination on pregnancy rate in mares. *Theriogenology* 35: 1111–1119.

26 Brinsko, S.P. (2001). How to perform uterine lavage: indications and practical techniques. *Proc. Am. Assoc. Equine Pract.* 47: 407–411.

27 LeBlanc, M.M. (2011). How to perform and interpret findings from a low-volume uterine flush. *Proc. Am. Assoc. Equine Pract.* 57: 32–36.

28 Ferris, R.A., McCue, P.M., Borlee, G.I. et al. (2014). In vitro efficacy of nonantibiotic treatments on biofilm disruption of Gram-negative pathogens and an in vivo mode of infectious endometritis utilizing isolates from the equine uterus. *J. Clin. Microbiol.* 54: 631–639.

29 Roszel, J.F. and Freeman, K.P. (1988). Equine endometrial cytology. *Vet. Clin. North Am Equine Pract.* 4 (2): 247–262.

30 Slusher, S.H., Freeman, K.P., and Roszel, J.F. (1985). Infertility diagnosed in mares using endometrial biopsy, culture and aspiration cytology. *Proc. Am. Assoc. Equine Pract.* 31: 165–170.

31 Couto, M.A. and Hughes, J.P. (1984). Technique and interpretation of cervical and endometrial cytology in the mare. *J. Equine Vet. Sci.* 4 (6): 265–273.

32 Card, C. (2005). Post-breeding inflammation and endometrial cytology in mares. *Theriogenology* 64: 580–588.

33 Troedsson, M.H.T., Lose, K., Alghamdi, A.M. et al. (2001). Interaction between equine semen and the endometrium: the inflammatory response to semen. *Anim. Reprod. Sci.* 68: 238–273.

34 Woodward, E.M. and Troedsson, M.H.T. (2015). Inflammatory mechanisms of endometritis. *Equine Vet. J.* 47: 384–389.

35 Zent, W.W., Troedsson, M.H.T., and Xue, J.L. (1998). Postbreeding uterine fluid accumulation in a normal population of thoroughbred mares: a field study. *Proc. Am. Assoc. Equine Pract.* 44: 64–65.

36 Slusher, S.H., Freeman, K.P., and Roszel, J.F. (1984). Eosinophils in equine uterine cytology and histology specimens. *J. Am. Vet. Med. Assoc.* 184: 665–670.

37 Ferris, R.A., Bohn, A., and McCue, P.M. (2015). Equine endometrial cytology: collection techniques and interpretation. *Equine Vet. Educ.* 27 (6): 316–322.

38 Reilas, T. and Katila, K. (2002). Proteins and enzymes in uterine lavage fluid of postpartum and nonparturient mares. *Reprod. Domest. Anim.* 37: 261–268.

39 Dascanio, J.J., Schweizer, C., and Ley, W.B. (2001). Equine fungal endometritis. *Equine Vet. Educ.* 13: 324–329.

17

Semen Evaluation

Camilo Hernández-Avilés[1], *Luisa Ramírez-Agámez*[2], *and Chelsea Makloski-Cohorn*[3]

[1] *Large Animal Clinical Sciences, College of Veterinary Medicine and Biomedical Sciences, Texas A&M University, College Station, TX, USA*
[2] *Animal Reproductive Services, Bogotá, Colombia*
[3] *Pinnacle Equine Veterinary Services, PLLC, Whitesboro, TX, USA*

The assessment of stallion fertility is a common cause for veterinary consulting in private practice. Due to the economic implications that reduced stallion fertility could have on the success of a breeding operation, a complete and thorough examination of the stallion reproductive health or breeding soundness becomes necessary. For this purpose, the Society for Theriogenology (SFT) has established a series of guidelines for the clinical evaluation of stallion fertility [1]. This manual considers several parameters that a stallion must meet to be considered as a "satisfactory breeding prospect."

- Have the physical capacity to copulate and deliver semen into the mare's reproductive tract or an artificial vagina (AV).
- Possess good libido.
- Have a pair of normal testes, consistent with their capacity for producing sperm.
- Test negative for venereal pathogens, such as *Klebsiella pneumoniae*, *Pseudomonas aeruginosa*, *Taylorella equigenitalis*, equine herpes virus-3, equine arteritis virus, and dourine.
- Ejaculate at least 1 billion progressively motile, morphologically normal spermatozoa in the second of two ejaculates collected one hour apart, preceded by one week of reproductive rest.

However, when the manual was published, most reproductive programs were focused on natural cover, and few clinical trials about the effect of cooling or cryopreservation on sperm quality and pregnancy rates were available. Currently, there is a whole body of knowledge related to the effects that storage procedures (cooling or cryopreservation) have on the spermatozoa [2, 3]. Thus, new methods for assessing those changes in the sperm have become available in clinical practice and research laboratories.

For these reasons, the evaluation of semen quality is important not only when establishing stallion fertility potential but also for determining whether the semen of a stallion could withstand the stresses related to the cooling or freezing process in programs of artificial insemination with cooled or frozen semen, as well as to determine the quality of a breeding dose before or after insemination. This chapter focuses on the common methods for stallion semen evaluation that practitioners should be familiar with, for assessing sperm quality and stallion fertility.

17.1 Semen Collection and Handling

Amongst the methods reported for stallion semen collection, the use of an AV is the most common and practical for veterinary practitioners. Many types of AVs are commercially available, the most common being the Missouri-type and Colorado-type AVs in North America, the Hanoverian type in Europe, and the Botucatu type in Brazil. Other methods reported for semen collection in stallions include the collection of dismount samples from the mare's vagina in Thoroughbred breeding programs or chemically induced ejaculation [4].

Before semen collection, the practitioner must prepare the collection equipment and the laboratory for sperm evaluation, taking care to keep all the plastic equipment, AV, collection bottles, and covers at 37 °C. Most laboratories and breeding farms use disposable plastic liners within the AV to reduce the probability of cross-contamination

Equine Hematology, Cytology, and Clinical Chemistry, Second Edition.
Edited by Raquel M. Walton, Rick L. Cowell, and Amy C. Valenciano.

of bacteria present in the smegma and stallion external genitalia. A nonspermicidal lubricating jelly must be used for the AV. Some commercially available brands of nonspermicidal lube in North America include Priority Care (First Priority, Inc., Elgin, IL), HR Lubricating Jelly (HR Pharmaceuticals, Inc., York, PA), Their Gel (Aptech, Inc., Manhattan, KS) and Clarity AI Lubricating Jelly (Aurora Pharmaceuticals, North Field, MN). Before semen collection, the stallion's penis must be washed with warm water (37–40 °C) and dried using paper towels, with emphasis on the glans penis, glans fossa, and fossa urethralis. This is particularly useful to reduce the amount of smegma and epithelial cells which can contaminate the ejaculate and reduce sperm longevity.

The semen is usually collected into plastic bottles, which are equipped with plastic liners for receiving the ejaculate and nylon micromesh filters to exclude the gel fraction from the ejaculate. It is recommended to protect the semen receptacle from direct sunlight and temperature changes by using a thermal cover, and to transport the ejaculate to the laboratory as quickly as possible, to avoid artefactual changes to the sperm quality and subsequently the sample's interpretation of quality.

17.2 Macroscopic and Physicochemical Analysis of the Ejaculate

After removing the gel fraction and placing the ejaculate into an incubator at 37 °C, the semen must be measured to determine its volume. Usually, the ejaculate volume is measured with prewarmed, sterile graduated cylinders. However, the most practical and accurate method for volume measurement is based on weighing the ejaculate on a scale, assuming an equivalence of 1 g to 1 mL. As a general procedure, the ejaculate should be split into two parts. One small aliquot can be kept as is (raw semen) and left inside an incubator, whilst the other part is mixed with at least an equal volume of prewarmed semen extender (1:1 dilution, v:v) and allowed to equilibrate to room temperature. This last aliquot will be used for estimation of sperm longevity after cooled storage (see Section 17.4). The ejaculate color must also be observed, being an indirect measure of sperm concentration. With higher sperm concentration, the ejaculate color tends to be more opaque-white, whilst with lower sperm concentration, the ejaculate will have a translucent or clear appearance.

Estimation of ejaculate color can be particularly useful when cases of urospermia or hemospermia are suspected. Urospermia and hemospermia are amongst the most commonly reported pathologies that can affect sperm motility and subsequently stallion fertility [5, 6]. This is mainly due to marked changes in semen pH and osmolarity (urospermia) or the presence of white blood cells which can impart oxidative stress to the spermatozoa (hemospermia). Although these pathologies cannot be ruled out just by assessing ejaculate color, marked changes of the color from yellow to greenish, or from pink to reddish are commonly seen in those cases. Normal pH and osmolarity of stallion semen have been reported as 7.2–7.8 and 300–334 mOsm/kg, respectively, within one hour of ejaculation [7, 8]. Some laboratories perform pH and osmolarity analysis of the ejaculate but in clinical practice, these procedures are only performed when pathologies such as urospermia or reproductive tract infections are suspected.

Although precise measurement of semen pH and osmolarity is usually obtained by using high-cost equipment, and the use of pH paper is not recommended due to the inaccuracy of the obtained results, some published research suggest that other diagnostic aids such as the measurement of creatinine and urea levels or the use of strip-paper kits for detection of metabolites (Azostix®, Siemens Healthcare Diagnostics, Tarrytown, NY) are particularly useful when cases of urine contamination are suspected [9, 10].

A relevant chemical marker of the stallion ejaculate that could be used in clinical practice for sperm quality assessment is the determination of alkaline phosphatase (AP) levels, particularly to differentiate between azoospermia (lack of sperm in the ejaculate), excurrent duct blockages (spermiostasis) and ejaculatory failure. AP is an enzyme which is active in several tissues, including testes and epididymides, and its presence in high concentrations in stallion ejaculatory fluid is associated with normal ejaculation (AP > 5000 IU/L) [11]. When no spermatozoa are observed in the ejaculate and high levels of AP are obtained from the semen, azoospermia should be considered as the cause whilst when no spermatozoa are observed in the ejaculate and low levels of AP are obtained, spermiostasis ("plugged ampullae") or retrograde ejaculation should be considered as differential diagnosis [12].

17.3 Routine Microscopic Analysis of Semen

17.3.1 Sperm Concentration

Determination of total sperm numbers in the ejaculate is fundamental to classify the reproductive potential of the stud, as well as to adequately prepare a breeding dose for artificial insemination, or to determine if a breeding dose contains sufficient sperm numbers. For this purpose, the total volume of the gel-free ejaculate must be multiplied by the sperm concentration, usually expressed in millions per mL (1×10^6 spermatozoa/mL).

Two methods are the most frequently reported in laboratories and breeding farms for analysis of sperm concentration: direct observation using hemocytometers and indirect determination using spectrophotometer-based counters. Several types of hemocytometers are commercially available, the most commonly used being the Improved Neubauer hemocytometer (Figure 17.1a), and the Makler chamber (Sefi Medical Instruments, Israel) (Figure 17.1b). A protocol commonly used in the authors' practice for estimation of sperm concentration using the hemocytometer is described in Box 17.1. However, despite the hemocytometer is considered the gold standard for sperm enumeration, and the analysis being relatively inexpensive and easy to conduct, it has become unpopular due to the time that analysis takes (~5–7 minutes) and the variation in results between technicians [13].

In the last 20 years, the hemocytometer has been replaced in breeding farms and private practice by semiautomated cell counters or spectrophotometers. Commercially available spectrophotometers are marketed as SpermaCue (Minitube, Tiefenbach, Germany) (Figure 17.2), Accuread (IMV Technologies, L'Aigle, France) and the Densimeter or "blue box" (Animal Reproduction Systems, Chino, CA) (Figure 17.3). These devices measure the changes in the opacity of a given fluid (i.e., semen) in comparison with a "zeroed" control (commonly buffered formalin saline); changes in fluid opacity between the control sample and the semen are assumed to be due to the presence of sperm.

Although these analyzers can offer estimations of sperm numbers in less than two minutes, some disadvantages with their use have been reported. For instance, as these devices measure the sperm concentration indirectly based on the opacity of the sample, they cannot be used for analysis of semen samples containing opaque extenders (milk or egg yolk-based extenders). Likewise, erroneous results can be obtained when ejaculates contaminated with cellular debris and smegma are analyzed. Lastly, their capacity to accurately estimate sperm concentration in an ejaculate is dependent on an optimal range of sperm concentration; thus, overestimation of sperm numbers is commonly seen with diluted ($<100\times10^6$ sperm/mL) or highly concentrated ($>300\times10^6$ sperm/mL) ejaculates [14].

More recently, an automated fluorescent-based cell counter, the NucleoCounter® SP-100™ (ChemoMetec A/S, Allerød, Denmark) (Figure 17.4), has been validated for estimation of sperm concentration in different domestic animal species, including the stallion [15]. This device uses disposable cassettes containing a fluorescent dye, propidium iodide, which crosses through the sperm plasma membrane and intercalates with DNA, generating a red-staining pattern over the entire sperm head. For the assessment of sperm concentration using the NucleoCounter SP-100, the sample must be diluted (usually 1:100 to 1:200 when raw semen is analyzed) with a detergent solution that permeabilizes all sperm membranes, allowing the propidium iodide to gain access to the sperm DNA. Studies have demonstrated a high statistical agreement level between the results obtained with the hemocytometer, the NucleoCounter, and flow cytometers in semen from boars, bulls, and stallions [15, 16]; thus, the use of the NucleoCounter has been widely

(a) (b)

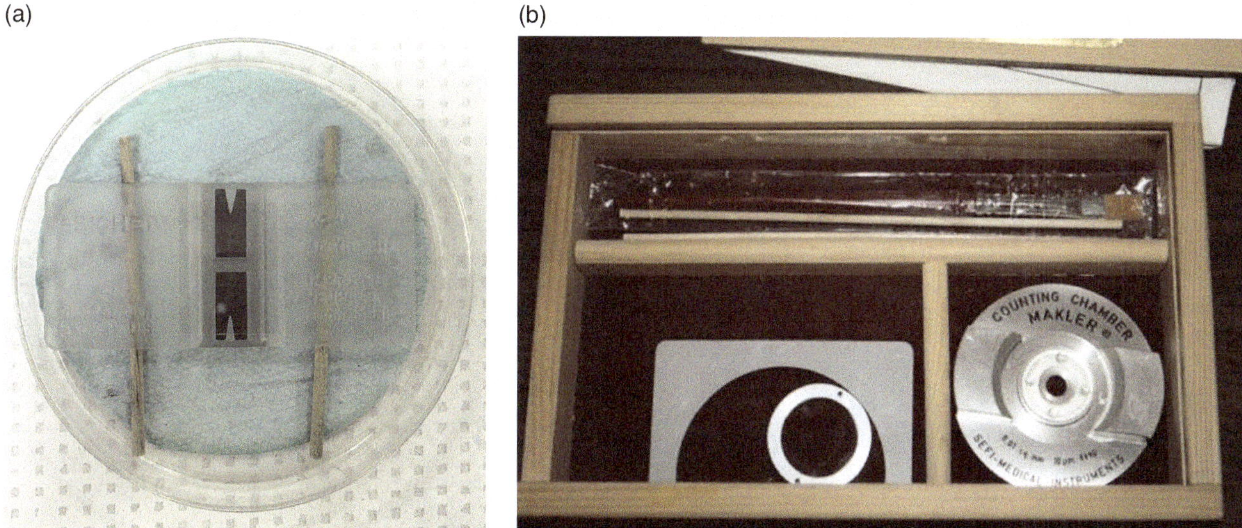

Figure 17.1 (a) Improved Neubauer hemocytometer, with V-shaped indentations on the top edges to help load the sample between the chamber grid and the coverslip. The hemocytometer is placed on top of a plastic Petri dish, with two wooden sticks to serve as supports of the slide, and a piece of humidified paper towel is kept beneath the hemocytometer to maintain the humidity whilst waiting before counting. (b) Makler counter.

Box 17.1 Hemocytometer method for evaluating sperm concentration in stallion semen

Equipment and supplies required

- Conventional light microscope with 10× and 40× objectives
- Improved Neubauer hemocytometer
- Mechanical pipettes (0.1–10, 10–100, 100–1000 μL) with plastic disposable tips
- Manual cell counter
- Plastic 2.0 mL microcentrifuge tubes (VWR International, Radnor, PA)
- Distilled water or 10% BFS
- Humidified chamber. Can be made by using a plastic Petri dish and two pieces of wooden sticks (as shown in Figure 17.1)
- KimWipes® (Kimberly-Clark, Irvine, TX)

Sample dilution

- Dilution factors commonly used for analysis of sperm concentration in raw equine ejaculates are 1:100 or 1:200.
- When samples are extremely diluted (i.e., <50 million sperm/mL), dilution factors such as 1:20 or 1:10 are recommended.
- Ideally between 100 and 300 spermatozoa should be counted in the large central grid of the hemocytometer for accuracy. Counting less than 100 or more than 300 spermatozoa may result in an error in calculation since the sample is too diluted or too concentrated, respectively.

Procedure for diluting samples (analysis of raw semen using a 1:100 dilution factor)

1) Using the 100–1000 μL mechanical pipette, measure 1.98 mL (1980 μL) of distilled water or BFS into a plastic microcentrifuge tube.
2) Mix the semen sample gently. Using the 0.1–10 μL mechanical pipette, measure 0.02 mL (20 μL) of the semen sample.
3) Use a KimWipe to dry the sides of the plastic tip, avoiding touching the end of the tip. Then, mix the sample with the diluent into the microcentrifuge tube.
4) To ensure that all the spermatozoa are rinsed from the plastic tip, flush the pipette by aspirating and expelling the solution 3–5 times.
5) Cap the plastic tube and mix the solution by gently inverting the container 10 times.
6) Using the 0.1–10 μL mechanic pipette, load the solution onto the hemocytometer.

Procedure to mount samples and counting spermatozoa using the hemocytometer

Hemocytometer preparation
It is recommended to use a Bright-Line, improved Neubauer hemocytometer. This instrument consists of a thick glass microscope slide with two rectangular indentations, or "chambers," aligned vertically in the center of the slide. The chambers are engraved with a laser-etched grid of perpendicular lines which divide each chamber into nine large grids. Each one of those grids is also subdivided into 25 medium-sized grids (each having 16 small squares). The hemocytometer comes with a special coverslip (20 × 26 × 0.4 mm), which rests not on the chamber area but on the "rails" to either side of the chamber. This is done to provide a volume of 0.01 mL for the semen sample in the counting area.

1) Make sure that the grid surface of the hemocytometer and the coverslip are clean.
2) Place the coverslip on the rails of the hemocytometer. Wetting the rails with a minimal amount of water will hold the coverslip in place, facilitating sample loading.
3) After gently mixing the plastic tube containing the diluted semen sample, load 10 μL of the solution between the coverslip and the chamber surface. Avoid touching the coverslip.
4) The sample will move between the chamber and the coverslip by capillarity. Thus, do not overload the chamber with more solution.
5) Both sides of the hemocytometer should be loaded with diluted sample.
6) Allow the sample to sit for approximately five minutes before counting spermatozoa, so the spermatozoa can settle into the hemocytometer counting grid.
7) The hemocytometer should be maintained in a humid environment during this five minutes, to prevent the chamber from drying out. To achieve this, the hemocytometer can be placed on top of two pieces of wooden sticks, within a plastic Petri dish, overlying a piece of wet paper towel.
8) After five minutes, the hemocytometer can be placed on top of the microscope stage for sperm counting.

Sperm counting using the hemocytometer

1) After placing the hemocytometer on the microscope stage, use the low-power objective (10×) to locate the center primary square of the counting grid (delimited by a triple-lined border).

2) Then, switch to the high-dry (40×) objective for counting. If spermatozoa are difficult to observe, the condenser can be lowered to increase the contrast.
3) Initiate the count from the left superior quadrant and progress using a horizontal pattern from left to right until the first five quadrants are counted. Then, the second line of quadrants is counted from right to left. This horizontal pattern is used until all 25 quadrants within the central grid are counted.
4) Keep track of all sperm within the quadrants using the manual counter. Only sperm heads are included in the count, not the tails.
5) If the sperm heads are lying on a bordering line, only count those sperm heads on the lower or left lines of the quadrant. This is done to prevent double-counting of the same spermatozoa when moving to the next quadrant.
6) The sperm counting procedure must be done in both hemocytometer chambers.
7) When the sperm concentration seems to be too high for counting, only five quadrants can be counted and the results obtained multiplied by 5. Use the same procedure for sperm counted as described above.

Calculating the sperm concentration after using the hemocytometer

1) The sperm concentration is expressed as sperm/mL of semen. This number is calculated as: sperm/mL = number of spermatozoa counted in the hemocytometer × hemocytometer factor × dilution factor used.
2) The hemocytometer factor is calculated as follows: the volume of liquid between the hemocytometer counting grid and the coverslip is 0.01 mL. By multiplying by 10, the obtained result will yield the number of sperm/mm^3/μL. This number is also multiplied by 1000, to yield the number of sperm/mm^3/mL. To shorten the calculations, the number of sperm counted in the hemocytometer is multiplied by 10 000 (when all 25 quadrants are counted) or 50 000 (when only five quadrants are counted).
3) The number obtained from the calculations made above is then multiplied by the dilution factor used, in this case 100. This calculation will yield the number of sperm (in millions)/mL. If other dilution factors are used, such as 1:200, 1:20 or 1:10, the results of multiplying the number of sperm counted in the hemocytometer by the hemocytometer factor will be multiplied by 200, 20 or 10, respectively.

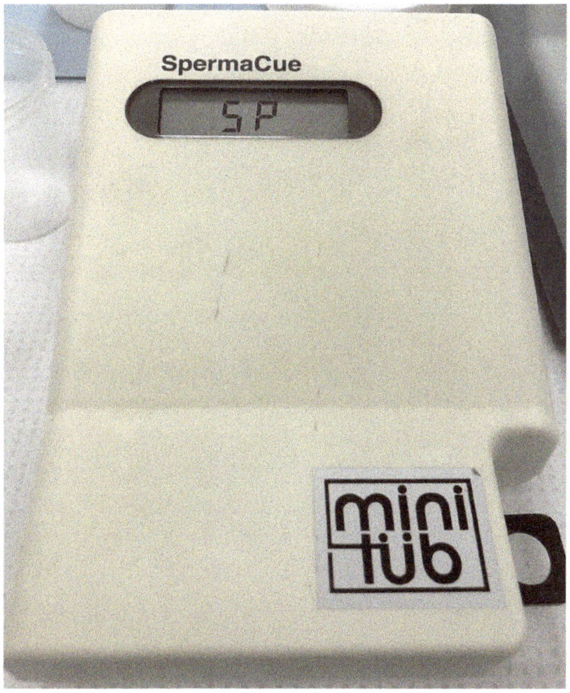

Figure 17.2 SpermaCue (Minitube, Tiefenbach, Germany) for spectrophotometric determination of sperm concentration. This device uses small cassettes (cuvette) to load a sample from the raw ejaculate.

accepted in research laboratories, breeding farms, and private clinics worldwide. Other automated methods for assessment of sperm concentration in equine ejaculates have also been reported, such as the use of computer-assisted sperm analyzers (CASA) coupled with fluorescent applications (Hamilton-Thorne IVOS–IDENT™) [17].

17.3.2 Sperm Motility

Estimation of sperm motility (or motion characteristics) is a fundamental test for the assessment of sperm quality and stallion fertility. Studies conducted in the late 1980s to early 1990s suggested that of all the conventional tests which can be performed to assess sperm quality, sperm progressive motility was the most correlated with stallion fertility [18]. Thus, the assessment of sperm progressive motility became a landmark when assessing semen quality and stallion fertility. Based on what the breeding industry expected at that time, threshold values of sperm progressive motility higher than 60% in freshly ejaculated semen or 30% in cooled semen (after 24–48 hours) and frozen/thawed semen were established.

However, practitioners must be aware that some stallions exhibiting "low" progressive motility in freshly ejaculated semen might be just as fertile as stallions with high

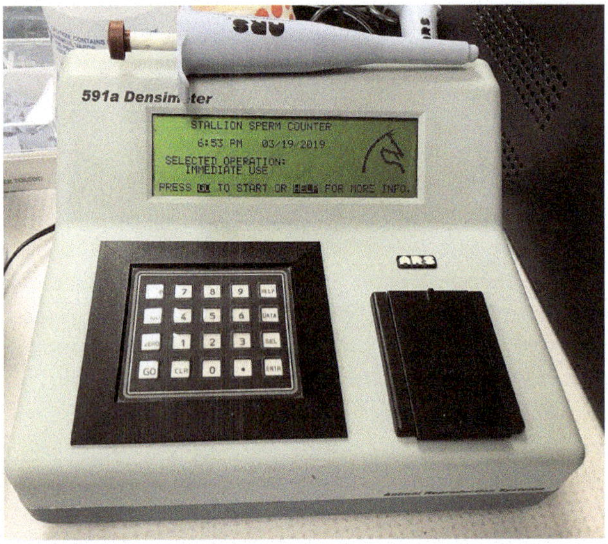

Figure 17.3 Densimeter ("Blue box," Animal Reproduction Systems, Chino, CA) for spectrophotometric determination of semen concentration. This device requires previous dilution of the raw semen with 10% buffered formalin before analysis.

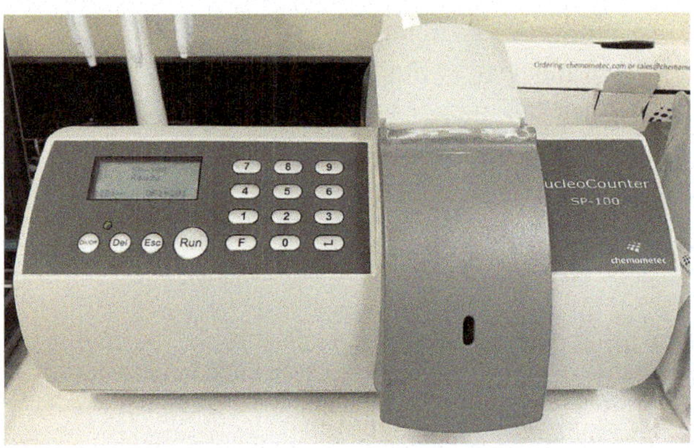

Figure 17.4 NucleoCounter SP-100 (ChemoMetec, Allerød, Denmark). This fluorescent-based counter uses small cassettes loaded with the fluorescent dye, propidium iodide, to determine the sperm concentration (in samples previously exposed to a detergent solution) and percentage of sperm plasma membrane intactness ("viability," in samples exposed to a physiological salt solution).

progressive motility, when other sperm quality characteristics such as sperm total motility, plasma membrane intactness or sperm morphology are normal. In fact, recent studies have shown that sperm total motility might be more associated with stallion percycle pregnancy rates and seasonal pregnancy rates, using both fresh (natural cover programs) and cooled-stored semen, than sperm progressive motility [19, 20]. Of particular interest is that semen from stallions with normal fertility (i.e., per cycle pregnancy rates >60%) may display a high incidence of sperm with circular movement, usually considered as abnormal in other species such as ruminants. This can be attributed to an abaxial attachment of the midpiece to the sperm head (see Section 17.3.3), as well as being caused by cooling or freezing procedures.

Under field conditions, sperm motility is commonly evaluated in both raw and diluted (extended) semen. Ideally, the semen sample should be evaluated using a phase-contrast microscope coupled to a warming stage. This is done to avoid temperature fluctuations in the sample that could induce an artefactual reduction on observed sperm motility. The use of phase-contrast optics instead of conventional light microscopy is desirable due to the inability to distinguish immotile spermatozoa, yielding false "high" motility estimates. Sperm motility is considerably susceptible to different environmental factors, such as excessive presence of lubricants, urine contamination, pH, and osmolarity unbalances, or low ambient temperature.

Commonly, sperm motility is assessed by placing a drop of raw semen onto a microscope slide and covering it with a coverslip. However, using this method, the practitioner cannot distinguish between individual motility patterns very well. Likewise, this method is commonly associated with overestimation of sperm motility, due to the accumulation of high quantities of spermatozoa in different planes of the vision field. Therefore, it is recommended to dilute the raw semen with an appropriate extender to a sperm concentration approximately between 25 and 30×10^6 sperm/mL, and then incubate it for at least 10 minutes at 37 °C before analysis (Box 17.2). With this concentration, the evaluator can assess sperm total and progressive motility in a more objective way, using either low- or dry-high power objectives (20–40×). When assessing sperm motility, the practitioner ideally determines the percentages of sperm total motility (spermatozoa displaying any form of movement), sperm progressive motility (spermatozoa displaying movement that follows a straight-line pattern), and sperm velocity classified on an arbitrary scale from 0 (static sperm) to 5 (fast-moving spermatozoa).

The use of computer systems for the assessment of sperm motion characteristics has become common in research laboratories and some veterinary hospitals. These systems, commonly termed CASA, are composed of a microscope with negative phase-contrast objectives coupled to a built-in stage warmer and a real-time video camera, and attached to a computer which displays the sperm observed through the microscope. The computer software uses algorithms to track each individual sperm based on their head size and movement, and expresses them in sperm velocity and displacement indices. These indices are used to determine the percentage of motile sperm and progressively motile sperm, as well as several sperm velocity indices. Commercially available CASA systems used widely in both clinical and research scenarios include CEROS and

Box 17.2 Analysis of sperm motility using conventional light or phase-contrast microscopy

Equipment and supplies required

- Conventional light, or preferably phase-contrast microscope with 10× and 40× objectives. It is desirable that a warming stage adjustable to 37 °C is attached to the microscope stage.
- Mechanical pipettes (0.1–10, 10–100, 100–1000 μL) with plastic disposable tips
- Plastic 1.5 mL microcentrifuge tubes (VWR International, Radnor, PA)
- Microscope slides and coverslips
- Water bath calibrated at 37 °C
- Stallion semen extender. Commercially available skim milk-based extenders such as EZ-Mixin (Animal Reproduction Systems, Chino, CA), INRA-96 (IMV Technologies, L'Aigle, France) or BotuSemen (Botupharma, Botucatu, SP, Brazil) are adequate.
- Slide warmer

Sample dilution

As mentioned, estimation of stallion sperm motility is best performed in an extended rather than a raw semen sample. Thus, the raw semen must be diluted as soon as possible to avoid sperm agglutination, cold-shock or artifactual changes on sperm motility. Semen extenders must be prewarmed before entering in contact with the raw semen. Under field conditions, one aliquot of raw semen is diluted at least 1:1 with prewarmed extender. This sample will be used for sperm motility and longevity analysis. Whilst the sperm concentration is calculated, the extended aliquot should be maintained at room temperature (20–22 °C) or incubated (37 °C, for no longer than 20 minutes).

1) After the sperm concentration in the raw semen is determined, one aliquot containing 1 mL (1000 μL) of semen extender must be pipetted into a plastic microcentrifuge tube and maintained warmed in the water bath.
2) To dilute the previously extended semen [1] to 25×10^6 sperm/mL, the following calculation can be used:

$$\frac{25\text{ million sperm/mL}}{\text{Sperm concentration in the raw semen}} \times 1000 = \textbf{microliters of raw (or extended) semen required to make an aliquot containing 25 million sperm in 1 mL of extender}$$

3) To properly dilute the semen to the desired concentration, it is necessary to discard the same volume of extender (in microliters) calculated previously from the microcentrifuge tube and replace it with the same volume of raw (or extended) semen.
4) This tube must be warmed for 10 minutes at 37 °C before analysis under the microscope.

For example, after collecting semen from one stallion, the following values of sperm concentration were obtained.

- Sperm concentration (using the hemocytometer): 235 million sperm/mL.

One aliquot of 10 mL of raw semen was diluted 1:1 with semen extender. This same aliquot is intended to be used for initial analysis of sperm motility. Thus, the calculation to properly dilute this sample to 25 million sperm/mL will be:

$$\frac{25\text{ million sperm/mL}}{235\text{ million sperm/mL (raw semen concentration)}} \times 1000 = 106\text{ microliters}$$

As the sample was previously diluted 1:1 with extender, then the number of microliters required to make a 1 mL aliquot containing 25 million sperm/mL will be 212 μL (twice diluted = twice volume required). Thus, 212 μL of the extender must be removed from the microcentrifuge tube and completed with 212 μL of the semen previously extended at 1:1 ratio.

Sample analysis

After 10 minutes of incubation at 37 °C, 6–10 μL of the extended semen should be pipetted onto a prewarmed microscope slide, covered with a 22 × 22 mm coverslip and visualized under the microscope. Although low-power objectives (10×) are commonly used in field situations, it is strongly recommended to analyze at least 10 microscopic fields at 40×. Percentages of total motility (any spermatozoal movement), progressive motility (sperm displaying a straight-line movement) and sperm velocity (in a scale from 0 to 4) need to be estimated and recorded.

IVOS (Hamilton-Thorne Biosciences, Beverly, MA), SpermVision, AndroVision (Minitube, Tiefenbach, Germany), and ISAS (ProISER, Valencia, Spain).

Although these analyzers offer repeatable and objective measurements of sperm motility, certain disadvantages associated with their cost and the lack of agreement amongst laboratories, CASA systems brands, and even within systems (when technical settings are changed) limit their use for research laboratories or large breeding operations. Users should be cautious when CASA analysis of stallion sperm is done, particularly when percentages of progressively motile sperm are evaluated, because the output of these values is highly influenced by the threshold values preset in the instrument settings, as well as the use of fixed-volume chambers, the volume of sample loaded into the analyzer, the type of extender used, and sperm concentration, amongst others [21, 22]. Likewise, although the use of CASA has become popular in recent years, the relationship of the different sperm motion parameters obtained with stallion fertility is relatively low, particularly sperm velocity indices. In fact, recent studies have found that the percentage of sperm total motility, compared to other measurements of sperm motility, is the most highly correlated to stallion per cycle and seasonal pregnancy rates when fresh, cooled, or frozen semen is used for artificial insemination (AI) [19, 20, 23, 24].

17.3.3 Sperm Morphology

Assessment of sperm morphology is intended to determine the proportion of spermatozoa with normal shape as well as the presence of abnormal sperm forms. Sperm morphology is considered a fundamental test when assessing stallion potential fertility, given that changes of sperm morphology reflect the stallion's intrinsic capacity to produce high-quality sperm. However, practitioners must be cautious that stallions with high sperm motility can also have high percentages of morphologically abnormal spermatozoa, and subsequently reduced fertility. In contrast, stallions with a high incidence of morphological defects may have normal fertility, when adequate numbers in the ejaculate or AI dose are included. Some morphological defects such as abnormal head forms, abnormal acrosomes or midpieces have a more profound effect on stallion fertility bred by natural cover, whilst other defects such as cytoplasmic droplets or bent tails have little or no effect on stallion pregnancy rates [19, 24]. Thus, it is important that veterinarians do not base their concepts regarding stallion potential fertility on only one test, such as sperm morphology. It is also important that practitioners become familiar with certain features of the stallion sperm structure that are considered abnormal in other species, particularly the abaxial attachment of the head and midpiece or the presence of certain head and shape sizes which could be normal for a given population of stallions.

Under field conditions, the evaluation of sperm morphology is commonly conducted by using air-dried stained slides. The most commonly used stains for this purpose are the eosin/nigrosin (Hancock stain), Papanicolaou, and Indian ink stains, which are termed background stains. Other stains such as Giemsa, Wright or Diff-Quik® are commonly used to assess the presence of somatic cells in the ejaculate, such as neutrophils. In both cases, a conventional light microscope equipped with either dry-high (40×) or immersion-oil objectives (100×) is used for estimation of sperm shape. For this purpose, it is highly recommended to have the samples, slides, and stains prewarmed to avoid artefactual changes in sperm morphology due to hypotonic or cold shock.

Other techniques available for assessment of sperm morphology includes fixation of sperm by dilution with buffered formalin saline solution (BFS) (Table 17.1) for posterior assessment using wet mounts and either phase-contrast or differential interference contrast (DIC) microscopy. In the authors' opinion and as reported by others, the use of wet-mount samples offers several advantages compared to evaluation of stained smears, particularly by eliminating artefactual changes of sperm morphology that may be created during the smearing and staining procedure (detached heads, bent midpieces and tails, or coiled tails), as well as allowing identification of the presence of subtle but fertility-limiting defects, such as acrosome, head or midpiece defects [25, 26]. Although the use of wet mounts requires access to the fixative solution and relatively more expensive pieces of equipment (phase-contrast or DIC microscopes), their use is more common in private hospitals or practices. Also, some laboratories in the US offer sperm morphology analysis and interpretation in fixed samples using DIC microscopy (i.e., Texas A&M University, College Station, TX; Colorado State University, Fort Collins, CO; University of California, Davis, CA), and good-quality phase-contrast microscopes can be purchased by private practitioners at relatively low cost (US $3000–5000, 2020 prices).

Table 17.1 Composition of buffered formol saline solution (1 L of solution).

Ingredient	Amount
Sodium phosphate monohydrate – Na_2HPO_4	4.93 g
Potassium phosphate monohydrate – KH_2PO_4	2.54 g
Sodium chloride – NaCl	5.41 g
36–38% Formaldehyde solution	125 mL
Deionized water	q.s. 1000 mL

As reported by Kenney et al. [1].

Table 17.2 Classification system for sperm morphological abnormalities, as reported by Kenney et al. [1]. The origin and possible implications of some of these morphological abnormalities are still unknown.

Sperm defect	Subclassification	Possible implications
Abnormal head	Microcephalic sperm Macrocephalic sperm Tapered head Pyriform head Nuclear vacuoles	Abnormal chromatin compaction, which can be associated with impaired early embryonic development
Acrosome defect	Lifted (partially reacted) acrosome "Knobbed" acrosome	Spontaneous acrosome reaction, impaired sperm – oocyte interactions
Detached heads	Normal detached head Abnormal detached head	Moderate to high numbers can reduce fertility. Commonly seen in stallions with spermiostasis, in conjunction with bent tails and distal droplets
Cytoplasmic droplets	Proximal droplet Distal droplet	Residue of cytoplasm not released during epididymal transit. Little to no effect on fertility in stallions
Abnormal midpieces	Segmental aplasia of the mitochondrial sheath Roughened midpiece Swollen midpiece Double midpiece/double head	Associated with mitochondrial dysfunction due to abnormal formation of the mitochondrial sheath. Related with low sperm motility or higher oxidative stress status
Bent midpieces	Single or double bends	Abnormal formation of the midpiece and tail during spermatogenesis. Impaired motility
Bent tail ("hairpin tail")	Single or double bends	Impaired motility
Coiled tails	Encircling the head	Abnormal formation of the midpiece and tail during spermatogenesis
Premature germ cells	Single or multiple nuclei	In high numbers, can be associated with impaired spermatogenesis (testicular dysfunction)

Several classification systems have been reported in the literature for analysis of stallion sperm morphology, which have been modified from systems used for morphological analysis of bovine spermatozoa. Historically, sperm morphological features were divided into primary, secondary, and tertiary abnormalities. Primary abnormalities include head and midpiece defects, which are associated with defects during spermatogenesis, and therefore considered as defects of testicular origin. Secondary abnormalities include detached heads, bent tails, and cytoplasmic droplets, which commonly occur during transport of the spermatozoa through the excurrent duct system. Tertiary abnormalities are considered iatrogenic in origin, due to improper semen collection or handling. Other classification systems classify sperm morphological abnormalities into major or minor abnormalities, where the major abnormalities (i.e., head or midpiece defects) are more related to fertility.

Using these classification systems, most practitioners tend to assume that the percentages of abnormal sperm are associated with reduced stallion fertility; however, it is instead recommended that fertility be based on the percentages of morphologically normal sperm. A preferred method for classifying stallion sperm morphology is to identify specific abnormalities [1], rather than packaging them into large categories (as the aforementioned), leading to erroneous assumptions in the possible origin or outcome of these abnormalities [25, 27]. Using the classification system of sperm abnormalities proposed by Kenney et al. [1], the most commonly observed abnormalities of stallion spermatozoa can be classified as shown in Table 17.2 (Figures 17.5–17.20).

17.4 Preparation of Cool-Stored Semen Doses and Estimation of Sperm Longevity

Given the widespread use of cool-stored stallion sperm in reproductive programs in North America, adequate preparation of seminal doses and estimation of sperm quality after cooling are necessary to determine if a stallion can be included in those programs. As a rule, a dose of cooled

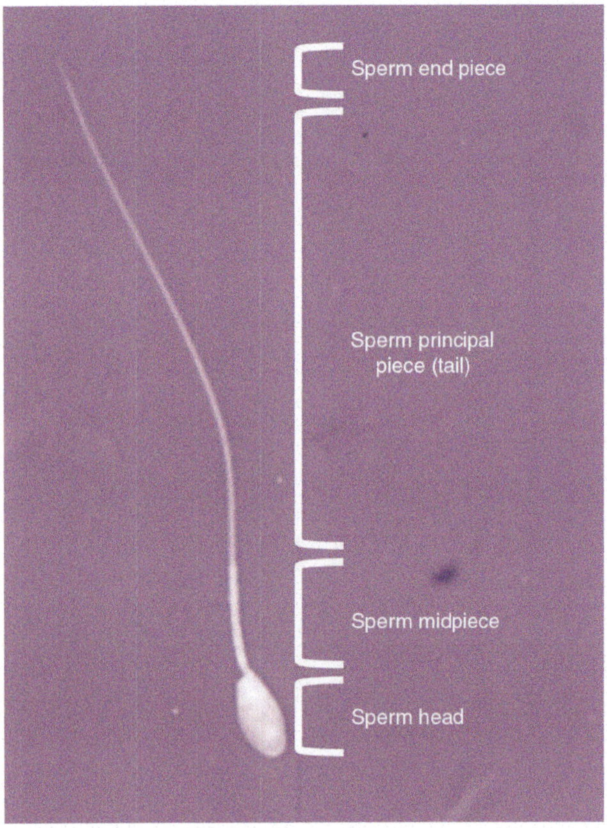

Figure 17.5 Morphologically normal stallion spermatozoa, as observed using eosin/nigrosin staining (Hancock stain). The different regions of the sperm are appreciated. Observe the abaxial attachment of the tail, which is considered normal for equine spermatozoa. Original magnification 1000×.

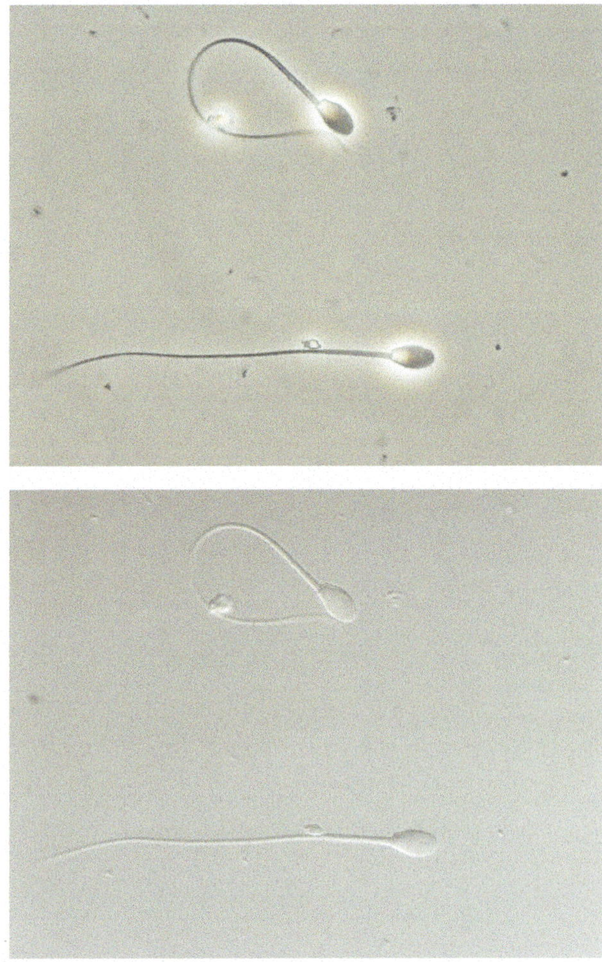

Figure 17.6 Stallion spermatozoa as observed under phase-contrast microscopy (*upper image*) and differential interference contrast microscopy (*lower image*). Spermatozoa in both images are morphologically normal. Original magnification 1000×.

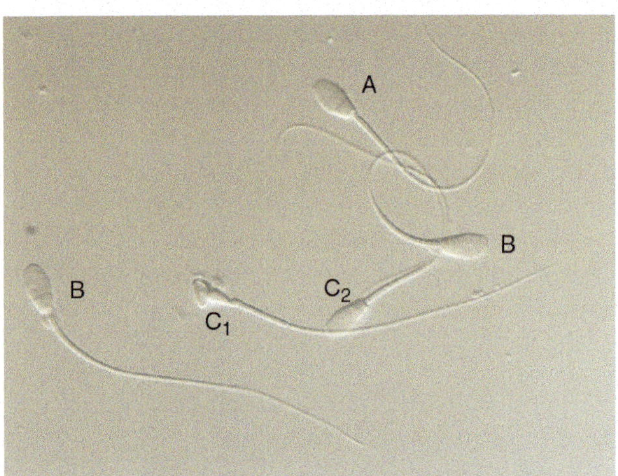

Figure 17.7 Stallion spermatozoa observed under DIC microscopy. A: Morphologically normal sperm. B: Spermatozoa with proximal cytoplasmic droplet. C_1: Abnormal head (observe the abnormally developed head and acrosome). C_2: Abnormal head (pyriform). Original magnification 1000×. In some of the sperm from this stallion, there is a prominent differentiation (ridge) between the acrosomal and postacrosomal regions, which is normal.

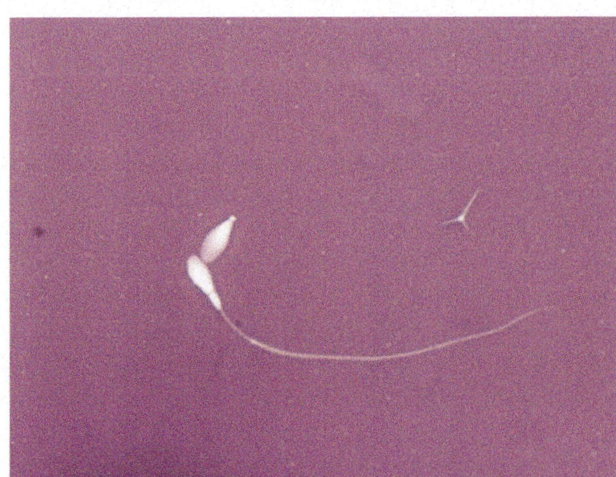

Figure 17.8 Sperm at the lower right has an abnormal head (pyriform), a "pseudodroplet" and segmental aplasia of the mitochondrial sheath. The detached head on the top also is abnormal (pyriform). Staining with eosin/nigrosin (Hancock stain). Original magnification 1000×.

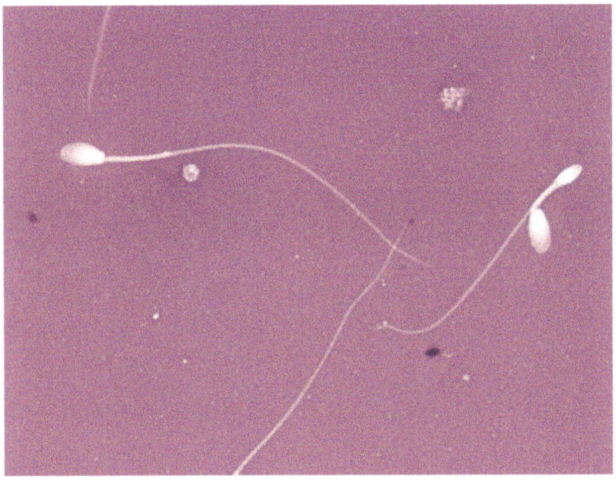

Figure 17.9 Sperm at the left is morphologically normal (observe the abaxial attachment of the midpiece). Spermatozoon on the right has a bent midpiece ("hairpin tail"). This defect is also known as distal midpiece reflex. Staining with eosin/nigrosin (Hancock stain). Original magnification 1000×.

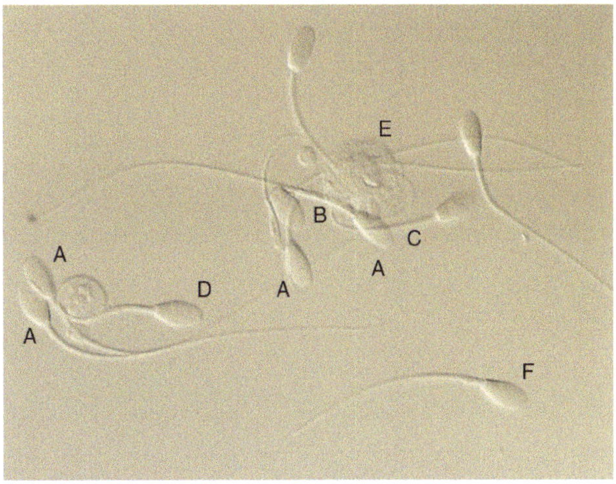

Figure 17.11 Stallion spermatozoa as observed under DIC microscopy. A: Morphologically normal spermatozoa. B: Detached head. C: Spermatozoon with abnormal midpiece (swollen mitochondrial sheath). D: Spermatozoon with coiled tail. E: Premature germ cell (one nucleus). F: Spermatozoon with broken tail. Original magnification 1000×.

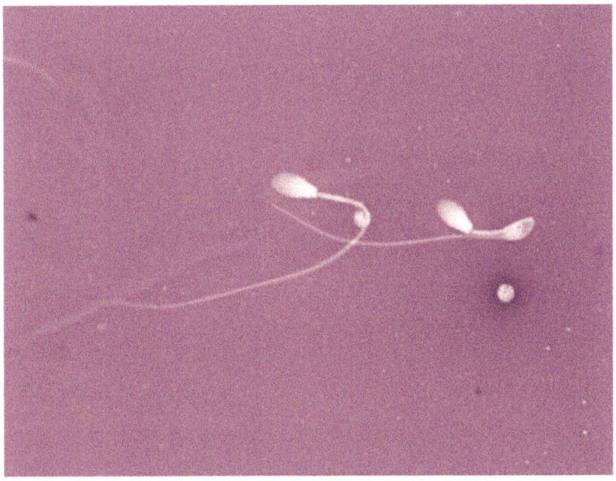

Figure 17.10 Spermatozoon on the left has a distal cytoplasmic droplet. Spermatozoon on the right has a bent midpiece ("hairpin tail") with a retained distal droplet. Staining with eosin/nigrosin (Hancock stain). Original magnification 1000×.

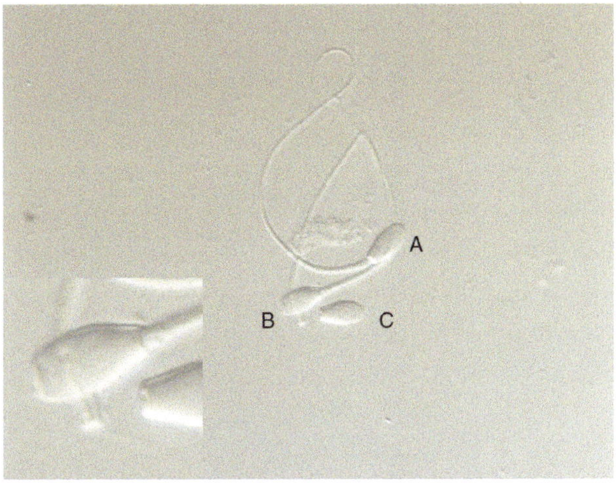

Figure 17.12 Stallion spermatozoa as observed under DIC microscopy. A: Morphologically normal spermatozoon. B: Spermatozoon with an abnormal acrosome ("knobbed"; observe the magnified image on the bottom left). C: Detached head. Original magnification 1000×.

semen must have at least 1 billion progressively motile sperm, with a sperm concentration between 30 and 50 million sperm/mL. The inclusion of 1 billion progressively motile sperm is intended to guarantee at least 500 million progressively motile sperm after cooling (assuming that half of the sperm would die due to cooling process); thus, estimation of sperm concentration and sperm progressive motility is necessary to calculate the amount of raw semen and extender required, as well as the number of doses that can be obtained from a given ejaculate. Likewise, the stallion semen must be diluted with an appropriate extender (i.e., milk-based extenders) at a minimal ratio of 1:4 semen:extender. This is done to reduce the deleterious effects that seminal plasma can have on sperm quality during cooling, when concentrations of 20% or higher are used [28, 29]. The calculations in Box 17.3 can be done to adequately prepare breeding doses for cooled storage.

After 24–48 hours of cooled storage (5 °C), it is expected that at least 30% of sperm progressive motility is retained. Use of the methods described above to determine sperm motility, concentration, and morphology is indicated when doses of cool-stored semen are prepared to be shipped or received to breed a mare. Sperm longevity during cooled storage is stallion dependent, and certain stallions can have

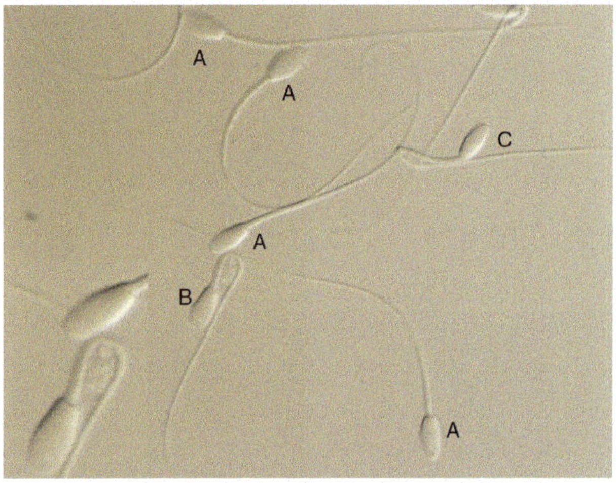

Figure 17.13 Stallion spermatozoa as observed under DIC microscopy. A: Morphologically normal spermatozoa. B: Spermatozoon with a bent midpiece ("hairpin tail" and retained cytoplasmic droplet – see bottom left). C: Spermatozoon with abnormal head (tapered head) and bent midpiece. Original magnification 1000×.

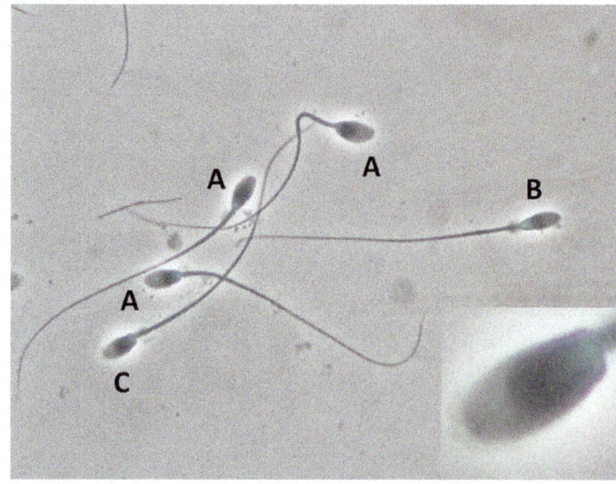

Figure 17.15 Stallion spermatozoa as observed under phase-contrast microscopy. A: Morphologically normal spermatozoa. B: Spermatozoon with abnormal head ("pyriform") and proximal cytoplasmic droplet. C: Spermatozoon with abnormal head (tapered) and abnormal acrosome ("lifted" or partially reacted acrosome – observe the halo around the acrosomal region in the image at the bottom right). Original magnification 1000×.

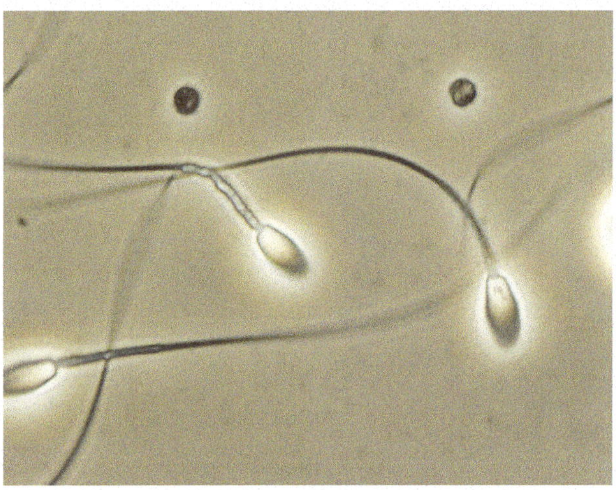

Figure 17.14 Stallion spermatozoa as observed under phase-contrast microscopy. Sperm on the right is morphologically normal, whilst the sperm on the left has an abnormal midpiece (swollen or roughened mitochondrial helix). These types of abnormalities can be seen in semen after freezing/thawing due to osmotic stress. Original magnification 1000×.

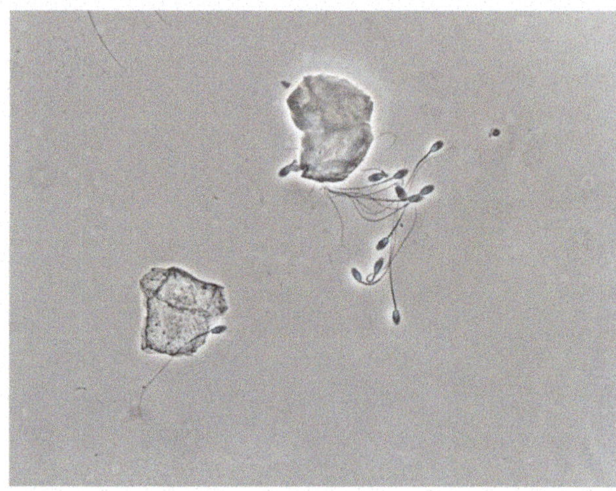

Figure 17.16 Stallion spermatozoa on phase-contrast microscopy. The presence of epithelial cells is commonly seen when the stallion penis is not appropriately washed before semen collection, or in cases when the ejaculate is collected after several mounts using the same artificial vagina. Original magnification 1000×.

higher values of sperm progressive motility after 48 or even 72 hours of cooling, particularly when appropriate extenders and dilution ratios are used. Likewise, other stallions may display lower sperm quality when semen is diluted using the technique described above, particularly in stallions where "seminal plasma toxicity" is suspected. In this case, techniques to completely remove the seminal plasma, such as cushioned centrifugation, should be performed [30]. The reader is referred to some excellent reviews on how to process stallion semen through cushion centrifugation and other techniques to enhance sperm quality after cooling [31, 32].

17.5 Ancillary Techniques for Stallion Sperm Quality Analysis

17.5.1 Sperm Viability

The term "viability" has been used as a synonym for sperm plasma membrane intactness. Due to the complexity of

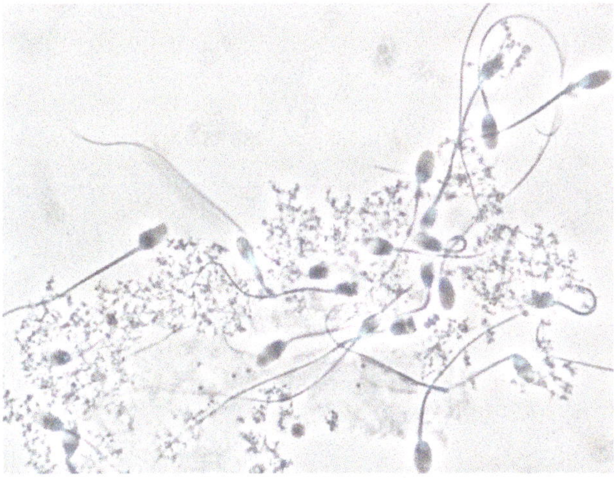

Figure 17.17 Stallion spermatozoa on phase-contrast microscopy. Observe the high quantities of debris, which in this case resulted from excessive use of lubricants in the artificial vagina before collection. Original magnification 1000×.

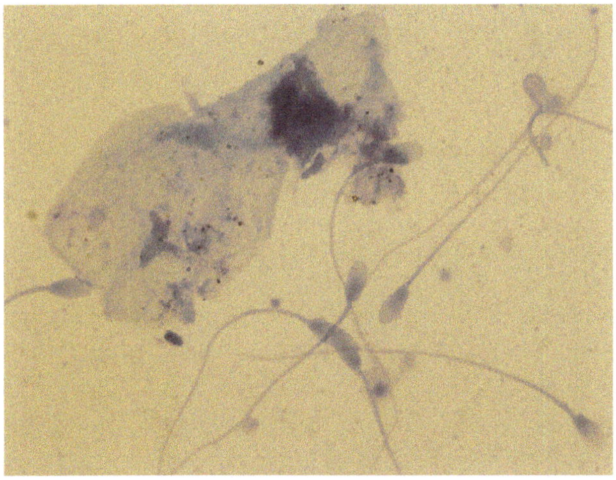

Figure 17.18 Stallion spermatozoa stained using Diff-Quik. The presence of other cell types, such as epithelial cells, can be enhanced by using this stain compared with Hancock stain. Note how the acrosomes of the sperm are easily differentiated with this stain. Original magnification 1000×.

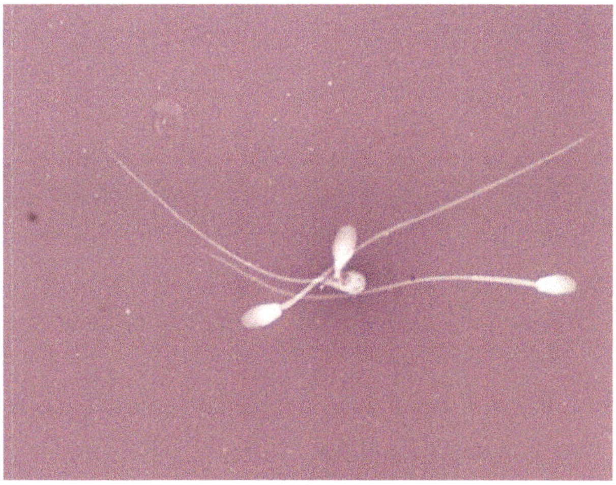

Figure 17.19 Stallion spermatozoa stained using eosin/nigrosin (Hancock stain). The sperm in the middle has an abnormal (tapered) head and an abnormal, bent midpiece. The other sperm are morphologically normal. Original magnification 1000×.

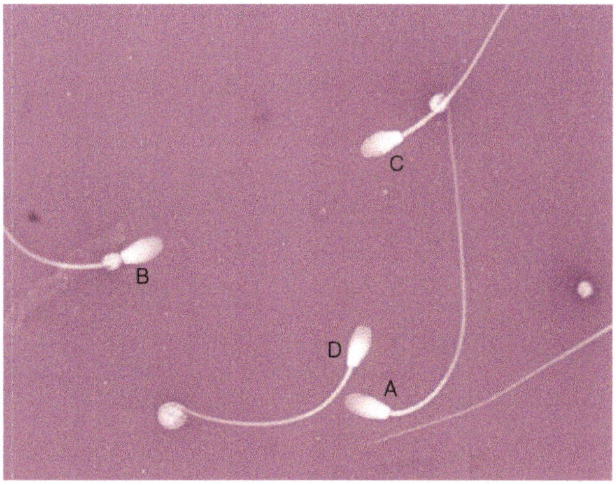

Figure 17.20 Stallion spermatozoa stained with eosin/nigrosin (Hancock stain). A: Morphologically normal sperm. Spermatozoa with (B) proximal and (C) distal cytoplasmic droplet. (d) Spermatozoon with coiled tail. Original magnification 1000×.

the processes related to sperm survival during cooling and cryopreservation, or during its transit through the female reproductive tract (i.e., capacitation, acrosome reaction), assessment of sperm plasma membrane integrity and function becomes necessary. Recent studies have demonstrated that the assessment of sperm plasma membrane in fresh, cool-stored, and frozen stallion spermatozoa is fundamental in predicting stallion fertility [23, 33].

Under field conditions, several techniques have been reported to determine the intactness of the stallion sperm plasma membrane, including the use of supravital stains such as eosin/nigrosin, trypan blue–Giemsa, or Chicago sky blue [34, 35]. The most commonly used stain for this purpose is eosin/nigrosin, where the exclusion of the stain in smears is related to an intact plasma membrane (Figure 17.21). However, its ability to accurately assess plasma membrane intactness is low compared with other techniques such as the use of fluorescent dyes and automated cell counters or flow cytometers. Foster et al. demonstrated that the eosin/nigrosin staining of stallion sperm yielded lower levels of agreement than flow cytometric analysis of plasma membrane intactness, particularly when reduced percentages of intact membranes were present in the samples; thus, eosin/nigrosin staining is more likely to overestimate the percentage of intact sperm in a sample, particularly in cooled semen [36].

Box 17.3 Calculations for preparing cool-stored semen doses

1) Assuming the following semen characteristics in the raw ejaculate:

- Semen volume: 45 mL
- Sperm concentration (hemocytometer): 187 million sperm/mL
- Sperm total motility/progressive motility: 80%/65%

2) Calculating the amount of raw semen required to prepare a cool-shipped semen dose:

$$\frac{1000 \text{ million progressively motile sperm (dose)}}{(\textit{raw} \text{ semen concentration} \times \text{percent progressive motility})} = \textit{Raw} \text{ semen required } \textit{per} \text{ dose}$$

a) Replacing the values obtained from the ejaculate in the equation

$$\frac{1000 \text{ million progressively motile sperm (dose)}}{(187 \text{ million } \textit{sp/mL} \times 0.65\%)} = 8.22 \ \textit{mL} \text{ of } \textit{raw} \text{ semen}$$

b) Each dose of cooled semen from this ejaculate must have 8.22 mL of raw semen, which have to be diluted at a dilution ratio 1:4 with an appropriate extender. Thus, the final volume of the dose will be = 8.22 mL × 5 = 41.1 mL total volume. The volume of extender required to dilute the raw semen will be 32.88 mL.

c) Diluting the raw semen (8.22 mL) with the extender (32.88 mL) will yield a final concentration per mL of 37.4 million sperm/mL = 8.22 mL × 187 million sperm/mL = 1587 million total sperm (dose) ÷ 41.1 mL (final volume/dose) = 37.4 million sperm/mL.

Using the above calculations, five doses of cool-stored semen can be obtained from the ejaculate, with at least 1.5 billion sperm per dose, at a dilution ratio at least 1:4 and a final sperm concentration between 30 and 50 million sperm/mL.

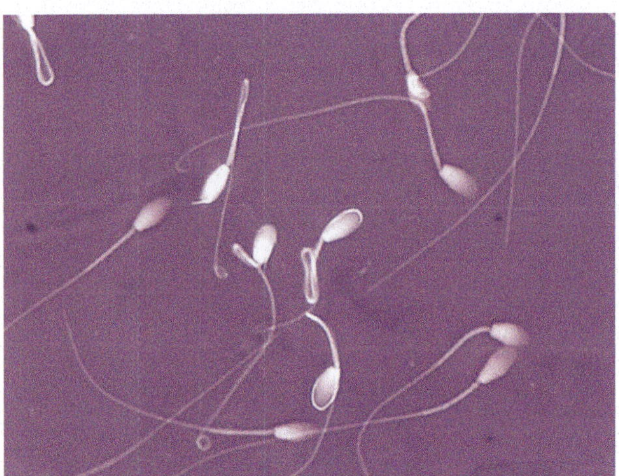

Figure 17.21 Stallion spermatozoa stained with eosin/nigrosin (Hancock stain) for assessment of sperm plasma membrane intactness ("viability"). Spermatozoa stained in pink are sperm with damaged plasma membranes ("dead"). Original magnification 1000×.

Another relatively simple technique commonly used under field conditions to assess the functional status of the sperm plasma membrane is the hypoosmotic swelling test (HOST). In this test, the sperm are incubated in a hypotonic solution (100 mOsm/L–1.72 g sucrose in 50 mL of deionized water) for one hour at 37 °C. Spermatozoa with functional plasma membranes (osmotically functional) will allow the entry of water into the sperm so a higher proportion of coiled tails will be observed after incubation (Figure 17.22). This test has been validated for use in stallion spermatozoa, and seems to be relatively associated with sperm motility, plasma membrane intactness (assessed by fluorescent methods), and fertility [33, 37, 38].

Most recently, the use of automated cell counters for assessment of sperm plasma membrane intactness has become widely accepted in research stations and large breeding operations. The NucleoCounter SP-100 can assess the percentage of intact plasma membranes in raw or extended stallion sperm, based on the use of the fluorescent dye propidium iodide, in samples previously diluted with an isotonic pH balanced salt solution. This method has been validated against more sophisticated methods for assessment of plasma membrane intactness (flow cytometry) with high reliability and agreement [36]. The use of high-throughput devices such as flow cytometers is commonly reserved for veterinary hospitals and research stations, where the combination of several fluorescent dyes, such as SYBR-14/propidium iodide (LIVE/DEAD Kit, Molecular Probes, Eugene, OR) (Figure 17.23) and Yo-Pro/Ethidium homodimer, amongst others, is intended to analyze up to 10 000 cells in a matter of minutes. These techniques can accurately determine the proportion of spermatozoa with damaged

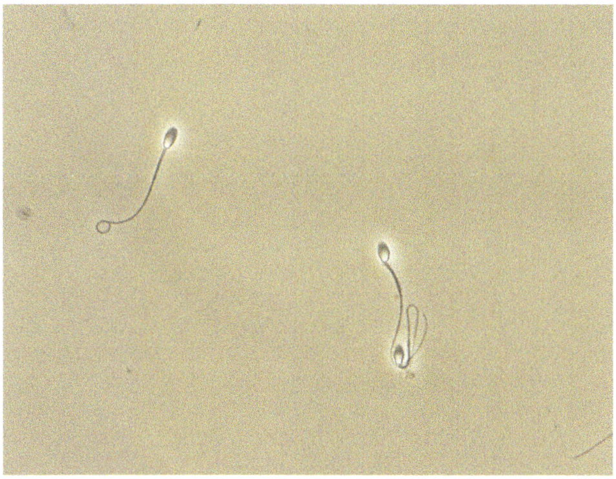

Figure 17.22 Stallion sperm plasma membrane function as assessed by the hypoosmotic swelling test (HOST). After incubation in the hypoosmotic solution (100 mOsm/L), the spermatozoon with a coiled tail (*left*) is considered to have a functional plasma membrane, due to the entry of water into the cell, which generates the coiling of the tail. Phase contrast microscopy at 400×.

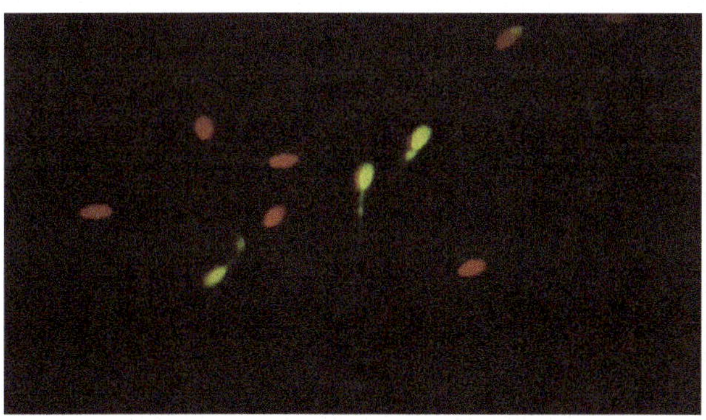

Figure 17.23 Frozen–thawed stallion spermatozoa stained using the combination of SYBR-14 and propidium iodide, for analysis of sperm plasma membrane intactness. Green spermatozoa are spermatozoa with intact plasma membranes (live sperm), whilst red spermatozoa are spermatozoa with damaged plasma membranes (dead sperm). 400× magnification.

plasma membranes in raw, cooled, and frozen/thawed stallion spermatozoa, and the potential relationship of these techniques with stallion fertility is described elsewhere [20, 23, 25, 33]. Laboratories in the US that offer these services include Texas A&M University, Colorado State University, and University of California, Davis.

17.5.2 Sperm DNA Quality

The relationship of sperm DNA quality and potential male fertility was established in the late 1980s and early 1990s, particularly when early embryonic death is observed after breeding using ejaculates with normal sperm motility or morphology. The estimation of sperm DNA quality using flow cytometry was initially established by Kenney and coworkers [39], and extensively used by Texas and French workers with fresh, cooled, or frozen/thawed semen [20, 23, 33, 40–42]. These techniques have demonstrated a clear association between stallion sperm DNA integrity (using the sperm chromatin structure assay – SCSA) and stallion fertility in breeding programs using natural cover and AI with cool-stored semen. Although the authors are not aware of other techniques that could be used in field situations for analysis of sperm DNA quality, practitioners can submit samples of raw, cooled, or frozen/thawed semen to reference laboratories, such as Texas A&M University for this test.

17.5.3 Acrosome Intactness and Function

In recent years, the assessment of acrosome intactness and function has become necessary in cases when other sperm quality tests, such as sperm motility, morphology or DNA integrity, cannot explain the causes of reduced fertility. The use of certain stains for assessment of acrosome intactness under field conditions has been reported [34, 35, 43]; however, in the authors' opinion their capacity to detect true acrosome reaction or acrosomal damage is limited, particularly when cooled or frozen semen is analyzed. The use of fluorescent stains for acrosomal assessment is superior to the use of conventional light microscopy, but this requires access to expensive equipment such as fluorescent microscopes or flow cytometers. Using fluorescent techniques, several combinations of dyes have been proposed to evaluate simultaneously the percentage of sperm with intact plasma membrane and acrosome membrane (Figure 17.24).

Under certain circumstances, the assessment of acrosomal function is done by stimulating the acrosome reaction with progesterone or calcium ionophore A23187 and staining the acrosome membrane with fluorescent probes. It has been demonstrated that sperm from a group of subfertile stallions was not able to acrosome-react after exposure to progesterone [44] or calcium ionophore A23187 [45], in comparison with fertile stallions. Furthermore, Brinsko et al. have reported a higher cholesterol-to-phospholipid ratio in semen and seminal plasma from subfertile stallions with impaired acrosome reaction, compared to fertile stallions [46], and have demonstrated a relationship between reduced fertility, impaired acrosome reaction after exposure to calcium ionophore A23187 and a single nucleotide polymorphism in the gene FKBP6, located in the chromosome 13 of a group of Thoroughbred stallions [47]. A genetic panel test is currently being offered by Texas A&M University for the diagnosis of this genetic abnormality.

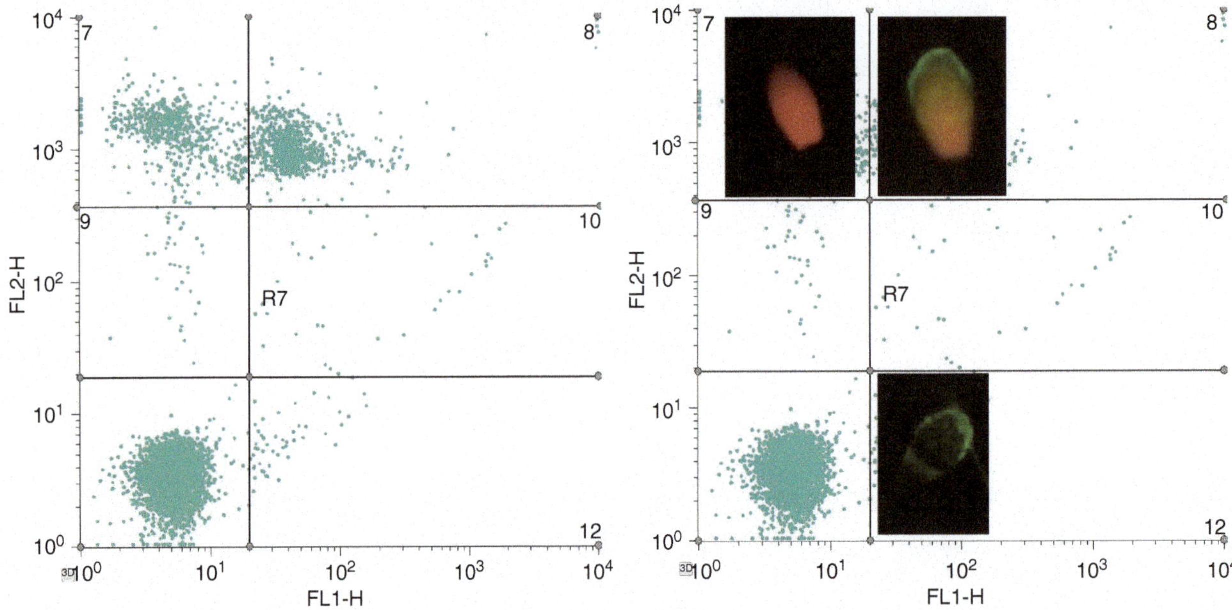

Figure 17.24 Flow cytometry scattergram representing the simultaneous assessment of sperm plasma membrane and acrosome intactness using the combination of FITC-PSA and propidium iodide in cooled stored stallion sperm, and the corresponding staining patterns after observation under fluorescence microscopy. (*Left lower quadrant*) Sperm with intact plasma membrane and acrosome. (*Right lower quadrant*) Sperm with intact plasma membrane and disrupted acrosome. (*Left upper quadrant*) Sperm with damaged plasma membrane and intact acrosome. (*Right upper quadrant*) Sperm with damaged plasma membrane and acrosome.

17.5.4 Mitochondrial Function, Oxidative Stress, and Apoptotic Markers in Sperm

Given recent advances in the understanding of spermatozoal damage during cooling or cryopreservation, attention has been paid to the relationship of mitochondrial function and stallion sperm quality [2]. Most of these assays are conducted using flow cytometry so their use in private practice is limited. However, practitioners must be aware that there is a direct relationship between abnormal mitochondrial function (which can be translated into low motility) and the overproduction of reactive oxygen species (ROS) or the presence of apoptotic markers in the sperm. All these molecular changes can be either a cause or a consequence of improper handling of semen during cooling or cryopreservation, as well as a susceptibility of some stallions to those procedures.

17.6 Conclusion

During the last 20 years, there has been an exponential growth in the methods designed to analyze semen quality under field conditions and in research situations. Practitioners need to be familiar with the commonly used techniques available to assess sperm quality in stallions, including assessment of sperm concentration, motility, morphology, and plasma membrane intactness. Most of these methods can be used to determine semen quality in fresh, cooled or frozen/thawed semen samples under field conditions, when appropriate equipment and methods are used. Other advanced techniques are currently available for veterinary practitioners when the previously mentioned tests cannot diagnose the reasons for impaired fertility in the stallion.

Acknowledgments

The authors would like to thank Drs. Dickson Varner, Charles Love and Steven Brinsko for their invaluable support whilst writing this chapter, as well as their generosity in sharing their perspectives about sperm evaluation in the stallion, and the use of their equipment to obtain some of the pictures illustrating the chapter. These individuals have established a cutting-edge program for the advancement of stallion reproduction at Texas A&M University, with masterful manuscripts and published works in this area. They can be considered as the current "fathers" of stallion reproduction worldwide.

References

1 Kenney, R.M., Hurtgen, J., Pierson, R. et al. (1983). *Theriogenology and The Equine, Part II: The Stallion*. Hastings: Society for Theriogenology.
2 Peña, F.J., Plaza-Dávila, M., Ball, B.A. et al. (2015). The impact of reproductive technologies on stallion mitochondrial function. *Reprod. Domest. Anim.* 40: 529–537.
3 Gibb, Z. and Aitken, R.J. (2016). Recent developments in stallion semen preservation. *J. Equine Vet. Sci.* 43 (Suppl): 29–36.
4 Love, C.C. (1992). Semen collection techniques. *Vet. Clin. North Am Equine Pract.* 8 (1): 111–128.
5 Griggers, S., Paccamonti, D.L., Thompson, R.A., and Eilts, B.E. (2001). The effects of pH, osmolarity and urine contamination on equine spermatozoal motility. *Theriogenology* 56 (4): 613–622.
6 Turner, C.E., Walbornn, S.R., Blanchard, T.L. et al. (2016). The effect of two levels of hemospermia on stallion fertility. *Theriogenology* 86 (6): 1399–1402.
7 Mann, T. (1975). Biochemistry of stallion semen. *J. Reprod. Fertil. Suppl.* 23: 47–52.
8 Pickett, B.W., Faulkner, L.C., and Voss, J.L. (1975). Effect of season on some characteristics of stallion semen. *J. Reprod. Fertil. Suppl.* 23: 25–28.
9 Althouse, G.C., Seager, S.W.J., Varner, D.D., and Webb, G.W. (1989). Diagnostic aids for the detection of urine in the equine ejaculate. *Theriogenology* 31 (6): 1141–1148.
10 Ellerbrock, R., Canisso, I., Feijo, L. et al. (2016). Diagnosis and effects of urine contamination in cooled-extended stallion semen. *Theriogenology* 85 (7): 1219–1224.
11 Turner, R.M.O. and McDonnell, S.M. (2003). Alkaline phosphatase in stallion semen: characterization and clinical applications. *Theriogenology* 60: 1–10.
12 Blanchard, T.L., Brinsko, S.P., Varner, D.D., and Love, C.C. (2009). How to investigate azoospermia in stallions. *Proc. Am. Assoc. Equine Pract.* 55: 331–335.
13 Brito, L.F.C., Althouse, G.C., Aurich, C. et al. (2016). Andrology laboratory review: evaluation of sperm concentration. *Theriogenology* 85 (9): 1507–1527.
14 Rigby, S.L., Varner, D.D., Thompson, J.A. et al. (2001). Measurement of sperm concentration in stallion ejaculates using photometric or direct sperm enumeration techniques. *Proc. Am. Assoc. Equine Pract.* 47: 236–238.
15 Comerford, K.L., Love, C.C., Brinsko, S.P. et al. (2008). Validation of a commercially available fluorescence-based instrument to evaluate stallion spermatozoal concentration. *Proc. Am. Assoc. Equine Pract.* 54: 367–368.
16 Hanse, C., Vermeiden, T., Vermeiden, J.P. et al. (2006). Comparison of FACSCount AF system, improved Neubauer hemocytometer, Corning 254 photometer, SpermVision, UltiMate and NucleoCounter SP-100 for determination of sperm concentration of boar semen. *Theriogenology* 66: 2188–2194.
17 Wessel, M.T. and Althouse, G.C. (2006). Validation of an objective approach for simultaneous assessment of viability and motility of fresh and cooled equine spermatozoa. *Anim. Reprod. Sci.* 94: 21–22.
18 Jasko, D.J., Little, T.V., Lein, D.H., and Foote, R.H. (1992). Comparison of spermatozoal movement and semen characteristics with fertility in stallions: 64 cases (1987–1988). *J. Am. Vet. Med. Assoc.* 200 (7): 979–985.
19 Love, C.C. (2011). Relationship between sperm motility, morphology and the fertility of stallions. *Theriogenology* 76 (3): 547–557.
20 Love, C.C., Noble, J.K., Standridge, S.A. et al. (2015). The relationship between sperm quality in cool-shipped semen and embryo recovery rate in horses. *Theriogenology* 84 (9): 1587–1593.
21 Hoogewijs, M.K., Govaere, J.L., Rijsselaere, T. et al. (2009). Influence of technical settings on CASA motility parameters of frozen thawed stallion semen. *Proc. Am. Assoc. Equine Pract.* 55: 336–337.
22 Yesté, M., Bonet, S., Rodríguez-Gil, J.E., and Rivera del Álamo, M.M. (2018). Evaluation of sperm motility with CASA-Mot: which factors may influence our measurements? *Reprod. Fertil. Dev.* 30 (6): 789–798.
23 Barrier-Battut, I., Kempfer, A., Becker, J. et al. (2016). Development of a new fertility prediction model for stallion semen, including flow cytometry. *Theriogenology* 86: 1111–1131.
24 Love, C.C., Varner, D.D., and Thompson, J.A. (2000). Intra- and inter-stallion variation in sperm morphology and their relationship with fertility. *J. Reprod. Fertil. Suppl.* 56: 93–100.
25 Love, C.C. (2016). Modern techniques for semen evaluation. *Vet. Clin. North Am Equine Pract.* 32: 531–546.
26 Brito, L.F.C., Greene, L.M., Kelleman, A. et al. (2011). Effect of method and clinician on stallion sperm morphology evaluation. *Theriogenology* 76: 745–750.
27 Varner, D.D. (2016). Approaches to breeding soundness examination and interpretation of results. *J. Equine Vet. Sci.* 43: S37–S44.
28 Brinsko, S.P., Crockett, E.C., and Squires, E.L. (2000). Effect of centrifugation and partial removal of seminal plasma on equine spermatozoal motility after cooling and storage. *Theriogenology* 54: 129–136.

29 Love, C.C., Brinsko, S.P., Rigby, S.L. et al. (2005). Relationship of seminal plasma level and extender type to sperm motility and DNA integrity. *Theriogenology* 63: 1584–1591.

30 Bliss, S.B., Voge, J.L., Hayden, S.S. et al. (2012). The impact of cushioned centrifugation protocols on semen quality of stallions. *Theriogenology* 77 (6): 1232–1239.

31 Varner, D.D., Love, C.C., Brinsko, S.P. et al. (2008). Semen processing for the subfertile stallion. *J. Equine Vet. Sci.* 28 (11): 677–685.

32 Varner, D.D. (2016). Strategies for processing semen from subfertile stallions for cooled transport. *Vet. Clin. North Am Equine Pract.* 32 (3): 547–560.

33 Barrier-Battut, I., Kempfer, A., Lemasson, N. et al. (2017). Prediction of the fertility of stallion frozen-thawed semen using a combination of computer-assisted motility analysis, microscopical observation and flow cytometry. *Theriogenology* 95: 186–200.

34 Kutvolgyi, G., Stefler, J., and Kovacs, A. (2006). Viability and acrosome staining of stallion spermatozoa by Chicago sky blue and Giemsa. *Biotech. Histochem.* 81 (4–6): 109–117.

35 Serafini, R., Longovardi, V., Spadetta, M. et al. (2014). Trypan blue/giemsa staining to assess sperm membrane integrity in salernitano stallions and its relationship to pregnancy rates. *Reprod. Domest. Anim.* 49 (1): 41–47.

36 Foster, M.L., Love, C.C., Varner, D.D. et al. (2011). Comparison of methods for assessing equine sperm membranes. *Theriogenology* 76 (2): 334–341.

37 Neild, D., Chaves, G., Flores, M. et al. (1999). Hypoosmotic swelling test in equine spermatozoa. *Theriogenology* 51 (4): 721–727.

38 Nie, G.J. and Wenzel, J.G.W. (2001). Adaptation of the hypoosmotic swelling test to assess functional integrity of stallion spermatozoal plasma membranes. *Theriogenology* 55 (4): 1005–1018.

39 Kenney, R.M., Evenson, D.P., Garcia, M.C., and Love, C.C. (1995). Relationships between sperm chromatin structure, motility, and morphology of ejaculated sperm, and seasonal pregnancy rate. *Biol. Reprod. Monogr.* 1: 647–653.

40 Love, C.C. and Kenney, R.M. (1998). The relationship of increased susceptibility of sperm DNA to denaturation and fertility in the stallion. *Theriogenology* 50 (6): 955–972.

41 Love, C.C., Thompson, J.A., Lowry, V.K., and Varner, D.D. (2002). Effect of storage time and temperature on stallion sperm DNA and fertility. *Theriogenology* 57 (3): 1135–1142.

42 Love, C.C. (2005). The sperm chromatin structure assay: a review of clinical applications. *Theriogenology* 89 (1–4): 39–45.

43 Runcan, E.E., Pozor, M.A., Zambrano, G.L. et al. (2014). Use of two conventional staining methods to assess the acrosomal status of stallion spermatozoa. *Equine Vet. J.* 46 (4): 503–506.

44 Meyers, S.A., Overstreet, J.W., Liu, I.K., and Drobnis, E.Z. (1995). Capacitation in-vitro of stallion spermatozoa: comparison of progesterone-induced acrosome reactions in fertile and subfertile males. *J. Androl.* 16: 47–54.

45 Varner, D.D., Thompson, J.A., Blanchard, T.L. et al. (2002). Induction of the acrosome reaction in stallion spermatozoa: effects of incubation temperature, incubation time, and ionophore concentration. *Theriogenology* 58: 303–306.

46 Brinsko, S.P., Love, C.C., Bauer, J.F. et al. (2007). Cholesterol-to-phospholipid ratio in whole sperm and seminal plasma from fertile stallions and stallions with unexplained fertility. *Anim. Reprod. Sci.* 99 (1–2): 65–71.

47 Raudsepp, T., McCue, M.E., Das, P.J. et al. (2012). Genome-wide association study implicates testis-sperm specific FKBP6 as a susceptibility locus for impaired acrosome reaction in stallions. *PLoS Genet.* 8 (12): e1003139.

18

Pleural, Peritoneal, and Synovial Fluid Analysis

Raquel M. Walton

IDEXX Laboratories, Inc., Langhorne, PA, USA

Acronyms and abbreviations that appear in this chapter include: NCC, nucleated cell count; RBC, red blood cell; TP, total protein; TP_{Ref}, total protein by refractometer; TS, total solids; WBC, white blood cell.

18.1 Pleural and Peritoneal Fluid

Pleural and peritoneal fluids are ultrafiltrates of plasma that reduce friction by lubrication. The constituents of peritoneal fluid are affected by the integrity of the mesothelial lining, changes in vascular permeability and lymphatic flow, plasma oncotic pressure, and capillary hydraulic pressure. Thus, changes in the character of the fluid can be attributed to specific disease processes and may yield information in diagnosis, treatment, and/or prognosis. Pleurocentesis and abdominocentesis are valuable clinical tools whose sensitivity and specificity are highest when all components of fluid evaluation are considered together. Fluid evaluations should include assessment of gross appearance, total protein (TP) concentration, cell counts (or estimation of cellularity), and cytology. If this is not possible, the minimum testing for fluid evaluation should include measurement of TP and measurement (or estimation) of cellularity because effusions are defined by these parameters.

18.1.1 Pathogenetic Mechanisms of Body Cavity Effusions

An effusion is defined as an increase in the normal volume of peritoneal or pleural fluid, which may or may not have increased protein or cell concentrations. Pleural effusions within North American equids are most often associated with bacterial pleuropneumonia. Other etiologies include neoplasia, penetrating chest wounds, hemorrhage, and cardiac disease. The majority of abdominal effusions are associated with gastrointestinal disorders, especially those causing colic. The main categories of pleural and peritoneal effusions are formulated to provide insight into the general pathophysiological mechanism responsible for an increase in the volume of body cavity fluid. Effusions are caused mainly by transudative, exudative, or hemorrhagic processes (Table 18.1). A fourth category, which is uncommon in horses, is lymphorrhagic effusion caused by leakage of lymph from lymphatic vessels (e.g., chylothorax or chyloabdomen) [1].

18.1.1.1 Transudates

Transudates are caused by increased hydraulic pressure or increased hydraulic and decreased oncotic pressure. These effusions have low protein concentrations and nucleated cell counts (NCCs). In horses, normal peritoneal and pleural fluids are distinguished from a transudate only by documenting an increase in fluid volume. The most common causes of transudates are the peracute/acute phase of any lesion causing decreased venous/lymphatic drainage in the portal or pulmonary system (e.g., volvulus/torsion, neoplasia, granuloma), as well as acute uroabdomen, and protein-losing nephropathies and enteropathies. Diagnosis of uroabdomen in the horse is facilitated by the characteristic presence of calcium carbonate crystals in equine urine, which are present extracellularly and within neutrophils and/or macrophages (Figure 18.1). Calcium carbonate crystals should be distinguished from glove starch crystals, which are commonly seen in cytological preparations (Figure 18.2). Suspicion of uroabdomen should be confirmed by measuring fluid creatinine concentration.

Plasma protein permeability of vessels within the hepatic sinuses is higher than that for vessels elsewhere in the peritoneal cavity. Consequently, increases in hydraulic pressure

Equine Hematology, Cytology, and Clinical Chemistry, Second Edition.
Edited by Raquel M. Walton, Rick L. Cowell, and Amy C. Valenciano.

Table 18.1 Classification of pleural and peritoneal effusions.

Classification	TP_{Ref}	NCC	RBC	Mechanism	Disorder
Transudate	<2.0	$<5\times10^3$	$<4\times10^4$	Increased hydrostatic and/or decreased oncotic pressure	Nephrotic syndrome Cirrhosis Acute uroabdomen
High-protein transudate	≥2.0	$<5\times10^3$	$<4\times10^4$	Increased hydrostatic and/or decreased oncotic pressure in postsinusoidal/sinusoidal hepatic or pulmonary vessels	Congestive heart failure Portal hypertension Neoplasia Acute torsion/volvulus
Exudate	>2.0	$>5\times10^3$	$>4\times10^4<5\times10^5$	Inflammation-mediated increased vascular permeability	Septic: Bacterial, fungal, or parasitic infection Nonseptic: Neoplasia Ischemic necrosis Pancreatitis Bile peritonitis Chronic uroabomen
Hemorrhage (acute)	≥2.0	$\geq$ or $\leq 5\times10^3$	$\geq1\times10^6$	Loss of blood from vessels	Trauma Neoplasia Hemostatic defects Uterine artery rupture

TP_{Ref}, total protein by refractometry (g/dL); NCC, nucleated cell count/μL; RBC, red blood cells/μL.

that involve the hepatic sinuses (i.e., sinusoidal or postsinusoidal increases) will produce a high protein transudate with a normal NCC. Congestive heart failure and any lesion that produces postsinusoidal portal hypertension are the most common causes of high protein transudates in the peritoneal cavity. Similarly, the pulmonary vasculature has higher permeability for plasma proteins and high protein transudates may result from increased pulmonary hydraulic pressure.

18.1.1.2 Exudates

Exudates are characterized by increased vascular permeability due to inflammatory mediators and therefore are attributable to inflammation. Inflammation may be caused by infectious or noninfectious processes (see Table 18.1). The absence of microorganisms on cytological examination does not preclude an infectious process. If clinical findings are suspicious of an infectious process, biochemical evaluation of the fluid (for lactate, glucose, and pH) and bacterial culture are warranted.

18.1.1.3 Hemorrhagic Effusions

Uniformly bloody specimens or consistently bloody specimens from different sites suggest true body cavity hemorrhage, which may be confirmed via cytology and/or ultrasonographic evaluation of the chest or abdomen. A hemorrhagic effusion is defined by the fluid red blood cell (RBC) count (see Table 18.1); acute hemorrhagic effusions usually have RBC counts >1,000,000/μL and packed cell volumes >3% [1]. Erythrocytes and plasma from hemorrhage will be resorbed by lymphatics so the fluid TP and RBC counts vary with time; in dogs ~65% of RBCs are resorbed within two days of hemorrhage [2].

Because platelets (and coagulation factors) are consumed during hemorrhage, hemorrhagic fluid contains no platelets and does not clot, whereas fluid that contains blood from peripheral or visceral vessels will contain platelets and will clot. In fluids with high RBC counts, the presence of platelets upon cytological evaluation indicates a component of blood contamination since platelets are not present in hemorrhagic effusions. However, the absence of platelets does not preclude peripheral blood contamination if the sample was collected into a nonanticoagulant tube (e.g., red top) and subsequently clotted *in vitro*. Cytological findings that support an interpretation of hemorrhage include the presence of erythrocytes and/or hemosiderin within macrophages (Figure 18.3). Note that if there is a delay in sample processing (>3–4 hours), RBC phagocytosis can occur *in vitro* in the transport tube. Conversely, erythrophagocytosis can be absent in samples

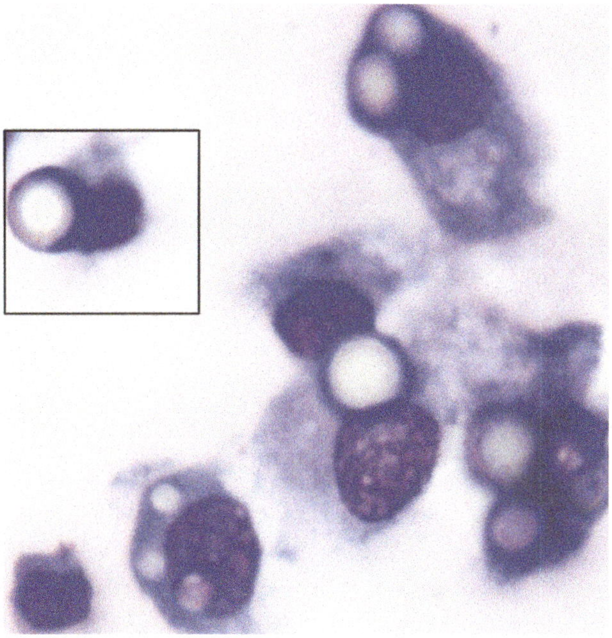

Figure 18.1 Calcium carbonate crystals within macrophages in peritoneal fluid. Note the concentric striations characteristic of the crystal (*inset*).

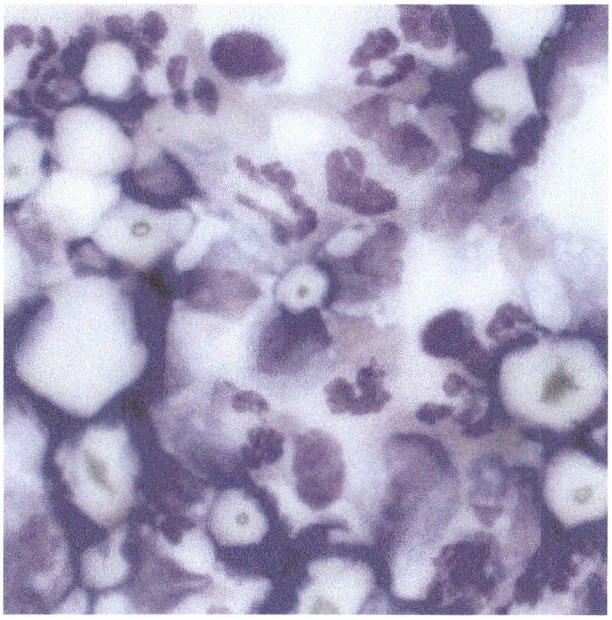

Figure 18.2 Glove talc (starch crystals) in a sample of peritoneal fluid. The crystals are round to rhomboid with a characteristic central divot.

from true hemorrhage if there has been insufficient time for RBC phagocytosis within the peritoneal cavity (i.e., peracute hemorrhage). In general, it takes several hours for erythrophagocytosis to occur; subsequent RBC breakdown into hemosiderin usually takes at least three days [3]. Thus, cytological interpretations of bloody fluid should be undertaken with knowledge of the type of collection tube used, as well as the amount of time before the sample was processed.

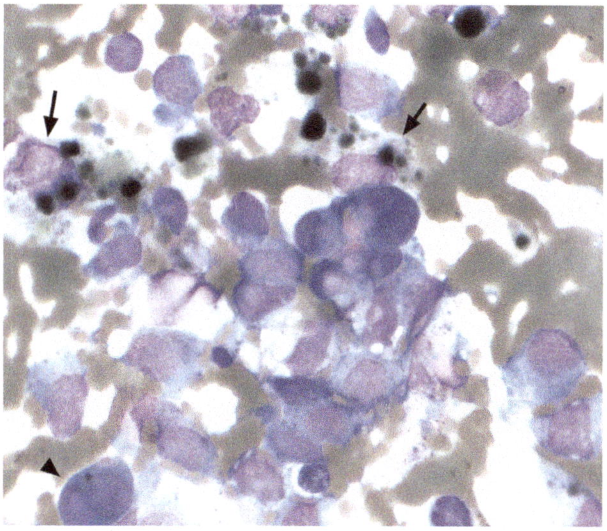

Figure 18.3 Hemorrhagic pleural effusion. Macrophages contain a globular green-black material consistent with hemosiderin (*arrows*). Note the presence of a binucleated mesothelial cell with hemosiderin (*arrowhead*). Mesothelial cells with hemosiderin can occasionally be seen in association with chronic hemorrhage.

18.1.1.4 Body Cavity Fluid Analysis

One of the first things to consider when evaluating body cavity fluid is whether the sample is representative. Two common causes of nonrepresentative fluid sampling include blood contamination and enterocentesis (for peritoneal fluid). Blood contamination may occur when a peripheral vein or abdominal organ (usually the spleen) is punctured. Blood contamination becomes apparent during centesis when the initial sample is clear and then becomes bloody or is bloody and then clears. As little as 0.05 mL blood in 1 mL of peritoneal fluid (5% contamination) can result in fluid RBC counts up to 449,000/μL, which is nearly10 times the upper limit of RBC reference values [4, 5]. However, WBC counts and TP concentration remain within reference intervals with up to 17% blood contamination [5].

Inadvertent enterocentesis has a reported frequency rate of 2–5% [4]. The incidence of complications directly related to inadvertent enterocentesis was reported to be 0.5% (four cases in 850 abdominocentesis samples) over a two-year period at one institution [6]. Enterocentesis may manifest grossly as a green to brown discoloration of peritoneal fluid, but contaminated fluid may also appear grossly normal with contamination only evident upon cytological evaluation. Presence of large ciliated protozoa, plant material, and a mixed bacterial population indicates enterocentesis or intestinal rupture (Figure 18.4). Peritoneal fluid evaluation alone cannot distinguish between enterocentesis and peracute intestinal leakage or perforation. This distinction is best accomplished in the context of the patient's clinical assessment.

18.1.1.5 Volume

Peritoneal fluid volume in health typically ranges from 100 to 300 mL, although it has been estimated that up to 2 L may be present [4]. While the equine peritoneal cavity normally contains a large volume of fluid, abdominal paracentesis typically yields <10 mL of fluid and most commonly 3–5 mL [7]. The pleural cavity often yields a similar volume of normal fluid (2–8 mL), but it may not be possible to retrieve pleural fluid from some healthy horses [8]. The amount of fluid obtained from paracentesis does not necessarily correlate with presence or absence of effusion. In seriously ill horses with effusion confirmed surgically or postmortem, abdominal paracentesis may yield only a small volume [7].

Diagnosis of mild to moderate effusions in equids, especially adults, can be difficult due to the constraints on palpation and large spaces that accommodates even moderate effusion volumes. Ultrasound is often necessary to diagnose effusion. In horses, it is convention to classify abnormal peritoneal and pleural fluid (i.e., increased protein concentration and/or cell count) as an effusion regardless of whether an increased volume is documented. In contrast, a fluid with a normal cell count and protein concentration is only classified as an effusion if there is a confirmed increase in volume.

18.1.1.6 Color and Clarity

The physical characteristics of body cavity fluid may provide hints as to its cellularity or biochemical composition. Normal body cavity fluid is yellow and transparent. Discoloration of the fluid may reflect hemorrhage (orange to red), enteric rupture (green or brown), bile peritonitis (dark green), infection (yellow-white), or vascular compromise (orange to reddish brown). Abnormal abdominal fluid color has been used in studies to predict the need for surgical treatment. The sensitivity and specificity of subjectively discolored fluid for predicting the need for surgical intervention vary in different reports: 92% and 74%, 78% and 48%, and 51% and 95%, respectively [9–11]. Weimann et al. [11] used hemoglobin concentration as an objective measurement of discoloration from hemolysis and found that when peritoneal hemoglobin concentration was >0.01 mmol/L (0.02 g/dL), the test was 80% sensitive and 82% specific for selecting surgical treatment. While discolored peritoneal fluid, especially serosanguineous, supports the

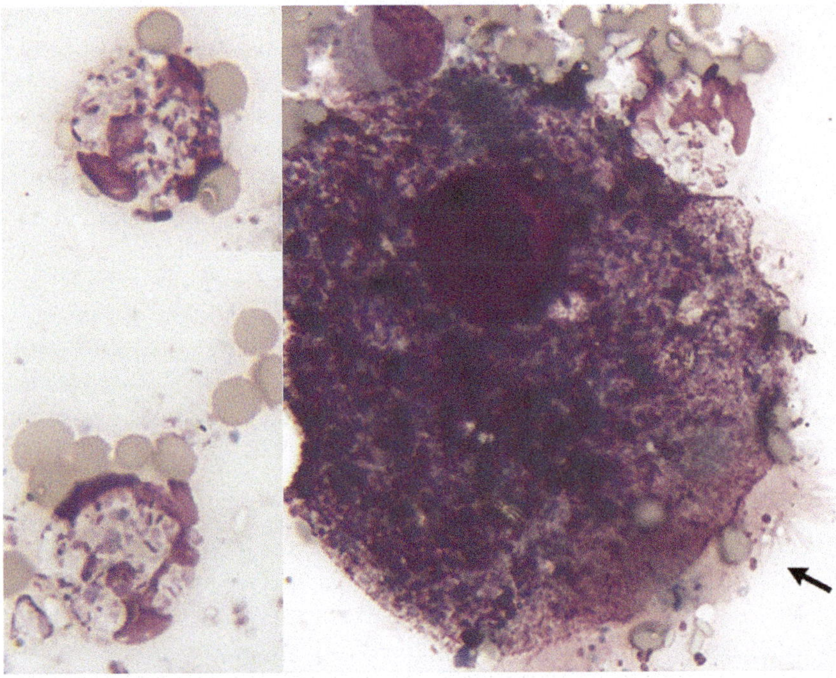

Figure 18.4 Peritoneal fluid with neutrophils containing abundant intracellular bacteria (*left panels*) and a ciliated protozoal organism (*right panel; arrow*). The protozoal organism indicates enteric contents are present. Neutrophils with intracellular bacteria suggest intestinal rupture/leakage and peritonitis rather than inadvertent enterocentesis. However, while less likely, these findings could be consistent with enterocentesis if suppurative enteritis were present.

need for surgical treatment, an interpretation of discolored fluid should only be made when the possibility of enterocentesis or blood contamination has been excluded and should be formulated in the context of physical exam findings.

The clarity of body cavity fluid in health reflects low cellularity. Increased turbidity is usually reported in terms of cloudy/hazy or opaque, and suggests increased cellularity, presence of plant material, or, rarely, lipid (i.e., chyloabdomen). While turbidity is abnormal, measurement of cell numbers and cytological evaluation of the fluid are necessary to determine its cause.

18.1.2 Biochemical Evaluation

18.1.2.1 Fluid Protein Concentration

Because body cavity fluid is an ultrafiltrate of plasma, protein concentrations are much lower than in plasma. Protein can be rapidly and accurately measured by hand-held refractometers. Protein measured by refractometer for body cavity fluids is linearly related to protein measured by biochemical methods and results are accurate to at least 0.6 g/dL [12]. Pleural fluid protein concentration runs slightly higher than for peritoneal fluid (0.2–4.7 g/dL), but the majority of healthy horses have pleural fluid protein concentrations <2.5 g/dL just as for peritoneal fluid [8]. Many studies cite the upper reference value for normal body cavity fluid protein concentration as <2.5 g/dL [4], which is the lowest protein reading on many refractometers. To report values below the lower end of the protein scale, the value measured using either refractive index, refraction, or urine specific gravity (SG) scales can be converted to TP with published conversion tables [13]. When abdominal fluid protein was calculated using conversion tables or measured biochemically, normal values were typically ≤2.0 g/dL in many studies [14–16]. Increases in fluid protein concentration above reference values indicate either increased permeability of the capillaries due to inflammatory mediators or increased hydraulic pressure within hepatic sinusoids or pulmonary vessels, which have higher permeability to protein. An increase in protein concentration due to inflammatory mediators is typically accompanied by an increase in NCCs.

Because refractometers measure protein via a total solids (TS)-based technique, the total dissolved solids in the sample affect light refraction [13]. In addition to protein, TS include electrolytes, glucose, urea, and lipids. While the altered refraction of body fluid is mostly due to protein content, increases in lipid, glucose, or urea content interfere with refractometric protein measurements. However, marked increases in urea or glucose (273 and 649 mg/dL, respectively) are needed to increase protein measurement by 0.4–0.5 g/dL [17]. Unlike glucose and urea, lipid does not freely diffuse into peritoneal fluid from plasma; increased concentrations of lipid in pleural or peritoneal fluid only occur in cases of chylous effusion.

Another potential cause of erroneous refractometer readings is the addition of EDTA from K_3EDTA anticoagulant tubes. At the standard concentration of EDTA (5 μmol/mL), K_3EDTA by itself has minimal effect on the fluid's refraction (≤0.1 g/dL increase). At higher concentrations of EDTA (10 and 20 μmol/mL), EDTA can increase refractometer total protein (TPRef) by 0.9–1.0 g/dL. Underfilling of EDTA tubes has the effect of increasing the EDTA concentration and will cause spurious increases in the TP_{Ref}. Some commercial tubes with K_3EDTA anticoagulant may also contain additives to prevent crystallization of the EDTA. Tubes that contain the additive may increase TP_{Ref} readings by up to 0.9 g/dL, even when properly filled [18]. It is recommended that TP_{Ref} readings should be performed either on fluid collected in serum tubes or in properly filled K_3EDTA tubes containing no additives. While sodium heparin anticoagulant has no effect on TP_{Ref} [18], heparin has deleterious effects on cellular morphology and is not recommended for samples that will be evaluated cytologically.

The term "total solids" has caused much confusion in the reporting of refractometric protein results. TP and TS are not synonymous. Currently, the vast majority of all refractometers incorporate a conversion factor in their design so that the scales report TP and not TS. Contributing to the confusion is the fact that at least one refractometer is named the "TS meter" (AO Corporation) when it is in fact calibrated to report TP [13]. Today, nearly all refractometers report TP and not TS, so comparisons between fluid samples are appropriate.

Specific gravity has also been used to estimate protein concentration in equine body cavity fluid. However, use of the refractometer SG scale will yield erroneous results because the SG scale is calibrated specifically for urine. Urea, not protein, is the principal constituent of urine, thus SG calibrated for urine gives falsely high results for body fluids [13]. A caveat applies to low protein fluid (<1.0 g/dL); in this instance, the urine SG scale more accurately estimates true SG because the fluid's refractive index is more similar to urine [1].

18.1.2.2 Other Biochemical Tests

18.1.2.2.1 Fluid Lactate, Glucose, and pH Most biochemical testing of body cavity fluid is performed on peritoneal rather than pleural fluid because of the importance of identifying severely diseased bowel and the ability to assess pulmonary disease via airway evaluation (see Chapter 20). Intestinal ischemia or infarction is one of the most common causes of mortality in colic cases because of subsequent circulatory collapse that can occur. Lactate is the endproduct of anaerobic glycolysis and has been used as a marker for ischemia in colic studies. Normal peritoneal fluid lactate concentrations vary with respect to methodology, but are usually <1.0 mmol/L [16, 19].

Studies of colic cases have shown that peritoneal lactate, TP, NCC, and glucose concentrations were significantly increased compared with peritoneal fluid from clinically normal horses. When the colic cases were subdivided on the basis of strangulating versus nonstrangulating obstructions, peritoneal lactate concentrations were significantly higher in strangulating lesions, with the exception of strangulating small colon obstructions [16, 19]. Increases in fluid lactate, decreases in fluid pH, and abnormal fluid color and/or turbidity were most strongly correlated with ischemic strangulating lesions. Peritoneal fluid lactate concentrations were shown to be more sensitive than blood lactate concentrations in detecting early ischemic lesions. The prognosis becomes progressively poorer for both strangulating and nonstrangulating lesions as peritoneal fluid lactate concentrations increase. One study showed the probability of death in nonstrangulating lesions to be 63% for peritoneal lactate concentrations of 12 mmol/L and 82% for lactate concentrations of 16 mmol/L; the same concentrations of peritoneal fluid lactate had 82% and 92% probabilities of death, respectively, in strangulating lesions [19].

Peritoneal glucose concentrations have been shown to be useful as a relatively rapid test for distinguishing septic from nonseptic exudates [20]. Positive bacterial culture or cytological identification of intracellular bacteria in abdominal fluid is a definitive indicator of abdominal sepsis, but false negatives do occur, especially with antimicrobial therapy. In one study of 36 peritonitis cases, peritoneal fluid glucose concentration and pH were significantly lower in horses with septic versus nonseptic peritonitis [20]. Serum to peritoneal fluid glucose concentration differences >50 mg/dL were most diagnostically useful in confirming sepsis.

18.1.2.2.2 Fluid D-dimer Concentration Mesothelial cells play a significant role in the initiation and resolution of inflammation by secretion of immunomodulatory mediators, which impact on coagulant and fibrinolytic factors such as D-dimer [21, 22]. D-dimer concentrations in normal peritoneal fluid are reported to be <88 ng/mL [22, 23], whereas in horses with colic, median peritoneal fluid D-dimer concentrations ranged from 2023 to 24,301 ng/mL depending upon diagnosis. Amongst colics, median fluid D-dimer concentrations were highest with enteritis, ischemic lesions, and septic peritonitis (8028, 16,181, and 24,301 ng/mL, respectively) compared with large colon obstructions (2023 ng/mL) [22]. Blood contamination up to 20% does not alter peritoneal fluid D-dimer concentrations in colic cases [23]. These studies show that peritoneal fluid D-dimer concentration appears to be a useful indicator of fibrinolytic activity and higher concentrations are correlated with greater disease severity.

18.1.3 Cells and Cell Counts

Cytological evaluation of body cavity fluid can yield important information that may even indicate the effusion's etiology (e.g., large cell lymphoma, carcinoma, uroabdomen, septic inflammation). Cytology should be interpreted in the context of clinical signs, cell counts, and biochemical evaluation.

18.1.3.1 Erythrocytes

Erythrocytes are not normally present in body cavity fluid in health, but blood contamination during thoracocentesis may produce RBC counts up to 540,000/μL, although the vast majority of horses have <370,000/μL [8]. Reported counts for paracentesis are lower, ranging from <5000 to <43,200/μL in healthy horses [4, 5, 24]. Visual assessment of discoloration attributable to RBCs was not detected for samples with <40,000 RBCs/μL [25], so typical amounts of blood contamination associated with paracentesis should not change the fluid color. Erythrocyte counts will increase above reference values because of minor blood vessel damage associated with necrosis and/or inflammation; true hemorrhagic effusions are discussed in the section on effusion classifications.

18.1.3.2 Nucleated Cells

Total NCCs for pleural and abdominal fluid are performed with automated blood count analyzers or manually with a hemocytometer. Reference values for pleural and peritoneal fluids are similar. The total NCC for pleural fluid for most horses is <8000/μL [8]. Generally, total NCC reference values in normal peritoneal fluid are reported as <10,000/μL [1, 4], and often <5000/μL [4, 14, 20]. Many equine practitioners and clinical pathologists consider values <5000/μL to be normal, values between 5000–10,000/μL to be ambiguous, and values >10,000/μL as abnormal. Reference values for peritoneal fluid in foals are <1500/μL [15].

The cells normally present within the pleural and peritoneal cavity include leukocytes and mesothelial lining cells. Nucleated cells in cytological differentials are categorized as neutrophils, lymphocytes, and monocyte/macrophages. Some practitioners will use a large mononuclear cell category that may include monocyte/macrophages and mesothelial cells but many cytopathologists and practitioners do not include mesothelial cells in the differential count.

In horses, mature neutrophils are the predominant cell type in the differential evaluation (typically 50–80% of nucleated cells). Because neutrophils age and die in body cavity fluid, pyknotic and hypersegmented neutrophils are normally noted in a proportion of the population. Increased numbers of neutrophils enter into the body cavity in response to chemotactic inflammatory mediators. During inflammation, the ability of neutrophils to respond to stimuli and migrate into tissue increases with maturation. Consequently, mature neutrophils arrive first and immature forms (i.e., bands, metamyelocytes) are only present in tissue when mature neutrophils have been severely depleted. Thus, the presence of band or earlier forms of neutrophils in fluid indicates severe inflammation; a caveat would be if the immature forms originate from blood and there is significant blood contamination of the sample. If blood contamination is not apparent, the presence of immature neutrophils in peritoneal fluid has been shown to have a poorer prognosis (i.e., need for surgical intervention and increased mortality rates) [26].

Degenerate change in neutrophils is characterized by swollen, pale-staining chromatin and loss of membrane integrity (Figure 18.5). While degenerate change is not pathognomonic for infection, the presence of degenerate neutrophils warrants a more thorough search for organisms. These changes occur *after* the cell has left the blood and indicate release of neutrophil enzymes and/or exposure to bacterial cytotoxins. In contrast, "toxic" neutrophils are characterized by the presence of cytoplasmic basophilia (often with Dohle bodies), foamy cytoplasm, less condensed chromatin, nuclear hyposegmentation, and larger cell size (see Chapter 2). These changes reflect maturational defects in the bone marrow that are associated with rapid neutropoiesis due to a strong systemic inflammatory stimulus. In contrast to degenerate change, toxic change exists in neutrophils *before* they enter the pleural or peritoneal cavity. Toxic change is often associated with severe bacterial infections or significant tissue necrosis.

Large mononuclear cells include both monocytes/macrophages and mesothelial cells. When monocytes exit the vasculature, they differentiate into macrophages; both forms will be present in body cavities (Figure 18.6). Macrophages will occasionally contain senescent neutrophils. As with neutrophils, increases in monocyte/macrophage concentrations in fluid are attributable to inflammation and usually accompany neutrophil increases; neutrophil proportions typically exceed those of monocyte/macrophages in acute inflammation, whereas mononuclear cells may predominate with chronic effusions and certain disease processes (e.g., fungal infection).

The lymphocytes in normal fluid are small to medium-sized (7–10 μm diameter) and constitute the smallest proportion of the three main cell types in normal cavity fluid. Increases in lymphocytes may be associated with chronic

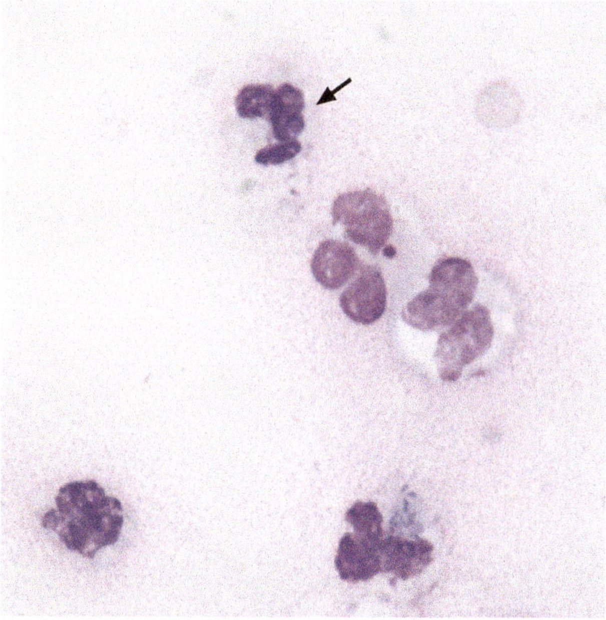

Figure 18.5 Degenerate changes in neutrophils from a suppurative pleural effusion. Two nondegenerate (*arrow*) and three degenerate neutrophils are present. Degenerate changes are characterized by loss of membrane integrity with nuclear swelling. One of the three degenerate neutrophils contains bacterial rods within the cytoplasm (*bottom right*).

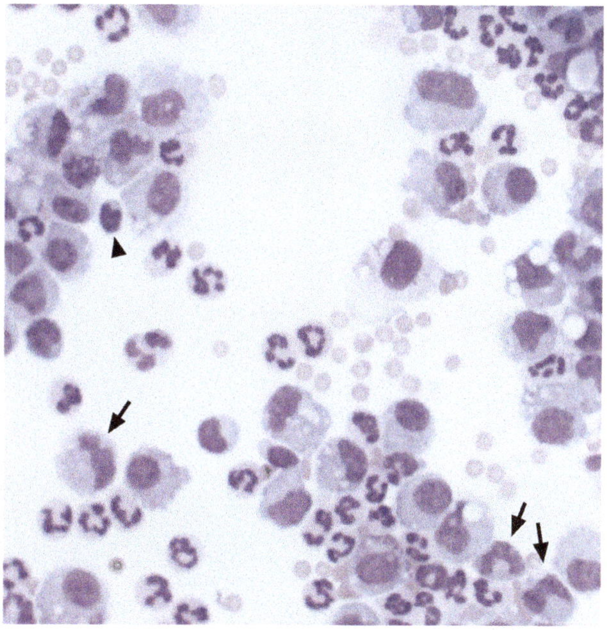

Figure 18.6 Concentrated preparation of normal peritoneal fluid. Monocytes (*arrows*), macrophages, neutrophils, and a single small lymphocyte (*arrowhead*) are present.

inflammatory conditions, parasitism, or chylothorax/abdomen. In chronic inflammation, the lymphocyte population is often a mixture of small lymphocytes, medium lymphocytes (prolymphocytes), reactive lymphocytes, and plasma cells. Reactive lymphocytes are usually slightly larger than small lymphocytes (9–11 μm diameter) and are characterized as having deeply basophilic cytoplasm and a mature chromatin. Lymphoblasts are large lymphocytes (12–16 μm diameter) whose nuclei have immature chromatin and usually contain a nucleolus or nucleoli. The presence of lymphoblasts in significant numbers is abnormal and is usually associated with large cell lymphoma. However, in the context of reactive lymphocytes and plasma cells, rare lymphoblasts may be part of the inflammatory response.

Eosinophils, basophils, and mast cells do not contribute to the cellular differential in normal body cavity fluid. The largest increases in eosinophil numbers can be associated with parasitic infections (including larval migration). Before routine deworming programs, it was not uncommon to find *Setaria equina* microfilariae in pleural or peritoneal fluid (Figure 18.7). The adults are harmless inhabitants of the pleural and peritoneal cavities and their presence is not associated with eosinophilia. Smaller increases in eosinophil numbers may be seen with inflammation due to any etiology. Eosinophilia in peritoneal fluid (Figure 18.8) may also be seen with focal eosinophilic enteritis and, rarely, lymphoma [27, 28]. Basophils and mast cells can increase concurrently with eosinophils, though both are rare findings, even in inflammation.

Mesothelial cells may be present individualized or in small clusters or sheets (Figure 18.9). They are readily identified when they are present in cohesive aggregates

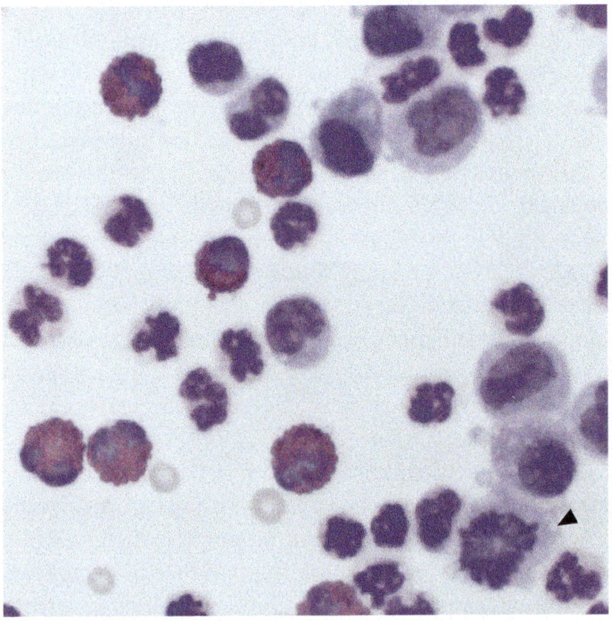

Figure 18.8 Eosinophilic peritoneal effusion of unknown etiology. The horse had a concurrent eosinophilia in the peripheral blood and eosinophilic hyperplasia in the bone marrow.

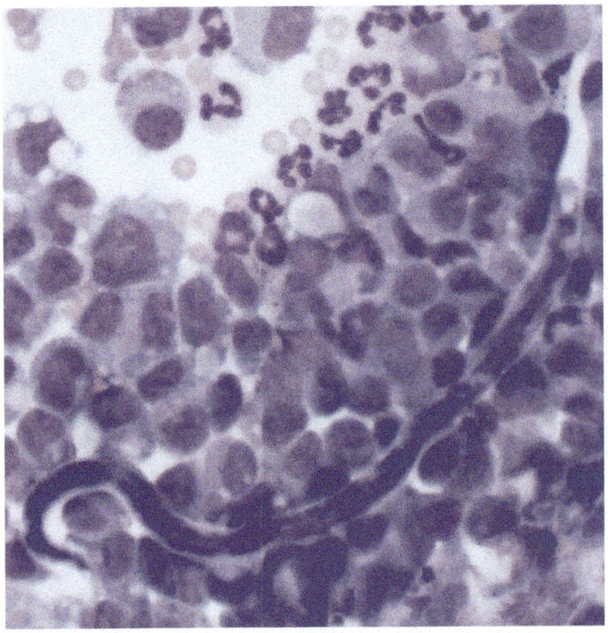

Figure 18.7 Concentrated preparation of peritoneal fluid containing microfilaria of *Setaria* species. The fluid cell count and protein concentration were within reference limits.

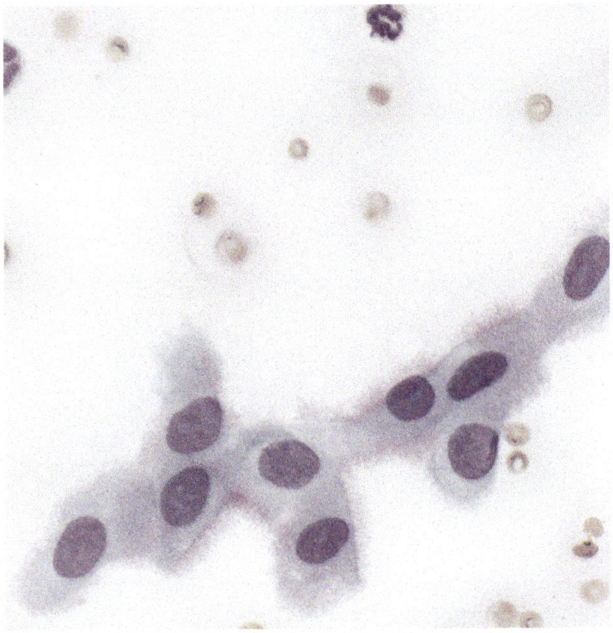

Figure 18.9 Mesothelial cells in pleural fluid. Mesothelial cells are rare in most body cavity samples from horses. Note the eosinophilic brush border, often referred to as a "glycocalyx."

and are rare in both normal fluid and effusions. Although sometimes included in the large mononuclear cell group, they comprise only a minor fraction of the large mononuclear cell differential. Mesothelial cells have round to oval nuclei with smooth chromatin, 1–2 small, variably distinct nucleoli, and a moderate rim of basophilic cytoplasm. Mesothelial cells may have a pink to red brush border that is variably prominent (see Figure 18.9).

Neoplastic cells can occasionally be found in body cavity fluid. Lymphoma (Figure 18.10) and carcinoma (Figure 18.11) are the most common neoplasms identified in cavity effusions. Since mesothelial cells are rarely noted in body cavity fluid, the presence of significant numbers of cohesive cells in body cavity effusions indicates either carcinoma or mesothelioma. It is difficult to distinguish between mesothelial and epithelial cells using morphology alone, but carcinoma occurs with more frequency than mesothelioma. Immunohistochemical staining of carcinoma is positive for cytokeratin markers and negative for vimentin, whereas staining of mesothelioma is positive for both cytokeratin and vimentin. Criteria of malignancy are often present with mesothelioma or carcinoma and include variability in nuclear size and shape (anisokaryosis), variability in cell size (anisocytosis), prominent and/or bizarre nucleoli, and multinucleation. The absence of criteria of malignancy does not preclude the possibility of carcinoma. The mere presence of epithelial cells in an effusion is diagnostic of carcinoma because epithelial cells are not normally present in body cavity fluid. The presence of mesothelial cells in body cavity fluid can be normal, however, so a very large number (especially with atypical morphology) must be present to permit an interpretation of mesothelioma.

An interpretation of lymphoma in body cavity effusion is based on the presence of significant numbers of large, immature lymphocytes. Criteria of malignancy are not taken into consideration, only the type of lymphocyte (lymphoblast, small lymphocyte or prolymphocyte). A predominance of lymphoblasts and/or prolymphocytes in body cavity effusion is abnormal and would be consistent with an interpretation of lymphoma. A predominance of small lymphocytes in an effusion could indicate an inflammatory response, chylothorax/chyloabdomen, or a small lymphocytic lymphoma. Identification and histological evaluation of an enlarged lymph node or mass would be necessary to establish a diagnosis of small cell lymphoma.

18.2 Synovial Fluid

Synovial fluid serves both to lubricate and nourish the articular cartilage. The fluid is an ultrafiltrate of plasma that is modified by hyaluronate (HA) and glycoproteins secreted by the synovial lining cells. Synovial fluid is filtered through the synovial membrane, a thin lining of tissue macrophage A-cells, fibroblast-like B-cells, and fenestrated capillaries. The cells of the synovium are discontinuous, separated by gaps several microns in width between cells. The extracellular matrix in these gaps contains collagen and other molecules such as HA and

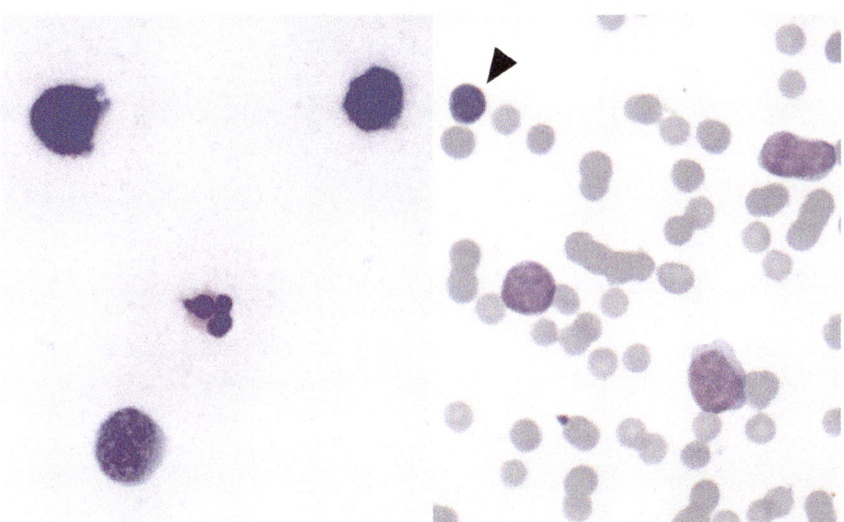

Figure 18.10 Pleural effusion (*left panel*) from a 14-year-old Thoroughbred horse. Lymphocytes are identified by the scant rim of basophilic cytoplasm. Although the chromatin is difficult to evaluate on this preparation because the cells are not spread out well, the lymphocytes are larger than a neutrophil, indicating that they are immature lymphocytes. The predominance of immature lymphocytes is consistent with an interpretation of lymphoma. The peripheral blood also contained large, immature lymphocytes (*right panel*). The arrowhead points to a small, mature lymphocyte.

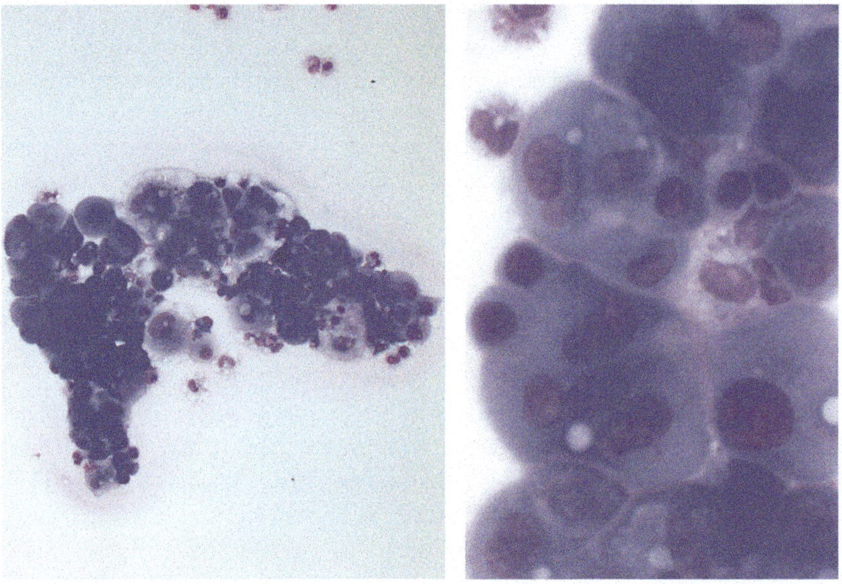

Figure 18.11 Peritoneal effusion from a 20-year-old Standardbred horse. The cytology showed many large aggregates of cohesive round cells (*left panel*). High-magnification evaluation of the cells shows moderate to marked anisokaryosis and marked anisocytosis. Note the prominent basophilic nucleoli in many nuclei. Differential interpretations for the cytology would include carcinoma or mesothelioma. Immunohistochemical staining of the neoplastic cells was positive for cytokeratin and negative for vimentin, consistent with a diagnosis of carcinoma.

glycoproteins that permit molecules such as glucose and electrolytes to pass, but restrict most proteins.

18.2.1 Fluid Analysis

Inflammatory, traumatic, and degenerative arthropathies are reflected in the composition and properties of joint fluid. As with body cavity effusions, a complete fluid evaluation should include assessment of gross characteristics, protein concentration, cell counts, and cytology. When there is a limited quantity of fluid, cytological examination is the single most useful test. With small sample volumes, the color and turbidity can be noted and the viscosity assessed as the sample is expelled onto a glass slide for preparation of a direct smear for cytological examination. In the absence of cell counts, an estimation of cellularity may suffice. A mean of 0–2 WBCs per 10 high-power fields (40× objective) corresponds with an actual WBC count <1300/μL [29].

Synovial fluid should be evaluated and interpreted in the context of physical examination and radiographic and/or MRI findings. The most common application of synovial fluid analysis in horses is to distinguish between septic and degenerative arthropathies. The main categories of equine arthropathies and their associated fluid characteristics are listed in Table 18.2. These values are generally accepted for articular joints as well as for the digital flexor tendon sheath synovial fluid [30].

18.2.1.1 Physical Characteristics

18.2.1.1.1 Color and Clarity In health, synovial fluid varies from colorless to straw colored and is clear. Changes in color and clarity reflect increases in cell count and decreases in HA concentration (see Table 18.2). Increased turbidity is usually reported in terms of cloudy/hazy or opaque, and suggests increased cellularity. A red color to the fluid reflects the presence of RBC, from either hemarthrosis or blood contamination. Blood contamination becomes apparent during arthrocentesis when the initial sample is clear and then becomes bloody or is bloody then clears. Blood contamination will adversely affect fluid analysis and interpretation and should be avoided.

18.2.1.1.2 Viscosity Viscosity is assessed by the length of the intact string of fluid when suspended between fingertips or pulled with an applicator stick. A fluid with normal viscosity should produce fluid strings 2–3 cm in length before breaking. Synovial fluid may become gelatinous upon standing, a property known as thixotropism. When this occurs, the sample can often be put back into suspension by simple agitation. If there is any blood contamination, the sample should be immediately placed into EDTA to avoid actual clotting. Note that EDTA will interfere with the mucin clot test and heparin should be used if a mucin clot test is desired.

Table 18.2 Synovial fluid characteristics[a].

	Normal	Degenerative	Inflammatory	Hemarthrosis
Color, clarity	Colorless to yellow, clear	Colorless, clear	Whitish, turbid to opaque	Red or xanthochromic, cloudy
Viscosity	High	Normal to decreased	Normal to decreased	Decreased
Mucin clot	Good	Normal to poor	Normal to poor	Fair to poor
Cellularity (/μL)	<500	<5000	>5000	High RBC count
Neutrophils	<10%	<10%	>10%	Proportional to blood
Mononuclear cells	>90%	>90%	<90%	Proportional to blood

[a] Includes the digital flexor tendon sheath synovial fluid. RBC, red blood cell.

18.2.1.1.3 Mucin Clot Test Samples for mucin clot evaluation should be submitted in a serum tube or one with heparin anticoagulant because EDTA interferes with the test. The mucin clot test provides a semiquantitative assessment of the degree of HA polymerization. The test is performed by mixing one part synovial fluid (centrifuged supernatant) with four parts 2.5% glacial acetic acid. Results are categorized as good, fair, poor, and very poor. A good mucin clot is characterized by the presence of a single clot that forms in a clear solution. A fair clot is present in a turbid solution, a poor clot is friable in cloudy solution, and a very poor clot consists of small flecks in a cloudy solution [31]. The mucin clot test is no longer performed as part of the routine synovial fluid analysis in many laboratories.

18.2.1.2 Protein Concentration

Protein can be rapidly measured by hand-held refractometers, but the most accurate measurement of synovial fluid protein concentration is performed using chemical methods. Refractometer readings provide values that are useful for clinical classification and interpretation of joint fluids and compare reasonably to biuret or Coomassie blue methods (see Chapter 8). Reference values for healthy synovial fluid using the biuret method range from 0.9 to 3.1 g/dL; the Coomassie blue method yields similar values [31]. Most reference values for equine synovial fluid are reported to be <2.5 g/dL.

18.2.1.3 Cells and Cell Counts

The cells normally present within the joint fluid comprise leukocytes and synovial lining cells. Nucleated cells in cytological differentials are categorized as neutrophils, small lymphocytes, and large mononuclear cells (Figure 18.12). The large mononuclear cell category includes both macrophages and synovial lining type B-cells. Individually, these cells cannot be distinguished morphologically unless the macrophages are activated (cytoplasmic vacuolization and/or phagocytic activity). Synovial type B-cells can be readily distinguished when they are present in sheets.

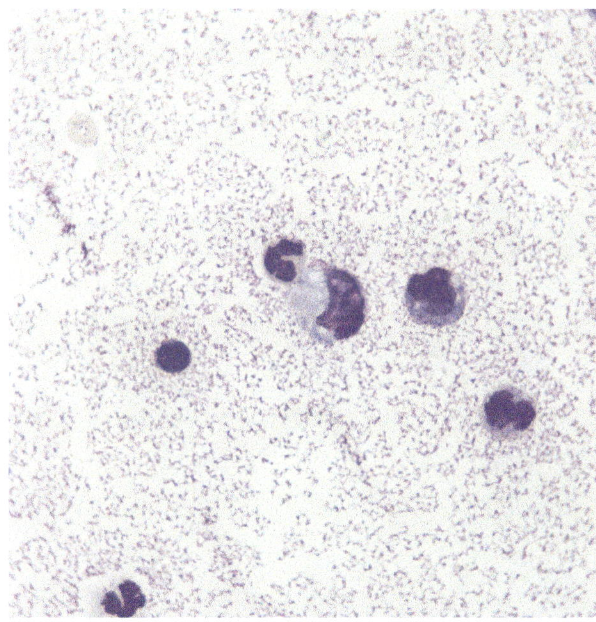

Figure 18.12 High-magnification view of synovial fluid from a horse with a resolving acute injury. Three large mononuclear cells, two neutrophils, and a small lymphocyte are present within a stippled eosinophilic glycosaminoglycan background.

Reference values for most joints in horses are typically <500 cells/μL (see Table 18.2). Cell counts may be performed manually or using an automated hematology analyzer. Sample viscosity often makes it difficult to perform cell counts, especially with automated analyzers. Fewer problems with sample aspiration and flow and more accurate counts were obtained using automated analyzers when samples were pretreated with hyaluronidase. Hyaluronidase is used at a final concentration of 0.01 mg/mL and incubated until the samples are sufficiently fluid (5–30 minutes) [32]. Automated point-of-care hematology analyzers for determining synovial fluid counts should be used only after the procedure has been properly validated by comparing with manual methods currently in use. Evaluation of viscosity and mucin clot should always be performed *before* hyaluronidase is added.

18.2.1.4 Cytology

Microscopic evaluation of synovial fluid should include assessment of cellularity (normal or increased) and the glycosaminoglycan background (normal or dilute and/or clumped). These evaluations are performed at both low power (10× objective) (Figure 18.13) and high power (40× or 100× objective). A differential count is performed at high power. The differential count in healthy synovial fluid is composed of >90% mononuclear cells, the majority of which are macrophages and type B synoviocytes, with the remainder represented by neutrophils. Increases in the proportion of neutrophils can be seen in both septic and nonseptic synovitis and with blood contamination or hemorrhage. In cases of blood contamination or hemarthrosis, interpretation of the neutrophil proportion can be difficult. The proportion of neutrophils can be compared to the amount of blood present to subjectively assess whether a component of suppurative inflammation exists; however, this method requires an experienced observer and knowledge of the peripheral neutrophil concentration, and is highly subjective. It is usually possible to distinguish between blood contamination and hemorrhage (see Section 18.2.5).

Cellular morphology is evaluated concurrently with the differential count. Neutrophil morphology is evaluated for degenerative changes or evidence of phagocytic activity (Figure 18.14). The presence of degenerative neutrophils is supportive of a septic process but is not pathognomonic, and the absence of detectable infectious agents does not preclude a septic process. In healthy joint fluid, the majority of macrophages are nonphagocytic with few vacuoles. Increased numbers of phagocytic macrophages or the presence of binucleated or multinucleated forms indicates histiocytic inflammation, even in the absence of increased cell counts (Figure 18.15). Some macrophages/synoviocytes may contain few magenta granules.

18.2.2 Degenerative Arthropathies

Degenerative processes that affect the joint have minimal to no inflammation as reflected in the synovial fluid, but inflammation of the synovium is recognized. The most common types of "degenerative" arthropathies in the horse include osteoarthritis and osteochondritis dissecans (OCD), both inflammatory processes. Osteoarthritis (OA) is one of the most common equine arthropathies. Currently, three type of OA are recognized: type 1 (primary) OA, type 2 (secondary) OA, and type 3 (nonprogressive) OA. Synovial fluid cell counts associated with OA are usually <5000/μL with TP concentrations

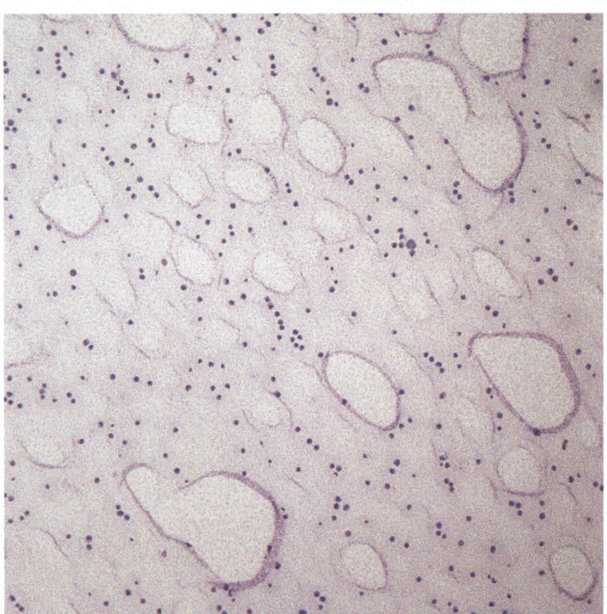

Figure 18.13 Low-magnification view of synovial fluid from a horse with an acute carpal chip injury. Cellularity is markedly increased. Note the presence of crescents in the glycosaminoglycan background, which are characteristic of synovial fluid cytology.

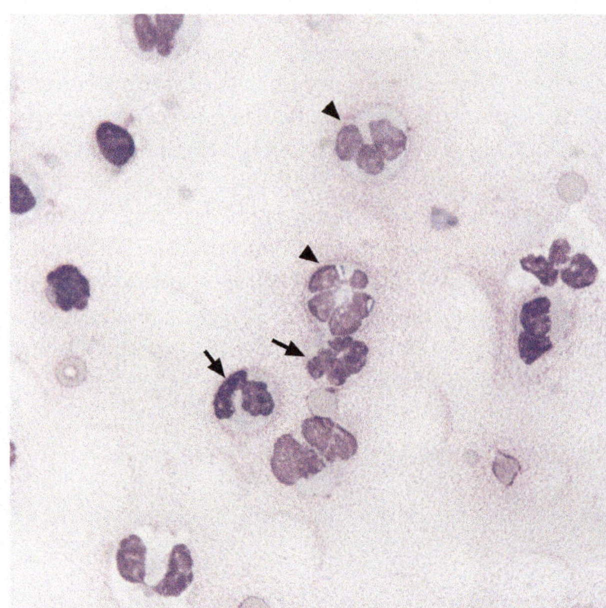

Figure 18.14 Degenerate neutrophils (*arrowheads*) and nondegenerate neutrophils (*arrows*) in a septic joint. Note the presence of basophilic bacterial rods within one of the degenerate neutrophils. The glycosaminoglycan background is dilute.

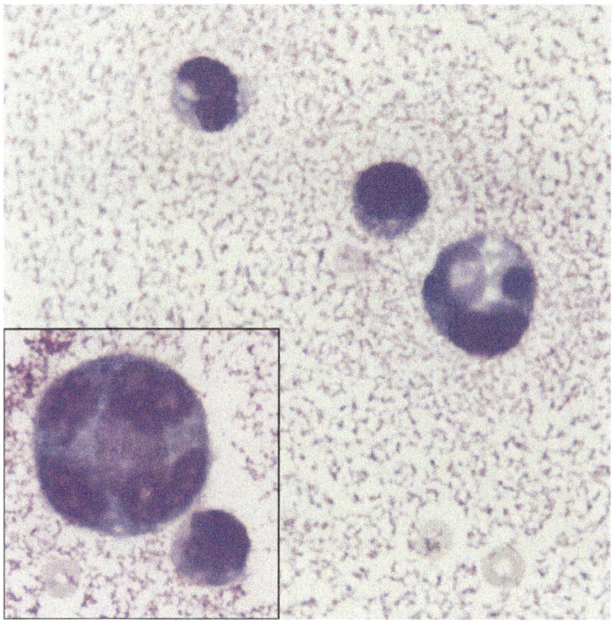

Figure 18.15 High-magnification view of a phagocytic macrophage and a multinucleated cell (*inset*) in a joint with a degenerative arthropathy subsequent to a chip fracture.

within normal limits or slightly increased and a mononuclear cell predominance. OCD is a defect in the subchondral bone with secondary effects on the articular cartilage that may result in osteoarthritis. Typical synovial fluid nucleated cells counts in OCD are <1000/μL and the TP concentration is often within reference limits or slightly increased. Similar to OA, the predominant cell type is mononuclear. Conventional synovial fluid analysis in joints affected with OA or OCD may reveal findings that are all within normal limits. However, in the context of clinical signs, this would support an interpretation of a degenerative, noninfectious arthropathy. Distinction between processes such as OA or OCD cannot be made using synovial fluid analysis alone; the fluid findings should be interpreted in the context of imaging findings, signalment, and clinical signs.

Synovial fluid and serum biomarkers show promise in the diagnosis of active cartilage damage, but most of these tests are not readily available in the clinical setting. Examples of fluid biomarkers include chondroitin and keratan sulfate epitopes, total glycosaminoglycans, matrix metalloproteinases, osteocalcin, and bone-specific alkaline phosphatase (BAP). BAP is an isoform of alkaline phosphatase that can be measured in most diagnostic laboratories. BAP concentrations in the synovial fluid from joints affected with OA or osteochondrosis are increased compared with normal joints [33, 34].

18.2.3 Inflammatory Arthropathies

18.2.3.1 Septic Synovitis

Diagnosis of a septic joint can be difficult in the absence of identifiable bacteria on cytological examination. Only about a quarter of cases demonstrate bacteria on gram stain. Moreover, the gold standard for the diagnosis of septic synovitis, a positive bacterial culture, is negative in almost half of clinical cases if enrichment medium is not used [35]. Use of enrichment media greatly improves culture success but even with enrichment media, 27% can still be negative [36]. Prior treatment with antibiotics and/or bacterial sequestration in the synovium may contribute to these results [37]. One study showed blood culture medium enrichment performed significantly better than conventional enrichment media for equine synovial fluid cultures [38]. Blood culture medium enrichment combined with 16S rRNA gene PCR had the highest sensitivity for detection of synovial infection (91.8%) [39].

Identification of intracellular bacterial organisms on cytological examination is a definitive indicator of septic synovitis, but their absence does not preclude infection. Identification of the organisms as cocci or bacilli with Romanovksy stains can aid in the preliminary antimicrobial treatment. Gram stains, when performed correctly, provide further information for antimicrobial selection. However, experience has shown that when the stain is old or the procedure done incorrectly, the stain may be misleading. Often all organisms will stain as gram negative in these instances.

In addition to cytology, fluid cell counts and differentials can help to distinguish septic from nonseptic inflammatory processes. Cell counts in septic joints typically exceed 10,000/μL and are often much higher [36, 40, 41]. However, septic joints with counts <10,000/μL can be seen in early sepsis, with corticosteroid administration, and with draining lesions [35]. Moreover, traumatic or chemical synovitis can have cell counts up to 90,000 and 30,000/μL, respectively, that are predominantly suppurative [42]. Despite the overlap in cell counts and protein concentrations for septic and nonseptic synovitis, cell counts >50,000/μL are highly suspicious for sepsis and >100,000/μL is considered diagnostic. Clinical signs, history, and radiographic and cytology findings should be interpreted in context. In cases where the cytology and fluid analysis fall within the "gray zone," the joint should be treated as if it were septic until proven otherwise.

Because synovial fluid is an ultrafiltrate of plasma, fluid glucose and pH are similar to plasma and may be useful in detecting bacterial infection. Glucose concentrations have been shown to be useful as a relatively rapid test for distinguishing septic from nonseptic effusions [43]. Differences between serum and fluid glucose concentrations of >2 mmol/L were reported in experimentally induced infectious arthritis. However, measurement of glucose concentrations using hand-held glucometers should be undertaken using only veterinary glucometers validated for use in horses (see Chapter 9). Synovial fluid glucose concentrations and pH both decrease and lactate increases relative to serum when there is bacterial infection. While these parameters are supportive of a septic process, they are not suitable to serve as primary diagnostic tests. These tests may help in confirming the diagnosis in cases that are clinically and cytologically suspicious for bacterial synovitis, but negative upon culture.

18.2.3.2 Nonseptic Suppurative Synovitis

18.2.3.2.1 Traumatic and Chemical Synovitis Synovitis resulting from traumatic or chemical causes may present with significantly high cell counts (>10,000/μL) with neutrophils as the predominant cell type. Traumatic synovitis usually causes mild mononuclear or suppurative inflammation with cell counts <5000/μL, but infrequently it may cause suppurative inflammation with counts exceeding 10,000/μL [31, 37]. Chemical synovitis, also known as a postinjection flare, can occur in response to injection of corticosteroids, local anesthetics, saline, antibiotics, and polysulfated glycosaminoglycans [30, 44, 45]. Intraarticular injection of 1 mL 0.9% saline alone may increase the NCC to values up to 14,000/μL [46]. Injection of polysulfated glycosaminoglycans, antibiotics, or anesthetics can produce NCCs >30,000/μL with a neutrophil predominance [47–50]. Prior sampling or treatment should be considered in the interpretation of synovial fluid findings. Because there can be overlap with findings for nonseptic and septic arthropathies, repeated lameness examination and follow-up sampling are necessary. Chemical synovitis usually occurs within hours after injection and resolves within 3–7 days.

18.2.3.2.2 Immune-Mediated Synovitis Nonseptic inflammation may be immune-mediated, often secondary to infection, gastrointestinal disease, or neoplasia. A noninfectious, nonerosive syndrome has been described in foals with *Rhodococcus equi* infection and usually resolves as the pneumonia resolves with antimicrobial therapy. Approximately a third of foals with *R. equi* infection develop synovitis [51, 52]. These foals have single or multiple joint distension but negative bacterial culture, no or mild lameness or stiffness, and a NCC of <8000/μL, with neutrophilic or mixed inflammation [53–55]. Synovial membrane biopsies of affected joints showed positive immunofluorescence for immune complexes, supporting an immune-mediated etiology. Similar findings have been described in a foal with bacterial endocarditis caused by *Escherichia coli* [54].

Lupus erythematosus (LE) is another immune-mediated nonerosive inflammatory arthropathy that may be present in horses [56, 57]. A LE-like syndrome was diagnosed in two horses based on the presence of a positive LE cell preparation and positive antinuclear antibody titers. Given the uncertainty of the significance of LE cells in horses, a definitive diagnosis of LE is questionable. Reported synovial fluid cell counts ranged from 25,200 to 46,000/μL with a predominance of neutrophils. Histologically, there was marked villous proliferation with infiltration of macrophages, lymphocytes, and plasma cells.

An idiopathic polysynovitis in four horses characterized by a suppurative, nonseptic synovitis in at least two different joints has been described [58, 59]. Immunoglobulins were detected in a synovial membrane biopsy from the only horse that was evaluated, but the horses were negative for antinuclear antibodies and LE cells. The horses presented with stiffness or lameness, fever, polysynovitis with a NCC <7000/μL with increased neutrophils (12–81%), and TP <3.6 g/dL. The cases showed response to immunosuppressive therapy and a microbial cause could not be identified on culture.

18.2.4 Eosinophilic Synovitis

Eosinophils are rare to absent (<1%) in equine synovial fluid in health. Eosinophilic synovitis is rare; only two clinical cases have been reported to date. In humans, eosinophilic synovitis has been reported post arthrography (dye or air) and can be associated with infectious diseases (e.g., Lyme disease, tuberculosis, and parasitism), rheumatoid arthritis, hypereosinophilic syndrome, neoplasia, or may be idiopathic. Eosinophilic synovitis has been experimentally induced in horses via intraarticular injection of streptococcal antigen in horses hyperimmunized with *Streptococcus equi* M protein vaccine [60]. The first reported equine clinical case was associated with prior intraarticular injections of methylprednisolone acetate into the affected joints [61]. No etiology was determined for the second clinical case [62]. NCCs in the reported cases range from 8300 to 12,800/μL with 11–76% eosinophils.

18.2.5 Hemarthrosis

A hemorrhagic effusion is defined by the fluid RBC count (Table 18.2); acute hemorrhagic effusions usually have RBC counts >1,000,000/μL. In one study, discoloration attributable to RBCs was not detected visually with <40,000 RBCs/μL [25]. Accordingly, a reddish synovial fluid should have >40,000 RBCs/μL. Erythrocytes and

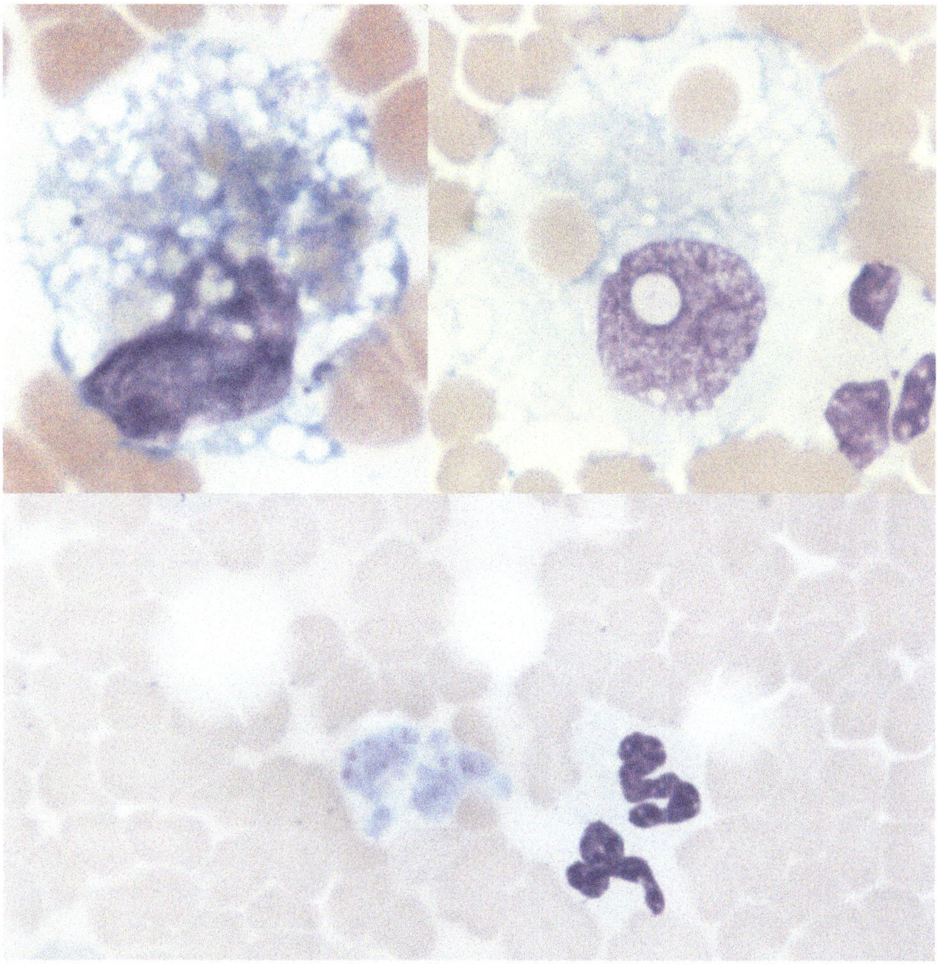

Figure 18.16 Macrophages containing golden-green hemosiderin (*upper left*) and erythrocytes (*upper right*) in a hemorrhagic effusion. The presence of platelet clumps (*lower center*) in another sample indicates peripheral blood contamination.

plasma from hemorrhage will be resorbed by lymphatics so fluid TP and RBC counts vary with time.

Hemarthrosis in horses is most often associated with joint trauma (e.g., fractures, intraarticular ligament tears). Cases of idiopathic hemarthrosis confined to the antebrachiocarpal and tarsocrural joints have been reported but this is an infrequent phenomenon. Idiopathic hemarthrosis of the antebrachiocarpal joint was associated with acute forelimb lameness, whereas hemarthrosis of the tarsocrural joint produced minimal lameness. RBC counts ranged from 4,100,000 to 11,100,000/μL with NCCs from 7400 to 16,000/μL and protein concentrations 4.0–5.6 g/dL [63].

Because platelets (and coagulation factors) are consumed during hemorrhage, hemorrhagic fluid contains no platelets and does not clot, whereas fluid that contains blood from peripheral vessels will contain platelets and will clot. In fluids with high RBC counts, the presence of platelets on cytological evaluation indicates a component of blood contamination since platelets are not present in hemorrhagic effusions (Figure 18.16). However, the absence of platelets does not preclude peripheral blood contamination if the sample was collected into a nonanticoagulant tube (e.g., red top tube) and subsequently clotted *in vitro*. Cytological findings that support hemarthrosis include the presence of erythrocytes and/or hemosiderin within macrophages (see Figure 18.16). Note that if there is a delay in sample processing (>3–4 hours), RBC phagocytosis can occur *in vitro* in the transport tube. Conversely, erythrophagocytosis can be absent in samples from true hemorrhage if there has been insufficient time for RBC phagocytosis within the joint space (i.e., peracute hemorrhage). In general, it takes several hours for erythrophagocytosis to occur; subsequent RBC breakdown into hemosiderin usually takes 2–3 days [3]. Thus, cytological interpretations of bloody fluid should be undertaken with knowledge of the type of collection tube used, as well as the amount of time before the sample was processed.

References

1 Stockham, S.L. and Scott, M.A. (2008). Cavitary effusions. In: *Fundamentals of Veterinary Clinical Pathology*, 2e (eds. S.L. Stockham and M.A. Scott), 831–868. Ames: Wiley-Blackwell.

2 Clark, C.H. and Woodley, C.H. (1959). The absorption of red blood cells after parenteral injection at various sites. *Am. J. Vet. Res.* 20: 1062–1066.

3 Epstein, C.E., Elidemir, O., Colasurdo, G.N., and Fan, L.L. (2001). Time course of hemosiderin production by alveolar macrophages in a murine model. *Chest* 120: 2013–2020.

4 DeHeer, H.L., Parry, B.W., and Grindem, C.B. (2002). Peritoneal fluid. In: *Diagnostic Cytology and Hematology of the Horse*, 2e (eds. R.L. Cowell and R.D. Tyler), 127–162. St Louis: Elsevier.

5 Malark, J.A., Peyton, L.C., and Galvin, M.J. (1992). Effects of blood contamination on equine peritoneal fluid analysis. *J. Am. Vet. Med. Assoc.* 201: 1545–1548.

6 Tulleners, E.P. (1983). Complications of abdominocentesis in the horse. *J. Am. Vet. Med. Assoc.* 182: 232–234.

7 Swanwick, R.A. and Wilkinson, J.S. (1976). A clinincal evaluation of abdominal paracentesis in the horse. *Aust. Vet. J.* 52: 109–117.

8 Wagner, A.E. and Bennett, D.G. (1982). Analysis of equine thoracic fluid. *Vet. Clin. Pathol.* 11: 13–17.

9 Freden, G.O., Provost, P.J., and Rand, W.M. (1998). Reliability of using results of abdominal fluid analysis to determine treatment and predict lesion type and outcome for horses with colic: 218 cases (1991–1994). *J. Am. Vet. Med. Assoc.* 213: 1012–1015.

10 Matthews, S., Dart, A.J., Reid, S.W.J. et al. (2002). Predictive values, sensitivity and specificity of abdominal fluid variables in determining the need for surgery in horses with an acute abdominal crisis. *Aust. Vet. J.* 80: 132–136.

11 Weimann, C.D., Thoefner, M.B., and Jensen, A.L. (2002). Spectrophotometric assessment of peritoneal fluid hemoglobin in colic horses: an aid to selecting medical vs. surgical treatment. *Equine Vet. J.* 34: 523–527.

12 George, J.W. and O'Neill, S.L. (2001). Comparison of refractometer and biuret methods for total protein measurement in body cavity fluids. *Vet. Clin. Pathol.* 30: 16–18.

13 George, J.W. (2001). The usefulness and limitations of hand-held refractometers in veterinary laboratory medicine: an historical and technical review. *Vet. Clin. Pathol.* 30: 201–210.

14 Brownlow, M.A., Hutchins, D.R., and Johnston, K.G. (1981). Reference values for equine peritoneal fluid. *Equine Vet. J.* 13: 127–130.

15 Grindem, C.B., Fairley, N.M., Uhlinger, C.A., and Crane, S.A. (1990). Peritoneal fluid values from healthy foals. *Equine Vet. J.* 22: 359–361.

16 Latson, K.M., Nieto, J.E., Beldomenico, P.M., and Snyder, J.R. (2005). Evaluation of peritoneal fluid lactate as a marker of intestinal ischemia in equine colic. *Equine Vet. J.* 37: 342–346.

17 McSherry, B.J. and Al-Baker, J. (1976). Comparison of total serum protein determined by t/s meter and biuret technique. *Vet. Clin. Pathol.* 5: 4–12.

18 Estepa, J.C., Lopez, I., Mayer-Valor, R. et al. (2006). The influence of anticoagulants on the measurement of total protein concentration in equine peritoneal fluid. *Res. Vet. Sci.* 80: 5–10.

19 Delesalle, C., Dewulf, J., Lefebvre, R.A. et al. (2007). Determination of lactate concentrations in blood plasma and peritoneal fluid in horses with colic by an Accusport analyzer. *J. Vet. Intern. Med.* 21: 293–301.

20 Van Hoogmoed, L., Rodger, L.D., Spier, S.J. et al. (1999). Evaluation of peritoneal fluid pH, glucose concentration, and lactate dehydrogenase activity for detection of septic peritonitis in horses. *J. Am. Vet. Med. Assoc.* 214: 1032–1036.

21 Collatos, C., Barton, M.H., Prasse, K.W., and Moore, J.N. (1995). Intravascular and peritoneal coagulation and fibrinolysis in horses with acute gastrointestinal tract diseases. *J. Am. Vet. Med. Assoc.* 207: 465–470.

22 Delgado, M.A., Monreal, L., Armengou, L. et al. (2009). Peritoneal D-dimer concentration for assessing peritoneal fibrinolytic activity in horses with colic. *J. Vet. Intern. Med.* 23: 882–889.

23 Delgado, M.A., Monreal, L., Armengou, L. et al. (2009). Effects of blood contamination on peritoneal D-dimer concentration in horses with colic. *J. Vet. Intern. Med.* 23: 1232–1238.

24 Stockham, S.L. and Scott, M.A. (2002). Glucose and related regulatory hormones. In: *Fundamentals of Veterinary Clinical Pathology* (eds. S.L. Stockham and M.A. Scott), 487–506. Ames: Blackwell.

25 Hunt, E., Tennant, B.C., and Whitlock, R.H. (1985). Interpretation of peritoneal fluid erythrocyte counts in horses with abdominal disease. Proceedings of the Second Equine Colic Research Symposium, University of Georgia, pp. 168–174.

26 Garma-Aviña, A. (1998). Cytology of 100 samples of abdominal fluid from 100 horses with abdominal disease. *Equine Vet. J.* 30: 435–444.

27 La Perle, K.M., Piercy, R.J., Long, J.F., and Blomme, E.A. (1998). Multisystemic, eosinophilic, epitheliotropic disease with intestinal lymphosarcoma in a horse. *Vet. Pathol.* 35: 144–146.

28 Southwood, L.L., Kawcak, C.E., Trotter, G.W. et al. (2000). Idiopathic focal eosinophilic enteritis associated with small intestinal obstruction in 6 horses. *Vet. Surg.* 29: 415–419.

29 Clayburne, G., Baker, D.G., and Schumacher, H.R. (1992). Estimated synovial fluid leukocyte numbers on wet drop preparations as a potential substitute for actual leukocyte counts. *J. Rheumatol.* 19: 60–62.

30 Dykgraaf, S., Dechant, J.E., Johns, J.L. et al. (2007). Effect of intrathecal amikacin administration and repeated centesis on digital flexor tendon sheath synovial fluid in horses. *Vet. Surg.* 36: 57–63.

31 Mahaffey, E.A. (2002). Synovial fluid. In: *Diagnostic Cytology and Hematology of the Horse*, 2e (eds. R.L. Cowell and R.D. Tyler), 163–170. St Louis: Elsevier.

32 Ekmann, A., Rigdal, M.-L., and Gröndahl, G. (2010). Automated counting of nucleated cells in equine synovial fluid without and with hyaluronidase pretreatment. *Vet. Clin. Pathol.* 39: 83–89.

33 Fuller, C.J., Barr, A.R., Sharif, M., and Dieppe, P.A. (2001). Cross-sectional comparison of synovial fluid biochemical markers in equine osteoarthritis and the correlation of these markers with articular cartilage damage. *Osteoarthr. Cartil.* 9: 49–55.

34 Trumble, T.N., Brown, M.P., Merritt, K.A., and Billinghurst, R.C. (2008). Joint dependent concentrations of bone alkaline phosphatase in serum and synovial fluids of horses with osteochondral injury: an analytical and clinical validation. *Osteoarthr. Cartil.* 16: 779–786.

35 Madison, J.B., Sommer, M., and Spencer, P.A. (1991). Relations among synovial membrane histopathologic findings, synovial fluid cytologic findings, and bacterial culture results in horses with suspected infectious arthritis: 64 cases (1979–1987). *J. Am. Vet. Med. Assoc.* 198: 1655–1661.

36 Schneider, R.K., Bramlage, L.R., Moore, R.M. et al. (1992). A retrospective study of 192 horses affected with septic arthritis/tenosynovitis. *Equine Vet. J.* 24: 436–442.

37 Steel, C.M. (2008). Equine synovial fluid analysis. *Vet. Clin. North Am. Equine Pract.* 24: 437–454.

38 Dumoulin, M., Pille, F., van den Abeele, A.-M. et al. (2010). Use of blood culture medium enrichment for synovial fluid culture in horses: a comparison of different culture methods. *Equine Vet. J.* 42: 541–546.

39 Pille, F., Martens, A., Schouls, L.M. et al. (2007). Broad range 16S rRNA gene PCR compared to bacterial culture to confirm presumed synovial infection in horses. *Vet. J.* 173: 73–78.

40 Lapointe, J.M., Laverty, S., and Lavoie, J.P. (1992). Septic arthritis in 15 standardbred racehorses after intra-articular injection. *Equine Vet. J.* 24: 430–434.

41 Steel, C.M., Hunt, A.R., Adams, P.L. et al. (1999). Factors associated with prognosis for survival and athletic use in foals with septic arthritis: 93 cases (1987–1994). *J. Am. Vet. Med. Assoc.* 215: 973–977.

42 Frees, K.E., Lillich, J.D., Gaughan, E.M., and DeBowes, R.M. (2002). Tenoscopic-assisted treatment of open digital flexor tendon sheath injuries in horses: 20 cases (1992–2001). *J. Am. Vet. Med. Assoc.* 220: 1823–1827.

43 Tulamo, R.M., Bramlage, L.R., and Gabel, A.A. (1989). Sequential clinical and synovial fluid changes associated with acute infectious arthritis in the horse. *Equine Vet. J.* 21: 325–331.

44 Wagner, A.E., McIlwraith, C.W., and Martin, G.S. (1982). Effect of intra-articular injection of orgotein and saline solution on equine synovia. *Am. J. Vet. Res.* 43: 594–597.

45 White, K.K., Hodgson, D.R., Hancock, D. et al. (1989). Changes in equine carpal joint synovial fluid in response to the injection of two local anesthetic agents. *Cornell Vet.* 79: 25–38.

46 Stover, S.M. and Pool, R.R. (1985). Effect of intra-articular gentamicin sulfate on normal equine synovial membrane. *Am. J. Vet. Res.* 46: 2485–2491.

47 Caron, J.P. (2005). Intra-articular injections for joint disease in horses. *Vet. Clin. North Am. Equine Pract.* 21: 559–573.

48 Kwan, C., Bell, R., Koenig, T. et al. (2012). Effects of intra-articular sodium pentosan polysulfate and glucosamine on the cytology, total protein concentration and viscosity of synovial fluid in horses. *Aust. Vet. J.* 90: 315–320.

49 Lloyd, K.C., Stover, S.M., Pascoe, J.R. et al. (1988). Effect of gentamicin sulfate and sodium bicarbonate on the synovium of clinically normal equine antebrachiocarpal joints. *Am. J. Vet. Res.* 49: 650–657.

50 Mills, M.L., Rush, B.R., St Jean, G. et al. (2000). Determination of synovial fluid and serum concentrations, and morphologic effects of intraarticular ceftiofur sodium in horses. *Vet. Surg.* 29: 398–406.

51 Bain, A.M. (1963). *Corynebacterium equi* infections in the equine. *Aust. Vet. J.* 39: 116–121.

52 Sweeney, C.R., Sweeney, R.W., and Divers, T.J. (1987). *Rhodococcus equi* pneumonia in 48 foals: response to antimicrobial therapy. *Vet. Microbiol.* 14: 329–336.

53 Kenney, D.G., Robbins, S.C., Prescott, J.F. et al. (1994). Development of reactive arthritis and resistance to erythromycin and rifampin in a foal during treatment for Rhodococcus equi pneumonia. *Equine Vet. J.* 26: 246–248.

54 Madison, J.B. and Scarratt, W.K. (1988). Immune-mediated polysynovitis in four foals. *J. Am. Vet. Med. Assoc.* 192: 1581–1584.

55 Paradis, M.R. (1997). Cutaneous and musculoskeletal manifestations of Rhodococcus equi infection in foals. *Equine Vet. Educ.* 9: 266–270.

56 Byars, T.D., Tyler, D.E., Whitlock, R.H. et al. (1984). Non-erosive polysynovitis in a horse. *Equine Vet. J.* 16: 141–143.

57 Vrins, A. and Feldman, B.F. (1983). Lupus erythematosus-like syndrome in a horse. *Equine Pract.* 5: 18–25.

58 Lumsden, J.M. (1990). Suspected immune-mediated polysynovitis and serositis in a horse. *Aust. Vet. J.* 67: 470–471.

59 Pusterla, N., Pratt, S.M., Magdesian, K.G., and Carlson, G.P. (2006). Idiopathic immune-mediated polysynovitis in three horses. *Vet. Rec.* 159: 13–15.

60 Madison, J.B. and Ziemer, E.L. (1993). Eosinophilic synovitis following the intra-articular injection of bacterial antigen in horses. *Res. Vet. Sci.* 54: 256–258.

61 Turner, A.S., Gustafson, S.B., Zeidner, N.S. et al. (1990). Acute eosinophilic synovitis in a horse. *Equine Vet. J.* 22: 215–217.

62 Climent, F., Carmona, J.U., Cuenca, R., and Prades, M. (2007). Eosinophilic synovitis of the tarsocrural joint in a horse. *Vet. Comp. Orthop. Traumatol.* 20: 142–145.

63 Vallance, S.A., Lumsden, J.M., Begg, A.P., and O'Sullivan, C.B. (2012). Idiopathic hemarthrosis in eight horses. *Aust. Vet. J.* 90: 214–220.

19

Cerebrospinal Fluid

Andrea Siegel

IDEXX Laboratories, Inc, New York, NY, USA

Cerebrospinal fluid (CSF) analysis combined with the history, physical and neurological exam, as well as other diagnostic tests, is an important component of the diagnostic evaluation of patients with central and peripheral neurological disease. CSF should be collected whenever an inflammatory, infectious, traumatic, neoplastic, or degenerative disorder of the brain and spinal cord is suspected. However, analysis of CSF often only supports the diagnosis of a central nervous system (CNS) disorder and is rarely definitively diagnostic. Similar to a complete blood count, CSF analysis has good sensitivity for disease detection but low specificity. However, CSF analysis is not always abnormal in a horse with central nervous disease if the lesion is extradural, collection occurred early or late in the course of disease, or the CSF collection site is far away from the lesion.

19.1 Formation, Circulation, Absorption, and Function

The CSF is a clear, colorless fluid that surrounds and permeates the entire CNS and therefore protects, supports, and nourishes it. The CSF is produced by ultrafiltration and active transport mechanisms in the choroid plexuses. Fluid formed in the lateral ventricles flows into the third ventricle and then into the fourth ventricle, where the majority exits into the subarachnoid space. The CSF also moves caudally, surrounding the spinal cord and leaving the CNS via the dural reflections of the spinal nerve roots. The CSF is absorbed by the arachnoid villi and ultimately directed into the venous system.

The CSF functions include physical support of the neural structures, excretion of potentially toxic by-products of cerebral metabolism, and intracerebral transport of biologically active substances [1].

19.2 Collection

The diagnostic quality of CSF depends on collection site and handling. CSF can be collected in horses from the atlantooccipital (AO) or lumbosacral sites depending on the neurological exam and location of the lesion. An intracranial or cervical lesion is more likely to yield a diagnostic sample if the CSF is obtained from an AO tap. In horses with clinical signs of brain herniation, the AO space should be avoided. Lumbosacral aspirates are indicated for lower spinal cord lesions. AO collection requires general anesthesia, whereas lumbosacral collection usually can be performed in standing horses. Ultrasound-guided thecal puncture techniques to collect CSF on the standing horse using the AO and C1–C2 locations have been described [2, 3]. In foals, CSF can be collected from either site with the animal in lateral recumbency [4]. Techniques of cerebromedullary cisternal and lumbosacral CSF collection are aptly covered in neuroanatomy and clinical neurology textbooks.

Specific risks of CSF collection include iatrogenic brainstem trauma or spinal cord trauma due to needle puncture, extradural hemorrhage, and herniation of the cerebrum or cerebellum through the foramen magnum in patients with increased intracranial pressure [5]. An aseptic technique is necessary due to the potential risk for introducing infectious agents into the CNS. A study that compared sequential samples of CSF in horses suggested that in order to minimize blood contamination, a minimum of three 2 mL samples should be collected before submitting the final sample for analysis, even if there is no gross evidence of blood contamination [6]. Artefacts like deteriorated cells and contaminants (including iatrogenic hemodilution) may affect the cytological interpretation.

Equine Hematology, Cytology, and Clinical Chemistry, Second Edition.
Edited by Raquel M. Walton, Rick L. Cowell, and Amy C. Valenciano.

19.3 Laboratory Analysis

The routine laboratory analysis of CSF includes gross inspection, cell counts, protein concentration, chemistry assays, and cytological examination (Table 19.1). Other tests, such as bacterial and fungal culture, serology, and polymerase chain reaction (PCR), are added depending on the results of the cytological examination, clinical presentation, and neurological exam.

Due to the low CSF protein and lipid concentrations, cells degenerate and lyse rapidly, causing distortion of cellular morphology and reduction of the total nucleated cell count. For this reason, cell counts and cytological preparations should be performed within 30 minutes of collection [7]. Cells can be preserved by mixing autologous serum with the sample, which will conserve cell morphology for 24 hours when stored at 4 °C [8]. The addition of hetastarch at a ratio of 1:1 (vol:vol) or fetal calf serum at a concentration of 20% volume can help to stabilize cells in CSF [7]. Samples containing additives to preserve cellular morphology should not be used to measure protein or for antibody titers.

Generally, 1 mL of fluid is sufficient for protein and cellular examination [9]. CSF samples should be collected in sterile plastic or silicon-coated tubes, especially when not processed immediately, because monocytes will adhere to glass and activate [1]. EDTA tubes are not recommended because the additive can falsely elevate the total protein concentration, although submission in an EDTA tube may be required if the sample is for PCR analysis [10, 11].

19.3.1 Gross Appearance

The normal CSF is clear and colorless, has a viscosity similar to water, and does not clot due to the absence of fibrinogen. Turbidity is measured subjectively from 0 or clear to +4, which is cloudy enough to preclude reading through the sample. Causes of CSF turbidity include elevated cell count (WBC or RBC or both), presence of microorganisms, markedly increased protein concentration, or aspiration of epidural fat [12]. Nucleated cell counts greater than 400–500 cells/μL are necessary to produce a slightly turbid CSF.

Table 19.1 Reference values for CSF in adult horses.

Macroscopic evaluation	Reference values
Color	Colorless
Turbidity	Clear
Erythrocytes	0 to small number
Total nucleated cell count	0–8 cells/L
Total protein	30–80 mg/dL
Microscopic evaluation	
Differential cell count	Small lymphocytes (70%) Monocytoid cells (30%) Rare erythrocytes

Source: Modified from [10].

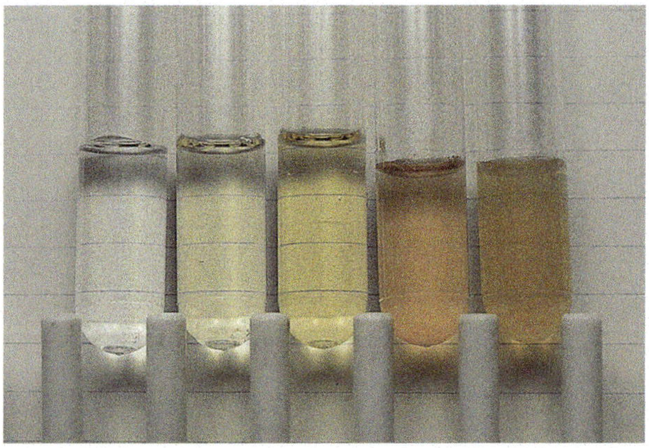

Figure 19.1 Macroscopic examination of CSF. Tubes are viewed against a lined white index card to assess colour and turbidity. (*Left to right*) Normal CSF, mildly xanthochromic CSF, moderately xanthochromic CSF, red-tinged turbid CSF caused by hemorrhage, and cloudy red-tinged fluid from a horse with bacterial meningitis.

Abnormal CSF colors on visual inspection include red-tinged, xanthochromic, and cloudy white (Figure 19.1). Pink or red discoloration suggests the presence of blood, which could result from iatrogenic blood contamination, intrathecal hemorrhage, or diapedesis secondary to blood–brain barrier (BBB) disruption. A clear supernatant after centrifugation indicates iatrogenic hemorrhage or peracute hemorrhage in the subarachnoid space. On the other hand, a red-tinged CSF with a xanthochromic supernatant (yellow-orange coloration) supports prior hemorrhage, likely associated with trauma, neoplasia, vascular disorders, or infectious disease [13]. Xanthochromia is caused by the erythrocyte degradation products oxyhemoglobin and bilirubin. Markedly increased CSF protein (>400 mg/dL) and severe icterus are other causes of xanthochromia. Normal neonates may have slightly xanthochromic CSF [5]. Cytological evidence of pathological hemorrhage includes the presence of hemosiderin, hematoidin, and/or erythrophagocytosis.

Increased fluid viscosity usually results from a very high protein concentration, especially fibrinogen. Cryptococcosis may increase the CSF viscosity due to the polysaccharide capsule of the yeast [1].

19.3.2 Protein Concentration

Reference intervals for CSF total protein concentration can vary with the laboratory and testing method used. Therefore, laboratory-established reference ranges should be used.

Normal CSF has very low protein concentration compared to plasma and other body cavity fluids. Most of the protein in normal CSF is albumin. Refractometric methods are not accurate for the measurement of CSF protein content. Refractive index of CSF can be artefactually increased by suspended particles (cells, bacteria), hemoglobin, or radiographic contrast media [13, 14]. Urine protein dipsticks have been used to estimate CSF protein concentration; however, they are highly specific for albumin detection and less specific for globulins [15]. The Pandy and Nonne-Apelt tests are qualitative methods that screen for the presence of globulins. These tests have been replaced by quantitative methods that measure immunoglobulins.

Quantitative methods that measure both albumin and globulin in CSF include turbidimetric procedures (trichloroacetic acid) and dye-binding assays (Coomassie brilliant blue, Ponceau S acid red, and pyrogallol red). Dye-binding protein methods are simple, rapid, and more accurate for the measurement of CSF protein concentration [1, 13]. The pyrogallol red assay gives a more uniform response to albumin and globulin and therefore is the preferred method [16]. Reported equine CSF protein values range from 10 to 120 mg/dL (generally 20–80 mg/dL), which are much higher than those reported in other domestic animals. CSF protein concentration in foals less than one week old ranges from 90 to 180 mg/dL, decreasing gradually to adult horse levels by two weeks of age [4]. Enhanced transport of albumin into CSF from blood or increased permeability of the BBB may be the reason for the difference between adult and neonatal CSF concentration [4, 17].

Nonpathological elevation of protein in CSF occurs with blood contamination during collection. Pathological causes of elevated CSF protein include damage to the BBB, intrathecal hemorrhage, increased local synthesis of immunoglobulins, degeneration of neural tissue, or obstruction of the CSF circulation (e.g., cervical vertebral malformations, abscess, or tumor).

Because albumin is not synthesized intrathecally, increased CSF albumin indicates damage to the BBB, iatrogenic blood contamination, or intrathecal hemorrhage. If hemorrhage or blood contamination is not present, the ratio between CSF albumin and serum albumin (albumin quotient) can be used to assess the functionality of the BBB:

$$\mathbf{AQ}\left(\text{albumin quotient}\right) = \frac{\text{CSF albumin}}{\text{Serum albumin}} \times 100 \qquad (19.1)$$

BBB damage in horses is suggested by CSF albumin concentration greater than 2.45 with an albumin quotient greater than 2.35. However, due to the normal variability of CSF albumin in horses, the use of this index is limited [17].

Electrophoretic techniques define the gamma-globulins as a heterogeneous group of proteins with similar migration rates; this fraction contains the immunoglobulins. High-resolution agarose gel electrophoresis (HRE) produces sharper bands and definition of CSF protein fractions [18]. Electrophoresis should be performed on CSF and serum simultaneously to compare the distribution of proteins. Three major immunoglobulins are found in CSF: IgG, IgM, and IgA. IgG is the major CSF immunoglobulin present in normal CSF. Since CSF IgG originates from plasma, elevated concentrations of IgG in CSF may indicate an abnormal BBB or increased intrathecal synthesis by inflammatory cells. An IgG index is used to determine whether the IgG present is due to local synthesis or originates from the plasma (alteration in the blood–brain CSF barrier, intrathecal hemorrhage, or iatrogenic blood contamination):

$$\mathbf{IgG\ index} = \frac{\text{CSF IgG/Serum IgG}}{\text{CSF albumin/serum albumin}} \qquad (19.2)$$

An IgG index greater than 0.3 with a normal albumin quotient suggests intrathecal IgG production, which is generally caused by infectious inflammatory diseases [19]. The IgG index may be useful in differentiating inflammatory lesions from noninflammatory diseases.

Other techniques such as the antibody index and C-value, that use antigen-specific antibody titers rather than total IgG, are believed to be more accurate than the IgG index [20]. The antibody index relates a specific IgG titer to the total IgG concentration, allowing the detection of a fraction of specific antibody made in the CNS. Movement of a specific antibody into the CSF due to leakage across a porous barrier or blood contamination during sample collection would not be expected to affect the antibody index [21, 22]. The C-value theory is that the ratio of antigen-specific antibody to total IgG in CSF is equal to the ratio in the serum. Values >1.7 are suggestive of intrathecal antibody production [19].

The presence of IgM is an abnormal finding in the CSF and is considered more specific than IgG or total immunoglobulin levels for detection of active or recent infectious disease [14]. Serum IgM capture ELISA (MAC-ELISA) is the preferred method for the diagnosis of West Nile virus infection in vaccinated and unvaccinated horses due to high sensitivity and specificity. Because there is 100% agreement between serum and CSF results, there is no clear advantage in testing CSF rather than serum. However, future introduction of live attenuated vaccines that may elicit a serological IgM response suggests that CSF testing may become the gold standard for diagnosing West Nile disease in vaccinated horses [23].

Elevated CSF protein concentration may be found in cases of encephalitis, neoplasms, meningitis, and trauma. Typically, neoplasms or trauma produce an increase of albumin, because of disruption of the BBB. In contrast, in inflammatory diseases such as encephalitis and meningitis, globulins are the primary protein increased, due to intrathecal production [23]. The CSF nucleated cell count and CSF protein concentration tend to increase proportionately. However, in some disorders the cell count remains normal, whereas the total protein concentration may be increased. This condition is called albuminocytological dissociation, which has been described in viral nonsuppurative encephalomyelitis such as equine herpes virus meningoencephalitis (EHV-1), neoplastic disease, and with traumatic, vascular, degenerative, and compressive spinal cord lesions [14].

19.3.3 Antibody Titers

A variety of antibody and antigen tests are available for viruses, fungi, rickettsia, protozoa, and parasites [24]. In order to evaluate antibody titers, two samples taken two weeks apart should be analyzed. Antibodies detected in CSF may be derived from vaccination, antigen exposure, or actual disease. Interpretation of CSF antibody titers should be done in light of the vaccination history, serum titers, BBB integrity, intrathecal immunoglobulin production (IgG index), and CSF IgM levels.

Antibody titers for EHV-1, togavirus, West Nile virus, and equine protozoal myelitis (EPM) (*Sarcocystis neurona*) can be measured in CSF [5, 25, 26]. Titers can be measured using Western blot, a semiquantitative antibody-based test, or indirect immunofluorescence indirect fluorescent antibody test (IFAT), which is a quantitative antibody test. Because there is evidence of passive movement of antibodies across the blood–CSF barrier, CSF antibody titers can be influenced by serum antibody titers and yield a false-positive result [27]. Moreover, even minimal iatrogenic blood contamination during collection (8 RBC/μL of CSF) has been shown to be the source of positive CSF Western blot for antibodies against *S. neurona* in equine serum and CSF [28]. Therefore, the Western blot test for *S. neurona* antibodies has low specificity but high sensitivity. While a positive result does not necessarily indicate active EPM, a horse with a negative CSF Western blot is probably not infected with *S. neurona*, ruling out the disease [29]. The IFAT for *S. neurona* antibodies is more specific and accurate than the Western blot test for diagnosis of EPM [24].

As discussed previously, to differentiate exposure from infection, the intrathecal production of an antigen-specific antibody can be evaluated via the antibody index and C-value. These antibody coefficients showed high specificity and sensitivity in one study using an ELISA based on the *S. neurona* SnSAG2 surface antigen, substantially improving the diagnosis of equine protozoal meningoencephalitis [12]. More recently, ELISA assays based on the trivalent SnSAG (2/4/3) surface antigens of *S. neurona* (parasitic-specific antibodies), performed in both serum and CSF, have been used to assess intrathecal antibody production and thus CNS infection [30]. In contrast, calculation of the CSF to serum ratio using the Lyme Multiplex yielded low sensitivity and fair specificity for the diagnosis of equine neuroborreliosis associated with *Borrelia burgdorferi* infection [31]. Therefore, identifying this rare disease, although caused by an endemic organism with widespread exposure, remains challenging.

19.3.4 Cell Counts

Because the cellular concentration of normal and sometimes abnormal CSF is too low to be detected by standard hematological analysis, red and white blood cell counts are performed using a hemocytometer. Undiluted CSF is added to the counting chamber. After 10–15 minutes the cells settle and are visible in the same plane of focus. Then, RBCs and WBCs are counted in both chambers (18 squares) and the average total count of each cell type is multiplied by 1.1 to obtain the number of cells per μL. Erythrocytes are recognized as small, refractile, light tan, and are generally crenated (Figure 19.2). White blood cells have irregular cell borders with a granular texture. Small lymphocytes may be difficult to differentiate from erythrocytes.

Normal CSF does not contain erythrocytes, but they may be present due to subarachnoid hemorrhage or, more commonly, with iatrogenic blood contamination. Blood contamination may affect the leukocyte and differential counts. A formula using the RBC count in blood and CSF along with the peripheral blood WBC count to correct the measured white blood cell count in the CSF has been used [6]. However, this formula is controversial and studies have shown that white blood cells are often overcorrected in blood-contaminated CSF, obscuring an underlying inflammatory process [6, 32]. In dogs, erythrocyte counts in blood-contaminated CSF correlate poorly with total nucleated cell counts and protein concentrations; using formulae to correct total nucleated cell count and protein concentration for the number of RBCs in CSF is inappropriate [33]. In two studies, no significant changes were detected in the total nucleated cell count of contaminated CSF aliquots containing up to 8480 RBC/μLand 13 200 RBC/μL, respectively [33, 34].

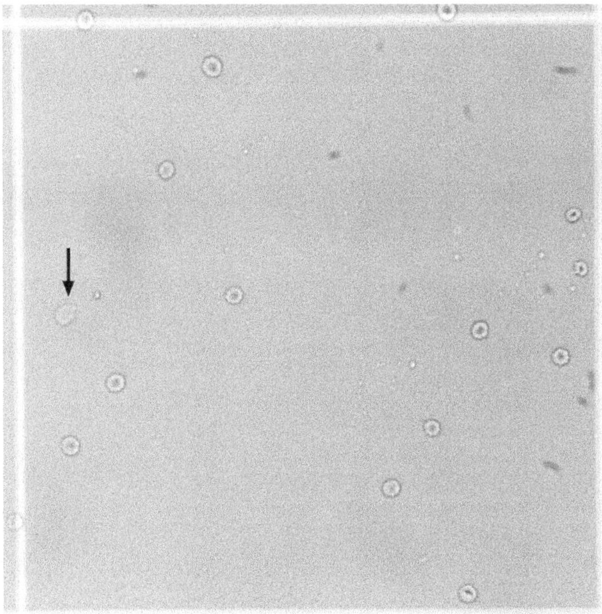

Figure 19.2 Microscopic identification of WBCs and RBCs in the hemocytometer chamber. The light tan, round, crenated cells are RBCs. There is one WBC (*arrow*) that has irregular borders and a granular opaque cytoplasm (magnification ×400).

The total white cell count in CSF of normal horses ranges from 0–8 depending on the reference. A normal hemocytometer count does not necessarily reflect normal CSF; abnormalities in cell types or cell proportions may be present [35]. Pleocytosis is the term used to indicate increased cellularity in CSF. The severity of pleocytosis is determined by the etiology and location of the lesion with respect to the subarachnoid space or ventricular system. Therefore, although often severe, deep parenchymal lesions that do not communicate with the subarachnoid space generally have CSF nucleated cell counts within reference limits.

19.3.5 Glucose

Cerebrospinal fluid glucose concentration varies proportionally with blood glucose values. Normal glucose cerebrospinal concentration in horses ranges between 30 and 70 mg/dL (30–75% of plasma glucose concentrations) [5, 13]. Therefore, CSF results must be interpreted in light of the serum glucose values. However, since CSF equilibration with plasma glucose requires 1–2 hours, CSF glucose concentration reflects serum glucose values one hour prior to CSF collection [1]. The main differential diagnoses for decreased CSF glucose are increased glucose utilization (associated with bacterial meningitis or marked neutrophilic pleocytosis) and hypoglycemia. Due to the lack of specificity of glucose measurement, more specific tests such as cytological evaluation and bacterial culture are recommended to assess for evidence of sepsis in the CSF.

19.3.6 Enzymes

Enzymes in the CSF may originate from the blood, neural tissue, or CSF cellular components. Therefore, interpretation of enzyme results should consider the integrity of the blood–brain–CSF barrier, blood contamination, and the cytological examination. Creatine kinase (CK) concentration is very low in normal CSF. Because CK is a large macromolecule and does not cross the BBB, the most likely source of increased activity of this enzyme in the CSF is nervous tissue damage. One study suggests that CK is often increased with protozoal myelitis, helping to differentiate this condition from compressive neurological disease [36]. However, other studies in horses have failed to demonstrate a correlation between nucleated cell counts, serum CK, or CSF protein concentration and a specific disease. Moreover, contamination of CSF with epidural fat or dura during CSF collection may falsely increase CSF CK activity [37].

19.3.7 Lactic Acid

Lactic acid is produced during anaerobic glycolysis by the enzymatic conversion of pyruvic acid. Because lactic acid diffuses very slowly through the intact blood–brain–CSF barrier, increased CSF lactate levels indicate anaerobic glycolysis in the brain. In a study of horses with confirmed neurological disease, CSF lactate concentrations were significantly elevated in several diseases. Thus, although sensitive for neurological disease, this assay lacks specificity [1].

19.3.8 Polymerase Chain Reaction

Polymerase chain reaction is a very sensitive molecular genetic test that amplifies short sequences of DNA (or RNA). In horses, PCR for bacteria, protozoa, and viruses is available in many diagnostic laboratories [27]. PCR testing for *S. neurona* in the CSF is highly specific for the diagnosis of EPM; however, many false-negative results have been reported, probably because intact merozoites rarely enter the CSF and free-parasite DNA is destroyed rapidly by enzymatic action [20]. In contrast, PCR testing of neural tissue has been shown to be useful as a postmortem test for EPM. The diagnostic sensitivity of West Nile virus PCR in the CSF is very low probably because viremia is often very short-lived. Collecting the sample early during the disease process may increase the sensitivity of this test [38]. EHV-1 real-time PCR testing of whole blood is able to differentiate neuropathogenic from nonneuropathogenic strains [39].

19.3.9 Lymphocyte Phenotyping

Immunophenotypic markers can be used to characterize the lymphocyte subpopulations in CSF and their association with disease. However, individual variation and the large volume of sample necessary make this test clinically impractical [40]. In horses, T-cells comprise about 80% of the lymphocyte population in CSF, which is similar to that found in humans.

19.4 Cytological Examination

Cytological assessment of the CSF provides information regarding cellularity, types of cells, and presence or absence of infectious agents or inclusions. Due to the low cellularity of normal CSF, concentration of cells by cytocentrifugation, sedimentation, simple centrifugation, or membrane filtration is necessary for morphological evaluation [41]. The diagnostic quality and cell recovery of slides made by simple centrifugation are generally poor, so this technique is not recommended. Membrane filtration methods produce the best cellular recovery (90–100%) and addition of 40% ethanol after collection eliminates the need for immediate processing [42]. Membrane filtration methods are not recommended, however, because they produce poor cellular morphology and are technically difficult. Sedimentation is the recommended technique when there is limited access to a laboratory or when a cytocentrifuge is not available. With this technique, the cellular yield is adequate and cellular morphology is well preserved. An inexpensive chamber has been described for in-house use [43]. Cytocentrifugation is the ideal method in human and veterinary medicine because it preserves cellular morphology, thereby facilitating cellular identification; however, it requires special equipment and the cellular yield is relatively low [35].

Slides containing sample are stained with Romanowsky stains (Wright's, Wright–Giemsa and Diff-Quik®). The use of special stains like gram, India ink, and luxol fast blue may be helpful in identifying bacteria, *Cryptococcus* organisms, and myelin, respectively. Cytological examination of the CSF is recommended even if the cell count is not increased because abnormalities in cell proportions or cell type may still be present.

19.4.1 Normal Findings

Most of the cells in normal CSF are mononuclear (80–90%), composed predominantly of small lymphocytes with fewer monocytoid cells (Figure 19.3). Lymphocytes (small mononuclear cells) are 9–15 μm in diameter and have a scant amount of pale-blue cytoplasm and a dark, dense, round to slightly oval or indented nucleus. Monocytoid cells (large mononuclear cells) are large (12–15 μm) with oval, sometimes kidney-shaped, nuclei. They have moderate to abundant light-blue cytoplasm, which may be foamy or finely vacuolated.

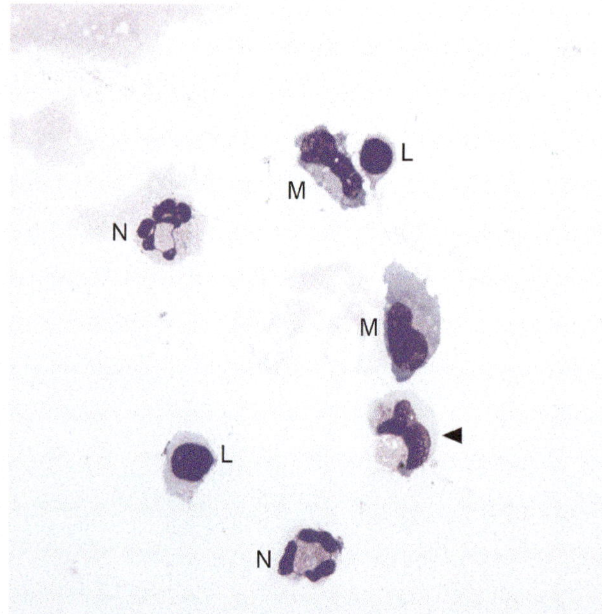

Figure 19.3 Mixed inflammatory cell response from a CSF from a foal with head trauma. Two neutrophils (N), two lymphocytes (L), two monocytoid cells (M), and one ruptured cell (*arrowhead*) are present (magnification ×1000). *Source:* Courtesy of Dr Theresa E. Rizzi, Oklahoma State University.

Eosinophils are not found in normal CSF, whereas the presence of a few neutrophils is controversial. While some authors suggest that rare neutrophils may be normally present, others propose that finding neutrophils is indicative of an abnormality [13, 35, 44, 45]. Occasionally, ependymal cells, choroid plexus cells, and meningeal lining cells are seen (Figure 19.4).

19.4.2 Abnormal Findings

A marked pleocytosis with predominance of neutrophils is suggestive of bacterial meningitis (Figure 19.5). Cytological identification of the bacteria or a positive culture result is confirmatory of septic meningitis. However, neutrophilic pleocytosis in the absence of degeneration and bacteria does not rule out sepsis, even if the gram stain and culture are negative [4, 46]. Neutrophils may also be found in noninfectious processes such as necrosis, early stages of Eastern equine viral meningoencephalitis, CNS hemorrhage, and post myelography with iodinated contrast agents [45].

In pathological conditions, monocytes are transformed into macrophages that contain varying amounts of

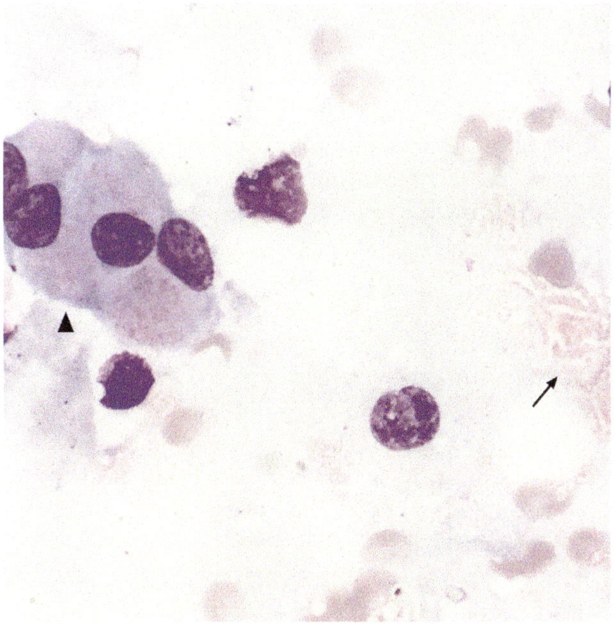

Figure 19.4 Ependymal or choroid plexus lining cells (*arrowhead*) from a touch preparation of tissue in the cerebellomedullary cistern. These, along with extracellular eosinophilic myelin (*arrow*), can be present in normal CSF as procedural contaminants.

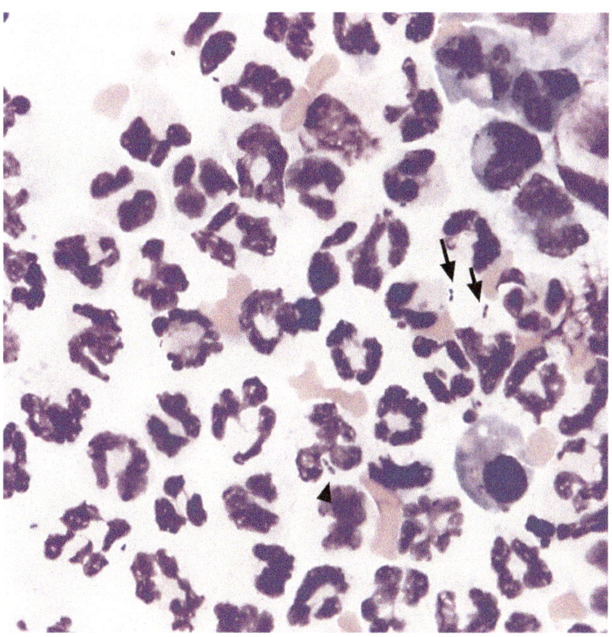

Figure 19.5 CSF from a foal with septic meningitis. The field shows numerous degenerative neutrophils, one of which contains a phagocytized bacillus (*arrowhead*). Extracellular bacterial bacilli are also present (*arrows*). *Source:* Courtesy of Dr Robin W. Allison, Oklahoma State University.

phagocytized material such as lipid droplets, erythrocytes, microorganisms, or cellular debris in various stages of digestion (Figure 19.6). Activated monocytoid cells and macrophages may appear in clusters mimicking epithelial cells. Phagocytic cells might be expected where there is extensive damage to nervous tissue.

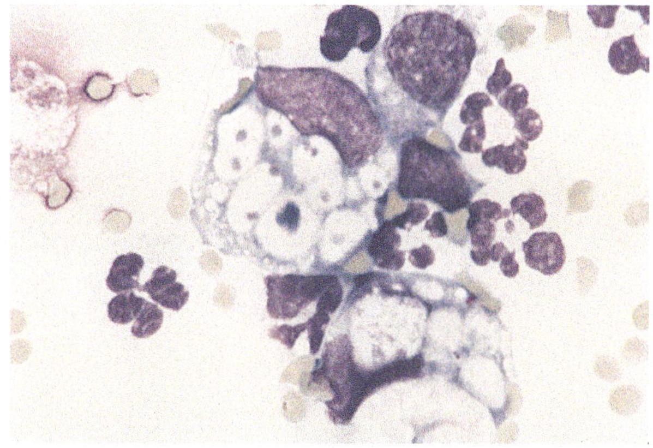

Figure 19.6 Cytophagia in CSF from a horse with resolving septic meningitis. A mixture of neutrophils, macrophages, and a lymphocyte is present. Macrophages at center and bottom contain phagocytized cellular debris, which should not be confused with fungal organisms. Original magnification ×1000, Wright stain.

Lymphocyte counts may be elevated in cases of spinal cord compression, axonal degeneration, infections, and immune-mediated disorders such as polyneuritis [25, 45]. Plasma cells are not a normal finding and may be observed with reactive lymphocytes in viral encephalitis, chronic protozoal or rickettsial infections, and immune-mediated diseases when there is a humoral response to inflammation. When a mixed pleocytosis with eosinophils is present, fungal or protozoal infection or parasite migration should be included in the differential diagnosis.

Cerebrovascular accidents can be suspected with a xanthochromic sample, increased protein concentration, presence of erythrocytes, and erythrophagocytosis (Figure 19.7). Hemorrhage can occur secondary to trauma, infection, parasite migration, coagulopathy, or neoplasia. In horses, CNS neoplasia is uncommon, with the exception of pituitary adenoma. Therefore, finding neoplastic cells in the CSF is rare. Melanin pigment and lymphoblasts are occasionally seen with CNS melanomas and lymphomas, respectively [47].

19.5 Cerebrospinal Fluid in Specific Diseases

19.5.1 Viral Infections

[fo]Many viral diseases of the CNS are associated with mononuclear pleocytosis, high protein concentration, or both. However, the CSF of acute Eastern and Venezuelan equine encephalomyelitis is typically neutrophilic initially, becoming predominantly monocytic within 2–3 days [48].

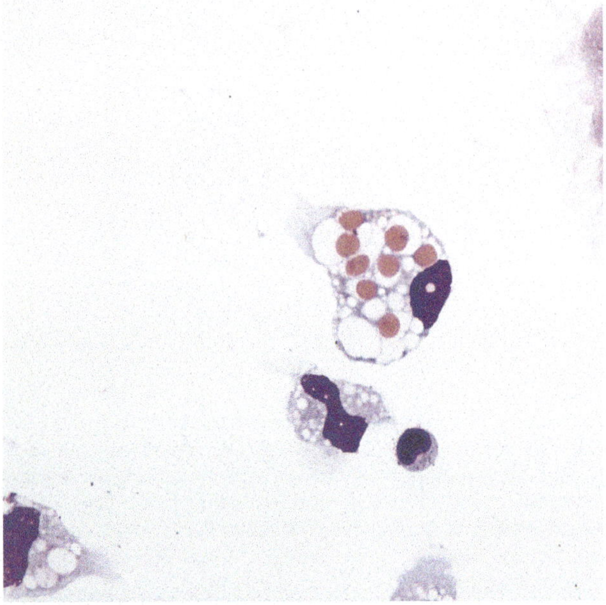

Figure 19.7 Erythrophagia in CSF from a foal with head trauma. Two monocytoid cells and one small lymphocyte are also present (magnification ×1000). *Source:* Courtesy of Dr Theresa E. Rizzi, Oklahoma State University.

CSF changes in equine herpesvirus encephalomyelopathy are consistent with a vasculopathy, and are characterized by marked xanthochromia and albuminocytological dissociation [38]. CSF findings in horses with West Nile meningoencephalitis are more likely to be abnormal when collected from the lumbosacral site, and consist of a predominantly lymphocytic, mononuclear pleocytosis with mildly increased protein concentration [49].

19.5.2 Bacterial Infections

Bacterial meningoencephalitis occurs most frequently in foals, secondary to neonatal septicemia. Hence, gram-negative enterobacteria predominate in foals, while gram-positive bacteria (*Streptococcus*) are more common in adult horses [50]. The CSF analysis is characterized by moderate to marked elevations of the nucleated cell counts, with a predominance of degenerative or nondegenerative neutrophils. Nevertheless, some foals may only have a mild pleocytosis, which should not preclude careful cytological examination of the CSF to search for bacteria. Protein concentration is generally elevated. Although bacteria are occasionally seen on cytological preparations, bacterial culture of CSF may be negative, especially if antibiotic therapy had been already initiated [51].

Despite the reported low sensitivity of microbial CSF cultures in horses with meningoencephalitis, an attempt to isolate the microbial organism is encouraged [46]. In neonates, blood and CSF cultures are indicated to increase the likelihood of isolating the organism [50]. PCR assays may be used to detect bacterial DNA. Compared to blood cultures, biomolecular assays are more sensitive and faster at identifying the organism, which is crucial for critically ill patients, but these assays do not provide information on antimicrobial sensitivity [52].

19.5.3 Fungal Infections

Rarely mycotic encephalitis may occur secondary to guttural pouch mycosis via hematogenous spread. In one report, a focal area of encephalitis caused by *Aspergillus* spp. was attributed to direct transfer from the frontal sinuses, rather than hematogenous spread from the guttural pouch [53]. In two horses with cryptococcal meningoencephalitis, the CSF findings were characterized by markedly increased protein concentration and profound neutrophilic pleocytosis [46, 54]. Increased CSF viscosity has been reported with cryptococcosis due to the polysaccharide capsule of the yeast [1].

19.5.4 Parasitic Infections

Cerebrospinal fluid changes in horses with equine protozoal encephalomyelitis are not consistent. There may be a mild to moderate mononuclear pleocytosis with increased total protein or the fluid may be normal. CSF analysis is more useful in differentiating other neurological diseases from EPM [55]. The CSF of horses with parasitic migration through the CNS, such as cerebrospinal nematodiasis (*Halicephalobus gingivalis*, previously *Micronema deletrix*), may be xanthochromic with a mixed pleocytosis and a normal to increased protein level [56].

19.5.5 Other Diseases

The CSF of horses with equine motor neuron disease may be normal or show albuminocytological dissociation, which may reflect necrosis of motor neurons and degeneration in the spinal roots [57, 58]. The CSF appearance in horses with cauda equina neuritis (polyneuritis equi) may be xanthochromic or cloudy with a moderate mixed (predominantly lymphocytic) pleocytosis and moderately increased protein concentration [25]. CSF analysis was normal in a report of four horses with cervical vertebral spinal hematomas [59].

Although CSF findings may help to formulate a differential diagnosis, abnormalities are often not specific and can also occur with other disease processes. Therefore, other diagnostic tests such as imaging, serology, and PCR are often necessary to identify the etiological agent or disease present.

References

1 Vernau, W. and Vernau, K.A. (2008). Cerebrospinal fluid. In: *Clinical Biochemistry of Domestic Animals*, 6e (eds. J.J. Kaneko, J.W. Harvey and M.L. Bruss), 769–819. Burlington: Elsevier.

2 Depecker, M., Bizon-Mercier, C., and Courouce-Malblanc, A. (2014). Ultrasound-guided atlanto-occipital puncture for cerebrospinal fluid analysis on the standing horse. *Vet. Rec.* 174 (2): 45.

3 MacKay, R.J. (2014). Developments in ultrasound-guided thecal puncture in horses. *Vet. Rec.* 174 (2): 43–44.

4 Adams, R. and Mayhew, I.G. (1985). Neurologic diseases. *Vet. Clin. North Am. Equine Pract.* 1 (1): 209–234.

5 Johnson, P.J. and Constantinescu, G.M. (2000). Collection of cerebrospinal fluid in horses. *Equine Vet. Educ.* 12 (1): 7–12.

6 Sweeney, C.R. and Russell, G.E. (2000). Differences in total protein concentration, nucleated cell count, and red blood cell count among sequential samples of cerebrospinal fluid from horses. *J. Am. Vet. Med. Assoc.* 217 (1): 54–57.

7 Fry, M.M., Vernau, W., Kass, P.H., and Vernau, K.M. (2006). Effects of time, initial composition, and stabilizing agents on the results of canine cerebrospinal fluid analysis. *Vet. Clin. Pathol.* 35 (1): 72–77.

8 Bienzle, D., McDonnell, J.J., and Stanton, J.B. (2000). Analysis of cerebrospinal fluid from dogs and cats after 24 and 48 hours of storage. *J. Am. Vet. Med. Assoc.* 216 (11): 1761–1764.

9 Cook, J.R. and DeNicola, D.B. (1988). Cerebrospinal fluid. *Vet. Clin. North Am. Small Anim. Pract.* 18 (3): 475–499.

10 Di Terlizzi, R. and Platt, S.R. (2009). The function, composition and analysis of cerebrospinal fluid in companion animals: Part II – analysis. *Vet. J.* 180 (1): 15–32.

11 Rand, J.S., Parent, J., Percy, D., and Jacobs, R. (1994). Clinical, cerebrospinal fluid, and histological data from thirty-four cats with primary noninflammatory disease of the central nervous system. *Can. Vet. J.* 35 (3): 174–181.

12 Furr, M., Howe, D., Reed, S., and Yeargan, M. (2011). Antibody coefficients for the diagnosis of equine protozoal myeloencephalitis. *J. Vet. Intern. Med.* 25 (1): 138–142.

13 MacWilliams, P.S. (2002). Cerebrospinal fluid. In: *Diagnostic Cytology and Hematology of the Horse* (eds. R.L. Cowell and R.D. Tyler), 171–179. St Louis: Mosby.

14 Chrisman, C.L. (1992). Cerebrospinal fluid analysis. *Vet. Clin. North Am. Small Anim. Pract.* 22 (4): 781–810.

15 Jacobs, R.M., Cochrane, S.M., Lumsden, J.H., and Norris, A.M. (1990). Relationship of cerebrospinal fluid protein concentration determined by dye-binding and urinary dipstick methodologies. *Can. Vet. J.* 31 (8): 587–588.

16 Marshall, T. and Williams, K.M. (2000). Protein determination in cerebrospinal fluid by protein dye-binding assay. *Br. J. Biomed. Sci.* 57 (4): 281–286.

17 Andrews, F.M., Geiser, D.R., Sommardahl, C.S. et al. (1994). Albumin quotient, IgG concentration, and IgG index determinations in cerebrospinal fluid of neonatal foals. *Am. J. Vet. Res.* 55 (6): 741–745.

18 Furr, M., Chickering, W.R., and Robertson, J. (1997). High resolution protein electrophoresis of equine cerebrospinal fluid. *Am. J. Vet. Res.* 58 (9): 939–941.

19 Furr, M. (2007). Humoral immune responses in the horse after intrathecal challenge with ovalbumin. *J. Vet. Intern. Med.* 21 (4): 806–811.

20 Furr, M., MacKay, R., Granstrom, D. et al. (2002). Clinical diagnosis of equine protozoal myeloencephalitis (EPM). *J. Vet. Intern. Med.* 16 (5): 618–621.

21 Heskett, K.A. and MacKay, R.J. (2008). Antibody index and specific antibody quotient in horses after intragastric administration of *Sarcocystis neurona* sporocysts. *Am. J. Vet. Res.* 69 (3): 403–409.

22 MacKay, R.J., Tanhauser, S.T., Gillis, K.D. et al. (2008). Effect of intermittent oral administration of ponazuril on experimental *Sarcocystis neurona* infection of horses. *Am. J. Vet. Res.* 69 (3): 396–402.

23 Porter, M.B., Long, M., Gosche, D.G. et al. (2004). Immunoglobulin M-capture enzyme-linked immunosorbent assay testing of cerebrospinal fluid and serum from horses exposed to west nile virus by vaccination or natural infection. *J. Vet. Intern. Med.* 18 (6): 866–870.

24 Duarte, P.C., Ebel, E.D., Traub-Dargatz, J. et al. (2006). Indirect fluorescent antibody testing of cerebrospinal fluid for diagnosis of equine protozoal myeloencephalitis. *Am. J. Vet. Res.* 67 (5): 869–876.

25 Aleman, M., Katzman, S.A., Vaughan, B. et al. (2009). Antemortem diagnosis of polyneuritis equi. *J. Vet. Intern. Med.* 23 (3): 665–668.

26 Miller, M.M., Sweeney, C.R., Russell, G.E. et al. (1999). Effects of blood contamination of cerebrospinal fluid on western blot analysis for detection of antibodies against *Sarcocystis neurona* and on albumin quotient and immunoglobulin G index in horses. *J. Am. Vet. Med. Assoc.* 215 (1): 67–71.

27 Pellegrini-Masini, A. and Livesey, L.C. (2006). Meningitis and encephalomyelitis in horses. *Vet. Clin. North Am. Equine Pract.* 22 (2): 553–589.

28 Murphy, J.E., Marsh, A.E., Reed, S.M. et al. (2006). Development and evaluation of a *Sarcocystis neurona*-specific IgM capture enzyme-linked immunosorbent assay. *J. Vet. Intern. Med.* 20 (2): 322–328.

29 Daft, B.M., Barr, B.C., Gardner, I.A. et al. (2002). Sensitivity and specificity of western blot testing of cerebrospinal fluid and serum for diagnosis of equine protozoal myeloencephalitis in horses with and without neurologic abnormalities. *J. Am. Vet. Med. Assoc.* 221 (7): 1007–1013.

30 Yeargan, M., de Assis Rocha, I., Morrow, J. et al. (2015). A new trivalent SnSAG surface antigen chimera for efficient detection of antibodies against *Sarcocystis neurona* and diagnosis of equine protozoal myeloencephalitis. *J. Vet. Diagn. Investig.* 27 (3): 377–381.

31 Johnson, A.L., Johnstone, L.K., and Stefanovski, D. (2018). Cerebrospinal fluid Lyme multiplex assay results are not diagnostic in horses with neuroborreliosis. *J. Vet. Intern. Med.* 32 (2): 832–838.

32 Wilson, J.W. and Stevens, J.B. (1977). Effects of blood contamination on cerebrospinal fluid analysis. *J. Am. Vet. Med. Assoc.* 171 (3): 256–258.

33 MacNeill, A.L., Andre, B.G., Zingale, Y. et al. (2018). The effects of iatrogenic blood contamination on total nucleated cell counts and protein concentrations in canine cerebrospinal fluid. *Vet. Clin. Pathol.* 47 (3): 464–470.

34 Hurtt, A.E. and Smith, M.O. (1997). Effects of iatrogenic blood contamination on results of cerebrospinal fluid analysis in clinically normal dogs and dogs with neurologic disease. *J. Am. Vet. Med. Assoc.* 211 (7): 866–867.

35 Christopher, M.M., Perman, V., and Hardy, R.M. (1988). Reassessment of cytologic values in canine cerebrospinal fluid by use of cytocentrifugation. *J. Am. Vet. Med. Assoc.* 192 (12): 1726–1729.

36 Furr, M.O. and Tyler, R.D. (1990). Cerebrospinal fluid creatine kinase activity in horses with central nervous system disease: 69 cases (1984–1989). *J. Am. Vet. Med. Assoc.* 197 (2): 245–248.

37 Jackson, C., de Lahunta, A., Divers, T., and Ainsworth, D. (1996). The diagnostic utility of cerebrospinal fluid creatine kinase activity in the horse. *J. Vet. Intern. Med.* 10 (4): 246–251.

38 Pusterla, N., Madigan, J.E., and Leutenegger, C.M. (2006). Real-time polymerase chain reaction: a novel molecular diagnostic tool for equine infectious diseases. *J. Vet. Intern. Med.* 20 (1): 3–12.

39 Johnson, A.L. (2011). Update on infectious diseases affecting the equine nervous system. *Vet. Clin. North Am. Equine Pract.* 27 (3): 573–587.

40 Furr, M., Pontzer, C., and Gasper, P. (2001). Lymphocyte phenotype subsets in the cerebrospinal fluid of normal horses and horses with equine protozoal myeloencephalitis. *Vet. Ther.* 2 (4): 317–324.

41 Deisenhammer, F., Bartos, A., Egg, R. et al. (2006). Guidelines on routine cerebrospinal fluid analysis. Report from an EFNS task force. *Eur. J. Neurol.* 13 (9): 913–922.

42 Freeman, K.P., Brewer, B., and Slusher, S.H. (1989). Membrane filter preparations of cerebrospinal fluid from normal horses and horses with selected neurologic diseases. *Compend. Contin. Educ. Pract. Vet.* 11 (9): 1100–1109.

43 Garma-Aviña, A. (2004). An inexpensive sedimentation chamber for the preparation of cytologic specimens of cerebrospinal fluid. *J. Vet. Diagn. Investig.* 16 (6): 585–587.

44 Beech, J. (1983). Cytology of equine cerebrospinal fluid. *Vet. Pathol.* 20 (5): 553–562.

45 Hayes, T.E. (1987). Examination of cerebrospinal fluid in the horse. *Vet. Clin. North Am. Equine Pract.* 3 (2): 283–291.

46 Toth, B., Aleman, M., Nogradi, N., and Madigan, J.E. (2012). Meningitis and meningoencephalomyelitis in horses: 28 cases (1985–2010). *J. Am. Vet. Med. Assoc.* 240 (5): 580–587.

47 Paradis, M.R. (1998). Tumors of the central nervous system. *Vet. Clin. North Am. Equine Pract.* 14 (3): 543–561.

48 Smith, J.M., DeBowes, R.M., and Cox, J.H. (1987). Central nervous system disease in adult horses. III. Differential diagnosis and comparison of common disorders. *Compend. Contin. Educ. Pract. Vet.* 9 (10): 1042–1054.

49 Wamsley, H.L., Alleman, A.R., Porter, M.B., and Long, M.T. (2002). Findings in cerebrospinal fluids of horses infected with West Nile virus: 30 cases (2001). *J. Am. Vet. Med. Assoc.* 221 (9): 1303–1305.

50 Viu, J., Monreal, L., Jose-Cunilleras, E. et al. (2012). Clinical findings in 10 foals with bacterial meningoencephalitis. *Equine Vet. J. Suppl.* 44 (41): 100–104.

51 Smith, J.J., Provost, P.J., and Paradis, M.R. (2004). Bacterial meningitis and brain abscesses secondary to infectious disease processes involving the head in horses: seven cases (1980–2001). *J. Am. Vet. Med. Assoc.* 224 (5): 739–742.

52 Stefanetti, V., Beccati, F., Passamonti, F. et al. (2016). Detection and DNA quantification of *Enterococcus casseliflavus* in a foal with septic meningitis. *J. Am. Vet. Med. Assoc.* 249 (1): 96–100.

53 Hunter, B. and Nation, P.N. (2011). Mycotic encephalitis, sinus osteomyelitis, and guttural pouch mycosis in a 3-year-old Arabian colt. *Can. Vet. J.* 52 (12): 1339–1341.

54 Hart, K.A., Flaminio, M.J.B.F., Leroy, B.E. et al. (2008). Successful resolution of cryptococcal meningitis and optic neuritis in an adult horse with oral fluconazole. *J. Vet. Intern. Med.* 22 (6): 1436–1440.

55 MacKay, R.J., Granstrom, D.E., Saville, W.J., and Reed, S.M. (2000). Equine protozoal myeloencephalitis. *Vet. Clin. North Am. Equine Pract.* 16 (3): 405–425.

56 Darien, B.J., Belknap, J., and Nietfeld, J. (1988). Cerebrospinal fluid changes in two horses with central nervous system nematodiasis (*Micronema deletrix*). *J. Vet. Intern. Med.* 2 (4): 201–205.

57 Cummings, J.F., de Lahunta, A., George, C. et al. (1990). Equine motor neuron disease; a preliminary report. *Cornell Vet.* 80 (4): 357–379.

58 Divers, T.J., Mohammed, H.O., Cummings, J.F., and de Lahunta, A. (1992). Equine motor neuron disease: a new cause of weakness, trembling, and weight loss. *Compend. Contin. Educ. Pract. Vet.* 14 (9): 1222–1226.

59 Gold, J.R., Divers, T.J., Miller, A.J. et al. (2008). Cervical vertebral spinal hematomas in 4 horses. *J. Vet. Intern. Med.* 22 (2): 481–485.

20

Cytology of the Respiratory Tract

Martina Piviani

Department of Small Animal Clinical Science, University of Liverpool, Liverpool, UK

Acronyms and abbreviations that appear in this chapter include: BAL, bronchoalveolar lavage; TW, tracheal wash; RAO, recurrent airway obstruction; IAD, inflammatory airway disease; EIPH, exercise-induced pulmonary hemorrhage; PCR, polymerase chain reaction; THS, total hemosiderin score

20.1 Cytology of the Nasal Cavity and Paranasal Sinuses

20.1.1 Indications

Cytology of the upper respiratory tract is infrequently performed in horses but can be useful in cases of nasal discharge, presence of intranasal masses, and suspected pathological conditions of the paranasal sinuses, especially if findings are combined with the results of bacterial and fungal culture. Nasal discharge and foul breath can be seen with both nasal and sinonasal disease. The latter may cause dullness on percussion of the affected sinus as well as facial deformity. Endoscopy to look for the presence of nasal discharge originating from the caudal portion of the middle meatus and radiography can be used for confirmation of primary sinus involvement prior to centesis.

20.1.2 Collection Techniques and Sample Processing

Cytological samples from the nasal cavities can be obtained by collecting secretions through the nares or via endoscopic examination and also by percutaneous fine needle apiration (FNA). Lesions localized near the external nares can be sampled via imprints or FNA. In addition, a squash technique can be used to prepare cytology slides from biopsies obtained through endoscopy. Paranasal sinuses can be aspirated using a urinary or intravenous catheter after skin incision followed by trephination with a small Steinmann pin. In many cases, sampling from the caudal maxillary sinus is sufficient to establish a diagnosis as the frontal sinus drains ventrally into the caudal maxillary sinus [1]. Nasal discharge and fluid aspirated from sinuses can be used directly to prepare smears to be stained or placed in a plain sterile tube for culture.

20.1.3 Cytological Findings

The cells lining the nasal cavity include several types of epithelia: keratinized and nonkeratinized stratified squamous epithelium in the rostral portion of the nasal passages and stratified squamous epithelium caudal to the vestibulum to progressively pseudostratified ciliated and nonciliated columnar epithelium containing numerous goblet cells. Gergeleit et al. [2] have summarized the main cytological features of secretions from the paranasal sinuses. The latter are lined by transitional epithelium and simple ciliated columnar or cuboidal epithelium containing goblet cells. All of these cells can be found in swabs and washes and can appear hyperplastic with an increase in Goblet cells and mucus, which appears as pink slightly granular amorphous material (Figure 20.1) [2].

Mixed types of saprophytic bacteria and "barn mold" are often present. With inflammation due to foreign bodies, trauma, or infection, an increase of inflammatory cells is noted. The presence of food material and a mixed population of extracellular bacteria can help to differentiate primary sinusitis (Figure 20.2) from sinusitis secondary to dental disease (Figure 20.3) [2, 3]. With bacterial infection, the inflammation is typically neutrophilic, while with mycotic rhinitis and sinusitis there is more often a mixed neutrophilic and histiocytic inflammation with an eosinophilic component. Fungal infection can be due to both

Equine Hematology, Cytology, and Clinical Chemistry, Second Edition.
Edited by Raquel M. Walton, Rick L. Cowell, and Amy C. Valenciano.

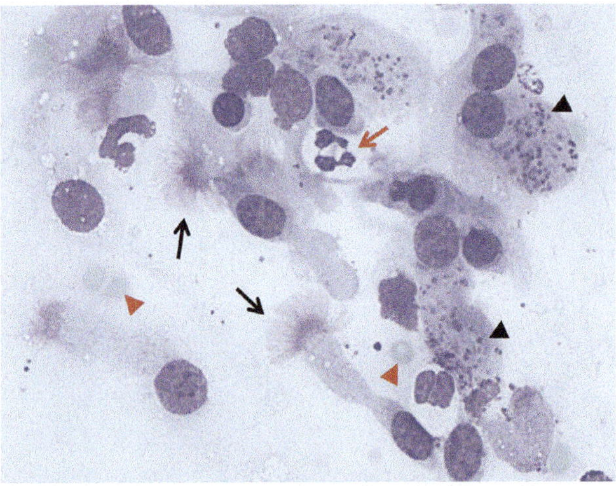

Figure 20.1 Smear from the paranasal sinus of a horse containing goblet cells with cytoplasmic mucin granules (*black arrowheads*), ciliated columnar epithelial cells (*black arrows*), rare neutrophils (*red arrow*), and few erythrocytes (*red arrowheads*). *Source:* Gergeleit et al. [2], Figure 5.A, p. 65. Reproduced with permission of Elsevier.

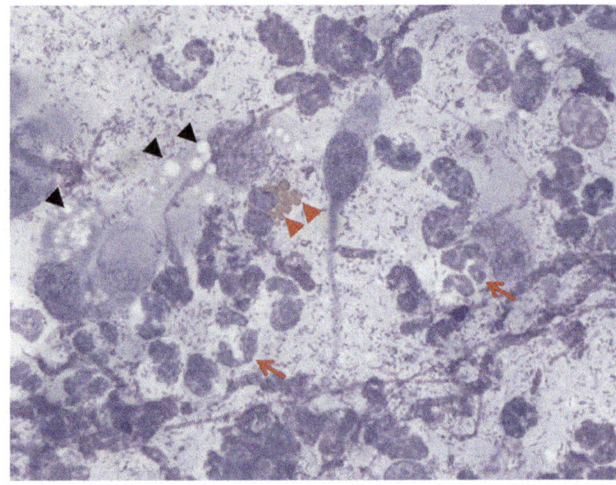

Figure 20.3 Secretion from the paranasal sinus of horse with dental sinusitis. Many degenerate neutrophils (*red arrows*), occasional eosinophils (*double red arrowheads*), and vacuolated epithelial cells (*black arrowheads*) surrounded by many extracellular bacteria. *Source:* Gergeleit et al. [2], Figure 2.B, p. 63. Reproduced with permission of Elsevier.

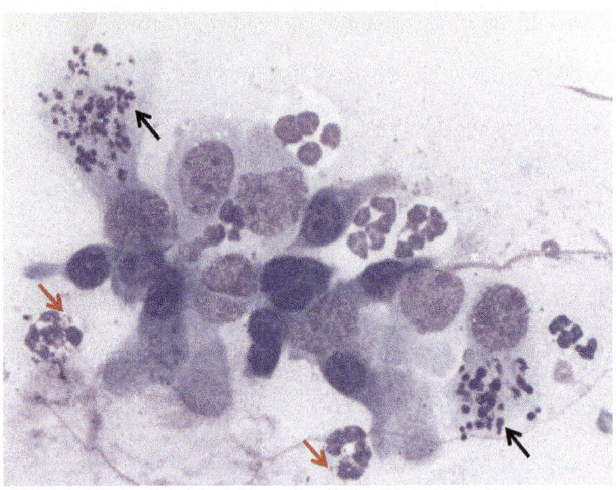

Figure 20.2 Squamous and ciliated epithelial cells, goblet cells with cytoplasmic granules (*black arrows*), neutrophils with intracellular bacteria (*red arrows*) and low numbers of extracellular bacteria in a smear of sinonasal secretion from a horse with primary sinusitis. *Source:* Gergeleit et al. [2], Figure 1.A, p. 63. Reproduced with permission of Elsevier.

primary pathogenic (e.g., *Cryptococcus neoformans*) and opportunistic fungi (e.g., *Aspergillus* spp., *Pneumocystis carinii*, *Pythomyces chartarum*, *Pseudallescheria boydii*) [4] and, rarely to algae (*Prototheca* spp.) [5]. Mycotic granulomas involving the nasal cavities and other organs due to *Coccidiodes immitis*, *Condiobolus coronatus*, *Entomopthora coronata*, *Condiobolus lamprauges*, and *Hyphomyces destruens* have also been reported [6]. Rhinitis due to *Rhinosporidium seeberi*, an organism previously classified as a fungus but regrouped into the class Mesomycetozoa (family Rhinosporideacae), has been infrequently reported in the United States, South America, South Africa, and the United Kingdom [7].

Aspiration of sinus cysts typically yields a paucicellular bright yellow fluid, whereas epidermoid cysts of the nasal diverticulum (formerly incorrectly called atheromata) contain abundant squamous cells, keratin debris, and cholesterol crystals.

Neoplasia is rare overall, but more frequently affects the paranasal sinuses than the nasal cavity in horses. Squamous cell carcinoma is the most frequent tumor and occurs predominantly in the maxillary sinus, similarly to sarcomas. Adenocarcinomas occur more frequently in the ethmoidal region and nasal cavity; bone and dental tumors, fibrosarcomas, hemangiosarcomas, mastocytomas, hemangiosarcomas, and lymphoma have also been recorded, albeit rarely [8]. Progressive ethmoid hematoma is cytologically characterized by macrophages with phagocytosed erythrocytes or hemosiderin (Figure 20.4) [2].

20.2 Cytology of the Lower Respiratory Tract

20.2.1 Indications

Lower airway disease is one of the major causes of poor performance in horses. The clinical diagnosis of equine pulmonary disorders is largely dependent on obtaining an accurate history and performing a thorough clinical examination. Depending on the cause, clinical signs of lower

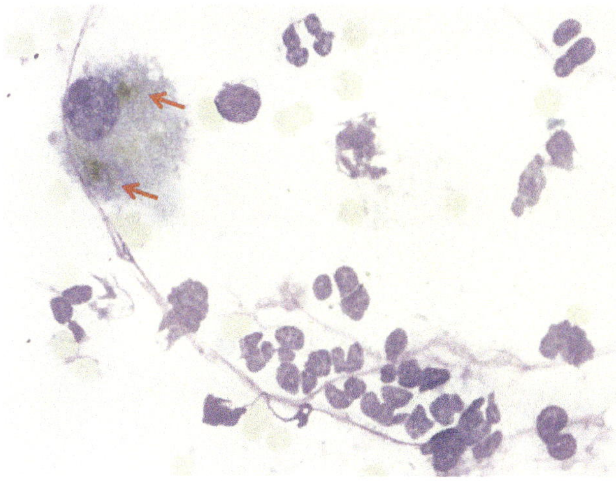

Figure 20.4 Cytology of a progressive ethmoidal hematoma containing macrophages with intracytoplasmic pigment, probably hemosiderin (*red arrows*) and several necrotic neutrophils amid a background of frequent erythrocytes. *Source:* Gergeleit et al. [2], Figure 3.A, p. 64. Reproduced with permission of Elsevier.

respiratory tract disease may include dyspnea, tachypnea, cough, stridor, nasal discharge, and fever. Auscultation may reveal abnormal sounds. When possible, additional diagnostic steps include radiographic examination and thoracic ultrasound. Other data, such as a hemogram and serum biochemistry, would add valuable information about the patient's general health status and may point towards a septic inflammatory process if leukocytosis or hyperfibrinogenemia is present. Specific tools for the diagnosis of lower airway disease in horses include bronchoscopy and cytological analysis of the fluid recovered from the respiratory tract by bronchoalveolar lavage (BAL) and tracheal wash (TW).

20.2.2 Collection Techniques

20.2.2.1 Bronchoalveolar Lavage

Bronchoalveolar lavage is a method for the recovery of respiratory secretions that line the lower airways and alveoli. It is usually performed during bronchoscopic evaluation of the lower respiratory tract and requires chemical restraint and the use of topical lidocaine solution during the procedure.

The endoscope is passed through the nares, nasopharynx, and trachea to be wedged into the most distal small bronchus. The procedure can also be performed "blindly" by passing a BAL catheter through the nostril into the lower airways until it appears wedged, and inflating the cuff with approximately 5 mL of air to seal the airway. Volumes of 250–500 mL of warm physiological saline or phosphate-buffered saline are then instilled and immediately reaspirated with the suction channel of the endoscope [9–11]. A significant difference in neutrophil percentages has been found between methods using different volumes, highlighting the importance of a standardized technique [12]. The fluid is then pooled and submitted for analysis.

Variations between different sequential aliquots have been reported in some studies but not in others [13–17]. Jean et al. [13] found higher percentages of neutrophils and lower percentages of macrophages in the first aliquot than in the second aliquot, both in healthy horses and horses with recurrent airway obstruction (RAO). Based on these results, the second aliquot is thought to contain less bronchial material, reach broader areas of the lung, and in general be more representative of the bronchoalveolar area in horses. Pickles et al. [15] showed that sequential aliquots of saline (100 mL each) did not significantly differ from a pooled sample (300 mL). Pooling all aliquots is still advised by most authors [10].

Several studies have shown no difference in most cell types between samples from the left and right lungs, with the exception of mast cells that were more numerous in the left lung in one study [16, 17] and in the right lung in another study [13]. However, a more recent study involving a larger number of horses found a statistically significant, albeit minimal, difference in the neutrophil percentage between left and right lung, leading the authors to recommend sampling both lungs to increase the sensitivity of the test for diagnosing airway inflammation [18].

Because the unprotected tube lumen is likely to be contaminated with bacteria found in the upper airways, BAL is used primarily for cytological examination of nonseptic conditions. It is especially helpful when a diagnosis of diffuse lower airway inflammation, such as in asthma or exercise-induced pulmonary hemorrhage (EIPH), is sought. The strength of BAL interpretation depends on the assumption that the pulmonary pathology is diffuse in nature rather than localized. In cases of pleuropneumonia, the lesions may be localized to one area of the lungs, thus BAL samples obtained from areas other than the affected bronchus may not be representative of the lung pathology and fail to detect cytological abnormalities. In addition, the area of lung lavaged depends greatly on the outer diameter of the bronchoscope. The use of a very small bronchoscope or a catheter passed through the lavage channel results in sampling of a small area of alveoli and bronchioles since wedging occurs in a peripheral bronchiole.

20.2.2.2 Tracheal Wash

A TW may be performed during endoscopic evaluation (e.g., prior to BAL) or with a transtracheal approach, which provides a sterile sample that can be used for culture. A sterile catheter is passed through a cannula or large hypodermic needle previously inserted between tracheal rings in the tracheal lumen. Once the catheter reaches the tracheal bifurcation, 10–30 mL of fluid are infused and rapidly reaspirated [19]. The major indication for TW compared to BAL is a suspected bacterial respiratory process since the sample is collected in a sterile fashion and can be submitted for culture. The association between TW neutrophilic inflammation and cough is acknowledged but historically, TW has been considered less sensitive and specific than BAL in detecting inflammation of peripheral airways [9, 10, 13, 20]. There is good agreement between BAL cytology and histopathology results, whereas cytology of BAL and TW correlate poorly [21–23]. Most established reference intervals for cell differentials refer to BAL samples. However, a recent study found that TW and BAL neutrophil percentages correlated well and suggested that TW may actually be more sensitive and specific than BAL in detecting neutrophilic airway inflammation [24].

20.2.3 Sample Processing

Bronchoalveolar lavage and TW fluid can be placed in either glass or EDTA tubes to avoid clotting if there is blood contamination, and should be refrigerated if immediate processing is not possible [10, 25]. In general, the use of additives should be avoided but if refrigeration is not possible, 40% ethanol at a ratio of 1:1 can be added to the sample in case of delayed processing. Formalin can be used but would likely cause a greater alteration of cell morphology. For fixated samples, best results are obtained through staining with hematoxylin and eosin, Papanicolaou, or Sano's modification of Pollack trichrome [25]. If the sample is to be sent to an external laboratory, sediment or direct smears should be prepared and submitted for evaluation along with the fluid. This may help the clinical pathologist distinguish between *in vivo* and *in vitro* changes (e.g., neutrophil degeneration versus aging; bacterial infection versus contamination and overgrowth). BAL and TW samples are diluted by the saline used during sample collection, so usually contain low numbers of cells and a low concentration of protein. Cells tend to rupture more easily in low-protein samples. For this reason, some authors recommend adding one or two drops of serum or commercial bovine serum albumin to the pellet obtained by centrifugation in order to obtain higher numbers of viable cells.

Bronchoalveolar lavage and TW sample processing include macroscopic evaluation, cell count, and the preparation of slides of the cytocentrifuged fluid and/or sediment smears. Normal fluid should appear clear or mildly turbid. BAL samples can contain a layer of foamy surfactant indicating that the alveoli have been sampled. Presence of flocculent material instead of foamy surfactant reflects mucus and cellular debris. The fluid may appear pink-red or yellow-brown in cases of recent or chronic hemorrhage, respectively.

Direct smears may be helpful if the fluid contains visible aggregates of mucus that can be smeared directly onto a slide for cytological evaluation. In our experience, this can increase the possibility of finding larvae, eggs, or aggregates of eosinophils entrapped within mucus. Due to the overall low cellularity of BAL and TW fluids, concentration of the sample is advised and can be performed through centrifugation of the fluid at 300 g for 10 minutes and smearing of the pellet obtained after removal of the supernatant. In direct and sedimented smears, cells tend to be rounder, smaller, and darker, making their morphological classification more difficult.

Cytocentrifugation is associated with significantly higher percentages of macrophages, mast cells, and eosinophils but lower lymphocyte counts compared to direct smear preparation, so reference intervals specific for the method used should be adopted [26]. Slides are then rapidly dried before staining to avoid cell crenation using a fan or manually by waving the slides in the air. Wright–Giemsa and May–Grunwald–Giemsa are superior in detecting mast cells compared to quick aqueous Romanowsky stains (e.g., Diff-Quik®, Baxter Scientific Products). If Diff-Quik is used, an additional slide should be stained with toluidine blue for more sensitive mast cell enumeration [27].

The cell count can be performed using an automated analyzer or a hemacytometer. Nucleated cell counts represent an estimate of the true cellularity within airway secretions; the accuracy and precision of the count are limited by the variability of the volume infused and fluid retrieved. The automated count may underestimate the cell count if cell size variation exceeds the window setting of the instrument. Both automated and manual counts are markedly affected by the presence of cell aggregation within the sample. For these reasons, the total cell count is not performed in our laboratory although reference intervals for BAL from healthy horses have been published, with reported cell counts lower than 1000 cells/μLfor healthy horses in most studies (Table 20.1) [19].

In most laboratories, the leukocyte differential is performed by counting a minimum of 400 nucleated cells. In one study, Fernandez et al. [40] demonstrated that this method is adequate for counting neutrophils, macrophages, and lymphocytes, while the reliability for mast cells and eosinophils was acceptable only when using a method in which five microscopic fields with high cellular density (more than 100 cells) were evaluated at high magnification (50× objective). Epithelial cells often tend to aggregate unevenly throughout the slide. For this reason, in our laboratory a leukocyte differential count is reported instead of a nucleated cell differential count.

Table 20.1 Reference values (mean ± SD) for TW and BAL in asymptomatic horses.

					Differential cell count (%)					
	Reference	No. of horses	Vol of saline (mL)	TNCC (× 10^6/L)	Neutro	Eos	Lymph	Macro	Mast	EC
BAL	[37]	10	300	182 ± 578	8.9 ± 3.8	< 1.0	43.0 ± 8.5	45.0 ± 8.8	1.2 ± 0.9	3.5 ± 2.2
	[28]	11	120	ND	7.0 ± 3.3	0.0 ± 0.0	28.0 ± 5.8	65.0 ± 6.2	0.2 ± 0.6	ND
	[29]	62	65	832 ± 578	8.8 ± 6.4	0.5 ± 3.1	31.3 ± 9.3	59.0 ± 9.7	ND	0.4 ± 0.8
	[11]	6	300	153 ± 17	3.8 ± 0.7	1.2 ± 2.0	28.3 ± 2.9	64.8 ± 11.2	0.3 ± 0.7	ND
	[30]	10	200	92.1 ± 142	5.9 ± 4.6	0.5 ± 0.9	36.7 ± 14.8	56.0 ± 13.0	ND	ND
	[31]	10	250	445 ± 142	3.8 ± 5.5	2.0 ± 1.0	22.9 ± 7.4	68.8 ± 8.8	1.5 ± 0.3	ND
	[32]	9	250	321 ± 100	6.8 ± 2.7	0.3 ± 0.5	31.4 ± 13.0	57.1 ± 10.3	1.5 ± 0.8	ND
	[10] (pasture)	14	300	94 ± 47	3.6 ± 3.5	0.7 ± 1.7	42.6 ± 11.5	41.0 ± 10.8	6.6 ± 5.1	8.1 ± 6.5
	[10] (stable)	14	300	89 ± 39	10.3 ± 8.1	1.2 ± 2.2	37.0 ± 9.8	41.4 ± 9.7	4.4 ± 3.9	8.4 ± 9.0
	[33]	14	120	517 ± 229	15.1 ± 2.8	0.0 ± 0.0	26.2 ± 6.5	50.2 ± 10.4	2.1 ± 1.4	3.4 ± 5.4
	[34]	26	ND	105 ± 40	9.1 ± 7.9	1.3 ± 5.1	33.9 ± 8.3	47.8 ± 10.3	5.0 ± 2.7	3.8 ± 2.5
	[23]	15	500	ND	2.5 ± 1.5	0.6 ± 0.7	44.2 ± 12.5	49.4 ± 9.5	1.2 ± 0.5	ND
	[19]	15	250	255 ± 81	5.1 ± 2.0	0.3 ± 0.5	20.4 ± 9.9	61.9 ± 16.9	0.6 ± 0.5	0.0 ± 0.0
	[35]	5	500	150 ± 20	8.5 ± 6.7	0.1 ± 0.0	52.3 ± 3.9	37.6 ± 3.9	1.5 ± 0.2	6.1 ± 1.5
	[36] (endoscopy)	42	30	ND	4.6 ± 4.9	0.7 ± 0.4	2.2 ± 2.4	43.0 ± 10.7	0.1 ± 0.2	49.1 ± 11.5
TW	[36] (transtrach)	15	30	ND	6.4 ± 5.5	1.2 ± 1.4	7.4 ± 3.8	65.0 ± 13.7	0.2 ± 0.4	19.8 ± 6.1
	[37]	10	20	ND	32.0 ± 28.1	<1.0	8.2 ± 6.0	24.0 ± 12.7	ND	34.0 ± 20.9
	[38]	66	20	ND	17.8 ± 21.8	0.7 ± 2.2	5.4 ± 4.1	44.1 ± 23.2	0.1 ± 0.2	34.0 ± 24.4
	[39]	9	20	ND	10 ± 10.8	1.9 ± 1.2	13.0 ± 3.6	74.2 ± 11.1	ND	ND
	[19]	12	30	ND	9.3 ± 4.9	0.2 ± 0.6	9.3 ± 5.8	79.6 ± 8.2	0.0 ± 0.0	ND

TW, tracheal wash; BAL, bronchoalveolar lavage; Neutro, neutrophils; Eos, eosinophils; Lymph, lymphocytes; Macro, macrophages; Mast, mast cells; EC, epithelial cells; ND, not determined.
Source: Adapted from [19].

20.2.4 Normal Findings

20.2.4.1 Cellular Elements

Cells present in respiratory fluid include epithelial cells, macrophages, small lymphocytes, neutrophils, eosinophils, and mast cells. BAL fluid samples from healthy animals are predominantly composed of macrophages and small lymphocytes admixed with only rare neutrophils. However, the first aliquot aspirated, especially if only a small amount of fluid is instilled, may contain a higher percentage of neutrophils due to bronchial sampling.

Reference intervals for BAL fluid are published (Table 20.1) [19]. In general, based on published references using an infusion volume of 250 mL, BAL samples from clinically healthy horses should contain 50–70% macrophages, 30–50% small lymphocytes, <5% neutrophils, <2% mast cells, and <1% eosinophils. The macrophage and lymphocyte percentages have been shown to decrease and increase with age, respectively [41–43]. In a recent study by Hostetter et al. [41], mast cell and eosinophil percentages also tended to increase slightly with age but the difference was not statistically significant. Epithelial cells, usually present in small numbers, may include a few nonciliated bronchial epithelial and goblet cells, but only rare ciliated epithelial cells [10, 44]. Predominance of epithelial cells in a BAL fluid with low numbers of leukocytes may indicate poor technique with inadequate sampling of the alveolar space (Figure 20.5). Goblet cells are nonciliated columnar to pyriform cells with a basally located nucleus and moderate to abundant cytoplasm with many round magenta mucin granules in the apical region (Figure 20.6). Goblet cells produce mucus and may be seen in increased numbers with chronic pulmonary irritation.

There are no accepted published reference intervals for TW differential leukocyte counts, although higher percentages of neutrophils (up to 20%) are normally seen compared to BAL cytology (Table 20.1) [16, 17, 44, 45]. Similarly, there are no published reference intervals for the differential

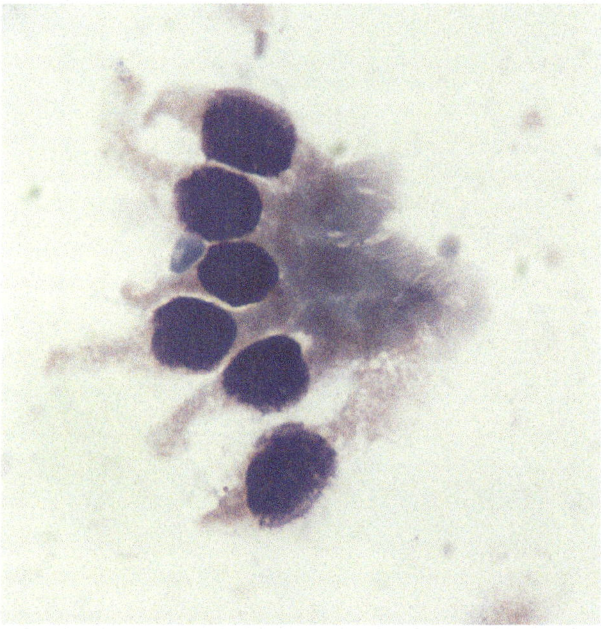

Figure 20.5 Cytocentrifuged BAL preparation. Ciliated columnar epithelial cells. In a BAL, low cellularity and predominance of ciliated epithelial cells may indicate poor technique with inadequate sampling of the alveolar space.

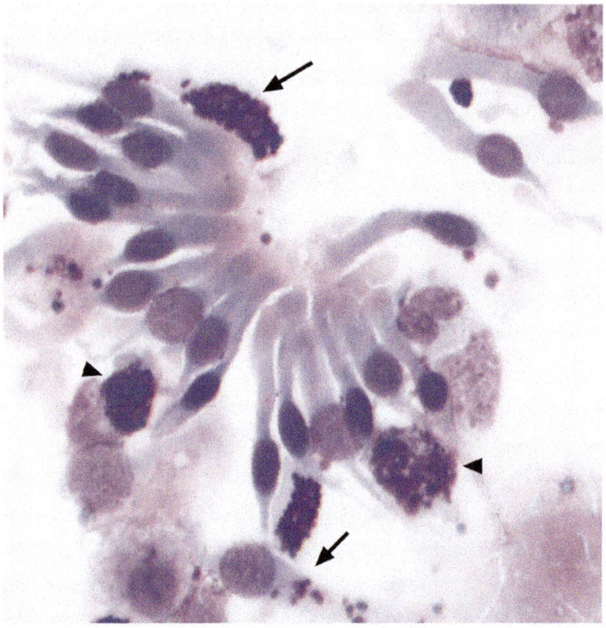

Figure 20.6 Ciliated columnar respiratory epithelial cells with admixed goblet cells (*arrows*) in a transtracheal wash. The apical portion of goblet cells containing mucin granules may break off and round up, mimicking a mast cell (*arrowheads*).

cell counts of BAL and TW obtained from foals. Based on old references, TW of healthy foals have a higher number of eosinophils, inflammatory cells, and mast cells than those of adults [46].

20.2.4.2 Acellular Elements

Bronchoalveolar lavage and TW typically contain some mucus, which appears as finely stippled to streaming, pink to lavender material in the background of the slide. Mucus can also form tight spirals called Curschmann's spirals (Figure 20.7), which are said to represent plugs of inspissated mucus that form within small bronchioles. However, Curschmann's spirals can be present in any sample with abundant mucus, including nasal washes, as a result of persistently increased mucus production or reduced mucus clearance. Occasionally, coarse round magenta granules (typically 1.5 μm in diameter) resulting from rupture of goblet cells may be present free in the background and entrapped within mucus. Occasionally, the apical portion of goblet cells can detach from the basal portion and nucleus, releasing round cytoplasmic fragments filled with magenta granules that resemble mast cells (Figure 20.6).

Free cilia or the ciliated apical portion of respiratory epithelial cells may be noted. This finding can be artefactual or represent ciliocytophthoria. This term was introduced in 1956 by Papanicolaou to indicate a severe lesion of the columnar epithelial cell characterized by the detachment of the apical portion of the cytoplasm containing cilia from the remainder of the cell. The process was originally associated with viral infections but later was observed with other diseases and lost pathognomonic significance.

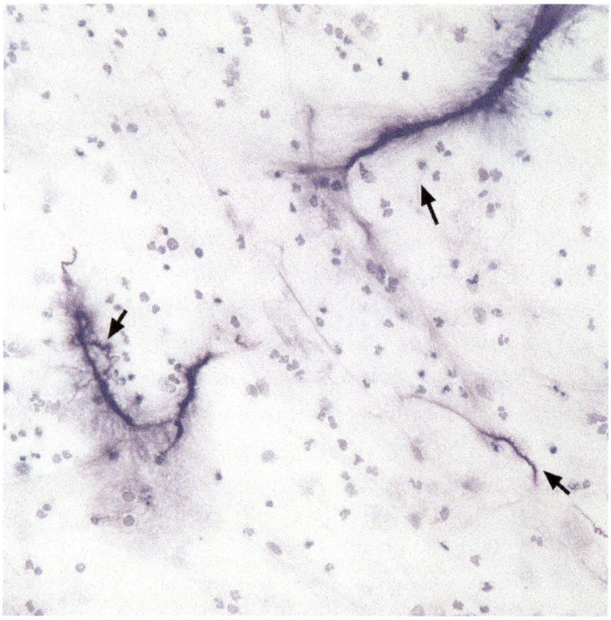

Figure 20.7 Tracheal wash from horse with IAD. Three Curschmann's spirals (*arrows*) are present in this field. The background contains numerous variably preserved neutrophils and streaming eosinophilic mucus.

20.2.4.3 Contaminants

Foreign materials can be found in BAL and TW fluids due to contamination during or after sample collection (e.g., oropharyngeal contamination, starch granules from gloves), but they may also represent inhalants from the environment. The latter include pollen, elements of saprophytic fungi such as *Alternaria* species, carbonaceous material (e.g., due to pollution or smoke inhalation), and silica crystals [47]. BAL cytology is considered a window on the environment of the horse and the frequency of mold spores is an indicator of particulate exposure from forage [10]. Inhalants are often noted within the cytoplasm of macrophages and multinucleated cells as a result of phagocytosis (Figure 20.8), while procedural contaminants are usually extracellular (provided that the sample has been processed immediately).

Oropharyngeal material that may be seen in BAL and TW includes squamous epithelial cells and various types of bacteria, often adherent to the squamous cell surface. *Simonsiella* bacteria are normal inhabitants of the oral cavity that divide lengthwise, forming large colonies that appear as a single large cigar-shaped organism with parallel light and dark stripes (Figure 20.9) [47]. The presence of oropharyngeal material may just reflect procedural contamination from the mouth, nasal passages, or oropharynx or it may reflect the horse having aspirated oropharyngeal contents into the airway (especially if associated with neutrophilic inflammation).

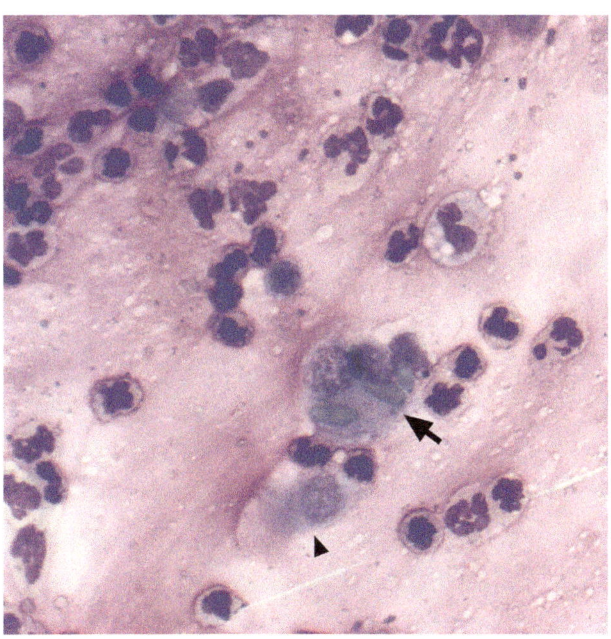

Figure 20.8 Neutrophils, few macrophages, and a nonciliated columnar epithelial cell (*arrowhead*) amid a pink background of mucus in a BAL from a horse; note the green fungal elements (likely barn inhalants) phagocytized by a macrophage (*arrow*).

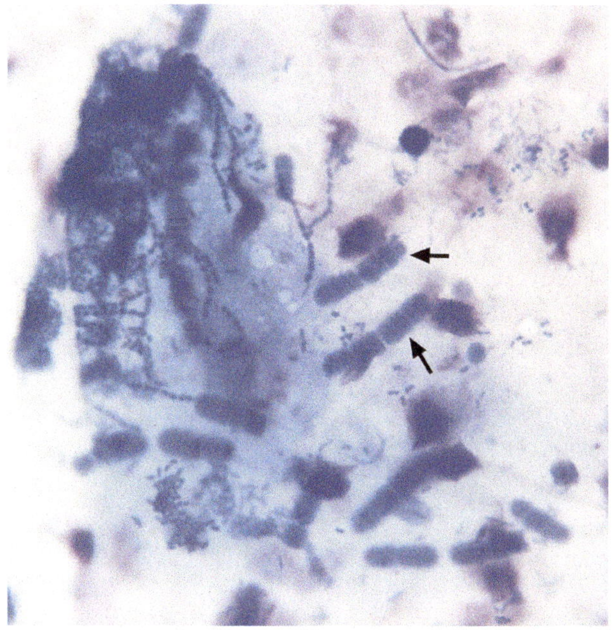

Figure 20.9 Transtracheal wash. Squamous epithelial cell with adherent *Simonsiella* (*arrows*) and other mixed bacterial bacilli. This horse coughed during acquisition of the sample, causing the catheter to become displaced into the oropharynx.

20.2.5 Interpretation of Cytological Patterns

20.2.5.1 Neutrophilic Inflammation

Neutrophils are rare in BAL samples from healthy horses (typically <5% of total nucleated cells) and an increased proportion indicates suppurative (neutrophilic) inflammation. Suppurative inflammation is generally considered an acute process, but it may also persist for a long time when there is an active stimulus. Neutrophilic inflammation can be seen with septic and nonseptic causes. In septic exudates, neutrophils tend to show degenerative changes such as nuclear swelling and cytoplasmic vacuolation or may appear necrotic. However, evaluation of cell morphology is not considered highly reliable in raising suspicion for a bacterial etiology in BAL and TW fluids because degenerative changes can also occur secondary to collection and handling. Conversely, a well-preserved neutrophil morphology does not rule out a septic process. Samples characterized by neutrophilic predominance should be cultured to rule out infection. Since any microbes detected usually belong to the normal flora of the upper airway, isolation of bacteria in TW may represent infection, transient lower airway colonization, or contamination of the sample [19].

20.2.5.1.1 Septic Etiologies Septic suppurative inflammation may be due to bacterial, fungal (e.g., *Aspergillus* spp.) or, less commonly, viral infection. Often bacteria may be found by microscopic examination of cytological samples and the presence of intracellular bacteria within neutrophils (or, less commonly, macrophages) is strongly supportive of infection as opposed to contamination, provided that the sample has been processed quickly (ideally within 30 minutes, since phagocytosis can also occur *in vitro*).

Bacteria found in BAL may include rod-shaped bacilli, round cocci, or microorganisms with a more distinctive morphology, such as *Rhodococcus equi*. *R. equi* organisms are small and pleomorphic, similar to watermelon seeds, rod-shaped to coccoid, with a thin peripheral halo (Figure 20.10). *R. equi*, a gram-positive facultative intracellular pathogen, is one of the most common causes of pneumonia in foals. This microorganism has the ability to survive and replicate within macrophages by suppression of phagosome–lysosome fusion or phagolysosome acidification [48, 49]. This pathogen can be seen cytologically within both neutrophil and macrophage phagosomes [35]. In one study [50], BAL cytology had higher neutrophil percentages in foals with *R. equi* infection compared to other bacterial etiologies.

The diagnosis of bronchopneumonia caused by *R. equi* should be confirmed on bacteriological culture or by amplification of the vapA gene using polymerase chain reaction (PCR) from a tracheobronchial sample. Amplification of vapA using PCR may be done in conjunction with (but should not replace) bacterial culture because it does not permit identification of other bacterial pathogens or antimicrobial susceptibility testing of *R. equi* isolates. The use of PCR assays based on genes other than vapA is not recommended as these assays would also detect environmental isolates lacking the virulence plasmid, which are not known to cause disease in foals. Both tests may have false-positive and false-negative results, thus culture or PCR amplification of *R. equi* from tracheobronchial fluid should be interpreted in the context of cytological and clinical findings. In addition, detection of *R. equi* from a foal without clinical signs of respiratory disease, cytological evidence of septic airway inflammation, or ultrasonographic or radiographic evidence of pulmonary lesions may be an incidental finding [51].

A severe neutrophilic inflammation, often associated with oropharyngeal elements, characterizes BAL fluids obtained from horses with aspiration pneumonia. A secondary bacterial infection, often mixed, is a common sequelum, thus intracellular bacteria may be found and bacterial culture and sensitivity testing are indicated.

Less often, suppurative inflammation can be due to fungal infections, which are usually secondary to immunosuppression or associated with other severe pulmonary and extrapulmonary diseases [52]. Fungal infections may be due to opportunistic fungi, such as *Aspergillus* and *Pneumocystis* spp., or more rarely caused by systemic yeasts, including *C. immitis*, *Histoplasma capsulatum*, *Blastomyces dermatitidis*, and *Cr. neoformans*. The most common fungal pathogen identified in the lower respiratory tract of horses is *Aspergillus* (Figure 20.11), but other etiologies are possible, including *Penicillium*, *Mucor*, and *Acremonium* spp.

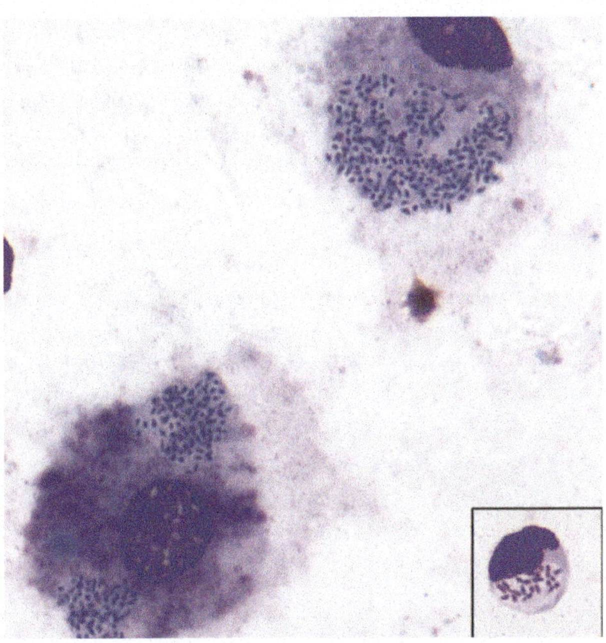

Figure 20.10 Small and pleomorphic, *Rhodococcus equi* coccobacilli are present within lysosomes in macrophages and a moderately degenerate neutrophil (*inset*).

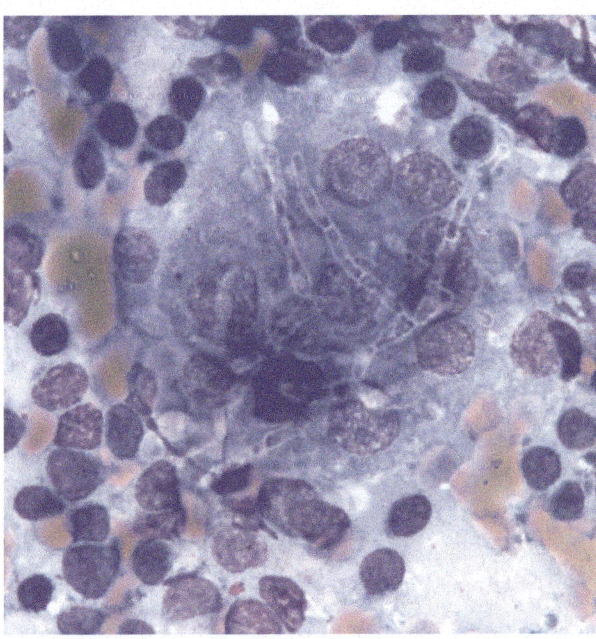

Figure 20.11 A multinucleated giant cell containing septated, branching fungal hyphae surrounded by a mixed neutrophilic and histiocytic inflammation in a TW from a horse with pulmonary aspergillosis. Modified Wright–Giemsa stain.

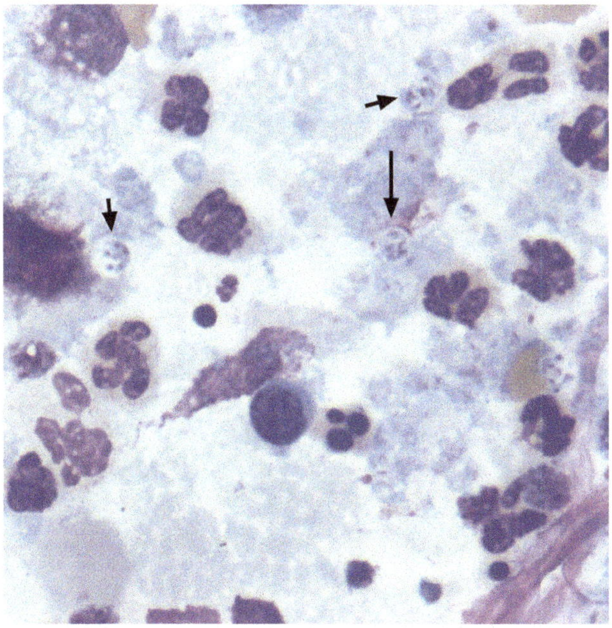

Figure 20.12 Neutrophils and a foamy macrophage amid a background of blue-gray material and chromatin debris in a sediment smear of BAL fluid from an Arabian foal with *Pneumocystis jirovecii* infection. Several cysts with up to eight internal spores are present extracellularly (*arrows*).

[53]. Cytology does not permit reliable identification of the specific fungus, so culture or fungal-specific PCR is required. However, fungal culture results should always be interpreted in light of BAL or TW cytologies because opportunistic fungi can also be cultured in a small percentage of TW samples collected from healthy horses [38].

Pneumocystis carinii is an opportunistic fungal pulmonary pathogen that can cause pneumonia in immunosuppressed foals or secondary to bacterial infection. *Pneumocystis* has a complete life cycle within alveoli that includes cyst and trophozoite forms. Cysts are round, measure 5–10 µm and contain up to eight intracystic bodies (Figure 20.12). Trophozoites are small (2–3 µm in length), pyriform to elongated, light staining, and difficult to distinguish from cellular debris. The associated inflammatory response can be suppurative, predominantly histiocytic, or mixed. *P. carinii* was long thought to be a protozoal organism based on the presumption that cystic and trophic forms represented distinctive phases of a protozoan life cycle and on its sensitivity to antiprotozoal drugs. However, mounting evidence, including the identification of genetic sequence homologies with fungi, led to the recategorization of this pathogen as a fungus, and its renaming as *Pneumocystis jirovecii*.

20.2.5.1.2 Nonseptic Etiologies The most common causes of poor performance and nonseptic airway inflammation, formerly known as RAO and inflammatory airway disease (IAD), are now considered two phenotypes of the same syndrome and, in the current literature, preferably indicated with the terms mild to moderate (IAD) and severe (RAO) equine asthma [54–56]. In this chapter, the new terminology has been adopted, but the old terms are maintained in brackets as used in most of the references and because readers may not be familiar with the new terms.

Severe asthma (RAO) is a common condition in stabled mature and old horses, which accounts for over 50% of all respiratory cases referred and has a reported prevalence of 10–20% in regions with cold or temperate climates [57, 58]. The disease is characterized by variable recurring airflow obstruction, increased mucus, bronchial hyperresponsiveness, and airway inflammation resulting in increased respiratory efforts at rest, coughing, and exercise intolerance. Clinical signs are triggered in susceptible horses by inhalation of dust particles, aerosolized allergens, and endotoxins that are present in stables, especially those associated with hay feeding. Severe asthma (RAO) likely results from complex interactions between innate and acquired immune responses, the environment, and genetic susceptibility [59]. It is characterized by increased mucus and neutrophilia (>25% neutrophils) in respiratory fluids, with the percentage of neutrophils in the BAL usually increasing with the severity of the condition [36, 56].

Mild to moderate asthma (IAD) is also characterized by poor performance, cough, and variably increased mucus but, in contrast to severe asthma (RAO), horses of any age may be affected and clinical signs at rest are usually subtle [9]. The pathogenesis of mild to moderate asthma (IAD) is still poorly defined, but environmental and stable factors may be involved [9]. BAL fluids from horses with mild to moderate asthma (IAD) are characterized by increased total nucleated cell count with mild neutrophilia (>5%), lymphocytosis, and monocytosis. BAL mastocytosis (>2%) and eosinophilia (>1%) are also compatible with a diagnosis of mild to moderate asthma (IAD). These thresholds for neutrophils and mast cells were found to be performance relevant in a recent study by Ivester et al. [60]. However, the lack of a standardized technique used to acquire, process, and analyze BAL samples and the intra- and interobserver variability for cell counting (especially for mast cell and eosinophils) may limit the reliability of these cut-off values in different clinical settings.

Cytological findings should always be interpreted in combination with the history, clinical examination, and endoscopic findings. Severe cases of asthma (RAO) may have clinical signs similar to chronic pneumonia, and early stages of severe asthma (RAO) may be difficult to distinguish from mild to moderate asthma (IAD) and other respiratory causes of poor performance. A neutrophilic inflammatory component is common to all these diseases. However, BAL neutrophilia is usually less pronounced with mild to moderate asthma (IAD) (<20%) compared to severe asthma (RAO) (>25%). In addition, increased respiratory effort at rest is present in severe (RAO), but not in mild to moderate (IAD), asthma. Signs of systemic inflammation observed in cases of pneumonia, such as fever and leukocytosis, are usually lacking in equine asthma [56].

20.2.5.2 Mixed Neutrophilic and Histiocytic Inflammation

All the aforementioned diseases can also elicit a histiocytic inflammatory component, which can predominate in chronic phases or with specific etiological agents (e.g., some fungi). Alveolar macrophages are resident within the alveoli and they constitute the main cell type in BAL fluids from healthy horses. Thus, increases in macrophages due to proliferation or recruitment from peripheral blood monocytes secondary to inflammation are difficult to recognize, especially if there is a concurrent increase in neutrophils. Assessment of the overall cellularity or phagocytized pathogens may help in these cases.

20.2.5.3 Eosinophilic and Mastocytic Inflammation

The differential diagnosis for eosinophilic inflammation includes migrating parasite larvae (e.g., *Dictyocaulus arnfieldi*) and allergic bronchitis. Hypersensitivity seems to be involved in the pathogenesis of both mild to moderate (IAD) and severe (RAO) asthma. Thus, an increase in eosinophil and mast cell percentages in BAL fluids may be expected in both conditions, although eosinophilia and mastocytosis seem to be described in mild to moderate (IAD) more often than in severe (RAO) asthma, and are currently not included in the proposed systems for severe asthma (RAO) diagnosis and staging [9, 58].

Eosinophils may be focally distributed and are often entrapped in mucus, so careful examination of the entire smear may be required to find concentrations of eosinophils (Figure 20.13). It should be noted that in some samples mast cell granules do not stain with aqueous-based Romanovsky stains (e.g., Diff-Quik), whereas eosinophil granules stain similarly with either methanol or aqueous-based Romanovsky stains. The interobserver agreement for mast cells enumeration is below acceptable limits although a slight improvement can be achieved using toluidine blue [27]. When evaluating BAL or TW cytologies, care should also be taken to avoid confusing fragments of goblet cell cytoplasm with mast cells. As mentioned previously, the apical portion of goblet cells can detach from the basal portion and nucleus, releasing round cytoplasmic fragments filled with magenta granules (see Figure 20.6). Like mast cell granules, goblet cell granules are metachromatic. The two can be distinguished based on the more globular appearance of goblet cell granules and absence of a discernible nucleus.

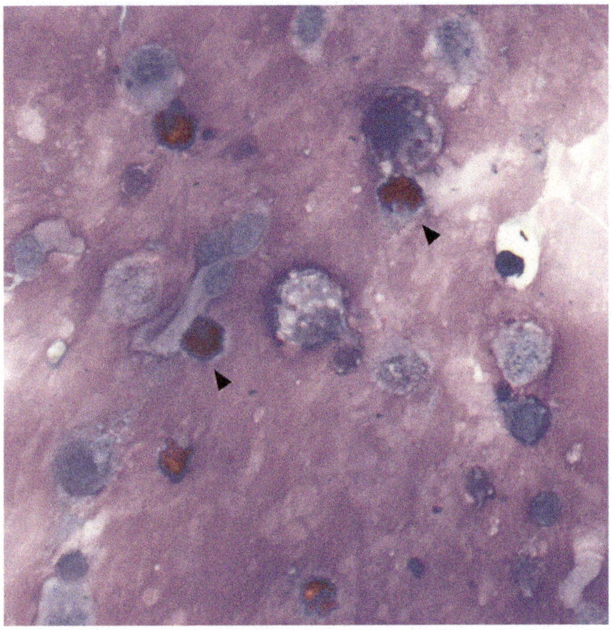

Figure 20.13 Eosinophils (*arrowheads*) and macrophages admixed with few columnar epithelial cells amid a background of abundant mucus in a sediment smear preparation of BAL fluid.

20.2.5.4 Hemorrhage

The presence of hemosiderin- or hematoidin-laden macrophages indicates previous hemorrhage into the airways. The presence of erythrophagocytosis indicates more recent hemorrhage. Staining cytocentrifuged slides with Perl's Prussian blue facilitates the detection of hemosiderophages (Figure 20.14). The primary causes of hemosiderophages in BAL and TW fluids are EIPH, inhalation of blood due to epistaxis, and bleeding from an ulcerated neoplasm within the respiratory system. The presence of erythrocytes in TW and BAL fluids can also be a consequence of trauma caused by the bronchoscopy or fluid collection procedure.

20.2.5.4.1 Exercise-Induced Pulmonary Hemorrhage Exercise-induced pulmonary hemorrhage occurs as a consequence of strenuous exercise and is a common cause of poor performance in racehorses [61]. While no clinical or laboratory gold standard method has been established, in the most recent consensus statement [62] EIPH is defined as the presence of

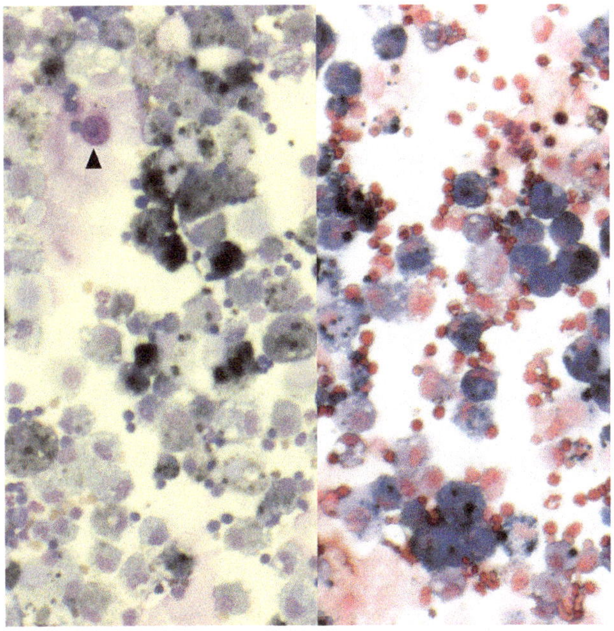

Figure 20.14 Cytocentrifuged preparation of BAL fluid from a horse with EIPH. (*Left panel*) Macrophages, small lymphocytes, occasional neutrophils, and a mast cell (*arrowhead*) amid a background of few erythrocytes. Note that most macrophages contain scant to abundant dark green to black pigment consistent with hemosiderin (hemosiderophages). Modified Wright–Giemsa stain. (*Right panel*) Most macrophages contain bright blue to black staining material consistent with hemosiderin. Prussian blue stain.

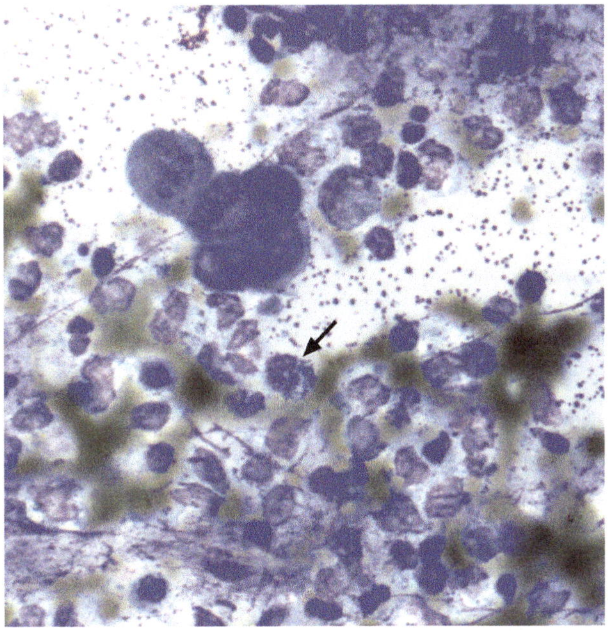

Figure 20.15 Sediment preparation of BAL fluid from a horse with septic suppurative inflammation. A cluster of atypical epithelial cells admixed with degenerate neutrophils and few small lymphocytes amid a background of chromatin debris (pink granular to linear material) and many erythrocytes. Small bacterial cocci in short chains are seen within the cytoplasm of degenerate neutrophils (*arrow*). Epithelial cells are mildly pleomorphic, with low cuboidal to round shape, increased nuclear to cytoplasmic ratio, immature chromatin, prominent nucleoli, and moderate anisocytosis and anisokaryosis. These features are interpreted as hyperplasia and dysplasia secondary to the inflammatory process.

blood detected by tracheobronchoscopic examination, or by enumeration of red blood cells or hemosiderophages in tracheal aspirates or BAL fluid. Cytology has probably higher sensitivity compared to tracheobronchoscopy, especially if the latter is not performed immediately after strenuous training exercise or racing, but the concentration of erythrocytes or macrophages containing erythrocytes in BAL fluid that is clinically relevant has not been determined. A cut-off of >1000 RBCs/μL has been used by Gold et al. [63] in a recent study, while Newton and Wood [64] used a cut-off point of >50% hemosiderophages as a second criterion in the diagnosis of EIPH to overcome the risk of underestimating EIPH by using solely the evidence of blood on endoscopy. A total hemosiderin scoring (THS) system based on scoring 300 macrophages by their hemosiderin content was assessed in one study [65] and found to be promising, but this method is not currently used in a routine diagnostic setting as it is very time-consuming.

20.2.5.5 Cellular Atypia

Bronchoalveolar lavage and TW samples may occasionally contain a few clusters of epithelial cells with a cuboidal rather than columnar shape, increased cytoplasmic basophilia, increased nuclear to cytoplasmic ratio, and some degree of anisocytosis (Figure 20.15). When associated with the presence of inflammatory cells, these findings are usually interpreted as respiratory epithelial cell hyperplasia and dysplasia secondary to chronic irritation. If marked atypia is present (e.g., pleomorphism, prominent multiple nucleoli or marked anisocytosis), an epithelial neoplasm may be suspected. However, primary lung tumors are rare in horses and difficult to diagnose on BAL and TW cytology unless the neoplasm has extensively invaded trachea, bronchi, and bronchioli.

Other nonepithelial primary and metastatic lung neoplasms reported in horses include pulmonary granular cell tumor, pulmonary chondrosarcoma, bronchial myxoma, malignant melanoma, and fibrosarcoma amongst others. Neoplastic cells from these neoplasms do not tend to exfoliate easily in respiratory fluids and in cases of suspected pulmonary neoplasia, percutaneous lung aspirates or biopsy is preferable.

References

1 Hoffman, A.M. and Viel, L. (1997). Techniques for sampling the respiratory tract of horses. *Vet. Clin. North Am. Equine Pract.* 13: 463–475.

2 Gergeleit, H., Bienert-Zeit, A., Seemann-Jensen, A. et al. (2019). Cytological examination of secretions from the paranasal sinuses in horses. *J. Equine Vet. Sci.* 78: 60–68.

3 Mair, T.S. (2010). Respiratory diseases. In: *Diagnostic Techniques in Equine Medicine*, 2e (eds. F.G.R. Taylor, T.J. Brazil and M.H. Hillyer), 217–248. St Louis: Saunders Elsevier.

4 Stewart, A.J. and Cuming, R.S. (2015). Update on fungal respiratory disease in horses. *Vet. Clin. North Am. Equine* 31: 43–62.

5 Schöniger, S., Roschanski, N., Rösler, U. et al. (2016). *Prototheca* species and *Pithomyces chartarum* as causative agents of rhinitis and/or sinusitis in horses. *J. Comp. Pathol.* 155: 121–125.

6 Tremaine, W.H. and Freeman, D.E. (2007). Disorders of the paranasal sinuses. In: *Equine Respiratory Medicine and Surgery* (eds. B.C. McGorum, P.M. Dixon, N.E. Robinson and J. Schumacher), 403–404. Philadelphia: Saunders Elsevier.

7 Leeming, G., Smith, K.C., Bestbier, M.K. et al. (2007). Equine rhinosporidiosis in United Kingdom. *Emerg. Infect. Dis.* 13: 1377–1379.

8 Head, K.W. and Dixon, P.M. (1999). Equine nasal and paranasal sinus tumours. Part 1: review of the literature and tumour classification. *Vet. J.* 157: 261–279.

9 Couëtil, L.L., Hoffman, A.M., Hodgson, J. et al. (2007). Inflammatory airway disease of horses. *J. Vet. Intern. Med.* 21: 356–361.

10 Hoffman, A.M. (2008). Bronchoalveolar lavage: sampling technique and guidelines for cytologic preparation and interpretation. *Vet. Clin. North Am. Equine Pract.* 24: 423–435.

11 Miskovic, M., Couëtil, L.L., and Thompson Hoffman, C.A. (2007). Lung function and airway cytologic profiles in horses with recurrent airway obstruction maintained in low-dust environments. *J. Vet. Intern. Med.* 21: 1060–1066.

12 Orard, M., Depecker, M., Hue, E. et al. (2016). Influence of bronchoalveolar lavage volume on cytological profiles and subsequent diagnosis of inflammatory airway disease in horses. *Vet. J.* 207: 193–195.

13 Jean, D., Vrins, A., Beauchamp, G. et al. (2011). Evaluation of variations in bronchoalveolar lavage fluid in horses with recurrent airway obstruction. *Am. J. Vet. Res.* 72: 838–842.

14 Mair, T.S., Stokes, C.R., and Burne, F.J. (1987). Cellular content of secretions obtained by lavage from different levels of the equine respiratory tract. *Equine Vet. J.* 19: 458–462.

15 Pickles, K., Pirie, R.S., Rhind, S. et al. (2002). Cytological analysis of equine bronchoalveolar lavage fluid. Part 1: comparison of sequential and pooled aliquots. *Equine Vet. J.* 34: 288–291.

16 Sweeney, C.R., Humber, K.A., and Roby, K.A. (1992). Cytologic findings of tracheobronchial aspirates from 66 thoroughbred racehorses. *Am. J. Vet. Res.* 53: 1172–1175.

17 Sweeney, C.R., Rossier, Y., Ziemer, E.L. et al. (1992). Effects of lung site and fluid volume on results of bronchoalveolar lavage fluid analysis in horses. *Am. J. Vet. Res.* 53: 1376–1379.

18 Depecker, M., Richard, E.A., Pitel, P.-H. et al. (2014). Bronchoalveolar lavage fluid in Standardbred racehorses: influence of unilateral/bilateral profiles and cut-off values on lower airway disease diagnosis. *Vet. J.* 199: 150–156.

19 Richard, E.A., Fortier, G.D., Lekeux, P.M. et al. (2010). Laboratory findings in respiratory fluids of the poorly-performing horse. *Vet. J.* 185: 115–122.

20 Christley, R.M., Hodgson, D.R., Rose, R.J. et al. (1996). Coughing in thoroughbred racehorses in training: the relationships between disease and viruses, bacteria and environment. *Vet. Rec.* 139: 308–313.

21 Fogarty, U. (1990). Evaluation of a bronchoalveolar lavage technique. *Equine Vet. J.* 22: 174–176.

22 Hughes, K.J., Malikides, N., Hodgson, D.R. et al. (2003). Comparison of tracheal aspirates and bronchoalveolar lavage in racehorses. 1. Evaluation of cytological stains and the percentage of mast cells and eosinophils. *Aust. Vet. J.* 81: 681–684.

23 Malikides, N., Hughes, K.J., Hodgson, D.R. et al. (2003). Comparison of tracheal aspirates and bronchoalveolar lavage in racehorses 2. Evaluation of the diagnostic significance of neutrophil percentage. *Aust. Vet. J.* 81: 685–687.

24 Rossi, H., Virtala, A.M., Raekallio, M. et al. (2018). Comparison of tracheal wash and bronchoalveolar lavage cytology in 154 horses with and without respiratory signs in a referral hospital over 2009–2015. *Front. Vet. Sci.* 5: 61.

25 Pickles, K., Pirie, R.S., Rhind, S. et al. (2002). Cytological analysis of equine bronchoalveolar lavage fluid. Part 3: the effect of time, temperature and fixatives. *Equine Vet. J.* 34: 297–301.

26 Pickles, K., Pirie, R.S., Rhind, S. et al. (2002). Cytological analysis of equine bronchoalveolar lavage fluid. Part 2: comparison of smear and cytocentrifuged preparations. *Equine Vet. J.* 34: 292–296.

27 Hansen, S., Fjeldborg, J., Hansen, A.J. et al. (2019). Reliability of cytological evaluation of mast cells from bronchoalveolar lavage fluid in horses: intraobserver agreement and mast cell identification. *Equine Vet. Educ.* epub before press, https://beva.onlinelibrary.wiley.com/doi/abs/10.1111/eve.13112.

28 Fogarty, U. and Buckley, T. (1991). Bronchoalveolar lavage findings in horses with exercise intolerance. *Equine Vet. J.* 23: 434–437.

29 Mazan, M.R., Vin, R., and Hoffman, A.M. (2005). Radiographic scoring lacks predictive value in inflammatory airway disease. *Equine Vet. J.* 37: 541–545.

30 Clark, C.K., Lester, G.D., Vetro, T. et al. (1995). Bronchoalveolar lavage in horses: effect of exercise and repeated sampling on cytology. *Aust. Vet. J.* 72: 249–252.

31 Couëtil, L.L. and Denicola, D.B. (1999). Blood gas, plasma lactate and bronchoalveolar lavage cytology analyses in racehorses with respiratory disease. *Equine Vet. J.* 30: 77–82.

32 Couëtil, L.L., Rosenthal, F.S., DeNicola, D.B. et al. (2001). Clinical signs, evaluation of bronchoalveolar lavage fluid, and assessment of pulmonary function in horses with inflammatory respiratory disease. *Am. J. Vet. Res.* 62: 538–546.

33 Courouce-Malblanc, A., Pronost, S., Fortier, G. et al. (2002). Physiological measurements and upper and lower respiratory tract evaluation in French Standardbred Trotters during a standardised exercise test on the treadmill. *Equine Vet. J. Suppl.* 34: 402–407.

34 Gerber, V., Robinson, N.E., Luethi, S. et al. (2003). Airway inflammation and mucus in two age groups of asymptomatic well-performing sport horses. *Equine Vet. J.* 35: 491–495.

35 Hylton, P.K., Rizzi, T.E., and Allison, R.W. (2006). Intracellular success: cytologic findings in an ulcerated submandibular mass from a cat. *Vet. Clin. Pathol.* 35: 345–347.

36 Leguillette, R. (2003). Recurrent airway obstruction-heaves. *Vet. Clin. North Am. Equine Pract.* 19: 63–86.

37 Derksen, F.J., Brown, C.M., Sonea, I. et al. (1989). Comparison of transtracheal aspirate and bronchoalveolar lavage cytology in 50 horses with chronic lung disease. *Equine Vet. J.* 21: 23–26.

38 Sweeney, C.R., Divers, T.J., and Benson, C.E. (1985). Anaerobic bacteria in 21 horses with pleuropneumonia. *J. Am. Vet. Med. Assoc.* 187: 721–724.

39 Christley, R.M., Hodgson, D.R., Rose, R.J. et al. (1999). Comparison of bacteriology and cytology of tracheal fluid samples collected by percutaneous transtracheal aspiration or via an endoscope using a plugged, guarded catheter. *Equine Vet. J.* 31: 197–202.

40 Fernandez, N.J., Hecker, K.G., Gilroy, C.V. et al. (2013). Reliability of 400-cell and 5-field leukocyte differential counts for equine bronchoalveolar lavage fluid. *Vet. Clin. Pathol.* 42: 92–98.

41 Hostetter, S.J., Clark, S.K., Gilbertie, J.M. et al. (2017). Age-related variation in the cellular composition of equine bronchoalveolar lavage fluid. *Vet. Clin. Pathol.* 46: 344–353.

42 Pacheco, A.P., Paradis, M.R., Hoffman, A.M. et al. (2014). Age effects on blood gas, spirometry, airway reactivity, and bronchoalveolar lavage fluid cytology in clinically healthy horses. *J. Vet. Intern. Med.* 28: 603–608.

43 Zink, M.C. and Johnson, J.A. (1984). Cellular constituents of clinically normal foal bronchoalveolar lavage fluid during postnatal maturation. *Am. J. Vet. Res.* 45: 893–897.

44 Robinson, N.E. (2003). Inflammatory airway disease: defining the syndrome. Conclusions of the Havemeyer workshop. *Equine Vet. Educ.* 15: 61–63.

45 Christley, R.M., Hodgson, D.R., Rose, R.J. et al. (2001). A case-control study of respiratory disease in thoroughbred racehorses in Sydney, Australia. *Equine Vet. J.* 33: 256–264.

46 Crane, S.A., Ziemer, E.L., and Sweeney, C.R. (1989). Cytologic and bacteriologic evaluation of tracheobronchial aspirates from clinically normal foals. *Am. J. Vet. Res.* 50: 2042–2048.

47 Zinkl, J.G. (2002). Lower respiratory tract. In: *Diagnostic Cytology and Hematology of the Horse* (eds. R.L. Cowell and R.D. Tyler), 73–86. St Louis: Mosby.

48 Fernandez-Mora, E., Polidori, M., Luhrmann, A. et al. (2005). Maturation of *R. equi*-containing vacuoles is arrested after completion of the early endosome stage. *Traffic* 6: 635–653.

49 Toyooka, K., Takai, S., and Kirikae, T. (2005). Rhodococcus equi can survive a phagolysosomal environment in macrophages by suppressing acidification of the phagolysosome. *J. Med. Microbiol.* 54: 1007–1015.

50 Vitale, V., Sgorbini, M., Cuteri, V. et al. (2019). Cytological findings in bronchoalveolar lavage fluid of foals with pneumonia caused by *Rhodococcus equi* and other bacteria. *J. Equine Vet. Sci.* 79: 9–12.

51 Giguère, S., Cohen, N.D., Keith Chaffin, M. et al. (2011). Diagnosis, treatment, control, and prevention of infections caused by Rhodococcus equi in foals. *J. Vet. Intern. Med.* 25: 1209–1220.

52 Sweeney, C.R. and Habecker, P.L. (1999). Pulmonary aspergillosis in horses: 29 cases (1974–1997). *J. Am. Vet. Med. Assoc.* 214: 808–811.

53 Pusterla, N., Holmberg, T.A., Lorenzo-Figueras, M. et al. (2005). *Acremonium strictum* pulmonary infection in a horse. *Vet. Clin. Pathol.* 34: 413–416.

54 Bond, S., Léguillette, R., Richard, E.A. et al. (2018). Equine asthma: integrative biologic relevance of a recently proposed nomenclature. *J. Vet. Intern. Med.* 32: 2088–2098.

55 Bullone, M. and Lavoie, J.-P. (2015). Asthma, 'of horses and men' – how can equine heaves help us better understand human asthma immunopathology and its functional consequences? *Mol. Immunol.* 66: 97–105.

56 Couëtil, L.L., Cardwell, J.M., Gerber, V. et al. (2016). Inflammatory airway disease of horses – revised consensus statement. *J. Vet. Intern. Med.* 30: 503–515.

57 Hotchkiss, J.W., Reid, S.W., and Cristely, R.M. (2007). A survey of horse owners in Great Britain regarding horses in their care. Part 2: risk factors for recurrent airway obstruction. *Equine Vet. J.* 39: 301–308.

58 Tilley, P., Sales Luis, J.P., and Branco, F.M. (2012). Correlation and discriminant analysis of clinical, endoscopic, thoracic X-ray and bronchoalveolar lavage fluid cytology scores, for staging horses with recurrent airway obstruction (RAO). *Res. Vet. Sci.* 93: 1006–1014.

59 Leclere, M., Lavoie-Lamoureux, A., and Lavoie, J.P. (2011). Heaves, an asthma-like disease of horses. *Respirology* 16: 1027–1046.

60 Ivester, K.M., Couëtil, L.L., and Moore, G.E. (2018). An observational study of environmental exposures, airway cytology, and performance in racing thoroughbreds. *J. Vet. Intern. Med.* 32: 1754–1762.

61 Hinchcliff, K.W., Jackson, M.A., Morley, P.S. et al. (2005). Association between exercise-induced pulmonary hemorrhage and performance in thoroughbred racehorses. *J. Am. Vet. Med. Assoc.* 227: 768–774.

62 Hinchcliff, K., Couetil, L., Knight, P. et al. (2015). Exercise induced pulmonary hemorrhage in horses: American College of Veterinary Internal Medicine Consensus Statement. *J. Vet. Intern. Med.* 29: 743–758.

63 Gold, J.R., Knowles, D.P., Coffey, T. et al. (2018). Exercise-induced pulmonary hemorrhage in barrel racing horses in the Pacific northwest region of the United States. *J. Vet. Intern. Med.* 32: 839–845.

64 Newton, J.R. and Wood, J.L. (2002). Evidence of an association between inflammatory airway disease and EIPH in young thoroughbreds during training. *Equine Vet. J. Suppl.* 34: 417–424.

65 Doucet, M.Y. and Viel, L. (2002). Alveolar macrophage graded hemosiderin score from bronchoalveolar lavage in horses with exercise-induced pulmonary hemorrhage and controls. *J. Vet. Intern. Med.* 16: 281–286.

Index

Equine Hematology, Cytology, and Clinical Chemistry, Second Edition.
Edited by Raquel M. Walton, Rick L. Cowell, and Amy C. Valenciano.

b

c

n